Genital Tract Infection in Women

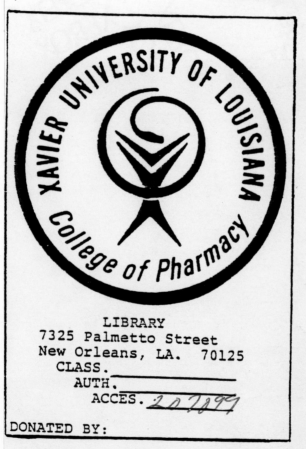

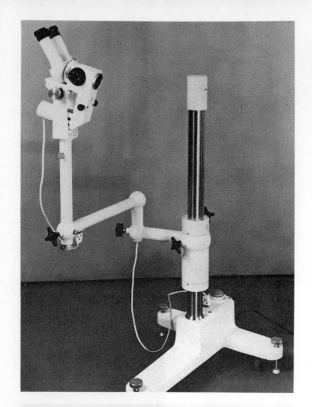

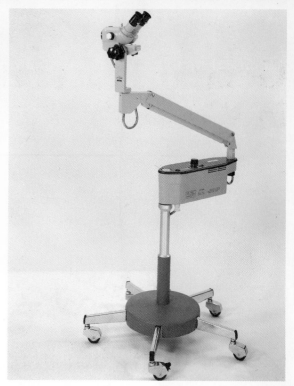

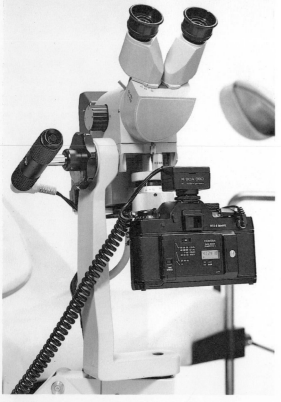

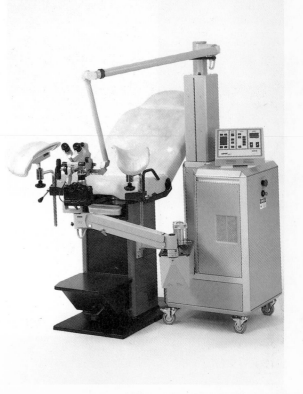

Originally developed in the 1920's for detection of pre-malignant disease of the uterine cervix, colposcopy has recently been shown to be of great value in the study of lower genital tract infection. The colposcope itself has also changed from the effective but clumsy and heavy instrument in the upper left corner to the simple light and streamlined model shown in the upper right corner. All modern colposcopes will take camera attachments to allow high quality photography (lower left). Many models may be used in conjunction with a laser to allow accurate micro-destruction of abnormal tissue (lower right).

All the colpo-photographs in this volume were taken using equipment from Carl Zeiss (Oberkochen) Ltd, and the editor is indebted to that company for sponsorship which allowed the colour plates to be published.

Genital Tract Infection in Women

EDITED BY

M.J. Hare

MA MD MRCOG

Consultant Obstetrician and Gynaecologist, Hinchingbrooke Hospital, Huntingdon; Senior Member (*formerly* Fellow),
Hughes Hall, Cambridge; *Formerly* University Lecturer in Obstetrics and Gynaecology, University of Cambridge;
Honorary Consultant Obstetrician and Gynaecologist, Addenbrooke's Hospital, Cambridge.

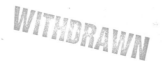

CHURCHILL LIVINGSTONE
EDINBURGH LONDON MELBOURNE AND NEW YORK 1988

CHURCHILL LIVINGSTONE
Medical Division of Longman Group UK Limited

Distributed in the United States of America by Churchill
Livingstone Inc., 1560 Broadway, New York, N.Y. 10036, and
by associated companies, branches and representatives
throughout the world.

First published 1988

ISBN 0 443 03485 0

British Library Cataloguing in Publication Data
Genital tract infection in women.
  1. Vagina—Diseases
  I. Hare, M.J.
  618.1'5   RG268

Library of Congress Cataloging in Publication Data
Genital tract infection in women.
  Includes index.
  1. Generative organs, Female—Infections.   I. Hare,
M.J. (Michael John) [DNLM: 1. Genital Diseases, Female.
WP 140 G3318]
RG218.G46   1988   618.1'42   87-13895

Produced by Longman Group (FE) Ltd
Printed in Hong Kong

Preface

The aim of this book is to break down barriers. Text-books dealing with infection of the female genital tract are written by a variety of doctors with backgrounds in a variety of branches of medicine, both clinical and laboratory based. Often the book will be written for, and confirm the beliefs of, doctors in the same group. Thus there will be a gynaecological approach to, for example, pelvic inflammatory disease, a venereological approach, a microbiological approach, an epidemiological approach and so on. Too often exchange of ideas between these groups is minimal.

I hope we have overcome this tendency in this book. The authors come from a wide range of disciplines: gynaecology, genito-urinary medicine, dermatology, microbiology, epidemiology, histo- and cytopathology, anatomy and psychology. Each is recognised as an expert within his or her professional subgroup, but also has a great deal to say to those in other disciplines. I asked each one to contribute because I thought he or she was the best person to deal with that subject, irrespective of clinical background. I am most happy and grateful to them for the contributions they produced, and, to be candid, humbled by the excellence of their work.

The other major question was on how to approach the subject, whether by syndrome and disease or by organism. The decision was to do both, because each approach has undeniable merit. This unavoidably led to some duplication and also to some controversy. This later I am sure is a good feature. The subject of female genital infection is much debated at present and is making rapid strides forward; new concepts are still to be clarified and some old and trusted beliefs must be re-examined.

To combine full time clinical work with medical editing is not easy, and without help and encouragement I would have not reached the end of this road. Most of all I would like to acknowledge the support of Sylvia Hull who commissioned the work for Churchill Livingstone; it is no exaggeration to say that on occasions when I fell flat on my face she picked me up, dusted me down and put me back on the right road. To all the contributors grateful thanks are due for chapters delivered on or nearly on time. Thanks also must go to my secretaries for their work; Judy Sansom for preparing my own and some other contributions and Sue Toseland for untiring and unceasing telephone communications. And lastly thanks to my wife and family for accepting a great deal of interference in their lives and loss of time that should have been theirs.

Huntingdon, Cambs.   M J H
1988

Contributors

Michael W Adler MD, FRCP, FFCM
Professor of Genito-Urinary Medicine, Middlesex
Hospital Medical School, London, UK

Ian McL. Brown MB, BS, FRCOG
Consultant Gynaecologist and Honorary Lecturer,
University of Zimbabwe, Zimbabwe

Pauline Cooper MA, MB, ChB, MRCPath
Consultant Cytopathologist and Histopathologist,
Addenbrooke's Hospital, Cambridge; Associate
Lecturer, University of Cambridge; Fellow of
Lucy Cavendish College, Cambridge, UK

Charles P Douglas MA, MB, FRCOG, FACS,
HonFACOG
Professor and Honorary Consultant, Cambridge
Clinical School, Rosie Maternity Hospital, Cam-
bridge, UK

Mark FitzGerald MA, MRCP, DRCOG
Consultant in Genito-Urinary Medicine, Adden-
brooke's Hospital, Cambridge; Associate Lecturer,
University of Cambridge, UK

Michael John Hare MA, MD, MRCOG
Consultant Obstetrician and Gynaecologist,
Hinchingbrooke Hospital, Huntingdon, UK

Edward O Hill PhD
Professor, Department of Pathology and Laboratory, and Director, Medicine and Clinical Microbiology, Emory University School of Medicine and
Emory University Hospital, Atlanta, Georgia, USA

William E Josey MD
Associate Professor of Gynecology and Obstetrics,
Emory University School of Medicine, Georgia,
USA

M H Kaufman MA, MB, ChB, PhD, DSc
Professor of Anatomy, University of Edinburgh,
UK

AS Latif MB, ChB, MFGP, DCH, DipVen, FCP
Consultant Physician and Venereologist, Senior
Lecturer, Department of Medicine, Godfrey Hug-
gins School of Medicine, University of Zimbabwe,
Zimbabwe

Peter J Lynch MD
Professor and Head, Department of Dermatology,
University of Minnesota School of Medicine,
Minnesota, USA

Nigel F Lyons DPhil
Lecturer, University of Zimbabwe, Department of
Medical Microbiology, Godfrey Huggins School of
Medicine, Zimbabwe

Janet Dorothy Milne MB, ChB, MD
Associate Specialist, Department of Genito-
Urinary Medicine, Bristol Royal Infirmary, UK

Adrian Mindel MB, BCh, MSc, MRCP
Senior Lecturer, Academic Department of Genito-
Urinary Medicine, James Pringle House, Mid-
dlesex Hospital, London, UK

P E Munday MD, MRCOG
Consultant Venereologist, The Praed Street Clinic,
St Mary's Hospital, London, UK

John K Oates MA, MB, FRCP
Consultant in Genito-Urinary Medicine, Addenbrooke's Hospital, Cambridge, and The Westmins-
ter Hospital, London, UK

Detlef Petzoldt ProfDrMed
Head of Dermatology and Venereology, University
of Heidelberg, West Germany

Julius Schachter PhD
Professor of Epidemiology, Department of Laboratory Medicine, University of California, San Francisco, USA

Renate Schroeter DrMed
AOR, Senior Physician of the Dermatologic Clinic, Heidelberg, West Germany

Pauline Slade PhD
Lecturer in Clinical Psychology, University of Manchester, UK

David C E Speller MA, BM, FRCP, FRCPath
Professor of Clinical Microbiology, Univesity of Bristol; Honorary Consultant Microbiologist, Bristol and Weston Health District, UK

David Taylor-Robinson MD, FRCPath
Head, Division of Sexually Transmitted Diseases, Clinical Research Centre, Harrow, Middlesex; Research Director, Jefferies Research Wing of the Praed Street Clinic, St Mary's Hospital, London, UK

R N T Thin DM, FRCP
Consultant Physician, Department of Genito-Urinary Medicine, St Thomas' Hospital, London, UK

Mary Turyk BS
Research Assistant, Rush Medical College, Rush University, Chicago, USA

David W Warnock BSc, PhD, MRCPath
Principal Mycologist, Bristol and Weston Health District; Honorary Lecturer in Medical Mycology, University of Bristol, UK

R E Warren MB, BChir, MRCPath
Consultant Bacteriologist, Addenbrooke's Hospital, Cambridge, UK

Lars V Weström MD
Associate Professor and Deputy Head, Department of Obstetrics and Gynaecology, University Hospital, Lund, Sweden

George D Wilbanks AB, MD
John M Simpson Professor and Chairman, Department of Obstetrics and Gynecology, Rush Medical College, Rush University, Chicago, USA

Ciaran B J Woodman MB, BCh, BAO
Registrar in Obstetrics and Gynaecology, Birmingham Maternity Hospital, UK

Contents

PART I

General concepts

1

The development of the female genital tract
M H Kaufman

INTRODUCTION

Until relatively recent times the gross morphology of the human female genital tract was shrouded in mystery and confusion, principally because few human bodies had been adequately dissected, and much information on reproductive tract anatomy was based on findings in animals, most of which had bicornuate uteri. Similarly, while embryological studies had been conducted by Aristotle and others, these related entirely to the development of non-human species such as the development of the chick embryo. Possibly the first anatomist to recognise and describe in detail the shape of the human uterus was Soranus in the second century AD, who compared its shape to that of a cupping vessel. He was also one of the first to recognise that the ovary played some role in the generative process, by calling it the female testis. Somewhat earlier, Rufus of Ephesus (working in the first century AD) correctly recognised that the oviducts or uterine tubes entered the uterus rather than the urinary bladder. Galen, in his turn, recognised that the oviducts had a large patent lumen through which the ova passed to the uterine cavity. After a gap of almost 1000 years, the Renaissance produced a wealth of medical texts, many of them illustrated by skilled artists showing clear evidence of firsthand knowledge obtained from carefully conducted dissections of the human body. Both Leonardo da Vinci and Berengario da Carpi were unequivocal in their belief that the uterus had a single chamber, contrary to the earlier notion that the uterus had seven chambers. Vesalius correctly described the shape and adnexa of the uterus, identified the muscular and decidual layers of the uterine wall, and employed the terms 'uterus' and 'pelvis' for the first time in his treatise 'De Humani Corporis Fabrica' of 1543.

Somewhat later his pupils named the labia and vagina (Colombo da Cremona), described the vasculature of the pelvis (Eustachio), and provided the definitive description of the uterine tubes (Fallopio da Modena) as well as accurately describing the corpus luteum, the hymen, and the clitoris, and observing that uterine prolapse was prevented by the integrity of the uterine ligaments. De Graaf subsequently provided a detailed description of the ovary, and a definitive account of the ovarian follicle, while Harvey wrote on the essential role of the ovary in reproduction (for further details, see Mettler & Mettler 1947; Garrison 1961; Singer & Underwood 1962; Tatarian 1962; and for recent review, see Ramsey 1977).

The development of initially simple lenses and somewhat later the availability of simple microscopes, combined with advances in tissue fixation and staining, greatly facilitated the study of embryology. The two scientists working at this time whose studies relate most closely to the development of the genital tract are Wolff, in about 1765, who provided a description of the ridge overlying the developing mesonephros and mesonephric ducts, and Müller, in about 1825, who studied and described the paramesonephric ducts.

The basic information presented here largely reflects current views on the development of the female genital tract to be found in all the standard embryology textbooks (for example, Hamilton & Mossman 1972; Moore 1982; Sadler 1985). These descriptions, and the account presented here, have in turn depended for their primary source material on the numerous important original articles, and the various reviews written on this complex topic (for example, Hunter 1930; Koff 1933; Bulmer 1957; Witschi 1970; O'Rahilly 1977; Edwards 1980). Many of the issues discussed here, particularly in relation to the factors that influence the development of the female genital tract, have yet to be fully resolved. Where several opinions have been expressed, for example in discussions on the development of the vagina, some of the relevant findings are described on which the various hypotheses have been based. It must also be emphasised at this stage that any detailed consideration of the development of the reproductive tract in either sex would be incomplete without a discussion on the sequential morphological changes that take place during the histogenesis of the gonads. This is essential because it provides the key to the critical role played by the gonads, both locally on the reproductive tract, and more distantly on the secondary sexual characteristics of the individual. Ultimately, of course, it is the genetic sex of the conceptus that controls both directly and indirectly, and in an active and a passive way, all of the events to be described in this chapter. The control of certain aspects of genital tract development is also achieved through the influence of hormones of extragonadal origin, namely from the fetal pituitary, the placenta, and from the mother, and these aspects will also be considered in the appropriate sections of the text.

THE DEVELOPMENT OF THE DEFINITIVE REPRODUCTIVE SYSTEM: URINARY DERIVATIVES

In the female, the definitive reproductive duct system develops from the intermediate mesoderm and adjacent coelomic epithelium, and is largely derived from the paramesonephric ducts. The latter develop in close proximity to the mesonephric ducts, but it is not clear whether they are in fact derived from them or not. However, a clear picture of the early development of the genital duct system in the female can only be obtained if it is considered in parallel with the associated components of the urinary system. Indeed, during the earliest stages of their development, the urinary and genital ducts open into a common cloaca which, initially at least, represents the dilated terminal part of the hindgut.

The components of the urinary system that need to be considered in relation to the development of the female genital duct apparatus are those that were originally derived from the nephrogenic cord.

While the latter gives rise to most of the excretory system, it is thought that the most cranial component, or pronephros, is only a transient structure and probably never functions in the human embryo (Torrey 1954), and it is principally the derivatives from the mesonephric ducts that need to be considered here. However, experimental studies in amphibian and in avian embryos have demonstrated that in these species at least, the pronephric duct plays an essential role in the induction of the mesonephros (Waddington 1938, O'Connor 1939). The segmentally arranged mesonephric tubules join to form the mesonephric ducts, which grow caudally and longitudinally and eventually open into the cloaca. Initially, the nephrogenic cords appear as solid masses of cells which eventually canalise to form the excretory organs and their ducts. The tubules which drain the mesonephros join the nephric duct, and the latter is then termed the mesonephric (or Wolffian) duct. The most caudal of the nephrogenic cord derivatives forms the metanephric blastema, and its excretory tubules connect with a special outgrowth or diverticulum from the mesonephric duct termed the ureter, or ureteric bud, which is first apparent on or about the 28th day of gestation. Within a matter of days, the cloaca is divided into two cavities, a dorsal rectal component, and a ventral primary urogenital sinus, by the caudal 'downgrowth' of the urorectal septum. During the seventh week of gestation, the urogenital and rectal derivatives of the cloacal membrane break down, thereby allowing the urogenital sinus and hindgut to communicate directly with the amniotic cavity.

While most of the mesonephric derivatives, apart from the ureter, probably regress in the female, a few remnants do persist to a variable degree (see Koff 1933). These are divided into cranial and caudal derivatives. Of the cranial or epigenital group, these are also subdivided into two groups. Excluding the first two tubules, these form the efferent ductules of the testis or their homologues in the ovary, whereas the first two pairs form the superior aberrant ductules (ductuli aberrantes superiores). The most caudal or paragenital mesonephric tubules may also persist, and often become separated from the mesonephric ducts to form the paradidymis in the male and the paroophoron in the female, while those that remain attached to the mesonephric ducts become the inferior ductules (ductuli aberrantes inferiores) in each sex. The mesonephric remnants may be located just lateral to the uterus and vagina (Gartner's ducts), or even within the substance of the cervix (Meyer 1909) as tubules or cysts. The cellular tissue sometimes proliferates, and may occasionally even undergo malignant transformation to form an adenocarcinoma. Mesonephric derivatives such as the epoophoron are quite frequently present in the broad ligament (Duthie 1925), though they do not appear to show evidence of secretory activity. The mesonephric ducts have a distinct muscular coat, and are lined by non-ciliated and cuboidal epithelium, while the mesonephric tubules have a generally less well defined muscular coat, and are lined with both ciliated and non-ciliated low columnar or cuboidal epithelium (O'Rahilly 1977).

THE CLOACAL DERIVATIVES AND UROGENITAL SINUS

The cloaca, as described earlier, is derived from the dilated caudal region of the hindgut, and is separated from the surface by the cloacal membrane. In this location, the ectoderm and endoderm remain in contact without an intervening layer of intraembryonic mesoderm. The cloacal membrane lies in a shallow depression termed the external cloaca or proctodaeum, and this is bounded on either side by a pair of elevations (the genital or labioscrotal folds). In the ventral midline between the cloacal membrane and the connecting stalk is a further elevation termed the genital tubercle which subsequently develops into the phallus. At an early stage in embryogenesis the cloaca is divided into a smaller dorsal hindgut or rectal compartment, and a more voluminous ventral urogenital sinus by the downgrowth of a transverse ridge termed the urorectal septum in the angle between the allantois and the hindgut. The urorectal septum also concomitantly divides the cloacal membrane into a dorsal anal membrane and a ventral urogenital membrane, and the site of fusion of the urorectal septum and the cloacal membrane is the location of the perineal body. Fusion in this region occurs in embryos measuring about 18 mm in crown–rump (C-R) length. At a later stage, both membranes break down to allow continuity to be made between the cloacal derivatives and the exterior. From its earliest appearance, the cloaca is in continuity with the allantois, both of which are endodermally lined, and only later (in late somite-containing embryos, on or about the 26th day of gestation) joined on either side of the urogenital sinus region by the downgrowing mesonephric ducts, which are of mesodermal origin.

The mesonephric ducts open into the cloaca on or about the 26th day of gestation, and effectively subdivide the urogenital sinus into cranial and caudal portions in relation to their site of entry. The cranial region is continuous with the allantois, and termed the vesicourethral canal. The latter subsequently develops into the bladder and the proximal part of the urethra, whereas the caudal part is termed the 'definitive' urogenital sinus (or urogenital sinus proper). Initially, the entrance of the mesonephric ducts into the urogenital sinus and the ureteric buds share a common site. As development proceeds, the ureteric openings enter the upper dorsolateral aspects of the urogenital sinus whereas, possibly due to differential growth of the intervening tissues (Frazer 1935), the mesonephric ducts open into the urethra in a much more caudal location. Alternatively, the mesonephric ducts may become absorbed into the dorsal wall of the urethra, and this may account for the widely held belief that the region of the primitive vesical trigone is of mesodermal origin. In the female, the primitive urethra forms most if not all of the definitive urethra, and eventually lies in close proximity to the ventral wall of the vagina. Epithelial buds arise from the primitive urethra and also from the almost adjacent pelvic part of the urogenital sinus in embryos of about 60 mm C–R length. These are thought to be the homologues of the prostate gland. The former develop in the female into the urethral glands, while the latter develop into the paraurethral glands of Skene, which are probably of complex origin, being derived from the epithelium in the region of the Müllerian tubercle (Glenister 1962).

DEVELOPMENT OF THE GONADS: MIGRATION OF THE PRIMORDIAL GERM CELLS

From about the 4–5 mm C-R length stage up to about the 17 mm C-R length stage, it is not possible, on histological or morphological analysis of the gonads, to distinguish between the two sexes. This is termed the 'indifferent' gonad stage, during which time very rapid changes take place in the histogenesis of the gonads, which are thought to be largely controlled by the genetic sex of the individual. Furthermore, the two sexes cannot be distinguished on the basis of the morphological appearance of their internal reproductive duct systems, as both sexes possess paired mesonephric and paramesonephric ducts. The latter develop slightly later than the former, and although the two systems are probably developmentally interrelated, they have quite different fates in the two sexes. The fate of these two systems will be considered in detail, after the histogenesis of the gonads is briefly described.

The gonadal or genital ridges are clearly apparent in embryos of 4–5 mm C-R length (on or about the 32nd day of gestation) as longitudinally running elevations which bulge into the coelomic cavity, and are located just medial to the mesonephros and lateral to the mesentery of the gut (Fig. 1.1). These ridges soon develop into circumscribed organs with a central core of mesenchymatous tissue surrounded by a thin layer of germinal epithelium of coelomic epithelial origin. The mesonephros and genital blastema are initially suspended from the posterior abdominal wall by the urogenital mesentery (Fig. 1.2) but with the regression of the mesonephros and enlargement of the gonad on the medial aspect of the urogenital ridge, this results in the formation of a gonadal mesentery (mesovarium, see Fig. 1.3, or mesorchium). At the same time as the gonad is enlarging, the cranial portion of the urogenital mesentery becomes displaced laterally. More caudally, the two ridges initially approach each other and subsequently fuse across the midline to form the urogenital ridge, which lies between the bladder and the hindgut.

Initially, the basement membrane separating the mesenchyme from the germinal epithelium on the surface of the gonad disappears, and this allows the progeny of the epithelial cells to invade the territory occupied by the mesenchyme tissue, and displace most of the latter cells. During the late somite stage of embryonic development, numbers of primordial germ cells (or gonocytes) migrate by amoeboid movement from the yolk sac into the hindgut mesentery, and thence into the gonadal ridges. In both sexes, the germ cells become associated with 'cortical' cords of cells which radiate in from the germinal epithelium into the medullary zone of the gonad. The cords are, however, much less well defined in the ovary than in the testis, and it is not entirely clear whether, in the female at least, they are indeed of cortical origin or derived from mesonephric cells which grow out from the rete ovarii. The pathway of migration of the primordial germ cells from their site of origin to the gonads can readily be traced, as these cells have a quite characteristic morphology, are spherical, and distinctly larger than the surrounding mesenchymal cells, and have a high level of cytoplasmic alkaline phosphatase activity (Chiquoine 1954; Ozdzeński 1967; Falin 1969; Clark & Eddy 1975; Snow & Monk 1983).

INFLUENCE OF THE GENETIC SEX OF THE FETUS AND HORMONES OF EXTRAGONADAL ORIGIN ON THE DIFFERENTIATION OF THE GONADS AND GENITAL DUCTS

After about the sixth week of development, in embryos of 17–20 mm C-R length, the morphological changes that have occurred in the definitive gonad now allow the ovary to be readily distinguished from the testis. It seems likely that it is the

Fig. 1.1 Representative transverse histological sections through the abdomen and pelvis of a 13 mm crown-rump length human embryo (Boyd reference no. H.1069) of approximately 6 weeks gestation. This embryo is at the indifferent gonad stage, and the gonadal ridges lie anteromedially in relation to the mesonephros. The latter contains degenerating tubules, but the mesonephric ducts are quite prominent. The metanephric blastema and ureter are clearly seen in E, as is the urogenital sinus. No evidence of a paramesonephric duct is seen.

1 Dorsal aorta; 2 lateral coelomic bay; 3 mesonephric glomerulus; 4 peritoneal cavity; 5 gonadal ridge; 6 medial coelomic bay; 7 segmental mesonephric artery; 8 degenerating mesonephric tubules; 9 mesonephric duct; 10 caudal pole of mesonephros; 11 dorsal mesentery of gut; 12 rectum; 13 umbilical artery; 14 allantois; 15 urachus; 16 genital tubercle; 17 metanephric blastema; 18 ureter; 19 urogenital sinus; 20 phallic part of urethra.

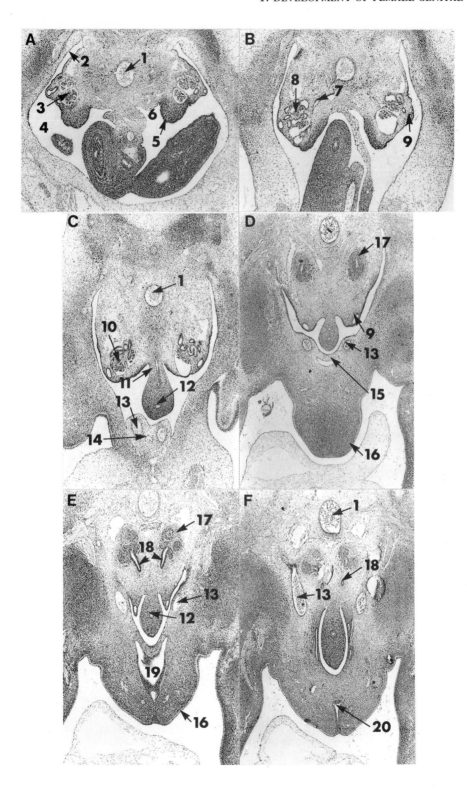

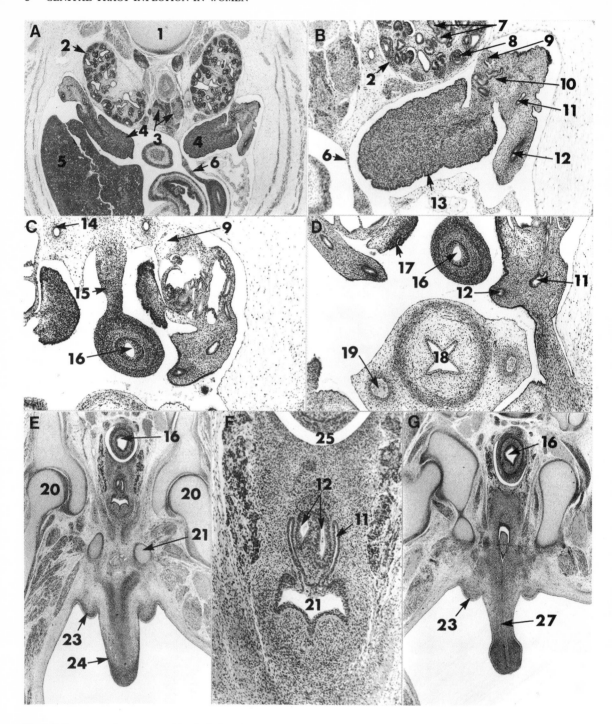

Fig. 1.2 Representative transverse histological sections through the abdomen and pelvis of a 28 mm crown-rump length human female embryo (Boyd reference no. H.585) of approximately 8 weeks gestation. The gonad now has the characteristic appearance of an ovary, with a prominent peripheral cortical layer, and absence of obvious medullary cords. The gonads are suspended by the urogenital mesentery from the posterior abdominal wall, and are at about the same level as the midpoint of the metanephros, the liver, and the physiological umbilical hernia (see Fig. 1.7A for more extensive view through the abdominal cavity of this embryo at the same level as A). Degenerating mesonephric tubules and the mesonephric ducts are all that remain of the mesonephric system.

genetic sex of the primordial germ cells, already established at fertilisation, that plays a critical role in inducing the differentiative changes that occur within the gonads during their 'indifferent' stage to take place. In genetically male embryos, with an XY-chromosome constitution, the presence of the Y-chromosome is thought to have a positive testis-determining effect, which induces the resultant changes to occur in the gonads that are clearly apparent during the succeeding few weeks of embryonic development. The underlying mechanism of action of the Y-chromosome in inducing the differentiation of the testis is unclear, though it is of interest to note that a similar effect can be induced in genetically female mice bearing the autosomal dominant mutation *Sxr* (sex reversal; Simpson 1976). Despite the presence of two X-chromosomes, these fetuses develop as males with testes, but have impaired spermatogenesis. Female goats bearing the *Polled* gene also show variable degrees of masculinisation (Soller et al 1969). Recent evidence has, however, been found which indicates that the Y-chromosome may induce maleness in the gonad and elsewhere via an immunological mechanism, possibly by the production of a histocompatibility antigen (H-Y antigen) which is determined by a gene on the Y-chromosome (Ohno 1977). Receptors for such an antigen are present on gonadal but not somatic tissues, and it is thought that testis differentiation only occurs in the presence of the antigen (Müller et al 1978).

It is equally unclear whether the maternal and placental oestrogens that circulate in the fetus also have a feminising role, only influencing the differentiation of the internal and external genital apparatus in female fetuses because of the absence of the more powerful male-inducing steroids produced by the fetal testis. While the precise influence of gonadotrophins secreted by the placenta (chorionic gonadotrophin and prolactin) and the fetal pituitary gland on sexual differentiation has yet to be fully evaluated, it seems likely that placental steroids may act as a source of androgens or their precursors. Indeed, it has been suggested that gonadotrophins may initiate steroidogenesis in the fetal testis, and this may be maintained by fetal pituitary hormones (Clements et al 1976). The fetal hypothalamus and pituitary have differentiated by about 3–4 months of gestation, and are probably capable of producing gonadotrophins at an even earlier stage (Winters et al 1974), though maximum levels of LH-RH activity in the hypothalamus are achieved by about 6 months (Kaplan et al 1976). This high level of gonadotrophin activity is only moderated when the hypothalamo-pituitary axis is established. This occurs during the second half of gestation, and the gonads can then exert an inhibitory effect via feedback mechanisms, though the latter only fully differentiate during the early childhood years. Highest levels of gonadotrophin activity occur in female fetuses, and this difference persists until after birth. The lower levels of activity observed in male fetuses are possibly accounted for by the inhibitory effects of testicular androgens. A similar though less marked inhibitory influence is observed in female fetuses due to the effect of oestrogens.

In the male, the mesonephric ducts amalgamate with the prominent cortical cords which radiate into the mesenchyme-derived substance of the testis. The germ cells are invariably located in close proximity to the cortical cords, and these eventually differentiate into the seminiferous tubules and become detached from the tunica albuginea and the cortex of the testis. At about the same time, the mesonephric tissue develops into the rete testis, through which the mature spermatozoa will eventually pass before progressing into the efferent ductules, the epididymis, and ductus (or vas) deferens.

In the female, the changes that take place during

Note that in E and F, which is a section from the pelvic region just below the site of entry of the ureters into the urogenital sinus, while the laterally located mesonephric ducts clearly enter the urogenital sinus, the medially located and as yet unfused paramesonephric ducts do not quite reach its dorsal wall. The latter site represents the location of the Müllerian tubercle. Note also the prominent phallus bounded on either side by the labial swellings.

1 lumbar vertebral body; 2 metanephros; 3 chromaffin tissue (prospective adrenal medulla); 4 ovary; 5 liver; 6 dorsal mesentery of gut; 7 metanephric tubules; 8 glomerulus; 9 urogenital mesentery; 10 degenerating mesonephric tubules; 11 mesonephric duct; 12 paramesonephric duct; 13 cortex of ovary; 14 ureter; 15 dorsal mesentery of hindgut; 16 rectum; 17 caudal pole of ovary; 18 urachus; 19 umbilical artery; 20 head of femur; 21 pubic bone; 22 urogenital sinus; 23 labial swelling; 24 phallus; 25 prospective location of pouch of Douglas; 26 location of Müllerian tubercle; 27 phallic part of urethra.

the histogenesis of the ovary are superficially at least altogether much simpler. The primordial germ cells become predominantly located in the superficial part or future cortex of the ovary, and are often in close contact with the coelomic epithelial cells. About 1000–2000 germ cells are present in the human ovary by about 30 days of gestation (Baker 1972). They initially differentiate into oogonia (Witschi 1963) and undergo a number of mitotic divisions, before becoming surrounded by a single layer of specialised presumptive granulosa cells, to form a discrete unit termed a primordial follicle. It is thought that the enclosure of the germ cells by the granulosa cells may act as a stimulus to induce the oogonia to enter meiosis (Byskov 1981).

The first oocytes are seen at about 3 months of gestation, while the first follicles are observed at about 4.5–5 months. The number of germ cells in the gonads increases from about 600 000 at 2 months up to a maximum of about 2 million oogonia and 5 million oocytes in meiosis in mid-pregnancy. A considerable proportion of the oogonia and oocytes, however, undergo atresia (Gondos et al 1971), effectively reducing the total number of germ cells in the ovary at birth to about 2 million, and this is further reduced to about 300 000 by 7 years of age (Baker 1972). It now seems clear that no additional germ cells are formed in the human ovary beyond the early neonatal period (Brambell 1956).

The exact origin of the granulosa cells is unclear. It was formerly believed that the granulosa cells were derived from the germinal epithelial tissue that invaded the ovary with the inward migration of the 'cortical' sex cords. More recent evidence, however, now tends to suggest that they may, in fact, originate from the medullary blastema of the mesonephric-derived rete ovarii tissue (Byskov 1981). Some granulosa cells resemble testicular Leydig cells, are possibly of medullary origin, and may be a source of androgens (Balboni 1976). Other authorities have suggested that the granulosa cells of the ovarian follicle may be homologous with the Sertoli cells of the testis (Zamboni 1976). It is thought that the interstitial cells, which are found in both the cortical and in the medullary stroma, may arise from the stromal mesenchyme (Gillman 1948). These are thought to be the precursors of

the thecal cells, and may also, in fact, originate from ovarian mesonephric derivatives (see Edwards 1980). The primordial follicles are loosely connected to each other through 'rete' cords. The latter are observed in mice after birth, and may occasionally be discerned in human ovaries and those of non-human primates in relation to the early Graafian follicles (Zamboni 1976). The formation of oocytes and primordial follicles, and observations on the embryological origin of ovarian somatic cells, with particular reference to the steroidogenic cells in the human ovary, have recently been reviewed by Edwards (1980).

In female fetuses, the mesonephric tubules degenerate and virtually completely disappear, leaving only remnants of rete ovarii tissue in the region of the mesovarium (see Fig. 1.2). The obvious absence of continuity between the sex cords and the mesonephric tubule derivatives, via the rete, explains in part why the mesonephric duct in the female fails to act as a means of egress from the ovary of the mature ova. In consequence, these have to escape from the gonad by the complex process of ovulation, mediated through the complex changes that take place during folliculogenesis. By contrast to the situation observed in the testis, where the cortical zone is particularly narrow, the cortical zone in the ovary eventually constitutes more than one-half of its thickness. The cortex contains all of the functional germ cells and their surrounding follicular cells, and is in addition the site of the majority of the ovarian hormone-producing activity.

THE FACTORS THAT INDUCE SEXUAL DIMORPHISM IN THE PARAMESONEPHRIC DERIVATIVES

During the embryonic period (up to about the ninth week of gestation, in embryos of about 35 mm C-R length) the paramesonephric ducts are identical in appearance and position in the two sexes (Glenister 1962). Only subsequent to this period do they show evidence of sexual dimorphism, possibly associated with the increasing influence of gonadally-derived sex hormones. The testis is thought to have a positive masculinising influence (Jost 1972), so that the mesonephric duct derivatives develop in the male, while the paramesonephric system largely regresses. Two complementary 'factors' are thought to be operating here. The first effect described above is likely to be due to the influence of androgens such as testosterone or dihydrotestosterone produced by the fetal testis, probably independent of any stimulation by gonadotrophins (George et al 1978), though the latter are obviously essential at a later stage when the testis becomes fully secretory (Wilson 1978). While the testis is first morphologically distinguishable from the ovary from about the sixth week of gestation, Leydig cells are first seen about 2 weeks later, and are present in large numbers between weeks 10 and 14. Testosterone production is first detected by weeks 8–10, and maximum levels are achieved by weeks 12–13 (Siiteri & Wilson 1974).

The influence of a second 'factor' has also been hypothesised, which induces the paramesonephric duct system to regress. This effect is first evident in male fetuses from about the 10th week of gestation, and is thought to be due to the anti-Müllerian 'hormone' (also termed Müllerian inhibiting substance, or MIS). It has been suggested that this may be secreted by the Sertoli cells of the fetal seminiferous tubules, and is a protein with a molecular weight of approximately 200 000 (Josso et al 1977; Price et al 1979). This factor appears to be produced by the fetal testis independent of the need for exogenous stimulation by hormones of fetal pituitary, maternal, or placental origin. It has been possible to demonstrate in an in vitro system that the paramesonephric ducts isolated from 30–32 mm C-R length human fetuses are sensitive to the effect of this 'hormone' over this relatively limited critical period of time, and show evidence of regression in culture (Josso et al 1977). Conversely, in the female, probably because of the absence of sufficiently high levels of androgens, the paramesonephric duct system is allowed to achieve its full potential, while the mesonephric duct derivatives largely regress.

It has been suggested that the ovary and testis may differentiate steroidogenically at about the same time, even though the ovary appears to develop later histologically (Gondos et al 1971). It seems more likely, however, that the precocious development of the testis compared to the ovary probably reflects an earlier onset of functional activity. In females, and in males with congenital absence of the testis, the current view is therefore that the mesonephric ducts largely degenerate (an example of programmed cell death) due to the absence of the 'positive' influence of sufficiently high levels of androgens, while the paramesonephric system persists because there are no 'factors' present to destroy it (Jost et al 1973; Edwards 1980). As indicated earlier, it is not entirely clear at the present time whether maternal and placental oestrogens might also have a feminising role, leading to the formation of a recognisable ovary, as well as inducing the characteristic changes which subsequently take place in the genital duct apparatus. A similar end result is observed in individuals with testicular feminisation where, due to the presence of the *tfm* gene, which is located on the X-chromosome in various mammalian species including man (Lyon & Hawkes 1970; Meyer et al 1975), male pseudohermaphroditism results. The target organs involved in male differentiation appear to be insensitive to the effects of otherwise adequate levels of masculinising hormones (Jost et al 1973). Female pseudohermaphrodites arise when female fetuses, with an XX-chromosome constitution, are exposed to androgens at critical stages of urogenital organogenesis, leading to varying degrees of masculinisation of the internal and external genitalia (Simpson 1976). A similar situation also arises in certain inherited disorders of steroid metabolism, due to the presence of abnormally high levels of androgens, such as testosterone, but the manifestations vary widely (for recent review see Edwards 1980). In these children, the external genitalia are often ambiguous. The most common cause of female pseudohermaphroditism, however, is the adrenogenital syndrome, where there is no ovarian abnormality, but masculinisation results from the excessive production of androgens of adrenal origin. Several genetic variants of this condition are known, and all are inherited as autosomal recessive traits. These are all characterised by a block in a specific step in cortisol biosynthesis, which results in an increased secretion of ACTH and hyperplasia of the fetal suprarenal glands (Thompson & Thompson 1980).

THE INITIAL CHANGES OBSERVED IN THE DERIVATIVES OF THE PARAMESONEPHRIC DUCTS

The embryological development of the specialised duct system that facilitates the passage of the unfertilised ovum from the ovary, provides a convenient site for fertilisation, and allows implantation and growth to maturity of the fertilised conceptus to take place, is reasonably well understood. The reproductive apparatus that differentiates in the female embryo to serve these various roles is derived from the paramesonephric (or Müllerian) ducts. In the male, this duct system virtually completely regresses during the early embryonic period (see Glenister 1962), and those components that remain soon lose their communication with the coelomic cavity. Indeed, the only derivatives to survive in the male are those that subsequently form the appendix of the testis, formed from the cranial component of the paramesonephric ducts (Rolnick et al 1968), and the utriculus masculinus (or prostatic utricle), neither of which have any ascribed function (Glenister 1962). Furthermore, some uncertainty exists as to whether the latter, which is possibly a derivative of the caudal part of the paramesonephric duct apparatus, is in fact derived from this source, or is of composite origin, possibly with a contribution from the urogenital sinus (for discussion see Hamilton & Mossman 1972).

The paramesonephric ducts are first seen in human embryos at about the 8–10 mm C-R length stage (on or about the 37th day of gestation) as invaginations of the coelomic epithelium into the underlying mesenchyme. These appear as two distinct longitudinally running entities, located just lateral to the cranial extremities of the mesonephric ducts. At a slightly earlier stage, however, it is just possible to recognise their site of origin in both sexes, as they initially develop in the mesonephric ridge in a localised placode-like area, which contains elongated columnar rather than the more characteristic flattened epithelial cells, and is said to be at the level of the third thoracic somite (Felix 1912). In the chick embryo, experimental studies have indicated that the paramesonephric duct system may be induced by factors emanating from the adjacent mesonephric ducts (Didier 1973). More caudally, they run more medially and ventrally in

relation to, and possibly under the guiding influence of, the mesonephric ducts (Gruenwald 1941, 1942). The paramesonephric ducts develop somewhat later than the mesonephros and its ducts, and some authorities (e.g. Gruenwald 1941) have proposed that they may even be derived from the longitudinal splitting of the latter. Certainly, the unilateral absence of a mesonephric duct is generally associated with the absence of the paramesonephric duct in the same general location, while the complete absence of the former is commonly associated with uterus unicornis and renal agenesis on the affected side. It is of equal interest that the rate of elongation of the paramesonephric ducts in the human embryo is said to provide an extremely accurate means of establishing the developmental age of any particular embryo over this period (Streeter 1948).

DEVELOPMENT OF THE PARAMESONEPHRIC DERIVATIVES INTO THE OVIDUCTS, UTERUS AND UTEROVAGINAL CANAL

The cranial extremities of the paramesonephric ducts open into the peritoneal cavity to form the abdominal ostia of the oviducts, and these are subsequently surrounded by a floret of fimbriae. Initially, at its caudal extremity, the two solid rods of paramesonephric tissue pass down towards the urogenital sinus within the mesenchyme tissue of the posterior abdominal wall, and in close proximity to the mesonephric ducts. In the human embryo, the medial direction of growth of the ducts from the two sides allows them to meet in the urogenital septum where they initially become closely apposed (23–28 mm C-R length stage, see Fig. 1.2) and then fuse to form a single median longitudinal derivative (27–31 mm C-R length stage). This takes place towards the end of the seventh week of gestation, even though their most caudal extremities have yet to reach the urogenital sinus (Koff 1933). In most mammalian species, however, fusion of the two paramesonephric duct derivatives does not occur, except in the prospective cervical region, and two distinct uterine horns are subsequently formed. At about this time a slight ventral projection becomes apparent on the dorsal wall of the urogenital sinus between the sites of entry of the two mesonephric ducts. This has been termed the Müllerian tubercle, and is said to overly a region in which connective tissue proliferation is occurring. The latter is thought to give rise to the urethrovaginal septum (Frutiger 1969). Other authorities, however, have suggested that the Müllerian tubercle may be produced at the site where the caudal tips of the paramesonephric ducts make contact with the dorsal wall of the urogenital sinus (see Koff 1933).

The paramesonephric ducts first become canalised at their cranial extremities, and the lumina thus formed gradually extend caudally. Initially, two separate canals are present in the region where the two paramesonephric ducts have previously fused, and these are separated by a temporary septum which generally breaks down by the middle of the 10th week of gestation, giving rise to a single and continuous uterovaginal canal (Fig. 1.3) which is lined with cuboidal epithelium. The uterovaginal canal has generally formed by the end of the eighth week of gestation, but evidence of incomplete resorption of the intervening septum is occasionally encountered at various sites within the uterine lumen, and may have important clinical sequelae. The latter may play a role in some individuals in inducing infertility by producing habitual abortions, or the premature onset of labour, depending on the location and extent of the intervening septum (Jarcho 1946).

The numerous types of gross anomalies involving the uterus and oviducts also arise during this period of embryonic development, for example, as a result of incomplete caudal migration of one or both paramesonephric ducts, leading to various degrees of complete or partial uterine aplasia. More commonly, however, anomalies arise as a result of a partial or complete failure of the ducts from the two sides to fuse together. The latter may be apparent externally, in the most extreme cases leading to bicornuate uteri each with their own distinct cervix and cervical canal, or, in less gross cases, their lumina may fail to amalgamate together after fusion of the two paramesonephric ducts has occurred. Very rarely, accessory or ectopic derivatives thought to be of paramesonephric duct origin are encountered, such as accessory oviducts, cysts and tubules. These are principally located along the course of caudal descent of these ducts (Jarcho 1946; Simpson 1976). Jarcho (1946) has estimated that lack of fusion of the paramesonephric ducts, either complete or incomplete, occurs once in about 15 000 obstetric, and about once in 2000 gynaecological cases, though other authorities have indicated that the incidence may be considerably higher.

Caudal to the most rostral site of fusion of the two paramesonephric ducts a definitive midline structure is formed which may now be termed the uterovaginal canal. This is present in 36–37 mm C-R fetuses during the ninth week of gestation, and consists of the prospective uterus and part of the vagina (Hunter 1930; Koff 1933). The two cranially directed tubular derivatives located between the abdominal ostia and the prospective corpus uteri, or 'body' of the uterus, are termed the uterine tubes or oviducts (Fig. 1.3), while the cranial site of fusion marks the location of the uterine fundus. Downward growth of the tissue at the caudal extremity of the uterovaginal canal results in the formation of a solid rod or cord of tissue which effectively increasingly distances the lumen of the uterovaginal canal from that of the urogenital sinus (Fig. 1.3G, H). The distance between the two is increased further, in embryos of about 63 mm C-R length, by the addition of cellular material of endodermal origin. This is derived from the region of the urogenital sinus, close to the site of insertion of the mesonephric ducts, and termed the sinovaginal bulbs. These extend cranially, and soon fuse with the caudally directed solid cord of tissue which develops from the uterovaginal canal, to form the vaginal plate (Fig. 1.3H). It has been suggested (Koff 1933) that the sinovaginal bulbs give rise to the lower part of the vagina, though other authorities have proposed that all of the epithelial lining of the vagina may in fact be derived from the endoderm of the urogenital sinus (Bulmer 1957). Whatever its source of origin, the vaginal plate becomes canalised by the caudal extension of the uterovaginal canal, and the eventual breaking down of the tissue derived from the sinovaginal bulbs.

While these changes are occurring in the major derivatives of the uterovaginal canal, a small component of the urogenital sinus termed the vesicourethral canal, located immediately cranial to the sinovaginal bulbs, becomes elongated and develops

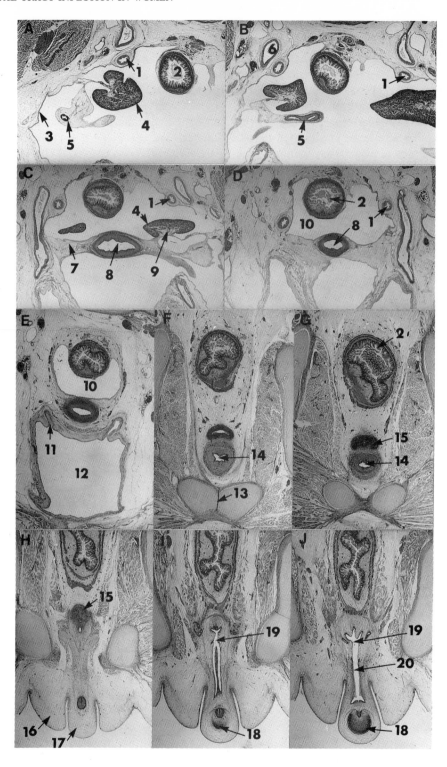

into the female urethra, while the caudal part of the definitive urogenital sinus enlarges and develops into the vestibule. The hymen is thought to represent the region between the urogenital sinus proper and the canalised derivatives of the sinovaginal bulbs. It contains an intermediate layer of mesoderm, and is lined externally by endodermal epithelium of urogenital sinus origin, and internally by vaginal epithelium (also endodermal in origin).

Curiously, little is known about the exact origin of the musculature of the female reproductive tract, but it seems reasonable to suggest that this is derived from the mesenchyme surrounding the paramesonephric ducts. Recent experimental evidence has, furthermore, clearly demonstrated that interactions between the mesenchyme, or the stromal tissue that is derived from it, and the subjacent epithelium, play an important part in the development of the ductal systems. The mesenchyme is effectively pluripotential, in that it has the ability to differentiate according to local needs. This is particularly evident when mesenchyme tissue is transferred to an appropriate location in a fetus of the opposite sex, where it would be exposed to a completely different hormonal environment, or when it is cultured in vitro under experimental conditions that mimic such a situation (Cunha 1976).

With the regression of the mesonephric ducts, and enlargement and transformation of the paramesonephric ducts, the urogenital mesentery that initially covered these structures on their dorsal aspect now expands and allows them to be suspended from the pelvic floor by transversely running folds of peritoneum termed the broad ligaments. The oviducts are located in its free edges. A summary of the sequential changes that take place in the development of the female genital tract with particular reference to the fates of the mesonephric and paramesonephric duct systems is illustrated diagrammatically in Fig. 1.4.

DEVELOPMENT OF THE VAGINA

As indicated earlier, various hypotheses have been proposed to account for the embryological origin of the vagina. Most authorities now consider that somewhere between the lower one-fifth (Koff 1933) and approximately the lower two-thirds of the vagina are probably endodermal in origin, and derived from the urogenital sinus (Cunha 1975; O'Rahilly 1977), though there are almost as many views on this topic as there are researchers who have investigated this particular problem. The confusion undoubtedly arises because no unequivocal cellular markers exist at the present time which would enable the fate of individual components to be traced during successive stages of embryonic development. Equally, it has yet to be established whether the endothelial lining of the various parts of the vagina has a similar origin to its other component parts.

Despite the considerable difficulties encountered in the interpretation of the histological evidence, most authorities now consider that the upper vagina is mesodermally-derived and of paramesonephric origin. The vaginal plate (Figs. 1.3 and 1.5), which forms where the caudal part of the uterovaginal canal becomes occluded at its site of contact with the upgrowth from the sinovaginal bulbs (of Müllerian tubercle origin), is initially of paramesonephric and sinovaginal origin (Koff

---

Fig. 1.3 Representative transverse histological sections through the lower abdomen and pelvis of a 65 mm crown-rump length human female fetus (Boyd reference no. H.118) of approximately 11 weeks gestation. Reference to Fig. 1.7B, in which a more extensive view through the mid-gonadal region of this fetus is presented, clearly demonstrates that the ovary is now located in the lower part of the abdominal cavity, at about the level of the iliac crests. While the mesonephric system has all but disappeared, the paramesonephric system is represented by the prospective uterine tubes or oviducts, and the midline uterovaginal canal which is oval in cross-section, being flattened dorsoventrally. Note that in C the gonad is suspended from the dorsal aspect of the broad ligament by the mesovarium, and that in C-E an obvious pouch of Douglas is now apparent. The lower part of the uterovaginal canal is very closely related to the dorsal surface of the wall of the urethra (in F and G). In addition, note that the lumen of the caudal part of the terovaginal canal is almost completely occluded (in G), and is in fact totally occluded (in H) in the region of the vaginal plate. The definitive pelvic and phallic parts of the urogenital sinus will subsequently form the vestibule.

1. Ureter; 2 hindgut (rectum); 3 peritoneum; 4 ovary; 5 paramesonephric duct (prospective oviduct); 6 common iliac artery; 7 broad ligament; 8 uterovaginal canal; 9 mesovarium; 10 rectouterine pouch of Douglas; 11 site of entry of ureter into bladder; 12 bladder; 13 pubic symphysis; 14 definitive urethra; 15 primitive vaginal plate; 16 labial swelling; 17 genital tubercle; 18 corpus cavernosum of clitoris; 19 definitive pelvic part of urogenital sinus; 20 definitive phallic part of urogenital sinus.

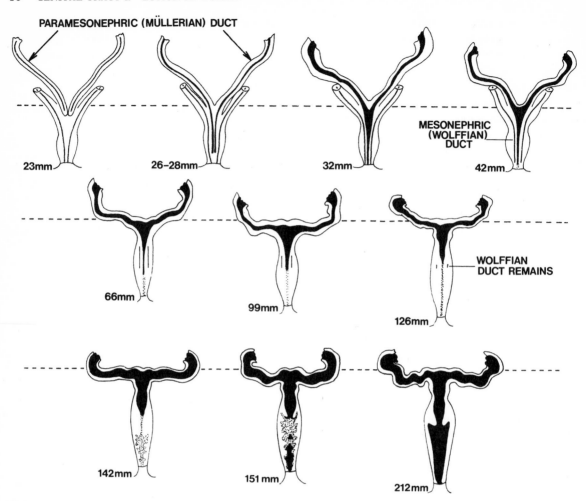

Fig. 1.4 A diagrammatic summary of the sequential changes that take place in the development of the female genital tract in human embryos and fetuses of between 23 and 212 mm crown-rump length, with particular reference to the fates of the mesonephric and paramesonephric duct systems (based on Hunter 1930).

Fig. 1.5 Representative transverse sections through the pelvis of a 112 mm crown-rump length human female fetus (Boyd reference no. H.226) of approximately 16 weeks gestation. Reference to Fig. 1.7C, in which a more extensive view through the mid-gonadal region of this fetus is presented, clearly demonstrates that the ovary is now located in the mid-pelvic region. The level of the prospective fundus region of the uterus is seen in B, though the lumen of the uterovaginal canal at this level, and more distally, is markedly narrower than at the earlier gestational stage illustrated in Fig. 1.3. It has been suggested by Witschi (1970) that the tissue comprising the tapered 'wings' observed on either side of the uterovaginal canal in E may be of mesonephric origin. Note that in F and G the urethra appears to have numerous glandular projections, and that in G and H the lumen of the primitive vaginal plate appears to be completely obliterated. More caudally, in I and J, the urogenital sinus opens out into the vestibule.

1 Common iliac artery; 2 rectum; 3 region of rete ovarii, with remnants of mesonephric tubules; 4 ovary; 5 paramesonephric duct (prospective oviduct); 6 bladder; 7 umbilical artery; 8 prospective fundus region of uterus; 9 rectus abdominis muscle; 10 ureter; 11 uterovaginal canal with cuboidal/columnar epithelial lining; 12 wall of bladder; 13 caudal end of uterovaginal canal with tapered 'wings'; 14 bladder; 15 urethra with numerous prominent glandular projections; 16 primitive vaginal plate with obliterated lumen; 17 level of sinovaginal bulbs; 18 urogenital sinus; 19 definitive pelvic part of urogenital sinus; 20 labial fold; 21 clitoris.

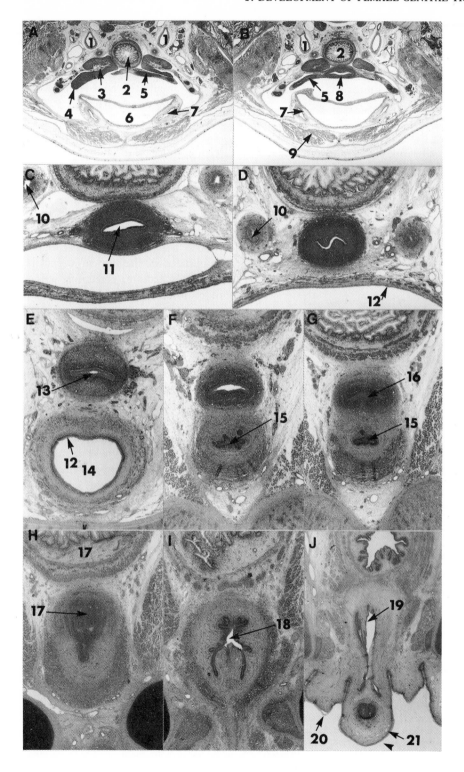

1933; Bulmer 1957). Histochemical studies (Forsberg 1963, 1965), however, suggest that the vaginal plate may, in fact, also have a mesonephric contribution, since the mesonephric ducts are close lateral relations of the uterovaginal canal in this location (Witschi 1970).

By about the 17th week of gestation, the central cells occluding the vaginal plate begin to degenerate (Fig. 1.6), allowing the formation of the vaginal lumen (Hunter 1930). The transitional zone between pseudostratified columnar epithelium (said to be of the uterus), and stratified squamous epithelium (said to be of the vagina) observed at this time is thought to represent the junctional zone between the uterine cervix and the vagina (Davies & Kusama 1962). However, the junctional zone between these two epithelia is very variable, even at term (O'Rahilly 1977).

The observations of Bulmer (1957) tend to support the view proposed by Zuckerman (1940) that, since the epithelium of the adult human vagina responds to oestrogenic stimulation by a stratified squamous type of response, it is likely to be a derivative of the sinus epithelium of the fetus. However, a large body of embryological evidence from other mammalian species would seem to indicate that the upper vaginal segment, at least, despite being lined by stratified squamous epithelium, and giving a squamous response to oestrogenic stimulation, is almost certainly a paramesonephric derivative. The possibility exists that paramesonephric cells in the vagina, but not in the uterus, respond to oestrogenic stimulation by forming stratified squamous epithelium, due to a local controlling 'factor' (Bulmer 1957). It is thought that the epithelium of paramesonephric origin may

be displaced during mid-gestation into the cervical canal. This suggests that the epithelial cells derived from the urogenital sinus probably extend to the level of the future cervical os, and uniformly displace cranially the epithelium of paramesonephric origin (Ulfelder & Robboy 1976). The fact that epithelium of sinus origin is of the squamous type and contains an abundance of glycogen, in common with epithelium of endodermal origin elsewhere in the body (Hashimoto et al 1966), has long been recognised, and has, in fact, been used as an alternative means of attempting to recognise those parts of the vagina that are thought to be of sinus origin (Ulfelder 1968).

It is also unclear to what extent the early development of the human vagina is influenced by hormonal factors, though it seems likely that in older fetuses (probably from about the 112 mm stage onwards) the enormous amount of epithelial activity seen here, and in the cervical region, results from their stimulation by maternal oestrogens (Fraenkel & Papanicolaou 1938). Bulmer (1957) has suggested that the very considerable enlargement that occurs in the lower end of the vaginal mass from about the 140 mm stage, associated with the formation of the hymen, may result from the influence of hormonal stimulation to which only the differentiated type of sinus epithelium is sensitive. Similarly, the upgrowth of the sinus may also be due to a selective response of its differentiated epithelium to appropriate hormonal stimulation. Bulmer (1957) tentatively speculated that some of the differences between vaginal development in different mammalian species may result from differences in the degree of hormonal stimulation they received at various critical periods during fetal life,

Fig. 1.6 Representative transverse sections through the pelvis of a 140 mm crown-rump length human female fetus (Boyd reference no. H.169) of approximately 18 weeks gestation. The midpoint of the gonads is at about the level of the sacral promontory, and the ovary is (in A-C) attached to the dorsal surface of the broad ligament by the mesovarium. The bladder is dilated, and occupies much of the pelvis, and the umbilical arteries are its lateral relations. The ureters are lateral relations of the uterovaginal canal within the broad ligament before they enter the dorsal aspect of the bladder. Note that the uterovaginal canal is closely related to the dorsal surface of the urethra in D-F, that there is some evidence of canalisation of the vagina (in G), and that no obvious cervical region is yet apparent. The various folds located on the dorsal aspect of the urogenital sinus (in I) are thought to represent the hymeneal folds.

1 Sacral promontory; 2 rectum; 3 ovary; 4 mesovarium; 5 paramesonephric duct (prospective oviduct); 6 cavity of the bladder; 7 umbilical artery; 8 common iliac artery; 9 ureter; 10 prospective fundus region of the uterus; 11 rectouterine pouch of Douglas; 12 uterovaginal canal; 13 urethra; 14 pubic symphysis; 15 canalisation in region of the prospective vagina; 16 labial swelling; 17 corpus cavernosum of clitoris; 18 junction between paramesonephric and urogenital sinus epithelia; 19 urogenital sinus; 20 hymeneal folds; 21 pelvic part of urogenital sinus; 22 definitive phallic part of urogenital sinus (urethral groove); 23 glans clitoridis.

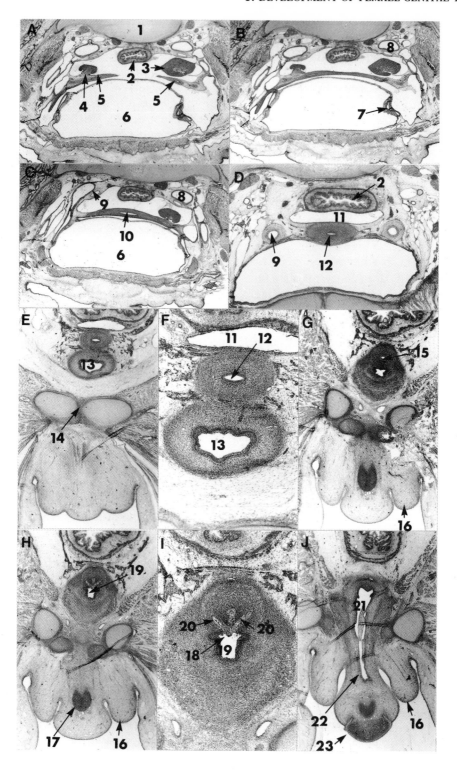

rather than being due to inherent differences in the structures which go to form the vagina. Alternatively, the histological differentiation of the epithelium of the sinus upgrowth in the human fetus may be due to a difference in its sensitivity to hormonal stimulation compared to that occurring in other mammals.

Studies of individuals with testicular feminisation, in which the paramesonephric ducts are suppressed during fetal life, should be instructive, as any vagina present would be expected to be a sinus derivative. Curiously, these studies have not been particularly instructive, as a complete spectrum is seen, varying between the complete absence of the vagina, to those in which a vagina of almost normal dimensions is present. Neither the cervix nor uterine body is seen in the majority of these individuals, though a small but recognisable oviduct, or region of uterine muscle, is occasionally found to be present (Ulfelder & Robboy 1976).

The feature observed most frequently in girls exposed to the hormone diethylstilboestrol (DES) in utero has been termed vaginal adenosis. It has been suggested that this condition may have an embryological basis, and may arise in individuals in which the normal development of the vagina has been interfered with during a critical stage of its organogenesis. This condition is characterised by the presence of small mucinous endocervix-like glands, or ciliated mucus-free tuboendometrium-like glandular epithelium, and poorly glycogenated metaplastic squamous epithelium which extends for variable distances below the cervical os (Robboy et al 1975). In some DES-exposed individuals, discrete patches or even quite large zones of adenosis are present. In others, while the morphological appearance of the vaginal epithelium may be grossly normal, patches of poorly glycogenated epithelium are often present, which fail to stain when Schiller's iodine test is performed.

Adenosis has also been described in individuals with varying degrees of vaginal agenesis (Ulfelder 1968). However, adenosis is not observed in individuals with testicular feminisation, in which the Müllerian contribution is largely absent. Ulfelder & Robboy (1976) have suggested that these observations support the hypothesis that, at any early stage in the development of the vagina, its entire luminal surface of cuboidal/columnar epithelium may be of paramesonephric origin, and that this is normally largely replaced by the advancing squamous epithelium of urogenital sinus origin. They have therefore proposed that exposure to a teratogenic agent, such as DES, probably interferes with the normal mechanism of endothelial replacement by sinus-derived cells. They believe that the localised areas of adenosis result from islands of unreplaced tissue of paramesonephric origin which may be left behind in the vagina in these individuals. In DES-exposed individuals, interference with the normal morphogenesis of the wall of the vagina and uterus apparently also occurs, and abnormal ridges, strictures and other deformities of the cervix are also commonly encountered.

DIFFERENTIATION OF THE CERVIX

While most authorities believe that the cervix is of paramesonephric duct origin (Koff 1933; Forsberg 1965; Witschi 1970), it has long been suggested that its mucous membrane may, in fact, be derived from the urogenital sinus (Fluhmann 1960). While it may be possible to recognise the prospective cervical canal region during the 9th–10th week of gestation, it is only by about the 16th week that the cervix becomes reasonably well defined. It has a narrow lumen, and extends throughout the lower two-thirds of the body of the uterus. It is also just possible to recognise at this time its mucosal, muscular, and serosal components. During the 17th week of gestation, glandular tissue is evident within the cervical region of the uterus. However, it is only by about the 18th–19th week of gestation that the glandular tissue within the body of the uterus is clearly recognisable (Koff 1933), as are the solid epithelial primordia of the anterior and posterior fornices of the vagina. The epithelium of the endocervix changes from cuboidal to cylindrical cells, and mucoid development is also first evident at this time (Witschi 1970). The fornices of the vagina hollow out by about the 21st week of gestation.

The rapid enlargement that occurs in the vagina and cervix compared to the body of the uterus in the second half of gestation, thought to be due to their differing and precocious sensitivity to maternal and placental hormonal stimulation, is halted when the levels of the latter decline after birth (Mossman 1973). Throughout the prenatal period, the cervical region occupies a disproportionately large part of the uterus compared to the situation seen in the adult. During the period between birth and puberty, the adult ratio of cervix: body of uterus is principally achieved by the reduced growth of the cervical region compared to that of the body of the uterus (Hunter 1930).

DESCENT OF THE GONADS

While the testis clearly 'descends' from its intra-abdominal site of origin to its eventual location in the scrotum by the process of differential growth of the surrounding structures, possibly facilitated by the action of the fibromuscular gubernaculum, it is of interest that the ovary also 'descends' from its site of origin in the upper abdominal region into the pelvis. There seems every reason to believe that the descent of the ovary and its adnexae is brought about by a set of factors similar to those thought to control the descent of the testis.

As in the male, the lower pole of the ovary is attached through a gubernaculum to the tissue of the genital ridge. The gubernaculum subsequently becomes attached to the lateral wall of the uterovaginal canal, close to the uterotubal junction. The ligamentous part of the gubernaculum that persists, which is located between the ovary and the uterus, is termed the round ligament of the ovary, and the part located between the uterus and the labium majus is termed the round ligament of the uterus. It has been suggested (Hamilton & Mossman 1972) that the attachment of the ovary to the uterus may prevent the extra-abdominal descent of the ovary. Instead, the ovary is usually retained within the 'true' pelvis, where its original caudal pole becomes directed medially. The ovary eventually lies as a posterior relation of the oviduct, on the dorsal surface of the broad ligament. On rare occasions, the ovary may 'descend' excessively through the inguinal canal and end up in the labial region. If the relationship between the ovary and the other abdominal and pelvic viscera is analysed by examining appropriate transverse histological sections through human fetuses taken at two- to four-weekly intervals, its descent from an abdo-minal to a pelvic position can be readily monitored. Representative histological sections taken through approximately the midpoint of the ovary in fetuses of about 8, 11 and 16 weeks gestation, which clearly demonstrate the 'descent' of the gonad, are illustrated in Fig. 1.7.

DEVELOPMENT OF THE EXTERNAL GENITALIA

The external genitalia in both sexes also pass through an 'indifferent' stage. Initially, mesenchyme cells migrate around the cloacal membrane to form a series of symmetrical cloacal folds. The folds unite ventrally to form the genital tubercle. By about the sixth week, when the cloacal membrane is divided into urogenital and anal membranes, the cloacal folds are correspondingly divided into urethral and anal folds. At about the same time, an additional more lateral pair of labioscrotal folds becomes evident. Within a week or two, the anal and urogenital membranes break down to form the anal canal and the urogenital orifice, respectively, which allows continuity to be made between the surface ectoderm and the endoderm of the cloacal derivatives. However, it is only by about the third month of gestation that it is possible on morphological grounds to recognise the sex of the fetus from the features of the external genitalia. The secondary sex characteristics appear earlier in the male than in the female fetus. This is probably related to the fact that functional activity is observed earlier in the testis than in the ovary.

It is thought that differentiation of the external genitalia in the female occurs because of the absence of the positive male-determining effect of the Y-chromosome. As indicated earlier, the presence of the Y-chromosome induces the gonad in the genetically male fetus to develop as a testis. The latter soon produces androgenic hormones and Müllerian inhibiting substance, and sets in train the sequence of events described in detail earlier in this chapter. At the same time, while the internal genital duct system in the female fetus develops principally from the paramesonephric duct system to form the oviducts and uterus, and the vagina develops largely from the urogenital sinus, the external genitalia change to the recognisably

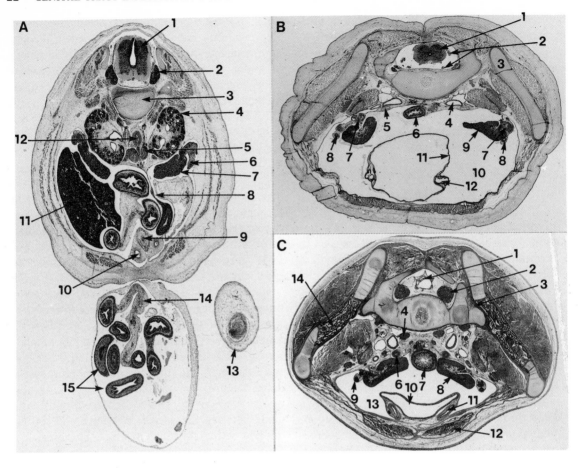

Fig. 1.7 Representative transverse sections through the mid-gonadal region of a 28 mm crown-rump length embryo (A), a 65 mm crown-rump length fetus (B), and a 112 mm crown-rump length fetus (C), being sections taken from the same conceptuses as those illustrated in Figs. 1.2, 1.3 and 1.5, respectively. These representative sections clearly illustrate the 'descent' of the ovary from its initial location in the mid-abdominal region to its final location in the middle of the pelvis.

In the 28 mm crown-rump length embryo, the section passes through the abdomen at the level of the metanephros, the liver, and just below the midpoint of the physiological umbilical hernia. In the 65 mm crown-rump length fetus, the midpoint of the ovary is at the level of the iliac crests. Note that the overall dimensions of the spinal cord in this embryo are considerably smaller than in the embryo illustrated in A, where the spinal cord occupies the whole of the vertebral canal. This section is just above the level of the conus medullaris. In the 112 mm crown-rump length fetus, the midpoint of the ovary is in the midpelvic region, as evidenced by the presence of the sacroiliac joints and appearance of the iliac bones in this section. Furthermore, the filum terminale, which has a small lumen, is the only neural element that is present within the sacral part of the vertebral canal, that is, except for the two large dorsal root ganglia. Note also that the overall dimensions of the pelvic part of the peritoneal cavity are considerably smaller in this section than the situation illustrated in the previous fetus sectioned at a comparable level with respect to the ovary.

A: 1 Spinal cord; 2 dorsal root ganglion; 3 vertebral body; 4 metanephros; 5 chromaffin tissue (prospective adrenal medulla); 6 paramesonephric duct; 7 ovary; 8 dorsal mesentery of gut; 9 urachus; 10 umbilical artery; 11 liver; 12 dorsal aorta; 13 glancing section through umbilical cord; 14 mid-gut mesentery; 15 loops of mid-gut in physiological umbilical hernia. **B:** 1 Spinal cord; 2 upper (proximal) components of cauda equina; 3 iliac crest; 4 common iliac artery; 5 ureter; 6 hindgut (rectum); 7 remnants of mesonephric system; 8 paramesonephric duct; 9 ovary; 10 pelvic part of peritoneal cavity; 11 wall of bladder; 12 umbilical artery. **C:** 1 Filum terminale; 2 dorsal root ganglion; 3 sacroiliac joint; 4 sympathetic trunk; 5 common iliac artery; 6 ureter; 7 rectum; 8 ovary; 9 paramesonephric duct; 10 wall of bladder; 11 umbilical artery; 12 rectus abdominis muscle; 13 pelvic part of peritoneal cavity; 14 ossification within the iliac bone.

female form. The latter differentiative changes occur, it is thought, largely because of the influence of placental and maternal oestrogens, and the absence of high circulating levels of male-determining androgens.

In females, the urethral groove remains open to form the vulva, the urethral folds form the labia minora, the genital swellings form the labia majora and anteriorly the mons pubis, and the genital tubercle forms the clitoris. The vestibule is said to be derived from the phallic part of the urogenital sinus, and into this region the urethra, the vagina, and ducts of the greater vestibular glands (of Bartholin) open. These glands are thought to be homologues of the bulbourethral glands of the male. Additionally, the lesser vestibular glands also open into the anterior part of the vestibule, and are thought to correspond to the glands of Littré of the male. In the lower part of the anal canal, a 'white line' (of Hilton) of relatively poor vascularity is said to mark the line of demarcation between surface ectoderm and gut endoderm, corresponding to the original location of the anal membrane. No clear and comparable line of demarcation is seen which exactly corresponds to the junctional zone where the urogenital membrane breaks down. This site is initially in a trough, and flanked on either side by the endoderm-covered primitive urethral folds. Ventrally, it is continuous with the primitive urethral groove, and is thought to be located on the inner aspect of the labia minora.

ACKNOWLEDGEMENTS

The photomicrographs used to illustrate this chapter are from histological sections of embryos and fetuses in the Boyd Collection in the Department of Anatomy, University of Cambridge. The author's embryological studies are supported by the National Fund for Research into Crippling Diseases.

REFERENCES

Baker T G 1972 Oogenesis and ovarian development. In: Balin H, Glasser S (eds) Reproductive biology. Excerpta Medica, Amsterdam, pp 398–437

Balboni G C 1976 Histology of the ovary. In: James V H T, Serio M, Giusti G (eds) The endocrine function of the human ovary. Academic Press, London, pp 1–24

Brambell F W R 1956 Ovarian changes. In: Parkes A S (ed) Marshall's physiology of reproduction. Vol 1, part 1, 3rd edn. Longmans Green, London, pp 397–542

Bulmer D 1957 The development of the human vagina. Journal of Anatomy 91: 490–509

Byskov A G 1981 Gonadal sex and germ cell differentiation. In: Austin C R, Edwards R G (eds) Mechanisms of sex differentiation in animals and man. Academic Press, London, pp 145–164

Chiquoine A D 1954 The identification, origin and migration of the primordial germ cells in the mouse embryo. Anatomical Record 118: 135–146

Clark J M, Eddy E M 1975 Fine structural observations on the origin and associations of primordial germ cells of the mouse. Developmental Biology 47: 136–155

Clements J A, Reyes F I, Winter J S D, Faiman C 1976 Studies on human sexual development. III. Fetal pituitary and serum, and amniotic fluid concentrations of LH, CG, and FSH. Journal of Clinical Endocrinology and Metabolism 42: 9–19

Cunha G R 1975 The dual origin of vaginal epithelium (I). American Journal of Anatomy 143: 387–392.

Cunha G R 1976 Alterations in the developmental propeties of stroma during the development of the urogenital ridge into ductus deferens and uterus in embryonic and neonatal mice. Journal of Experimental Zoology 197: 375–388

Davies J, Kusama H 1962 Developmental aspects of the human cervix. Annals of the New York Academy of Sciences 97: 534–550

Didier E 1973 Recherches sur la morphogénèse du canal de Müller chez les oiseaux. II. Étude expérimentale. Wilhelm Roux Archiv für Entwicklungsmechanik der Organismen 172: 287–302

Duthie G M 1925 An investigation of the occurrence, distribution and histological structure of the embryonic remains in the human broad ligament. Journal of Anatomy 59: 410–431

Edwards R G 1980 Sexual differentiation, infancy and puberty. In: Conception in the human female. Academic Press, London, pp 23–98

Falin L I 1969 The development of genital glands and the origin of germ cells in human embryogenesis. Acta Anatomica 72: 195–232

Felix W 1912 The development of the urogenital organs. In: Keibel F, Mall F P (eds) Manual of human embryology. Vol 2. Lippincott, Philadelphia, pp 752–979

Fluhmann C F 1960 The developmental anatomy of the cervix uteri. Obstetrics and Gynecology 15: 62–69

Forsberg J -G 1963 Derivation and differentiation of the vaginal epithelium. Institute of Anatomy, Lund (cited by O'Rahilly 1977)

Forsberg J -G 1965 Origin of vaginal epithelium. Obstetrics and Gynecology 25: 787–791

Fraenkel L, Papanicolaou G N 1938 Growth, desquamation and involution of the vaginal epithelium of human fetuses and children with a consideration of the related hormonal factors. American Journal of Anatomy 62: 427–451

Frazer J E 1935 The terminal part of the Wolffian duct. Journal of Anatomy 69: 455–468

Frutiger P 1969 Zur Frühentwicklung der Ductus paramesonephrici und des Müllerschen Hügels beim Menschen. Acta Anatomica 72: 233–245

Garrison F H 1961 An introduction to the history of medicine. 4th edn. Saunders, Philadelphia

George F W, Catt K J, Neaves W B, Wilson J D 1978 Studies on the regulation of testosterone synthesis in the fetal rabbit testis. Endocrinology 102: 665–673

Gillman J 1948 The development of the gonads in man, with a consideration of the role of fetal endocrines and the histogenesis of ovarian tumors. Contributions to Embryology 32: 81–132

Glenister T W 1962 The development of the utricle and of the so-called 'middle' or 'median' lobe of the human prostate. Journal of Anatomy 96: 443–455

Gondos B, Bhiraleus P, Hobel C J 1971 Ultrastructural observations on germ cells in human fetal ovaries. American Journal of Obstetrics and Gynecology 110: 644–652

Gruenwald P 1941 The relation of the growing Müllerian duct to the Wolffian duct and its importance for the genesis of malformations. Anatomical Record 81: 1–19

Gruenwald P 1942 Primary asymmetry of the growing Müllerian ducts in the chick embryo. Journal of Morphology 71: 299–305

Hamilton W J, Mossman H W 1972 Human embryology: prenatal development of form and function. 4th edn. Heffer, Cambridge

Hashimoto K, DiBella R J, Shklar G 1966 Electron microscopic studies of the normal human buccal mucosa. Journal of Investigative Dermatology 47: 512–525

Hunter R H 1930 Observations on the development of the human female genital tract. Contributions to Embryology 22: 91–108

Jarcho J 1946 Malformations of the uterus. Review of the subject, including embryology, comparative anatomy, diagnosis and report of cases. American Journal of Surgery 71: 106–166

Josso N, Picard J -Y, Tran D 1977 The antimüllerian hormone. Recent Progress in Hormone Research 33: 117–167

Jost A 1972 A new look at the mechanisms controlling sex differentiation in mammals. Johns Hopkins Medical Journal 130: 38–53

Jost A, Vigier B, Prépin J, Perchellet J P 1973 Studies on sex differentiation in mammals. Recent Progress in Hormone Research 29: 1–41

Kaplan S L, Grumbach M M, Aubert M L 1976 The ontogenesis of pituitary hormones and hypothalamic factors in the human fetus: maturation of central nervous system regulation of anterior pituitary function. Recent Progress in Hormone Research 32: 161–243

Koff A K 1933 Development of the vagina in the human fetus. Contributions to Embryology 24: 59–90

Lyon M F, Hawkes S G 1970 X-linked gene for testicular feminization in the mouse. Nature 227: 1217–1219

Mettler C C, Mettler F A 1947 History of medicine: a correlative text arranged according to subjects. Blakiston, Toronto

Meyer R 1909 Zur Kenntnis des Gartnerschen (oder Wolff-schen) Ganges besonders in der Vagina und dem Hymen des Menschen. Archiv für Mikroskopische Anatomie 73: 751–792

Meyer W J, Migeon B R, Migeon C J 1975 Locus on human X chromosome for dihydrotestosterone receptor and androgen insensitivity. Proceedings of the National Academy of Sciences of the United States of America 72: 1469–1472

Moore K L 1982 The developing human: clinically oriented embryology. 3rd edn. Saunders, Philadelphia

Mossman H W 1973 The embryology of the cervix. In: Blandau R J, Moghissi K (eds) The biology of the cervix. University of Chicago Press, Chicago, pp 13–22

Müller U, Aschmoneit I, Zenzes M T, Wolf U 1978 Binding studies of H-Y antigen in rat tissues: indications for a gonad-specific receptor. Human Genetics 43: 151–157

O'Connor R J 1939 Experiments on the development of the amphibian mesonephros. Journal of Anatomy 74: 34–44

Ohno S 1977 The original function of MHC antigens as the general plasma membrane anchorage site of organogenesis-directing proteins. Immunological Reviews 33: 59–69

O'Rahilly R 1977 Prenatal human development. In: Wynn R A (ed) Biology of the uterus. 2nd edn. Plenum, New York, pp 35–57

Ozdzeński W 1967 Observations on the origin of primordial germ cells in the mouse. Zoologica Poloniae 17: 367–379

Price J M, Donahoe P K, Ito Y 1979 Involution of the female Müllerian duct of the fetal rat in the organ-culture assay for the detection of Müllerian inhibiting substance. American Journal of Anatomy 156: 265–284

Ramsey E M 1977 History. In: Wynn R A (ed) Biology of the uterus, 2nd edn. Plenum, New York, pp 1–18

Rolnick D, Kawanoue S, Szanto P, Bush I M 1968 Anatomical incidence of testicular appendages. Journal of Urology 100: 755–756

Robboy S J, Scully R E, Herbst A L 1975 Pathology of vaginal and cervical abnormalities associated with prenatal exposure to diethylstilbestrol (DES). Journal of Reproductive Medicine 15: 13–18

Sadler T W 1985 Langman's medical embryology. 5th edn. Williams & Wilkins, Baltimore

Siiteri P K, Wilson J D 1974 Testosterone formation and metabolism during male sexual differentiation in the human embryo. Journal of Clinical Endocrinology and Metabolism 38: 113–125

Simpson J L 1976 Disorders of sexual differentiation. Academic Press, New York

Singer C, Underwood E A 1962 A short history of medicine. 2nd edn. Clarendon Press, Oxford

Snow M H L, Monk M 1983 Emergence and migration of mouse primordial germ cells. In: McLaren A, Wylie C C (eds) Current problems in germ cell differentiation. British Society for Developmental Biology Symposium 7: 115–135

Soller M, Padeh B, Wysoki M, Ayalon N 1969 Cytogenetics of Saanen goats showing abnormal development of the reproductive tract associated with the dominant gene for polledness. Cytogenetics 8: 51–67

Streeter G L 1948 Developmental horizons in human embryos. Description of age groups XV, XVI, XVII, and XVIII, being the third issue of a survey of the Carnegie Collection. Contributions to Embryology 32: 133–204

Tatarian G 1962 Historical aspects of the cervix. Annals of the New York Academy of Sciences 97: 530–533

Thompson J S, Thompson M W 1980 Genetics in medicine. 3rd edn. Saunders, Philadelphia

Torrey T W 1954 The early development of the human nephros. Contributions to Embryology 35: 175–198

Ulfelder H 1968 Agenesis of the vagina. A discussion of surgical management and functional and morphologic comparison of end results, with and without skin grafting. American Journal of Obstetrics and Gynecology 100: 745–751

Ulfelder H, Robby S J 1976 The embryologic development of the human vagina. American Journal of Obstetrics and Gynecology 126: 769–776

Waddington C H 1938 The morphogenetic function of a vestigial organ in the chick. Journal of Experimental Biology 15: 371–376

Wilson J D 1978 Sexual differentiation. Annual Review of Physiology 40: 279–306

Winters A J, Eskay R L, Porter J C 1974 Concentration and distribution of TRH and LRH in the human fetal brain. Journal of Clinical Endocrinology and Metabolism 39: 960–963

Witschi E 1963 Embryology of the ovary. In: Grady H G, Smith D E (eds) The ovary. Williams & Wilkins, Baltimore, pp 1–10

Witschi E 1970 Development and differentiation of the uterus. In: Mack H C (ed) Prenatal life. Wayne State University Press, Detroit, pp 11–35

Zamboni L 1976 Modulations of follicle cell-oocyte association in sequential stages of mammalian follicle development and maturation. In: Crosignani P G, Mishell D R (eds) Ovulation in the human. Academic Press, London pp 1–30

Zuckerman S 1940 The histogenesis of tissues sensitive to oestrogens. Biological Reviews 14: 231–271

The normal flora of the vagina
R E Warren

INTRODUCTION

Sampling and populations

The view that the vaginal flora, dominated by the bacilli originally described by Döderlein in 1892, is a simple one has been frequently repeated in text books and papers since the 1940s. In recent times, the resurgence of interest in human anaerobic microflora and the interest in perinatal and sexually transmitted infection has emphasised the complex interrelationship of the flora in health and disease but has so far provided neither an agreed synthesis of the normal flora's role in the pathogenesis of vaginitis nor the prediction, from microbial cultures, of the presence of genital tract sepsis. Equally we lack any profound understanding of factors involved in the stability or change in the flora. This chapter firstly examines general principles limiting our knowledge of the vaginal flora and then examines some of the species present in greater detail.

As in the urinary tract, infection of the upper genital tract is believed normally to arise from infection of the lower tract. The upper half of the endocervical cavity and the endometrium is usually sterile (Sparks et al 1977). Some bacteria may be present without infection up to 30 days after insertion of an intrauterine device (Mishell et al 1966). It seems likely that at parturition bacterial colonisation of the upper tract may also occur in the absence of overt infection. The mechanisms of resistance to bacterial infection in the corpus uteri and fallopian tubes are not well defined. This chapter concentrates on the normal bacterial flora of the vagina.

Little is known about the stability of components of the vaginal flora. The statistical analysis of the number of colonies of a species on an agar plate that must be examined by typing to give confidence that minority populations are not being overlooked has received almost no attention in the vaginal flora. Assessment, by typing isolates on consecutive examinations, has also been neglected on the assumption that the vaginal flora is a static population. By contrast, this approach to the faecal flora has revealed that methods that do not systematically examine a defined number of colonies grossly overestimate the stability of the flora (Hartley et al 1977). On the other hand, transient variations in numbers in the faecal flora and the innate insensitivity of plating methods may conceal stable members of the flora and falsely suggest instability (Hedges et al 1977). The vagina's proximity to the urethra, skin and rectum and their flora, and the additional factor of sexual transmission of microbes, suggests that repeated assessment of the vaginal flora might reveal similar instabilities in carriage of microbes that are regarded as stable and normal components of the flora. The vaginal flora differs from the gastrointestinal flora in lacking the constant introduction of new strains from food. The importance of appropriate adhesion mechanisms in converting transient to prolonged colonisation is well known from studies of pathogenicity in the gut, but this is another mechanism controlling the normal flora which workers are only now starting to investigate in the genital tract (Kallenius & Winberg 1978; Moi et al 1984).

There are few technical problems in obtaining samples for studies of the flora in the lower genital tract, but, as in the gut, this is not true for the upper genital tract. Quantitative studies of the vaginal flora based on dilution or selective media are essential as controls on the sensitivity of other methods. Assessments of the flora made in clinical laboratories are usually essentially qualitative, involving at best semiquantitative plating. These methods may miss minority populations just as liquid enrichment culture in research studies may overemphasise their clinical importance. Quantitative studies have been few until recently (Bartlett et al 1977, 1978; Levison et al 1977, 1979; Onderdonk et al 1977, Lindner et al 1978, Wilks et al 1982). Most studies assess the bacterial count in the vaginal secretions as some 10^9 organisms/gram. The study of Onderdonk et al (1977) showed that anaerobes outnumbered aerobes in 70% of samples, usually by 10-fold, although the patients studied may not represent a normal population.

It is not certain if the mucosal-associated flora differs from that in aspirated secretions but it is doubtful if the differences in flora between anatomical sites in the lower genital tract are significant. Aspirated secretions from the vaginal fornix appear to yield a different flora from aspirated secretions from the lower cervix, although the differences are small and inconsistent and only apparent with organisms present in low numbers (Bartlett et al 1978). Culture of cotton wool swabs of the secretion also appears to produce a different result from culture of aspirated secretion and similarly to underestimate the diversity of the Gram-positive flora (Onderdonk et al 1977). Some of these differences between sites and different groups of workers are probably caused by differences in the sensitivity and reproducibility of the sampling techniques, which have only recently been adequately assessed (Wilks et al 1982). Methodological approaches used by various authors are indicated in Table 2.1, as are the additional variables of whether samples are diluted prior to culture, or enriched, or cultured using selective media. The additional important variable of the duration of uninterrupted incubation of culture plates is not shown (Wren 1980). The different environments at the surface of the vaginal and endocervical cells suggest the endocervical flora requires further definition in relation to cervical ectropion, parity and mucosal-associated flora.

Practical aspects of defining the human population from which samples have been obtained have also been neglected in studies of the normal genital flora. Populations that are frequently examined include those attending clinics for contraceptive advice and clinics for sexually transmitted diseases, and volunteer populations such as college and medical students and nurses. These may constitute subtle and non-representative selections of the general population. Certainly assessment and definition of sexual activity is difficult and this may be important in considering the stability of the flora. Age and pathology may limit the availability of samples but also certainly affect the vaginal flora. Assessments of prepubertal (Hammerschlag et al 1978a, 1978b) and postmenopausal normal flora (Tashjian et al 1976; Larsen & Galask 1980) are few, since cultures are usually only taken in the presence of genital tract symptoms. Even these studies require careful assessment. Thus sampling a relatively excessive number of children wearing napkins, in a prepubertal group, gives the impression that the overall prepubertal flora is dominated by faecal flora such as *Escherichia coli* and *Bacteroides* sp. (Hammerschlag et al 1978a). Similarly, age alone is an inadequate criterion. After the menopause it appears that anaerobes are more frequent in those not treated with oestrogens (Larsen & Galask 1980).

During the reproductive period it is even more difficult to define a normal flora. Taking genital tract cultures from patients with conditions unrelated to the genital tract is usually impractical. Cyclical changes in the genital tract, with or without the use of tampons or sanitary towels, are believed to influence the flora (Onderdonk et al 1977) but very few studies define when samples were taken in relation to the menstrual cycle. Recent work (Larsen & Galask 1982) emphasises the increase in the number of species detected at the time of menstruation, and the significant decline in the prevalence of *Staphylococcus epidermidis*, coryneforms, faecal streptococci, *Bacteroides* sp. (in particular *B. vulgatus*), *Peptostreptococcus anaerobius*, and to a more doubtful extent *E. coli* after menstruation. Bacterial numbers also decrease after menstruation. Changes in the bacterial flora, particularly of anaerobes similar to those at menstruation, are seen in the postpartum period, in malignancy, and in the presence of *Gardnerella vaginalis* and *Trichomonas vaginalis*. This may depend on pH changes. Larsen and Galask (1982)

Table 2.1 Methodologies used in assessment of anaerobic vaginal flora

Authors	Sample	Culture of diluted sample	Primary selective solid media	Broth enrichment
Blackwell et al 1983	Aspirate (loop)	+	Nal	–
Blythe 1978	Swab	–	–	Thioglycollate
Bramley et al 1981	Swab	–	–	Paracresol
Brook et al 1979	Swab	–	Van/Kan	Thioglycollate
Corbishley 1977	Swab	–	Neo	–
De Louvois et al 1975a	Swab	–	–	–
Duerden 1980	Swab	–	–	–
Duignan & Lowe 1975	Swab	–	Van/Kan	–
Gibbs et al 1982	Amniotic fluid	–	Van/Kan Col/Nal	Cooked meat
Goldacre et al 1979	Swab	–	Neo	–
Goplerud et al 1976	Swab	–	–	Cooked meat
Gorbach et al 1973	Swab	–	Neo	–
Grossman & Adams 1979	Swab	–	Neo/Van	Thioglycollate
Hammann 1982	Swab	–	Van/Kan Nal	–
Hammerschlag et al 1978a, b	Swab	–	–	Cooked meat
Larsen & Galask 1982	Washings	+	Not specified	–
Levison et al 1977, 1979	Aspirate (loop)	+	–	–
Lindner et al 1978	Aspirate	+	Van/Neo	–
Mead 1978	Swab	–	Not specified	–
Moberg et al 1978	Swab	–	Gentian violet	–
Morris & Morris 1967	Swab	–	Crystal violet	–
Neary et al 1973	Swab	–	Neo	Cooked meat
Ohm & Galask 1975	Swab	–	–	Cooked meat
Osborne et al 1979	Swab	–	–	–
Ross & Needham 1980	Swab	–	–	–
Sautter & Brown 1980	Washings	–	Van/Kan Col/Nal	–
Sparks et al 1977	Swab } Biopsy }	–	Col/Neo	–
Spiegel et al 1980	Washings	+	–	–
Tashjian et al 1976	Aspirate (swab) } Washings }	–	Van/Kan	Thioglycollate
Taylor et al 1982	Aspirate (loop)	+	Nal	–
Thadepalli et al 1973	Swab	–	Neo	Cooked meat
Watt et al 1981	Swab	–	Neo	–

Incorporated selective agents:
Col = colistin;
Kan = kanmycin;
Neo = neomycin;
Nal = nalidixic acid;
Van = vancomycin.

point out that pH and redox potential (Eh) are directly related. A high hydrogen-ion concentration (low pH) produces a high redox potential which discourages anaerobic growth. The buffering capacity of the more alkaline vaginal fluid originating from the cervix and vestibular glands, and the factors which control the very small but critical changes in the usually very acid vaginal pH, require further study. The role of microbes in generating rather than surviving this acid environment is also unclear.

Other changes in the reproductive period also influence the flora. The use of local, rather than systemic humoral, contraception methods might be expected to influence the chances of new additions to the microbial flora. Physiological changes during pregnancy and the puerperium (Goplerud et al 1976; Lindner et al 1978) include changes not only in the opportunities for acquisition of new strains from the environment, but also in humoral status, and changes in the vaginal milieu associated with trauma at delivery. These disturbances are associated with dramatic changes in the vaginal flora which are important because they affect colonisation and infection of the neonate. In general terms lactobacilli increase in numbers and prevalence during pregnancy. Anaerobes and most aerobes become less prevalent during pregnancy but increase very rapidly in numbers and diversity in the first 3 days of the puerperium. By 6 weeks after delivery the flora is essentially normal.

The vaginal flora must also be assessed as normal, or otherwise, in relation to pathologies other than infection. Malignancy (Blythe 1978; Mead 1979) or, in our experience, chronically retained foreign bodies such as Shirodkar suture, seem to be associated with higher than expected rates of isolation of haemolytic streptococci and particularly anaerobes. The best example of an abnormal but not necessarily pathogenic flora is perhaps the association of plastic intrauterine devices with the presence in the vaginal flora of *Actinomyces israeli*.

Infections in adjacent organs such as the bladder may affect the vaginal flora. The vaginal flora of patients with indwelling urinary catheters is often dominated by the coliforms concurrently colonising the urinary tract. Urinary pH is usually considerably above vaginal pH. Changes in the vaginal flora consequent on urinary infection have received less attention than changes in periurethral flora in relationship to initiation of urinary infection. Studies of patients about to undergo genital tract surgery for conditions which predispose to urinary infection should not necessarily be accepted as studies of the normal vaginal flora (Gorbach et al 1973; Ohm & Galask 1975; Grossman & Adams 1979).

Treatment or prophylaxis may also affect the vaginal flora. Topical applications to the vagina of iodophors (Osborne & Wright 1977) or chlorhexidine (Duignan & Lowe 1975) affect the flora, although topical applications have a lesser effect on the flora of the endocervix. In the intermenstrual period, antibiotics such as trimethoprim (Stamey et al 1977), and probably tetracyclines, but not sulphonamides (Stamey & Condy 1975), ampicillin, or nalidixic acid and other quinolones, are found in vaginal secretions in significant quantities after oral or parenteral administration. Antibiotics in the secretions may be expected to modify the vaginal flora directly. It is important to note that some antibiotics such as aminoglycosides and erythromycin are much less active at acid pH and this may vitiate conventional sensitivity tests for organisms colonising the vagina rather than infecting its wall (Durfee et al 1979). It is also important to note that some members of the flora are intrinsically resistant to certain antibiotics, e.g. lactobacilli are resistant to trimethoprim and sulphonamides. Parenteral or oral antibiotics also influence the composition of the gastrointestinal flora which subsequently may colonise the genitourinary tract, particularly in the menstrual period. Incomplete absorption of antibiotics when they are given by mouth, or biliary excretion when they are given by either route, are important in these selective effects on the gut flora.

In adults, resistance to new, permanent, rather than transient, colonisations of the faeces with enterobacteriaceae depends particularly on the anaerobic flora although it is not clear which component is responsible. This resistance is termed colonisation resistance (Van der Waiij et al 1972). Although antimicrobial probes such as vancomycin (with an exclusively Gram-positive spectrum) have been used to examine this, their use in combination with gentamicin (to which bacteroides are resistant) has not answered the question of whether colonisation resistance resides in the mucosal associated gram-positive bacteria. Although permanent colonisation with Gram-negative aerobes was increased, *Bacteroides* sp. were also unexpectedly reduced in numbers (Bodey 1981). There is no described association of colonisation resistance with faecal or caecal pH and the mechanism of suppression of new colonisations requires further elucidation. Potential analogies of faecal and vaginal colonisation resistance are evident. It is tempting to predict that specific organisms will mediate resistance to vaginal colonisation and restrict the range of the vaginal flora. Indeed there is some tantalising evidence that lactobacilli produce substances that inhibit other aerobes (Mardh & Soltesz 1983). The mechanism and species involved in this vaginal 'colonisation resistance' would probably vary with vaginal pH. By analogy with the gut, description of such species mediating colonisation-resistance and their antimicrobial susceptibility in the vagina would have important implications both for choice of antimicrobial therapy in infections in the genitourinary tract and also for eliminating vaginal carriage of potential pathogens. (Wiegersma et al 1982)

The normal flora and the pathogen

The definition of a pathogen in the vaginal flora is difficult. Components of the normal flora may assume a pathogenic role but this poses problems in the assessment of cultures. It is well recognised that the normal flora is often replaced on mucosal surfaces by a pathogen in infective states, and that pure growths are frequently an apparent accompaniment of adhesion associated infection, sometimes associated with invasion or local toxin production. The limitations of assumptions about pathogenicity based solely on observations on the purity of any growth on culture or the consistency of any association must be clearly recognised. Four points merit consideration.

Firstly, the purity of the growth may reflect no more than the failure to culture or examine the specimen obtained under appropriate environmental conditions or with appropriate selective media. In the 1950s and 1960s bacteria that could only be grown with anaerobic techniques were neglected. The comparatively recent recognition of *Campylobacter* sp. in gastrointestinal infections, *Actinomyces* sp. in the genital tract of women with intrauterine contraceptive devices, and of *Haemophilus ducreyi*-like bacilli in some genital ulcers (Ursi et al 1982) perhaps should remind us both that anaerobiasis is a relative term and that intermediate microaerophilic environments may be as important as the habitually studied, extreme anaerobic and aerobic environments. Inadvertent neglect of parts of the flora is reflected in the failure, until recently, to recognise the close association between high counts of *Gardnerella* sp., or the presence of *Trichomonas vaginalis*, in the vagina and isolation of non-sporing anaerobes.

Secondly, it is unjustified to assume that a pathogen will uniformly quantitatively suppress other flora or indeed that elements of the normal flora that are present play no part in the pathogenic process. Infections due to synergic interactions between bacteria are well recognised in animals but with some exceptions, such as the synergistic bacterial gangrenes associated with the names of Meleney (1931) and Fournier, have seldom been studied in man. Synergic infection between aerobes and anaerobes in surgical wounds has been increasingly acknowledged. It has been suggested that *Gardnerella* sp. is not responsible for the decarboxylation of amino acids which liberates the characteristic amine odours that are the major source of patient complaint in Gardnerella genital tract colonisation. The occurrence of non-sporing anaerobes and *Mycoplasma hominis* in this condition suggests both that similar synergistic relationships may exist in the genital tract and that abnormal mixed colonisation on the flora, both qualitative and quantitative, may produce disease in the vagina without invasion. Other indirect effects of a changed flora on luminal metabolites are seen in the gastrointestinal tract in the jejunal bacterial overgrowth syndromes (Gorbach & Tabaqchali 1969). It may be difficult when assessing the importance of mixed microbial growths to disentangle double infections, concurrent sexual transmission and the common selective effects of one environment. Changes in the genital tract's microbial ecology in infection may be non-random and attribution of pathogenic interactions based on observation of association is difficult without experimental evidence with pure cultures. The contrast on the one hand of a poor anaerobic flora with frequent persistence of lactobacilli in the acid pH of candidal vaginitis and on the other hand the frequent coincidence of an extensive anaerobic flora with few lactobacilli in vaginitis due to the anaerogenic protozoon *Trichomonas vaginalis* perhaps exemplifies the difficulty posed by association alone, particularly when lactobacilli are considered.

Thirdly, it must be recognised that deciding whether a single organism is a pathogen in the flora cannot easily be done by resort to Koch's postulates. Some workers, overcoming ethical difficulties, have attempted to assess pathogenicity by inoculating pure cultures into the human vagina. This approach must be treated with much greater suspicion when applied to inoculation of putative pathogens into sites with a normal flora than to direct inoculation into sterile tissues (Criswell et al 1969). This is further demonstrated by work with *Mobiluncus* sp. and *Gardnerella* sp. in animal models where the production of a discharge depends on inoculation of the two species on a background of normal anaerobic flora (Mardh et al

1984). Unsuspected minority members of the flora may not be detected in preinoculation samples. These organisms could be essential for production of disease and their growth could conceivably be selectively enhanced by synergic interactions with the inoculated microbe. Antimicrobials with specific spectra have been used as probes to elucidate the role of *Chlamydia trachomatis* and *Ureaplasma urealyticum* in non-specific urethritis (Bowie et al 1976; Coufalik et al 1979) and a similar approach could, perhaps, with advantage also be applied to synergic interactions in the vaginal flora.

Finally, it is important to make the point that one should attempt to define any pathological entity on many parameters to allow for difficulties associated with the sensitivity and specificity of any single laboratory or clinical test. The use of other tests in addition to classical microscopy and culture, for example vaginal pH and the presence, identity or ratios of volatile branched-chain fatty acids, may permit better definition of disease states and a more accurate assessment of sensitivity and specificity of more usually assessed parameters.

In addition to these interpretative problems it is important to analyse cultural results in clinical terms. The carriage state must be distinguished from subclinical infection, which implies damage to the host. For many genital pathogens it has become clearer over recent years that subclinical infection is commoner than carriage. However, merely because an organism may cause a pathological process in a sexual partner or a neonate, it is illogical to deny the existence of a carrier state in another individual, or to imply that the carrier state for any pathogen represents any process other than its integration into a normal flora.

This completes this brief survey of difficulties with defining and assessing the vaginal flora as normal.

The practical problem facing the microbiologist and the clinician is the interpretation of the significance of a named species in a particular patient. For this reason, in the rest of this chapter, the flora of the vagina is considered group by group so that some assessment of the variation that is normal can be made. It should be clear from the considerations earlier in this introduction that clear definitions are needed of the population being examined before any differences in the vaginal flora can be considered significant. Such definition has seldom been made in published studies and it is correspondingly difficult to generalise accurately about the normal flora. Normality can be defined only in terms of the population being examined and is subject additionally to methodological variations between laboratories. In the consideration of the normal flora which follows it is all too frequently obvious that the portrait of the flora sketched by one group of workers at one time and place is not recognisably the same as that painted by others.

MEMBERS OF THE FLORA

Lactobacilli and bifidobacteria

These genera of Gram-positive bacilli are included together since they are frequently confused in discussions on the normal vaginal flora. *Bifidobacterium* (formerly known as *Lactobacillus bifidus*) or 'anaerobic lactobacilli' is a genus of obligate anaerobic bacteria, whereas the familiar *Lactobacillus* sp. often referred to as Döderlein's bacilli are aerobes and only facultatively anaerobic.

Lactobacilli are acid-tolerant bacilli and are found in the gastric and dental flora as well as in the vaginal flora at all ages. Lactobacilli are usually the dominant flora of the vagina under the acid conditions found early in the neonatal period, and between puberty and the menopause, times when the cervical epithelium is laden with glycogen under oestrogenic stimulus (Cruickshank & Sharman 1934). Cruickshank & Sharman noted that on the first day of life the vaginal secretion already had a mean pH of 5.7, although lactobacilli were absent. By the third day of life, vaginal pH had fallen to a mean of 4.9 and aerobic lactobacilli had assumed a dominant role in the flora. Lactobacilli are regularly the dominant flora in women attending clinics for sexually transmitted disease or family planning, from whom no pathogens are isolated and in whom the vaginal pH is less than 4.5. By contrast lactobacilli are seldom dominant if the vaginal pH is above 4.5. This higher pH is usual in the presence of nonsporing anaerobes including *Mobiluncus, Gardnerella* or *Trichomonas* (Karnaky 1959; Taylor et al 1982) Lactobacilli are present in numbers of $>10^4$/ml in 75% of normal women or those with candidiasis compared with 25% in those with *Trichomonas* or non-specific vaginitis (Taylor et al 1982). Davies and Pearl (1938) reported floras dominated by lactobacilli at a 'normal' adult pH of 4.8–5.7, a pH considered abnormal in the study of Taylor and colleagues. This sort of difference emphasises the difficulty of critical pH measurement on small volumes of secretion over such a narrow range.

It is interesting that lactobacilli are not uncommon members of the flora prior to puberty or after the menopause when the vaginal pH is commonly above 6.0 and the epithelium contains little glycogen. Cruickshank & Sharman (1934) drew the conclusion from the common dominance of lactobacilli that they fermented any glycogen present in the secretions and that the lactic acid which was produced lowered the pH of the secretions. They were aware that evidence of glycogen fermentation by lactobacilli was scanty and conflicting. They acknowledged that enzymes from other bacterial or human sources might be responsible for the initial attack on glycogen even if lactobacilli subsequently metabolised the products of this attack. It has since become clear that usually the aerobic lactobacilli do not ferment glycogens (Rogosa & Sharpe 1960), including glycogen obtained from the human vagina (Wylie & Henderson 1969). Only 3 out of 32 strains isolated from the vagina fermented glycogen in one study (Wylie & Henderson 1969) and only about half the *Lactobacillus acidophilus* strains, representing 30% of all strains, in another (Rogosa & Sharpe 1960). *L. fermentus*, *L. casei*, *L. brevis*, *L. lactis*, and *L. cellobiosus* do not ferment glycogen. *L. salivarius* and *L. leichmanii*, which are rare in the vagina, may ferment glycogen occasionally. Thus although lactobacilli are undoubtedly acid-tolerant there is no evidence that they produce acid from glycogen. Indeed there is evidence that glycogenolytic enzymes are derived from endogenous genital secretion, although the subsequent metabolism may be mediated by bacteria (Fienberg & Cohen 1967; Gregoire et al 1967).

Aerobic lactobacilli are not stable members of the faecal flora of infants in the first year of life (Stark & Lee 1982) despite, if anything, their increased dominance in the normal vaginal flora during pregnancy which might predispose to neonatal colonisation. By contrast bifidobacteria are common in infant faecal flora and may be involved in control of the normal flora in the neonate.

Bifidobacteria (anaerobic lactobacilli), like their aerobic counterparts, are acid-tolerant. Their ability to ferment glycogen is uninvestigated. The metabolic activities of bifidobacteria in an acid environment have been closely studied both in vitro and in the neonatal gut and may be relevant to the maintenance of the vaginal pH. In lactose-containing culture media in vitro bifidobacteria can generate a pH of 3.9 before entering a stationary phase, compared with a pH of 5.2 generated by *E. coli*. Inoculation of the relatively unbuffered medium of human (rather than cow's) milk with bifidobacteria produces similar acidity which curtails the growth of, but does not eliminate, a concurrent inoculum of *E. coli* (Bullen & Willis 1971).

Bifidobacterium bifidum produces large quantities of acetate and generates, in the breast-fed infant's faeces, a stable acetate buffer system maintaining a low pH (5.2). This is associated with counts of *Bacteroides* sp. of 10^8/ml compared with 10^{10}/ml in infants fed on reconstituted milk formulations. Growth of bifidobacteria in the gut also suppresses the appearance in faeces of the branched-chain volatile fatty acids, characteristic metabolic products of non-sporing anaerobes (Bullen et al 1977). This reflects the suppression of non-sporing anaerobes. Colonisation with clostridia is also suppressed, and coliform counts tend to fall after 4 weeks of age. This suppression of acquisition of a complex flora by a low pH, associated with bifidobacterial growth, resembles the exclusion of anaerobes and coliforms from the vaginal flora of the premenopausal adult. Indeed some workers have found that bacteroides are unable to become stable members of the neonatal faecal flora until weaning, when facultative aerobes such as coliforms and enterococci also increase in numbers (Stark & Lee 1982).

Bifidobacteria in the female genital tract have received comparatively little attention. Distinguishing these bacteria amidst the facultatively anaerobic lactobacilli may be difficult, but the consistency of the reported rate suggests that bifidobacteria are genuinely uncommon in the vagina, unlike the neonatal gut. Goplerud et al (1976) report an isolation rate of 2 to 6% from cultures during and immediately after pregnancy and a similar rate is recorded in the prepubertal period (Hammerschlag et al 1978a), in pre- and postmenopausal private clinic patients (Osborne et al 1979) and pre-hysterectomy samples (Ohm & Galask 1975). Repeating cultures does not increase the isolation rate (Sautter & Brown 1980). A note of caution is necessary about the conclusion that these organisms are rare. Two reports cite respectively a recovery of 29 isolates from 112 samples in normal patients (Crociani et al 1973) and a 24% rate from the mixed anaerobic flora seen in invasive carcinoma of the cervix (Mead 1979). In the normal patients bifidobacteria were present in considerable numbers but not as the dominant organism. *B. bifidum* was the species in only 9/85 isolates. *B. breve*, *B. adolescentis* and *B. longum* were more commonly identified.

Corynebacteria

These aerobic gram-positive rods are difficult to speciate and classify, and seldom, in the vagina, conform to the type species of *Corynebacterium xerosis* and *C. hofmani* commonly found in the upper respiratory tract. These atypical corynebacteria are common in the vagina and are frequently referred to as diphtheroids or coryneforms. Reports of isolation rates are further confused by the brief respite offered in the genus *Corynebacterium* to *Gardnerella vaginalis* in its taxonomic travels from the genus *Haemophilus*. Like lactobacilli, but unlike *Gardnerella*, unclassified coryneforms morphologically similar to *G. vaginalis* are usually resistant to 5 mg/l trimethoprim (Piot et al 1980). Corynebacteria are usually distinguished from lactobacilli by their possession of catalase, but in some papers a category of unclassified catalase-negative coryneforms is introduced.

In general in the vagina corynebacteria are present in lower numbers than lactobacilli (Onderdonk et al 1977). Numbers in the fornix (10^8/ml) are at least 100-fold higher than in the endocervix. Both in normal adults and those with cervicitis, this quantitative difference in flora at the two sites is much more striking than for any other species (Lindner et al 1978). Although strains of *C. xerosis* from the vagina are unusual in their saccharolytic power and produce large amounts of acid (Laughton 1950), isolation rates are higher at menstruation when vaginal pH is higher. The acid tolerance of coryneforms is limited (Larsen & Galask 1982).

Isolation frequences of 15–30% are usual in adults both before and after the menopause (Morris & Morris 1967; Bartlett et al 1977; Osborne et al 1979). During pregnancy corynebacteria can be isolated from 30–40% of specimens (Goplerud et al 1976; Ross & Needham 1980). Much higher rates (60–85%) have been reported from similar cultures of the fornix in adults (De Louvois et al 1975b, Tashjian et al 1976; Corbishley 1977) and from premenarchal cultures (Hammerschlag et al 1978a). It seems unlikely that this relates to confusion with *G. vaginalis* but the reasons for these differences are not clear.

Non-sporing anaerobes in the vaginal flora

General assessment

Modern anaerobic techniques were applied to cultures of genital tract infections before they were applied to cultures in normal patients, especially in the postoperative and postpartum periods. Many medical staff assume that *Bacteroides fragilis*, *B. melaninogenicus* and *Peptostreptococcus anaerobius* are associated only with infection and do not appreciate that these organisms are usually present at these times and contribute as part of the normal flora to any local infection. This may lead to unnecessary chemotherapy. Relative changes probably occur in anaerobic populations in the menstrual cycle and this needs to be assessed when considering the presence of anaerobes at other times. The aerobic species—*Staphylococcus epidermidis*, *Streptococcus faecalis*, coryneforms and *E. coli*—as well as the anaerobes, *Peptostreptococcus anaerobius* and *Bacteroides* sp., are commoner at the time of menstruation than 7 to 9 days later, according to Larsen & Galask (1982). By contrast, whilst essentially confirming the changes with aerobes, Bartlett et al (1977) felt that anaerobic counts remained essentially constant throughout the menstrual cycle.

In no other area of clinical laboratory practice is interpretation of anaerobic isolates more difficult than in vaginal and cervical cultures taken for assessment of suspected pelvic sepsis. Using unsheathed swabs isolation rates respectively of 16–78% for *B. fragilis*, 21% for *B. melaninogenicus*, and 54% for *Peptostreptococcus* have been reported in genital tract sepsis (Swenson et al 1973; Thadepalli et al 1973). Major authorities (Sutter et al 1980) have recorded their advice that vaginal swabs should not be cultured anaerobically and that a double-plugged catheter with contained brush similar to the Wimberley brush or cannula (Wimberley et al 1979) used for obtaining bronchoscopic samples free of contaminating upper respiratory flora should be used to obtain uterine samples free of contaminating vaginal flora, regardless of whether the ectocervix is treated with antiseptics. In the United Kingdom this excellent advice is seldom heeded by research workers, and never in the clinical setting. Obtaining meaningful samples postpartum is even more problematic because of changes in the cervix. Nevertheless refinements on the described techniques should be possible (Eschenbach et al 1986; Pezlo et al 1979; Knuppel et al 1981). Unfortunately, almost all the data on infection in the literature are open to the criticism that samples are contaminated with normal flora.

Isolation of anaerobes in the preoperative period is not always associated with sepsis in the postoperative period, but isolation rates increase markedly after hysterectomy. Larsen & Galask (1980) report evidence that the isolation rate of *B. fragilis* from preoperative vaginal cultures of those undergoing respectively vaginal or total abdominal hysterectomy increased from 4.3 and 17.4% to 31.8% and 35% in the postoperative period. Similar increases are seen for *E. coli*. In a similar study, with a comparable preoperative percentage of cultures positive for *Bacteroides* sp. (Neary et al 1973), only 4/19 patients with preoperative bacteroides developed postoperative sepsis and in only one of these cases was *Bacteroides* sp. isolated.

An accurate description of the normal anaerobic flora of the vagina has been made more difficult by recent findings. Isolation of anaerobes is very significantly associated with the frequently unrecognised condition of non-specific vaginitis and *Gardnerella vaginalis* (Taylor et al 1982). The association may actually be with the rather higher vaginal pH typical of this condition, *Trichomonas vaginalis* and the postpartum period. Non-specific vaginitis has only recently gained widespread bacteriological acceptance and definition. Since little information about its prevalence in sexually active populations is available, it is difficult to assess in retrospect the incidence of anaerobes in allegedly 'normal' populations where mild degrees of vaginal discharge associated with *G. vaginalis* have not been excluded. Irrespective of the presence of an intrauterine contraceptive device, anaerobes were isolated from 124/693 women with an abnormal discharge in one large series of patients attending a family planning clinic and from 14/145 without discharge, a significant difference ($P \leqslant 0.05$). Some of this association could be with unrecognised nonspecific vaginitis for which full diagnostic criteria have only recently been described (Amsel et al 1983).

The association of *Gardnerella* sp. with nonsporing anaerobes is an interesting one since anaerobes may play a part in the pathogenesis of this condition. The fishy odour of the vaginal discharge in non-specific vaginitis is intensified if 10% potassium hydroxide is added to the secretions. Odorous amines (methylamine, isobutylamine, putrescine, cadaverine, histamine, tyramine, and phenethylamine) are present in these secretions until the patient is treated with metronidazole or ampicillin (Chen et al 1979). These amines are not volatile at the pH of the secretions, but become volatile under more alkaline conditions which may be produced by introduction of semen into the vagina. Putrescine is the most constant of these amines. This can be produced either by decarboxylation of ornithine or by decarboxylation and hydrolysis of arginine. Chen et al (1979) have shown that the metronidazole-sensitive flora of nonspecific vaginitis, in the absence of *G. vaginalis*, is capable of synthesising putrescine from arginine but did not show that arginine was synthesised by *Gardnerella* sp. The precise organisms responsible for the amine synthesis have not been identified. Recently anaerobic curved (vibrio-like) gramnegative rods have been described and isolated in this condition in some 58% of patients (Blackwell et al 1983). These are of two distinct sorts, long (4μ) and short (1.5μ) rods. The short forms are not susceptible to 8 mg/l metronidazole but do hydrolyse arginine; the long forms do not hydrolyse arginine but are metronidazole-susceptible (Fox & Phillips 1984). These organisms, which are often associated, have been classified in a new genus—*Mobiluncus*.

Eubacteria and propionibacteria

These Gram-positive anaerobic rods are seldom reported by most clinical laboratories and for such common members of the anaerobic flora they receive scant attention. *Eubacterium* and *Propionibacterium* are probably usually dismissed as part of the mixed flora of unidentified facultatively anaerobic lactobacilli, coryneform bacilli and bifidobacteria, and assumed to be non-significant isolates.

Isolation rates of *Eubacterium* sp. vary widely, perhaps reflecting variations in interest in, and familiarity with, this genus. In a comparison of paired cervical and vaginal swabs, taken from premenopausal patients admitted for elective hysterectomy, Bartlett et al (1978) recovered eubacteria from 5/14 vaginal and 2/14 cervical swabs in counts of 10^8/g. By contrast, in a comparable study, Osborne et al (1979) isolated eubacterium only from 2/50 cervical swabs but not from vaginal samples until the postmenopausal period. Overall Bartlett et al (1977) isolated eubacteria from 8/22 (36%) of patients and found *E. lentum* as the commonest species.

Eubacterium sp. is present in the vaginal flora of 32% of prepubertal girls. A variety of species, including *E. tenue*, *E. rectale*, *E. lentum*, *E. moniliforme*, *E. cylindroides*, and *E. alactolyticum* are found (Hammerschlag et al 1978a). In a study of serial samples in seven sexually active women, *Eubacterium* sp. was the dominant anaerobic species in 25% of cultures where anaerobes were found. *Eubacterium* sp. was only intermittently detectable in at least one woman studied (Sautter & Brown 1980). A much lower isolation rate of 1% was reported from a sexually active group with a high incidence of *Gardnerella* sp., *Candida* sp. and *Trichomonas* sp. (Taylor et al 1982). A similar isolation rate of 5 to 7% is reported in patients with infertility (Moberg et al 1978), before hysterectomy (Ohm & Galask 1975) and in pregnancy or labour (Gorbach et al 1973; Moberg et al 1978). Isolation of *Eubacterium* sp. is unusual postpartum (Brook et al 1979). In a study of the bacteriology of amniotic fluid, *Eubacterium* sp. was grown from 4% of patients without infection and 12% of those with intra-amniotic infection (Gibbs et al 1982).

Propionibacteria isolation rates from the vagina seem consistent with the changes in the numbers of propionibacteria on the skin, these being hormonally influenced. *Propionibacterium* sp. is isolated from only 4% of cultures from prepubertal girls (Hammerschlag et al 1978a). A similar low rate of isolation of propionibacteria is usual in sexually active adults (Taylor et al 1982). In premenopausal patients admitted for hysterectomy, propionibacteria were isolated from 14% of patients in counts of 10^8/l (Bartlett et al 1977). Propionibacteria are present in up to 25% of cultures taken in pregnancy but this varies with the stage of pregnancy. More patients carry *Propionibacterium* sp. in the second trimester (Goplerud et al 1976), but the proportion of carriers declines significantly to 2% 3 days postpartum. Interestingly, *Propionibacterium acnes* was the commonest anaerobe isolated from the cervix immediately postpartum in one series (Brook et al 1979).

Anaerobic streptococci

Two genera of anaerobic streptococci, *Peptococcus* and *Peptostreptococcus*, are common. Peptococci can be distinguished both easily and relatively reliably in the clinical laboratory from peptostreptococci by their resistance to a 5 μg novobiocin disc but speciation is substantially more difficult (Wren et al 1977). Indeed the allocation of the species between the two genera is sometimes questioned (Ezaki et al 1983). Extraordinary differences are quotable in the rates of isolation of these two genera from the genital tract and the differences in the isolation rates of their respective species are equally great. One species of anaerobic streptococcus, *Peptostreptococcus putridus*, has been claimed to be particularly associated with puerperal thrombophlebitis and metastatic infection (Smith 1975). This species is now regarded as synonymous with *Peptostreptococcus anaerobius*, a common species in the normal flora as well as infection, and this specific association should probably now be doubted.

The anaerobic coccal flora of the vagina changes widely during progress from cradle to grave. Hammerschlag et al (1978a) isolated peptostreptococci, almost exclusively *Peptostreptococcus anaerobius*, from 56% of prepubertal girls and peptococci from 76%. Larsen & Galask (1982) showed that numbers of *Peptostreptococcus anaerobius*, but not peptococci, increased during menstruation. Bartlett et al (1978) studied 14 adult patients before hysterectomy and recovered peptostreptococci from only 2 patients and peptococci from 10. There was no significant difference in the isolation rates from vaginal and endocervical cultures and counts were similarly high (10^7–10^9 ml) in both sites. Osborne et al (1979) in a similarly selected group of patients grew peptococci from only 18% of patients but peptostreptococci from 32%. It is likely that the difference reflects the use of dilution of the sample and selective media containing aminoglycosides in the study reported by Bartlett and his colleagues. Isolation rates reported by Bartlett from younger adults were similar (1977).

Lindner et al (1978) reported that the isolation rate of anaerobic streptococci declines as pregnancy progresses. This finding, as a generalisation, has been confirmed (Goplerud et al 1976) although it is not true when individual species are considered. This might imply a decrease in the diversity of the anaerobic coccal flora as pregnancy progresses. Only some 73% of patients at term, compared with 90% in the first trimester, carry anaerobic cocci (Goplerud et al 1976). Three days postpartum there was an increase in the overall isolation rate to 97% with an isolation rate of approximately 60% for the peptococci and 40% for *Peptostreptococcus anaerobius*. Only 3 of 46 patients cultured at this time were febrile and these were diagnosed as having endometritis. This strongly suggests that isolation postpartum of these anaerobic streptococci, including *Peptostreptococcus anaerobius*, offers little extra support to a clinical diagnosis of postpartum infection. By 6 weeks postpartum the rates had declined slightly to those seen in the first trimester. In contrast to this report, Brook et al (1979) isolated peptococci and peptostreptococci from only 25% of patients in the immediate postpartum period. Other studies of anaerobic streptococci during pregnancy are less convincing. A study from Queen Charlotte's Hospital, London, reported an increase in the isolation of anaerobic cocci as pregnancy progresses (De Louvois et al 1975b). This may reflect a difference in study design as these authors did not sequentially culture patients and only performed cultures in the third trimester in 15 of 280 patients investigated. Another study records an isolation rate of only 1–2% from patients at various stages of pregnancy (Ross & Needham 1980), but these authors also failed to isolate bacteroides from any samples which might suggest less than optimal anaerobic techniques. Gibbs et al (1982) did not isolate anaerobic cocci from the amniotic fluid of any of 52 patients without amnionitis but peptococci and peptostreptococci were isolated respectively from 5/52 and 3/52 patients with amnionitis.

In general these isolation rates for anaerobic streptococci are very much higher than the 7.2% rate recorded (Watt et al 1981) from a population of 1498 attending a contraceptive clinic. In this study there was no significant difference in recovery rate by contraceptive method. Corbishley (1977) in a study of 40 women from a similar population recorded an isolation rate of about 50%. These differences in isolation rate are perhaps not surprisingly great when it is noted that small numbers were ignored in the study of Watt and his colleagues.

Differences in the distribution of species of peptococci with different conditions may reflect difficulties with the taxonomy of this genus or the number of strains identified from each specimen. Onderdonk et al (1977) isolated peptococci from 4/8 patients but in 3/4, multiple species were identified.

In the prepubertal period *Peptococcus prevoti* (which may be only a variant of *P. asaccharolyticus*) was isolated from 15/25 prepubertal girls: *P. asaccharolyticus* and the two species *P. magnus* and *P. variabilis*, which are particularly closedly related, were much less common (Hammerschlag et al 1978a). In a study on a population of reproductive age *P. prevoti*, *P. asaccharolyticus*, *P. magnus* and *P. variabilis* were equally common (25%) (Bartlett et al 1977). In prehysterectomy samples, *P. asaccharolyticus* was the commonest anaerobic coccus isolated, being found in 48% of patients, *P. prevoti* in 11% amd *P. magnus* in 7% (Ohm & Galask 1975). Taylor et al (1982) also found *P. magnus* and *P. variabilis* were less common in a population studied with a high incidence of non-specific vaginitis. One other study, with samples taken in pregnancy and 6 weeks postpartum, reports a high isolation rate of *P. prevoti*. *P. prevoti* was isolated from 20–40% of cultures in pregnancy, but *P. asaccharolyticus* was recovered from 42–52% of patients and *P. magnus* from 40–65% (Goplerud et al 1976).

The variation in recovery of *Peptostreptococcus* species is much less marked. A 15–30% rate of recovery for *P. anaerobius* is usual in prehysterectomy samples (Ohm & Galask 1975), in pregnancy (Goplerud et al 1976) and in the postpartum period (Goplerud et al 1976; Brooke et al 1979). Higher rates are recorded in the prepubertal period (Hammerschlag et al 1978a) and immediately postpartum (Goplerud et al 1976). *P. micros* (which is in fermentation characteristics not dissimilar from *Peptococcus magnus*) is usually found in only 2–7% of cultures.

Bacteroides species: taxonomy and pathogenicity

The picture of colonisation by anaerobic gram-negative bacilli, loosely termed bacteroides, has been complicated by studies of pathogenicity and taxonomy. Ten years ago most British laboratories would have reported all penicillin-resistant anaerobic gram-negative bacilli as *Bacteroides fragilis* and many still do. Studies in abdominal sepsis have revealed that infections are usually caused by *B. fragilis* subspecies *fragilis*, now confusingly elevated to specific status as *B. fragilis sensu strictu*, and to a lesser extent *B. thetaiotamicron* (formerly *B. fragilis* subsp. *thetaiotamicron*). Other former subspecies of *B. fragilis* now recognised as *B. ovatus*, *B. vulgatus* and *B. distasonis*, are present in much larger numbers than *B. fragilis sensu strictu* in the faecal flora, although rare in wound infections. Earlier assumptions that any penicillin-resistant, non-pigmented, anaerobic gram-negative bacillus was likely to be the bile-resistant *B. fragilis sensu lato* have proved to be false. In anaerobic pleuropulmonary infection it has become apparent that the usually quoted isolation rate for *B. fragilis* is about three times the true rate (5%; Kirby et al 1980). *B. fragilis* may also not be the usual penicillin-resistant species in the genital tract. Three new species of bacteroides that occur in the genital tract have been described in the last 10 years—*B. ruminicola*, *B. bivius* and *B. disiens*. These bile-sensitive species are uncommon in the faecal flora. All are commonly resistant to penicillins, often cephalosporins, and sometimes cephamycins (cefoxitin) or oxa-cephems (Moxalactam) (Hill & Ayers 1985). In vitro *B. bivius* can be distinguished from other bile-sensitive, saccharolytic bacteroides by its inability to hydrolyse aesculin

or ferment sucrose: *B. disiens* shares these properties and in addition does not ferment lactose.

Taxonomic turmoil prevails in other species of bacteroides. *B. melaninogenicus sensu lato* includes subspecies *melaninogenicus* and *intermedius*. Another subspecies of this black pigmented bacteroides has been separately speciated as *B. asaccharolyticus* and this species is commonly associated with sepsis. *B. melaninogenicus* and *B. asaccharolyticus* are occasionally penicillin-resistant. Other bacteroides, such as *B. oralis*, are closely related to *B. melaninogenicus* but do not produce the black porphyrin (with, under ultraviolet light, its characteristic red fluorescence which may also be detected instantly in pus from an infected patient).

Other bacteroides are reported both from genital tract sepsis and the normal vagina. *B. capillosus*, *B. coagulans*, *B. pneumosintes*, *B. putredinis*, and *B. ureolyticus* (syn. *B. corrodens*—a species susceptible to the aminoglycoside antibiotics such as neomycin or kanamycin, commonly used in the selective media in many studies) have all been reported from the genital tract (Kirby et al 1980).

It seems possible by analogy with gut-associated sepsis that only some *Bacteroides* sp. in the vagina are frequently associated with infection, whereas others are seldom present except as members of the normal vaginal or faecal flora. The assessment of the clinical significance of penicillin-resistant bacteroides in pelvic sepsis might be easier if species were formally identified to exclude *B. vulgatus* and *B. ovatus*, and if other species of low pathogenicity could be delineated. Studies carried out before 1980 on anaerobic genital tract sepsis need to be repeated using a modern taxonomic approach and a control population with a similarly high anaerobic isolation rate in the absence of clinical signs of sepsis. It is likely that such analysis will only produce a relative reduction in uncertainty about the pathogenic role of an organism, rather than an absolute statement that an organism is non-pathogenic. One recent study reported the isolation of bacteroides other than *B. fragilis*, *B. melaninogenicus*, and *B. asaccharolyticus* in 25% of patients with genital tract sepsis, including nine cases of acute salpingitis, and three cases of postpartum endometritis (Kirby et al 1980), although it is not clear how frequently other pathogenic organisms were present in these infections. Of the isolates, 14 of 16 belonged to the *B. bivius/B. disiens* complex. *B. bivius/B. disiens* have been reported from abdominal hysterectomy wound infection (Appelbaum et al 1978, 1980), Bartholin's abscess (Hill 1978) and obstetric infections (Gibbs et al 1980). These species may therefore possess some pathogenic potential. It is doubtful if penicillin-resistant bacteroides from endocervical swabs taken for investigation of pelvic sepsis need to be speciated at the present time for diagnostic rather than research purposes. Further information on the species involved in such sepsis, and present in comparably sampled uninfected controls, is highly desirable. In the following account an author's identification of *B. fragilis* should be treated with caution unless details of other speciation of bacteroides for the study are given. It is frequently not clear in publications or, indeed, in routine clinical laboratory reports, if identification has been carried far enough to distinguish different penicillin-resistant bacteroides even if the confusing specific name *fragilis* is used. Equal difficulty pertains to identifications of *B. melaninogenicus* which may or may not be used in a sense which includes *B. asaccharolyticus*.

Most earlier studies require reconsideration in the light of these findings.

With this background what species of bacteroides are recovered from the female genital tract? Duerden (1980), selecting, almost always, 10 colonies for identification from vaginal cultures of 20 patients attending a family planning clinic, isolated *B. fragilis sensu lato* from only one patient, who carried four of the former subspecies—an association of bile-resistant *fragilis* species also apparent in at least one other study (Onderdonk et al 1977). Members of the *B. bivius/B. disiens* group were isolated from 12 patients, *B. melaninogenicus* ssp. *intermedius* (or ssp. *melaninogenicus*) from 7, and *B. asaccharolyticus* and *B. oralis* each from 4 patients. Hammann (1982) in a less clearly defined patient group reported 26 *B. bivius*, 7 *B. disiens*, and 10 *B. oralis* isolated from 212 genital tract swabs. Only 16 isolates of *B. fragilis sensu lato* were made, 7 of which were either *B. fragilis sensu strictu* or *B. thetaiotamicron*. Only three strains of the *B. melaninogenicus/B. asaccharolyticus* group were recorded, with an additional 14 strains of unidentified non-fermentative *Bacteroides* sp. The dominance of *B. bivius* in the vaginal flora appears from these two studies to be established. Interestingly, there are now data suggesting that *B. bivius* will adhere to vaginal epithelial cells and that this adherence is increased at high vaginal pH (Moi et al 1984).

Bacteroides species: occurrence in the genital tract

In prepubertal girls Hammerschlag et al (1978a) found *Bacteroides fragilis* in 4/6 children who were less than 2 years old and 2/17 older premenarchal girls. This probably relates to the wearing of napkins with frequent faecal contamination of the vagina. Other faecal members of the *B. fragilis group* (*sensu lato*), *B. vulgatus*, *B. ovatus* and *B. thetaiotamicron* were isolated from 5, 4 and 2 patients respectively. Age-related data were not provided in the rest of the study. *B. melaninogenicus* was present in 14/56 of vaginal cultures, *B. oralis* in 2, and unidentified bacteroides in 11 patients. *B. bivius* and *B. disiens* were not recognised in this study.

Isolation of bacteroides from vaginal swabs varies widely in different groups of adults. Spiegel et al (1980) reported its isolation from 13/17 patients with non-specific vaginitis and 2/21 without this condition. Watt et al (1981) reported its isolation from 12% of a population attending a family planning clinic. Patients using the diaphragm or contraceptive pill had isolation rates of 8%, compared with 10.8% in patients not using contraceptives and 26.7% in those with intrauterine contraceptive devices in situ, the latter being a significant difference. The suggestion that bacteroides were present much more frequently in the first week of the menstrual cycle (Neary et al 1973; Larsen & Galask 1982) has not been confirmed (Bartlett et al 1977; Sautter & Brown 1980) but no penicillin-susceptible members of the *B. melaninogenicus* complex were reported in one of these studies (Neary et al 1973). Corbishley (1977), examining a group of 40 patients attending for fitting of a contraceptive device, grew bacteroides equally frequently (in approximately 20%) from vaginal and cervical cultures. Before hysterectomy bacteroides were isolated in two series from 50% of patients (Bartlett et al 1977; Osborne et al 1979), Gorbach et al (1973), Sanders et al (1975) and Tashjian et al (1976) isolated bacteroides from 16/50 premenopausal patients. Of these patients 11/50 had

Gardnerella vaginalis but the proportion of patients with both organisms is not stated. This group may not be representative of the general population. A similar rate of 29% is reported from a prehysterectomy population by Ohm & Galask (1975) with *B. fragilis* accounting for 4% and *B. corrodens* for 7%. In their series in younger patients Bartlett et al (1977) grew *B. melaninogenicus* in concentrations of 10^7/g from 36% of women but *B. fragilis* from only 5%. Members of the *B. oralis* group were present in 18% of women. Much lower rates of isolation of bacteroides—circa 5%—are reported by some groups. A rate of 12.1% was recorded by Watt et al (1981) in their study of an unselected population of 1498 women attending a family planning clinic. These authors comment that anaerobes present in small numbers (< 20/plate inoculated with a swab) were not recorded in their study. Tashjian et al (1976) isolated *B. fragilis* on only 1/100 cultures, in this case from a postmenopausal patient. The relative rarity of *B. fragilis* even in the presence of *Gardnerella* is confirmed by Taylor et al (1982) who isolated members of the *B. melaninogenicus* complex frequently, with *B. bivius*, *B. asaccharolyticus*, *B. intermedius*, *B. disiens* and *B. oralis* in descending order of frequency. *B. bivius* usually outnumbered, by 10–100-fold, *B. asaccharolyticus* and *B. intermedius* and was present at a mean count of 10^{10} cfu/ml.

In pregnancy Goplerud and colleagues (1976) found an initial isolation rate of 54% for anaerobic Gram-negative rods in the first trimester falling to some 30% and then rising to 73% at 3 days postpartum. *B. melaninogenicus* was present in 5–10% of cultures throughout pregnancy, rising to 30% postpartum. *B. fragilis* declined from 20% in the first trimester to 2% at term, rising to 35% after delivery. A similar pattern was seen with *B. corrodens* which was isolated surprisingly frequently on 10–20% of occasions, rising to 35% postpartum. Unidentified bacteroides were isolated very frequently in this study and may well have been members of the *bivius/disiens* or *oralis* group. Gibbs et al (1982) isolated *B. bivius* from 10/52 samples of amniotic fluid from women with amnionitis and 3/52 in both groups. Werner et al (1978) found *B. oralis* as the predominant anaerobic species postpartum. Brook et al (1979), in cultures taken immediately postpartum, isolated *B. melaninogenicus* from 8% of patients, *B. fragilis* from 8% and *B. distasonis* and *B. vulgatus* from a similar percentage. These figures presumably represent a combination of innate flora and a faecal inoculum added to the vaginal flora at parturition.

In patients with carcinoma of the cervix *B. fragilis* was isolated from 5/21 and *B. melaninogenicus* from 13/21 patients (Mead 1979). One or more bacteroides species were found in 67% of patients. Unusual species, including *B. coagulans*, *B. clostridiformis*, *B. capillosus*, *B. pneumosintes*, and *B. corrodens*, but surprisingly few unidentified isolates and no members of the *B. bivius/B. disiens*, and only *B. ruminicola* of the *B. oralis* groups, were described in this study.

Mobiluncus

The presence of fastidious motile curved gram-negative rods in vaginal secretions has been increasingly recognised since 1980 and their identity and significance, particularly in anaerobic vaginosis, has been intensively investigated. It is not clear if these are minority members of the normal flora. Although their DNA-relatedness is limited, two species of the genus *Mobiluncus* are recognised (Christiansen et al 1984) for which the specific names *Mobiluncus curtisii* and *M. muliensis*, for respectively the short and long forms, have been proposed (Spiegel & Roberts 1984). The long forms are susceptible to metronidazole and are about twice as common in patients with floras not dominated by lactobacilli from a gynaecological outpatient clinic. Short forms are seldom seen in the absence of long forms (Holst et al 1984a). In a further study (Holst et al 1984b) designed to investigate the relationship between these organisms and *Gardnerella vaginalis* in patients with symptoms including those of bacterial vaginosis, *Gardnerella* sp. was found in all patients with *Mobiluncus* sp. but was present in higher numbers in patients growing *Mobiluncus* sp. Complaints of vaginal malodour were commoner in those with *Mobiluncus* sp. and growth of *Mycoplasma hominis* was more significantly associated with growth of *Mobiluncus* sp. and other anaerobes. Some preliminary data (Pattman 1984) suggest that *Mobiluncus* sp., as assessed by microscopy, may be commoner in patients with intrauterine devices, multiple sexual partners and chlamydial infection but more data are required to establish the occurrence of *Mobiluncus* sp. in essentially normal patients.

Fusobacteria and veillonella

Fusobacteria, another genus of pathogenic gram-negative non-sporing anaerobes, are rare in the vaginal flora (George et al 1981). Hammann (1982) isolated only two strains from 212 genital tract samples. Sautter & Brown (1980) recorded a single isolate in 65 similarly examined samples from 7 normal subjects. Bartlett et al (1977) obtained 7 isolates from 52 samples. Interestingly, Bartlett et al (1977) reported fusobacteria from 23% of their patients. Taylor et al (1982) recovered 6 isolates from 82 samples in non-specific vaginitis. A similar isolation rate is reported in childhood (Hammerschlag et al 1978a), in pregnancy (Goplerud et al 1976), immediately postpartum (Brook et al 1979), and after the menopause (Osborne et al 1979).

Veillonella, a genus of anaerobic gram-negative cocci, was isolated by Bartlett et al (1977) from 9% of women and by Sautter & Brown (1980) from 10% of 65 sequential cultures of 7 normal women. Taylor et al (1982) reported *Veillonella* from 15/82 cultures in non-specific vaginitis and a single isolate of *Acidaminococcus*, a related genus. A similar isolation rate was recorded postmenopausally (Osborne et al 1979), and in pregnancy in one series (Goplerud et al 1976) but was lower in another survey in pregnancy (Ross & Needham 1980). These low rates are surprising since *Veillonella* utilises lactic acid, which is plentiful in the vagina, as a preferred substrate (Delwicha et al 1985).

A somewhat higher rate of 19% was recorded for both *Veillonella* and *Fusobacterium* from patients with carcinoma of the cervix (Mead 1979).

Clostridia

Of 25 girls examined by Hammerschlag et al (1978a), 12 carried *Clostridium* sp. in their vaginal flora and in 8 cases this included *C. perfringens*. Other species included *C. beijerincki*, *C. innocuum*, *C. ramosum*, *C. sartagoformum*, *C. glycolicum* (also recorded by Bartlett et al 1978), and *C. cochlearium*. In adults, slightly lower rates of 2–8% are normal (Morris & Morris 1967; Ohm and Galask

1975; Tashjian et al 1976; Osborne et al 1979). These recent figures agree with those in the older literature (Falls 1933; Bysshe 1938; Salm 1944). *C. perfringens* is rarely isolated from the amniotic fluid in amnionitis but Gibbs et al (1982) recorded the isolation of *C. sporogenes*, *C. ramosum* and *C. sordelli*. Goplerud et al (1976) reported the isolation of *C. perfringens* from 2% of patients in the first trimester of pregnancy and 3 days postpartum. Brook et al (1979) obtained a similar rate immediately postpartum. Rather higher rates are recorded in the older literature, and Salm (1944) noted that the rate was higher following manual or instrumental interference, but no recent literature addresses this point. Few clinicians would now expect to accumulate the experience of advanced uterine gas gangrene described by Hill (1964) and the rarity of the syndrome may now make its recognition difficult. Butler (1942, 1945) emphasised the importance of the gram-stained smear in differentiating colonisation from early or advanced gas gangrene. In colonisation bacilli are rarely seen, seldom capsulate and frequently intracellular, and leucocytes are rare. Culture of other clostridia from the vagina or cervix has much less clinical significance, although uterine gas gangrene due to *C. septicum* is recorded.

One rather fastidious anaerobes, *C. difficile*, which can produce cytotoxins and enterotoxins implicated in antibiotic-associated colitis, has been reported from a surprising 17% of 902 vaginal cultures from women attending a family planning clinic (Bramley et al 1981). This follows a report from one of the co-authors of an extraordinarily high recovery rate of 78% from women attending family planning and genitourinary medicine clinics (Hafiz et al 1975). This finding has been independently confirmed using a broth enrichment technique for isolation (O'Farrell et al 1984). These high rates are interesting in view of the recorded high incidence of *C. difficile* colonisation in infants.

Actinomycetes

Three human species of *Actinomyces*, *A. israeli*, *A. naeslundi*, and *A. odontolyticus*, and a close relative *Arachnia propionica* are relevant to discussion of actinomycetes in the genital tract. These bacilli are characteristically gram-positive and branching but can apparently occur as single bacilli looking not unlike coryneforms (Pine et al 1981). They are characteristically anaerobic or microaerophilic. Culture plates require incubation for more than 4 days (usually 10) for characteristic colonies to grow (Traynor et al 1981). Dilution of samples which usually contain other anaerobes, the use of media containing 2.5 mg/l metronidazole, or special selective media are useful in achieving successful isolation. Cultures are often unsuccessful because technique is poor and this has persuaded many American workers to rely solely on microscopy of stained smears of material, sometimes confirming their impression by using direct immunofluorescent techniques. With the very wide range of coryneforms and lactobacilli present in the vaginal flora, the specificity of such techniques is critically important if they are used as the sole means of diagnosis. It is probable that such differences underly a controversy as to whether actinomycetes are normal members of the vaginal flora.

Papanicolaou-stained cervical smears frequently show microcolonies of gram-positive rods which appear to branch. These are usually from patients with intrauterine contraceptive devices (IUCDs) in situ. Valicenti et al (1982) reported such findings in 212 of 6450 such patients in a community survey. Only 103/212 such smears fluoresced with a polyvalent antiserum. Higher rates were recorded from a family planning clinic with 9 fluorescent smears from 13 suspect smears taken from 170 patients. A higher rate of 40/128 from patients with plastic IUCDs is recorded from a British series (Duguid et al 1980). None of the 165 patients with copper IUCDs and none of the 300 patients on oral contraceptives had similar microscopic findings. This group has subsequently extended its findings using culture and confirmatory immunofluorescence using homemade polyvalent antisera (Traynor et al 1981). From these findings it may be concluded that actinomycetes are only found in the flora of those with IUCDs in situ.

However a number of studies have found a different picture. Grice & Hafiz (1983) isolated actinomycetes from the endocervical swabs of 12/58 women using contraceptives other than IUCDs, compared to 20/78 IUCD wearers. Pine et al (1981) reported, using direct fluorescence with a complex technique to avoid non-specific fluorescence, that this is not the case. In this and a subsequent report (Curtis & Pine 1981) they report positive fluorescent findings in 8/32 patients without IUCD, tampon, etc. in situ and 10/20 in those with an IUCD or similar foreign item in situ. Only 4/18 of the fluorescent bacteria were in branching form and only 3 were seen on review of Papanicolaou-stained smear. Their antibody reagents, however, were claimed to have species and genus specificity and only a third as many of the isolates in the non-IUCD group of patients were positive for *Actinomyces israelii*. Almost as many smears were reported as positive on fluorescence with *Arachnia propionica* and only two isolates appeared to react with *Actinomyces naeslundi* reagent. Only *Actinomyces israelii* was more frequent in the IUCD group. Other workers have not been able to repeat these findings (Jones et al 1983b). The presence of *Actinomyces odontolyticus* in the female genital tract has been investigated by Mitchell & Crow (1984), who isolated this species from 27 of 561 (4.8%) women fitted with IUCDs, 4/101 women with pelvic inflamatory disease without known IUCDs and 9/525 (1.8%) women without known IUCDs and without pelvic inflamatory disease. In only 5 of the patients were actinomyces-like bacteria seen in the smears.

Further work is needed to investigate the identity of the microcolonies, seen on smears, that are not *Actinomyces israelii* and to confirm or refute whether actinomycetes such as *Actinomyces propionica* can be grown from the vaginas of patients without an IUCD in situ. It seems proper to regard these actinomycetes as part of the normal flora of patients with an IUCD in situ. At most, 25% of these patients have symptoms of pelvic inflammation (Gupta & Woodruff 1982) and in some series the figure is lower (Aubert et al 1980, Curtis & Pine 1981).

Streptococci

Streptococci are important members of the normal vaginal flora but can behave as invasive pathogens.

The taxonomy of the genus leads to considerable confusion. The simplistic medical division of streptococci into alpha-(viridans or sometimes misleadingly abbreviated α-), beta-(sometimes abbreviated β-) or gramma-(non-)haemolytic strains according to their cultural characteristic on blood agar is unreliable as a guide to their pathogenicity, and depends on the constituents in the agar base, whether horse, human or sheep blood is used in culture plate preparation, and whether the plates are incubated under aerobic or anaerobic conditions. It is not usually a useful property to report on strains which have been further identified. Strains of *Streptococcus pyogenes*, *Str. milleri*, *Str. agalactiae*, and *Str. faecalis* which have atypical haemolytic reactions are within the experience of all clinical microbiologists who do not rely exclusively and dangerously on this character. The terms enterococci or faecal streptococci are frequently applied to bile- and heat-tolerant streptococci which possess the Lancefield Group D antigen. These strains may not be distinguished easily from other important species such as non-haemolytic *Str. agalactiae* unless they are assigned to Lancefield groups. Many laboratories do not speciate strains from all sites. *Str. bovis* strains (Lancefield Group D) are indistinguishable on blood agar from the viridans streptococci, such as *Str. sanguis* and *Str. mitis*.

Streptococci are also frequently reported by their Lancefield group antigens. This is more helpful as it frequently correlates with their behaviour as pathogens and with their species, and has the virtue of accurately describing the criteria most clinical laboratories rely on for their identification, since few additional characters are usually tested. *Str. pyogenes* carries the Lancefield Group A antigen, *Str. agalactiae* Group B, *Str. equisimilis* Group C, *Str. sanguis* sometimes Group H, *Str. salivarius* sometimes Group K, and *Str. mitis* sometimes Group K. Specific designation of streptococci bearing Lancefield Group G antigens has not been made. Species bearing Lancefield Group D antigens include *Str. faecalis* (often used inaccurately to include the whole group) *Str. faecalis* var. *zymogenes*, a variant which produces a plasmid-encoded beta-haemolysin (Jacob et al 1975), *Str. avium*, *Str. bovis*, *Str. equinus* and *Str. faecium*, which includes *Str. durans*. *Str. faecum* is frequently even more penicillin-resistant than *Str. faecalis* and is also more likely to be resistant to the usual synergic effects of aminoglycosides with penicillins (Moellering et al 1979). Group R strains also carry Group D antigens and, like *Str. agalactiae* for which we have mistaken it on blood agar cultures from adult cerebrospinal fluid, is relatively

penicillin-susceptible. *Str. milleri* usually carries the Lancefield Group F antigen when beta-haemolytic, although it may lack this or carry Lancefield Group G or A antigens. This species is commonly non-haemolytic or α-haemolytic. *Str. milleri* may be misidentified as an anaerobic streptococcus since its growth is usually enhanced by or is dependent on incubation in 10% carbon dioxide, a usual component of gases used for anaerobic incubation. *Str. intermedius*, *Peptostreptococcus intermedius* (an anaerobic genus), and *Str. anginosus-constellatus* are all 'species' which have proved to be synonymous with *Str. milleri* (Ball & Parker 1979).

The use of Linnaean binomials for streptococci based on fermentation, assimilation and tolerance tests has a chequered career for viridans strains other than *Str. pneumoniae*. There are two commonly used classifications—those of Facklam (1977) and of Colman & Williams (1972), which differ in significant respects, e.g. the inclusion of some *Str. sanguis* strains (designated 11) with *Str. mitis* in *Str. mitior* by Colman & Williams.

With haemolytic species, the strains of Group C streptococci originally described as animal pathogens which occasionally appear in human outbreaks appear to differ from the usual human strains in pathogenicity as well as biochemical parameters which define them as *Str. zooepidemicus*, *Str. equi* or *Str. equisimilis* (Facklam & Ruttledge 1985).

The recent recognition (Elliot et al 1966, Windsor & Elliot 1975) of *Str. suis* Type 1, which carries Group R and D antigens—a rare cause of human meningitis in adults and an important cause of meningitis and septicaemia in weaned pigs—and of *Str. suis* Type 2, which carries the S and D antigens—the cause of meningitis and septicaemia in unweaned piglets—emphasises the advantages and limitations of serological typing in studies of pathogenicity as well as providing interesting models for Group B streptococcal infections. Pathogenicity is not always delineated by a specific name or a single antigen. A number of species are further subdivided into serotypes on antigens other than the Lancefield group antigens and these serotypes, at least in *Str. pyogenes*, and probably *Str. agalactiae*, reflect antigens which generate a type-specific immune response. In Group B streptococci the prevalent antigenic subtype varies with locality (Huang & Diena 1982). Bovine Group B strains are more frequently untypable with current sera but only one species apears to exist (Nakkash & Jones 1982). Group B streptococci can survive sewage treatment and may appear in fresh water (Jensen & Berg 1982).

There is remarkably little information about the different species of alpha-haemolytic streptococci which make up such a common part of those vaginal floras not dominated by lactobacilli and no information, to my knowledge, in an adequately clinically-defined population. In a study (Haffar et al 1983) of strains from 'maternity' patients 53% of isolates were *Str. sanguis* II and 4% *Str. mitis* (both sometimes included in *Str. mitior*). Twenty-eight per cent of strains were from the *Str. MG-intermedius* group. *Str. salivarius* (7%), *Str. sanguis* I (5%), *Str. uberis* and *Str. mutans* (2% each) were less frequently encountered. In view of the increasing isolation of non-Group B and D alpha-haemolytic strains, especially *Str. mitis* from neonatal blood cultures (Haffar et al 1983), more work in this area is indicated. *Str. milleri* is commonly isolated from pus from the brain, liver, abdomen, and lower respiratory tree where it may be not uncommonly found in the absence of anaerobes. It has been reported as a cause of overwhelming neonatal sepsis (Spencer et al 1982) and two similar cases have been seen in Cambridge. The association of *Str. milleri* with genital tract sepsis and morbidity has not been explored.

Str. pyogenes is not a common member of the normal vaginal flora. However it is not uncommon for the perianal skin to become a site of carriage after streptococcal infection, particularly, in my experience, if the nose or skin is involved. Perineal carriage may be so heavy that a few colonies are grown from the vagina or the urine in the absence of infection and the presence of other flora. Penicillins seem not to be very effective in clearing this carriage, either because these antibiotics penetrate intact skin poorly, or because of beta-lactamase destruction or carriage on anal skin. Vaginitis caused by *Str. pyogenes* can occur in children and adults. It is usually associated with a heavy and often 'pure' growth on culture on blood agar if non-selective media are part of the diagnostic laboratory's routine. This infection, although rare, is more commonly encountered in our rural population than might be anticipated from some surveys.

It usually occurs where a number of members of the family have recently, and often repeatedly, suffered from streptococcal upper respiratory infection. Ascending streptococcal infections from this site should not be overlooked when seeking the source of streptococcal septicaemia. It is difficult to assess the significance of reports of this organism from the 'normal' vaginal flora. It seems safer never to consider it normal, although it may only reflect a source for other infections arising from perianal carriage. In a survey of 280 antenatal patients De Louvois et al (1975b) did not encounter Lancefield Group A streptococci. Isolation rates of 0.3% from 291 patients attending a family planning clinic and 1.4% from 1104 patients with discharge in general practice are reported by Morris & Morris (1967).

Lancefield Group G streptococci are more commonly isolated from the vagina than *Str. pyogenes* (isolation rate 0.3% (Morris & Morris 1967)) and in our experience also commoner than Lancefield Group C streptococci. They can cause local or, rarely, systemic sepsids and may also be carried chronically on the perianal skin. They are not infrequently isolated in small numbers as part of a mixed flora from the vagina of patients in our hospital before hysterectomy, curettage, or prolapse repair. These organisms often appear to be stable members of the vaginal flora without any perianal carriage or associated infection.

Lancefield Group C streptococci of the commoner *Str. equisimilis* variety resemble in their behaviour those of Lancefield Group G. Other biochemically distinguished strains can cause outbreaks of severe infection. Isolation rates of about 0.5–1% are recorded (Morris & Morris 1967; Moberg et al 1978).

Lancefield Group B streptococci are very major pathogens of neonates and also a very frequent cause of maternal bacteraemia in labour—often in association with amnionitis (Gibbs et al 1982)—and occasional causes of endocarditis after delivery (Fry 1938). This important and common species has been extensively reviewed (Baker 1977). The stability of carriage has been assessed to determine if antepartum screening is a worthwhile investigation for any form of selective prophylaxis at delivery. These studies are now being extended as serotyping and bacteriophage typing (Stringer 1982) have become available to assess whether this pathogen is commonly transmitted to other babies and mothers in hospital. From experience in other situations such typing schemes are essential to determine if chronic carriage occurs.

There is no evidence that carriage is particularly affected by whether patients are premenarchal (Hammerschlag et al 1978b), postmenopausal, or have concurrent disease. In a population with a high incidence of *Gardnerella* infection an isolation rate of 12% was reported with a mean count of 10^6 cfu/ml (Taylor et al 1982). A similar rate is reported from other series of normal women (Tashjian et al 1976), including one where repeated cultures were taken from a small group of normal women (Sautter & Brown 1980). Group B streptococci are isolated significantly more frequently in the first week of the menstrual cycle (Baker 1977; Bollgren et al 1978). Isolation rates are greatly affected by whether selective culture media are used for isolation (Fenton & Harper 1979) and by the number of swabs taken. Isolation from the introitus is commoner than from the cervical os (Feigin 1976). Rectal carriage is not uncommon (Mhalu 1977) but perianal skin rather than faeces may be the common site for colonisation, particularly for certain serotypes (Islam & Thomas 1980; Islam 1981). In a group attending a clinic for sexually transmitted diseases (Ross & Cumming 1982), Group B streptococci were isolated from cervical cultures in 40/373 patients. Urethral and particularly rectal cultures revealed a further 71 patients carrying the species. Had selective broth enrichment cultures not been used only 54% of cervical, 76% of urethral and 70% of rectal isolations would have been made: 2–13% of strains would have been missed if only the selective broth had been used. Isolation rates of 4–7% from the vagina are reported in early pregnancy and labour (Moberg et al 1978). Using selective liquid enrichment media Sanderson et al (1980) reported an essentially unchanging 7% isolation rate throughout pregnancy, although culture of the same specimens on non-selective solid media yielded an isolation rate which was only half this (Ross & Needham 1980). Earlier studies suggest an isolation rate from the vagina in early labour of 9% without enrichment culture, rising to 14% if broth enrichment is used. In only 4% of patients was the Group B streptococcus present in the rectum alone. Easmon et al (1982) took vaginal and anorectal cultures from women at antenatal booking clinic, at 28 and 36 weeks' gestation and on admission in labour. From 8000 swabs they concluded a 14% carriage rate on direct agar culture and 25% after broth enrichment. Carriage rate in labour at 15% was lower than earlier in pregnancy (26%). Sampling both sites and using enrichment media at 36 weeks identified 85% of mothers who had positive cultures in labour but the number of false predictions of carriage is not stated. Earlier studies (Ferreiri et al 1977) had reported identifying only 58% of patients with Group B streptococci prior to labour and missed 19%. This probably reflects a failure to identify earlier a rectal source for vaginal spread. Persistent vaginal carriage throughout pregnancy probably occurs in only 35% of patients (Anthony & Concepcion 1975). Easmon et al (1981) also cultured babies within 24 hours of birth and surveyed staff and older babies. They noted that vaginal carriage was the most important predictor of transmission to the baby. A total of 37/95 carrier mothers, of whom 17 were carriers of small numbers of organisms, transmitted organisms to their baby. On surveillance culture an additional 42 babies acquired Group B streptococci by nosocomial spread after delivery, although this was more transient than after maternal transmission. There seems little doubt that the early form of neonatal Group B streptococcal disease—respiratory distress and septicaemia—is associated with heavy maternal vaginal carriage (Lim et al 1982). This is detectable within 6 hours of admission to hospital in labour although the number of false positives is high. Rectal carriage is less important as a source for neonatal infection (Jones et al 1983a). By contrast, case to case transmission of Group B streptococci as colonists and infective agents in late onset disease is well recorded (Ancona et al 1980).

Lancefield Group D streptococci are frequent in the vaginal flora. Numbers appear to increase with menstruation (Larsen & Galask 1982). There is little information on the frequency with which the various species occur. They are isolated from some 20–25% of patients in early pregnancy or in labour (Ross & Needham 1980) and this isolation rate has also been reported from non-pregnant patients (Bartlett et al 1977). A similar rate of some 35% was recorded in prehysterectomy patients by Ohm & Galask (1975), in patients attending a clinic for fitting of an IUCD (Corbishley 1977) and in pre- and postmenopausal asymptomatic patients (Tashjian et al 1976). Cephalosporin usage as prophylaxis at hysterectomy selects less against this species than other streptococci (Ohm & Galask 1976) because faecal streptococci are innately more resistant to this class of antibiotics. A higher isolation rate (75%) in early pregnancy in those aged over 35 years was noted by De Louvois et al (1975b), although overall a similar 20% carriage was noted. Lower rates of 6–11% are recorded throughout pregnancy and in a non-pregnant population of various ages by Ross & Needham (1980) and also in premenarchal populations (Hammerschlag et al 1978b). There seems to be no variation in this lower rate of 6–11%, found by a number of other authors, according to tampon or contraceptive usage (Morris & Morris 1967) or with associated *Gardnerella* infection (Taylor et al 1982), although one group of authors did find a significant association with the concurrent presence of coliforms (Watt et al 1981). Relatively high mean counts of 10^9/ml (Taylor et al 1982) compared with Group B streptococci may make for difficulty in detecting Group B streptococci unless starch-containing agar bases (such as Columbia or Islam's media) with an anaerobic environment, which enhances pigment production by Group B strains, are used. This pigmentation is not however produced by all strains on first isolation (Fallon 1974) and is not found in non-haemolytic strains (Noble et al 1983).

Staphylococci and micrococci

Staphylococci, which do not produce coagulase, and micrococci are the commonest aerobic cocci in the vaginal flora but are present in variable numbers (Bartlett et al 1977, 1978; Onderdonk et al 1977). Coagulase-negative staphylococci as distinct from micrococci are present in the vaginal flora in some 60% of patients in early labour, a rather higher figure than in early pregnancy (De Louvois et al 1975b; Moberg et al 1978), and micrococci in some 35% of patients. They are not associated with any specific pathology in the vagina (De Louvois et al 1975b) but are of some interest, as one member of the group of closely related staphylococcal species *Staphylococcus saprophyticus*—formerly *Micrococcus* Type 3—is the second commonest causative organism in urinary tract infection in the sexually active female (Mitchell 1968; Meers 1974). Whilst one study of rectal swabs (Pead et al 1977) provided isolates of this species from 10% of women, others have been unrewarding (Gillespie et al 1978). Surprisingly, only one (negative) study of introital swabs has been published (Sellin et al 1975) but a study of 'urogenital' isolates did not produce a single isolate of *S. saprophyticus* from 78 women (Baldellon & Megraud 1985).

Interest in the biology of *S. aureus* in the vaginal flora is intense because of the recent description of the staphylococcal toxic shock syndrome, associated with a 90% isolation rate of *S. aureus* from the vagina. Initially described in the United States and estimated to have a prevalence of 8.9 cases/100 000 menstruating women (Peterson 1982), this syndrome is now widely recognised in Europe. In seems clear that a spectrum of disease occurs with the cases which can be formally designated as toxic shock syndrome—with hypotension, multisystem failure, and a high mortality, in addition to fever and a desquamating rash representing an extreme. From our own experience, we suspect that the condition is underdiagnosed and underreported and seems still to be unfamiliar to British clinicians. Our experience has emphasised the value of firstly, a vaginal examination in a female patient with shock without obvious cause—particularly if associated with conjunctival hyperaemia, myalgia, vomiting or profuse, watery diarrhoea, and secondly, the importance of the laboratory enquiring into the other symptoms of a patient where *S. aureus* is grown and the only clinical details given are 'vaginal discharge' before it is assumed to be a normal component of the vaginal flora. Clinicians should be aware that some laboratories restrict their examination of samples from patients with vaginal discharge and do not examine them for *S. aureus* or the much rarer *Streptococcus pyogenes*. A history of other associated factors such as conjunctivitis, diarrhoea, etc. is therefore invaluable.

About one-third of patients with staphylococcal toxic shock syndrome give a history of previous associated symptoms and 10% report multiple previous episodes (Davis et al 1982). This emphasises that chronic perineal staphylococcal carriage may be important in the condition, as does the decline in recurrences after a single course of antistaphylococcal therapy, even with continued tampon usage.

The staphylococci involved in the syndrome in the USA have been described by Altermeier et al (1982). They characteristically belong to the group of bacteriophage types usually referred to as phage Group 1, usually those lysed by typing bacteriophage 29 with or without 52. Some 60% of toxic shock syndrome strains belong to this group, compared in the same geographical areas with 12% of strains from other sources. Georgraphical variations in this percentage are likely and they will certainly vary from time to time in the hospital environment. There is no information on whether staphylococci of this group are more likely to be carried chronically on the perineum than staphylococci of other phage groups. It is important to note that 30% of strains from both toxic shock syndrome and other patients are not typable with the routine international bacteriophages, which suggests that this restriction to particular phage types may be modified in future, probably by the strains acquiring other prophages which modify their phage typing pattern. Many Group 1 strains have the potential to produce the pyrogenic toxin C (synonymous with enterotoxin F or toxic shock toxin) that has been implicated as another marker of strains that are associated with toxic shock syndrome (Schlievert et al 1982). It seems that strains involved in the syndrome are always toxigenic. Toxigenic staphylococci are not infrequent in vaginal strains from women without toxic shock syndrome. Schlievert et al (1982) reported its presence in 7/22 strains from non-menstruating women and 5/14 strains from menstruating women without the syndrome. Linneman et al (1982) reported a much lower incidence of toxin-producing strains of some 1% and Chow et al (1984) an intermediate rate of 2.6%. Altermeier and co-workers (1982) could find no trace of this toxin in staphylococcal strains from many sources saved from years prior to 1970. In strains saved from subsequent years they found a rate in Group 1 strains which fluctuated between 25 and 60%. It may be that acquisition of toxigenic potential is a new property of *Staphylococcus aureus* or that older strains have lost, on storage, the gene responsible. There is as yet no substantial information on whether this gene is plasmid-borne or can be mobilised by plasmids or bacteriophage. With a 50% carriage of the toxin in Group 1 staphylococci,

evidence of toxigenicity adds only twofold to the likelihood that a Group 1 strain from an individual could be involved in generating the syndrome. By contrast, the presence of neutralising antibody to the toxin (determined by radio-immunoassay) is of more interest. Vergeront et al (1983) reported that 88% of normal women have antibody titres of >100 by the age of 20, whereas only 15% of women with toxic shock syndrome have titres of >5 at the time of presentation. It is interesting to note that only 45% of women seroconvert within a year of their presentation with toxic shock syndrome. Others have made similar findings (Bonventre et al 1984).

The reason for the association of toxic shock syndrome with menstruation and tampons is not clearly established. A neutral rather than acidic pH increases the amount of toxin produced (Schlievert et al 1982) and tampon absorbency is related in some ill-defined way to the risk of toxic shock syndrome (Osterholm et al 1982). Other properties of the staphylococci implicated in toxic shock syndrome should not be neglected. Schlievert et al (1982) have described differences between the haemolysin and lipase production of strains from normal menstruating women and those with toxic shock syndrome.

In patients attending a family planning clinic, staphylococcal carriage rates were similar at 2–4% in those women who did or did not use tampons and also similar in those who did or did not use oral contraceptives (Morris & Morris 1967). Prior to the publicity associated with description of the syndrome, carriage rates of 1–7% seemed normal for most adult female populations, including patients prior to hysterectomy (Ohm & Galask 1976), with cervical cancer (Mead 1979), with amnionitis in labour (Gibbs et al 1982), and attending family planning clinics (Watt et al 1981). The latter series, the largest reported and which involved some 1500 patients, gives an isolation rate of just over 1% but specifically ignored some light culture growths. It now seems clear that staphylococci are more commonly found if samples are taken during the menstrual period, with maximal rates on the third day, although the difference is small. Schlievert et al (1982) isolated *Staphylococcus aureus* from 14/95 menstruating women and 22/205 non-menstruating women. Surprisingly, there appears to be a specific association of carriage of toxigenic *S. aureus* with co-carriage of *Escherichia coli* (Chow et al 1984). The apparent carriage rate is increased if labial as well as vaginal swabs are cultured. Linneman et al (1982) reported a 9% carriage rate overall with 5% positive vaginal cultures. Higher vaginal rates of 10 and 17% were reported in vaginal cultures during the reproductive period and postpartum. This paper provides important information on the dynamic relationship between labial and vaginal carriage and on the chronicity of vaginal carriage. Only 35% of 'positive' patients persistently carried *S. aureus* for three menstrual cycles. This figure is very close to the 40% persistence rate for perineal carriage of staphylococci reported from the older literature on the relationship of this to surgical wound infection (Ridley 1959; Boe et al 1964). Linneman et al (1982) noted that in 9/17 patients where the first culture showed that staphylococci were present on the labia but not in the vagina, repeated culture at subsequent menstruation yielded positive vaginal cultures. This suggests that perineal carriage of staphylococci constitutes a risk factor for vaginal colonisation with staphylococci and that the dynamics of perineal carriage require further examination.

A number of other series record high vaginal carriage rates of *S. aureus*—17% in one series of patients attending for fitting of a IUCD (Corbishley 1977); 16% in another series of patients with heterogeneous conditions (Osborne & Wright 1977). Variable rates according to contraceptive method are also recorded by other workers, although this is not reflected in an increased prevalence of toxic shock syndrome. Guinan et al (1982) recorded the following rates: diaphragm 18%, IUCD 16%, oral contraceptive hormones 10%, condom 6% and nil 8%—but this study did not take cultures always at the same point in the menstrual cycle. A rate of 4% is reported from children (Hammerschlag et al 1978b). The frequency of isolation of *S. aureus* in pregnancy or early labour has been reported to be as low as 0.7% (Moberg et al 1978) although De Louvois et al (1975b) and Ross & Needham (1980) report respectively rates of 4 and 15%. Goplerud et al (1976) in a sequential study reported an isolation rate of about 2% with a rise to 4–6% postpartum. From these reports it seems unlikely that *S. aureus* carriage rates vary widely and it is unclear what

would predispose patients to chronic vaginal carriage of staphylococci. It remains important to establish if there is any correlation between perineal carriage of staphylococci, which is well recognised from studies of wound infection, and vaginal carriage.

Gardnerella vaginalis

Controversy has surrounded this organism's role in non-specific vaginitis and its taxonomic position for many years. It still seems inappropriate to omit it from a discussion of normal flora since it may be that other microbes such as non-sporing anaerobes are necessary to join *Gardnerella* sp. in the flora responsible for this condition. In polymicrobial conditions such as this, it may be that the flora, although normal, predisposes to the condition by including one of the necessary components.

The taxonomic position of this wanderer from *Haemophilus* and *Corynebacterium*, whose very existence has long been doubted (Lapage 1961), now seems secure following numerical taxonomic studies (Greenwood & Pickett 1979, 1980; Piot et al 1980). A variety of selective differential media (Goldberg & Washington 1976; Totten et al 1982) and identification methodologies that go beyond the colonial morphology, catalase, and carbohydrate fermentation tests originally used to define this organism, have also now been described, reproduced, and refined (Greenwood et al 1977; Bailey et al 1979; Piot et al 1982; Yong and Thompson 1982). Immunofluorescent techniques for rapid methods await further exploitation and investigation (Redmond & Kotcher 1963; Tarlinton & D'Abrera 1974). Many early reports of isolation rates from normal populations (Dunkelberg et al 1962; Frampton & Lee 1964; McCormack et al 1977; Hammerschlag et al 1978b) must be treated with suspicion since there are closely related organisms which may be misidentified on the result of a too limited range of confirmatory tests. Microscopy for clue cells results in approximately a 15% false positive rate (Delaha et al 1964; Dunkelberg 1965).

In one study of a control population no *Gardnerella* strains were isolated in 60 matched controls. An isolation rate of 70% in non-specific vaginitis was reported but hippurate hydrolysis and antimicrobial susceptibilities were not used in the identification scheme (Teare et al 1981). A low carriage rate (3/23) in women with normal vaginas was reported by Taylor et al (1982). In this study, which did not use highly selective media, isolation rates of *Gardnerella* sp. in strictly defined non-specific vaginitis were 65%. By contrast, using rather similar identification criteria, another group (Spiegel et al 1980) isolated *Gardnerella* sp. from 25/60 normal controls and 52/53 patients with non-specific vaginitis. Many of these differences may be quantitative since in the later study 19/25 controls, compared with 5/53 non-specific vaginitis patients, had less than 10^7 organisms/ml of secretion, and selective media were used in this study, unlike those of Taylor et al (1982) and Teare et al (1981) or the original study by Gardner & Dukes (1955). Similar findings have recently been made by Amsel et al (1983). This quantitative difference did not appear to be the explanation for the low isolation rate in the patients compared by Levison et al (1979). Gardner (1980) criticised the clinical definition of the non-specific vaginitis group in this study but continued to insist that *Gardnerella* sp. is not found at all in normal populations. The organism is said not to occur in premenarchal children (Kummel 1963) although this has been denied (Hammerschlag et al 1978b).

Haemophilus sp.

Haemophilus influenzae is an uncommon member of the normal vaginal flora of adults (Tashjian et al 1976). Contrary views on the prevalence of *Haemophilus* sp. may reflect inadequate identification (Watt et al 1981). It may be encountered on blood agar media as a colony satelliting around another organism: commonly, but not exclusively, staphylococci. Biotyping of isolates from cases of perinatal and maternal invasive infection suggests that *Haemophilus influenzae* Killian biotype 4 may be specifically associated with a tendency to cause invasive infection from a genital source. Preliminary results on biotyping strains from the genital tract suggest that this biotype is uncommon (Wallace et al 1983). Other strains of *Haemophilus*, which are carbon dioxide-dependent on first isolation, designated as *H. aphrophilus* and *H. para-aphrophilus*, may be regarded as variants of *H. influenzae* and *H. parainfluenzae* respectively. *H. ducreyi*, the organism implicated in soft sore, may be

isolated from asymptomatic female partners of men with genital sores. It is unlikely to generate confusion in most diagnostic laboratories since it does not grow well on conventional horse blood-containing media, even when the blood has been 'chocolated' by heat. Supplements with Isovitalex are needed (McEntegart et al 1982).

Enterobacteriaceae and pseudomonadaceae

The assessment of finding these organisms in the vaginal flora is as difficult as the assessment of the finding of anaerobes, although with the current vogue for attributing all infections to anaerobes rather than recognising that mixed or aerobic infections can occur, it is perhaps more likely that a laboratory worker will dismiss them as non-significant and may not report their presence. Some 30% of vaginal swabs yield coliforms. It is important in the context of the vaginal flora to remember the close proximity of the vagina to the urethra. Some workers have suggested that periurethral coliform carriage in the normal patient may predispose to urinary infection but this association is denied by others (Cattell et al 1975; Stamey & Sexton 1975; Schaeffer & Stamey 1977). There is some evidence of differences between groups of patients with and without recurrent bacteriuria, not only in the proportion of patients carrying enterobacteriaceae (Stamey & Sexton 1975; Schaeffer et al 1981) but in the numbers of coliforms present in the premenstrual part of the cycle (Botta et al 1981) and in adherence of coliforms to preurethral epithelia (Kallenius & Wimberg 1978). This, with the low numbers and the cyclical variation present in normal patients according to this study, will considerably affect rates of reported carriage. Neary et al (1973) gave some information on isolation rates of coliforms from the vagina at different times in the menstrual cycle; there was no significant evidence of cyclical variation in the isolation rates in this study. However this group only included patients awaiting gynaecological surgery and it may be that associated urinary infection in these patients might obscure any variation seen in the normal patient.

It is important to recognise that urinary tract infection is a common accompaniment of anatomical disturbances of the pelvic floor and infected urine may provide a heavy inoculum of coliforms to the vaginal flora. In a recent study of patients in the immediate postpartum period in Cambridge, about half the patients with coliforms in their vaginal swabs had bacteriuria ($> 10^8/l$), either transient or maintained on repeat sampling. Few patients without vaginal coliforms had significant bacteriuria. Without suprapubic aspiration it is impossible to be certain whether vaginal coliforms contaminated the urine or urinary coliforms the vaginal in this study. Against this background we should perhaps consider that the urethral and bladder flora should particularly be assessed before accepting a 'coliform' as a member of the normal vaginal flora if there is any anatomical factor present that predisposes to urinary infection. This has seldom been done.

In a large family planning clinic survey no significant difference was found in the symptoms of dysuria, nocturia and frequency of micturition between those patients with and without coliform colonisation and this argues against any direct association with lower urinary tract infection (Goldacre et al 1979). Broadly similar findings with regard to discharge and isolation rate are reported in pregnancy (De Louvois et al 1975b). Similar rates of isolation for *Escherichia coli* (15%) are recorded for girls aged 3–10 years—a rate many times higher than that of urinary infection in this age group. Not surprisingly, very high rates are recorded for younger children wearing diapers (Hammerschlag et al 1978b). This raises the difficult assessment point of whether minor faecal contamination contributes to any of the figures quoted in other described series.

A good illustration of the interesting interpretative problems posed by the absence of information on urinary tract infection or quantitation of coliforms is provided by a study by Ohm & Galask (1976) on patients undergoing abdominal hysterectomy. This excellent study of the effect of prophylactic antibiotics on the vaginal flora gives no data on the source of superinfecting resistant organisms, or of antecedent or postoperative urinary infection in association with the condition for which hysterectomy was performed. Ohm & Galask report that 37% of preoperative vaginal cultures from patients contained aerobic gram-negative bacilli, a much higher than usual figure. The ranking order reported was *Escherichia coli* (30%), *Proteus mirabilis* (6%), *Klebsiella* sp. (4%),

Acinetobacter sp. (2%), *Proteus vulgaris* and *Enterobacter cloacae* (1% each). Colonisation with multiple gram-negative bacilli was not uncommon. Postoperatively vaginal cultures grew aerobic gram-negative bacilli from 65 and 85% of patients, depending on whether prophylactic cephalosporins had or had not been given to cover surgery. Some 24% of cultures contained exclusively gram-negative bacilli other than *Escherichia coli* in the cephalosporin group, compared with 10% in the placebo-treated group. In the placebo group each species increased in prevalence by about 2.5-fold but only one additional species, *Enterobacter aerogenes*, was noted. By contrast, in the cephalosporin group a greater diversity of species was recorded, including *Hafnia* sp., *Enterobacter agglomerans*, *Citrobacter freundi* and *C. diversus*, and *Pseudomonas aeruginosa*. Although in postoperative compared with preoperative cultures there was a 30–50% increase in *Escherichia coli*, *Proteus mirabilis*, and *Klebsiella* sp., *Enterobacter cloacae* appeared with a 15% and *Pseudomonas aeruginosa* with an 11% prevalence, a much greater increase. These species are intrinsically resistant to the cephalosporins used in this study and although data on antibiotic susceptibility are not given it is reported that the effect of antibiotics on the vaginal flora, as on the bowel flora, was to diminish the prevalence of susceptible and increase the prevalence of resistant microbes. It would be interesting to know if these changes represented urinary catheter superinfection spilling into the vaginal flora or faecal contamination of the vagina due to the change in vaginal colonisation resistance.

In almost all studies, the ranking order for frequency of species of enterobacteriaceae remains similar to that produced by Ohm & Galask in the preoperative period. However there is quite marked variation in the absolute recovery rate. A high rate of isolation, similar to that of Ohm & Galask, was reported by Neary et al (1973) who studied 68 specimens with coliforms from 246 vaginal swabs of patients awaiting gynaecological surgery. Specimens from 112 patients gave no growth and coliforms occupied a dominant position in the flora of the remaining patients. Eight out of 12 patients with cervical cancer in another series had *Escherichia coli* in their vaginal flora (Mead 1979). According to Tashjian et al (1976), similar high carriage rates of *E. coli* occur in pregnancy, and in the premenopausal and postmenopausal period, but a significant increase in other gram-negative bacteria does occur in the postmenopausal period. This increase after the menopause was not confirmed by another group (Osborne et al 1979). Watt et al (1981) reported from a large survey of a family planning clinic that coliforms were isolated in 30% of women using a diaphragm, compared with 16% using other contraceptive methods, and were also commoner in those who used sanitary towels as opposed to tampons. Both these differences were statistically significant. There was no significant difference in coliform isolation rate between those with and without discharge. Coliforms were also significantly more frequent in patients who had received antibiotics in the previous 4 weeks. Apart from in this small group of patients, faecal streptococci were more frequently isolated with coliforms than would be expected by chance. *E. coli* was isolated from 10.5% and *Proteus* sp. from 2.5% of patients in the series. *Klebsiella* sp. was identified in 0.3% and *Pseudomonas aeruginosa* in 0.1% but coliforms from 3% of women were not further identified. Rather similar findings have been reported from Canada. In one study there was an association between *E. coli* carriage and the phase of the menstrual cycle, the use of antibiotics within the preceding 2 weeks, the use of a diaphragm or cervical cap for contraception and a history of previous urinary infection (Percival-Smith et al 1983). These authors subsequently produced data showing that co-carriage of toxic shock toxin-producing *Staphylococcus aureus* and *E. coli* was more frequent than would be expected by chance (Chow et al 1984). This association did not extend to non-toxigenic strains.

The paucity of *Klebsiella* sp. and *Pseudomonas* sp. in the vaginal flora extends to pregnancy (De Louvois et al 1975b). A high isolation rate of 31% for lactose-fermenting coliforms, 3% for *Proteus* sp. and 17% for other enterobacteriaceae has been reported in women attending for fitting of an IUCD (Corbishley 1977). This was associated with a 54% isolation rate for faecal streptococci. Many of the coliforms were present in small numbers and no significant difference was found between vaginal and cervical swabs. A tendency for marginally more (16%) coliform isolates to be made from samples from the fornix compared with those from the cervix was noted by Watt et al (1981) in a series of 838 paired samples, but this difference was not statistically significant.

A much lower rate of isolation of enterobacteriaceae has been recorded by a number of authors. In another family planning clinic population, apparently similar to those already discussed above, an isolation rate for *E. coli* of 6% was recorded. Neither the apparent association of growth with the second half of the menstrual cycle, nor the increases noted with absence of tampon or oral contraceptive usage, were statistically significant in the study of Morris & Morris (1967). An isolation rate of 6% for all enterobacteriaceae was recorded in one large group of pregnant and premenopausal women not awaiting surgery (Lindner et al 1978). In this group enterobacteriaceae were present in counts of 10^6/ml of secretion. It was notable that *Streptococcus faecalis*, another species found in faeces but usually accepted as a normal component of the vaginal flora, was also not common. A similar 6% rate of isolation of *E. coli* in pregnancy is reported by other workers (Moberg et al 1978; Ross & Needham 1980). *E. coli* was isolated from 2/52 amniotic fluids of patients without amnionitis compared with 7/52 patients with amnionitis in one recent study (Gibbs et al 1982). Goplerud et al (1976) reported a sharp increase in the isolation rate of *E. coli* to > 30% at 3 days postpartum and this high rate was maintained 6 weeks later. In another series of premenopausal patients with a high incidence of *Gardnerella* sp., or other cause of vaginal discharge, a recovery rate of 6% for *E. coli* was recorded (Taylor et al 1982). *Proteus* sp., *Klebsiella* sp. and *Acinetobacter* sp. were proportionally rarer.

In summary, the rates of coliform isolation reported from the vaginal flora are surprisingly wide. Associations with cycle time and urinary infection are subtle and contraceptive type or usage also affect the rate.

Listeria

Listeria sp. are aerobic gram-positive bacilli which are difficult to isolate from mixed flora without selective media and prolonged enrichment in liquid media. Isolation rates from faeces vary from 1% to much higher figures in family contacts and those occupationally exposed to animals or wet silage (Bojsen Moller 1972). Some cases of neonatal listeriosis at term are clearly associated with the presence of *Listeria* sp. in the maternal vagina, although earlier in pregnancy maternal and associated fetal listeriosis clearly seems to be a haematogenous transplacental infection.

The true incidence of *Listeria* in the female genital tract is not clearly known. Rappaport et al (1960) reported its presence in 25/34 women who had had 2–6 abortions and 0/87 with uneventful obstetric history, although the criteria for identification of the organism in all cases may be criticised. The same group of authors was subsequently only able to demonstrate *Listeria* sp. in 4/300 patients (Rabinowitz et al 1963). Definite recurrence of perinatal infection has never been described with *Listeria* although it is now well described in the immunocompromised (McLauchlin et al 1986). Its role as a member of the vaginal flora is not established. There is some evidence for sexual transmission of the organism from one group of authors (Toaff et al 1962). It is now clear that *Listeria* sp. other than *L. monocytogenes* are ever found in the vaginal flora (Lamont & Postlethwaite 1986). Other species are rarely responsible for human infection. There is evidence that both lactobacilli and other aerobic and lactic acid may inhibit multiplication of *Listeria* sp. (Bojsen Moller 1972).

Genital mycoplasmas

This subject is dealt with more fully elsewhere. *Mycoplasma hominis* and *Ureaplasma urealyticum* can frequently be isolated from the genital tract with appropriate media. Vaginal cultures are more frequently positive than cervical cultures (McCormack et al 1973a, 1977). Ureaplasmas have been isolated from the genital tract of up to one-third of neonates, but this rate declines as children grow older (Klein et al 1969; Foy et al 1970, 1975; Braun et al 1971; Lee et al 1974). Ureaplasmas can be isolated from some 10–20% of prepubertal girls and *M. hominis* from some 8–9%. In the postpubertal period colonisation seems proportional to the number of sexual partners. It is not clear if the relationship to socioeconomic class, suggested by the study of McCormack et al (1973b), is independent of this. In this study *Mycoplasma* sp. and *Ureaplasma* sp. were isolated respectively from 54 and 76% of patients attending a US municipal hospital, compared with 21 and 53% attending a private clinic in the same area. It seems that after the menopause the carriage rate of mycoplasmas declines. There appears to be an association of carriage of *Mycoplasma* sp. with vaginal pH. Only 1% of women carry these organisms if the vaginal pH is < 4.4 (Freundt 1953; Edmunds 1959; Bercovici et al 1962). Perhaps not surprisingly there is a clear association of *M. hominis* carriage with anaerobic vaginosis, and it may be that it is associated in particular with the occurrence of *Mobiluncus* sp. rather than *Gardnerella*. *Ureaplasma* is not associated with non-specific vaginitis (Romano & Romano 1968). Pheifer et al (1978) reported an increased isolation rate in association with *Trichomonas*- or *Gardnerella*-associated vaginitis. It is not clear if the level of vaginal colonisation with mycoplasmas increases with vaginal pH postpartum, but certainly at this time bloodstream invasion with *Mycoplasma hominis* in association with fever is not uncommon, and always occurs in association with *Mycoplasma* sp. in the endometrium (Eschenbach et al 1984). An elucidation of the importance of mycoplasmas as pathogens or as normal flora in conditions with a raised vaginal pH seems overdue. *Mycoplasma* sp., unlike most non-sporing anaerobes and chlamydia, are resistant to rifampicin and this might therefore be used as an antimicrobial probe (Coufalik et al 1979).

Genital yeasts

The subject of vaginal candidiasis is dealt with fully in Chapter 10. There is a widespread assumption that yeasts cultured as a heavy growth from the vagina always play a pathogenic role. The position of yeasts other than *Candida albicans* as members of the normal vaginal flora has been examined on a number of occasions. Despite this many laboratories do not speciate their yeast isolates and may report all of them as *Candida* species or *C. albicans*.

A survey (Goldacre et al 1981) of 1498 women attending a family planning clinic revealed yeasts and fungi in 20.8%; only 72% of these were *C. albicans*. *Torulopsis glabrata* and *T. candida* comprised respectively 12 and 1% of the yeasts isolated and were the next commonest group. *C. parapsilosis*, a yeast that is most frequently recovered from skin-related sites, accounted for a further 6% of isolates. Three isolates of *C. tropicalis*, two of *C. intermedia*, and single isolates of *C. krusei* and *C. guilliermondi* were also made. *Trichosporon cutaneum* (the aetiological agent of piedra), *Aspergillus versicolor*, and *Rhizopus* sp. (a member of the mucorales) were also grown from specimens. Surprisingly, in this survey only a single fungal species was isolated from any one specimen. Yeasts other than *C. albicans* were no commoner in patients with abnormal discharge, but were commoner in women aged 35 years or over, or in those who used a diaphragm for contraception. Tampon usage and recent prescription of antibacterial drugs were not associated with a higher colonisation rate.

A prospective study of the yeast flora in pregnancy (Hurley et al 1974) also recorded that *Torulopsis glabrata* accounted for 11–15% of the yeasts isolated from all patients attending their first antenatal clinic. This fungus was rarer (5%) in a comparative group with symptoms and signs of vulvovaginitis. In these patients a positive association with pruritus but not with discharge or mycotic plaques was noted but does not seem to have been statistically significant. Recovery of more than one yeast strain

per patient was also uncommon in this study. Other differences from the quoted study in the family planning clinic population were a much lower recovery rate for *C. parapsilosis* and the fact that *Saccharomyces cerevisisae* was the third commonest yeast isolate.

C. albicans should probably never be regarded as a member of the normal vaginal flora (Carroll et al 1973). By contrast, it seems from the study of Goldacre et al (1981) that *Torulopsis* and other yeasts species may reasonably be so regarded. The factors involved in their establishment in the vaginal flora, their origin and relationship to the yeast flora of the rectum, urethra and skin, and the constancy or lability of carriage in an individual all await further study.

CONCLUSION

The normal microbial flora of the vagina is complex. The ecological niches found therein and the key control mechanisms for the ecosystem are still ill-understood. Further analyses of the flora require complete and methodologically critical descriptions. Experimental studies of microbial interactions created in pathological and physiological conditions provide insights of great importance to the future understanding of pathogenic mechanisms.

REFERENCES

Altermeir W A, Lewis S A, Schlievert P M et al 1982 Staphylococcus aureus associated with toxic shock syndrome. Annals of Internal Medicine 96: 978–982

Amsel R, Totten P A, Spiegel C A, Chen C K S, Eschenbach D A, Holmes K K 1983 Non-specific vaginitis: diagnostic criteria and microbial and epidemiologic associations. American Journal of Medicine 74: 14–24

Ancona R J, Ferrieri P, Williams P P 1980 Maternal factors that enhance the acquisition of Group B streptococci by newborn infants. Journal of Medical Microbiology 13: 273–280

Anthony B F, Concepcion N F 1975 Group B streptococcus in a general hospital. Journal of Infectious Diseases 132: 561–567

Appelbaum P C, Moodley J, Chatterton S A, Cowan D B, Africa C W 1978 Metronidazole in the prophylaxis and treatment of anaerobic infections. South African Medical Journal 54: 703–706

Appelbaum P C, Moodley J, Chatterton S A, Cowan D B, Africa C W 1980 Tinidazole in the prophylaxis and treatment of anaerobic infections. Chemotherapy 26: 145–157

Aubert J M, Gobeaux-Custodent M J, Boria M C 1980 Actinomyces in the endometrium of IUD users. Contraception 21: 577–583

Bailey R K, Voss J L, Smith R F 1979 Factors affecting isolation and identification of Haemophilus vaginalis (Corynebacterium vaginale). Journal of Clinical Microbiology 9: 65–71

Baker C J 1977 Summary of the workshop on perinatal infections due to Group B streptococcus. National Institutes of Health. Journal of Infectious Diseases 136: 137–152

Baldellon C, Megraud F 1985 Characterisation of Micrococcaceae strains isolated from the human urogenital tract by the conventional scheme and a micromethod. Journal of Clinical Microbiology 21: 474–477

Ball L C, Parker M T 1979 The cultural and biochemical characters of Streptococcus milleri strains isolated from human sources. Journal of Hygiene (Cambridge) 82: 63–78

Bartlett J G, Onderdonk A B, Drude E et al 1977 Quantitative bacteriology of the vaginal flora. Journal of Infectious Diseases 136: 271–277

Bartlett J G, Moon N E, Goldstein P R, Goren B, Onderdonk A B, Polk B F 1978 Cervical and vaginal bacterial flora: ecologic niches in the female lower genital tract. American Journal of Obstetrics and Gynecology 130: 658–661

Bercovici R, Persky S, Rozansky R, Razins 1962 Mycoplasma (pleuropneumonia-like organisms) in vaginitis. American Journal of Obstetrics and Gynecology 84: 687–691

Blackwell A, Fox A R, Phillips I, Barlow D 1983 Anaerobic vaginosis (non specific vaginitis): clinical microbiological and therapeutic findings. Lancet ii: 113–129

Blythe J G 1978 Cervical bacterial flora of patients with gynaecological malignancies. American Journal of Obstetrics and Gynecology 131: 438–445

Bodey G P 1981 Antibiotic prophylaxis in cancer patients: regimens of oral, nonabsorbable antibiotics for prevention of infection during induction of remission. Review of Infectious Diseases S: 259–268

Boe J, Solberg C O, Vogelsang T M, Wormines A 1964 Perineal carriers of staphylococci. British Medical Journal 2: 280–281

Bojsen Moller J 1972 Human listeriosis in diagnostic, epidemiological and clinical studies. Acta Pathologica et Microbiologica Scandinavica B Suppl 229: 1–157

Bollgren I, Vaclavinkova V, Hurvell B, Bergquist G 1978 Periurethral aerobic microflora of pregnant and non pregnant women. British Medical Journal 1: 1314–1317

Bonventre P F, Linnemann C, Weckbach L S et al 1984 Antibody response to toxic-shock-syndrome (TSS) toxin by patients with TSS and by healthy staphylococcal carriers. Journal of Infectious Diseases 150: 662–666

Botta G A, Pedulla D, Melioli G, Madoff S, Minuto F 1981 Absence of fluctuation in vaginal colonization by Enterobacteriaceae during the menstrual cycle in patients with recurrent cystitis. Lancet ii: 1116–1117

Bowie W R, Alexander E R, Floyd J F, Holmes K K, Miller Y 1976 Differential response of chlamydial and ureaplasma associated urethritis to sulphofurazole (sulfisoxazole) and aminocytolitols. Lancet ii: 1276–1278

Bramley H M, Dixon R A, Jones B M 1981 Haemophilus vaginalis in a family planning clinic population. British Journal of Venereal Diseases 57: 62–66

Braun P, Lee Y H, Klein J O et al 1971 Birth weight and genital mycoplasmas in pregnancy. New England Journal of Medicine 284: 167–171

Brook I, Barrett C T, Brinkman C R, William M D, Martin W J, Finegold S M 1979 Aerobic and anaerobic bacterial flora of the maternal cervix and newborn gastric fluid and conjunctiva: a prospective study. Pediatrics 63: 451–455

Bullen C L, Willis A T 1971 Resistance of the breast fed infant to gastroenteritis. British Medical Journal 2: 338–343

Bullen C L, Tearle P V, Stewart M G 1977 The effect of 'humanised' milks and supplemented breast feeding on the faecal flora of infants. Journal of Medical Microbiology 10: 403–413

Butler H M 1942 The examination of cervical smears as a means of rapid diagnosis in severe Clostridium welchii infection following abortion. Journal of Pathology and Bacteriology 54: 39–44

Butler H M 1945 Bacteriological studies of Clostridium welchii infections in man. Surgery, Gynecology and Obstetrics 81: 475–486

Bysshe S M 1938 Significance of Clostridium welchii in genital tract of pregnant and puerperal women. American Journal of Obstetrics and Gynecology 35: 995–999

Carroll C J, Hurley R, Stanley V C 1973 Criteria for diagnosis of Candida vulvovaginitis in pregnant women. Journal of Obstetrics and Gynaecology of the British Commonwealth 80: 258–263

Cattell R W, McSherry M A, Brookes H L, O'Grady F W 1975 Relation of bacteria isolated from the urethral area to bacteriuria. In: Koss E H, Brumfitt W (eds) Infections of the urinary tract: proceedings of the third international symposium on pyelonephritis. University of Chicago Press, Chicago, pp 69–73

Chen K C S, Forsyth P S, Buchanan T M, Holmes K K 1979 Amine content of vaginal fluid from untreated patients with nonspecific vaginitis. Journal of Clinical Investigation 63: 828–835

Chow A W, Bartlett K H, Percival-Smith R, Morrison B J 1984 Vaginal colonisation with Staphylococcus aureus positive for toxic-shock marker protein and Escherichia coli in healthy women. Journal of Infectious Diseases 150: 80–84

Christiansen G, Hansen E, Holst E, Christiansen C, Mardh P A 1984 Genetic relationships of short and long anaerobic curved rods isolated from the vagina. In: Mardh P A, Taylor Robinson D (eds) Bacterial vaginosis. Almquist and Wiksel, Stockholm, pp 75–78

Colman G, Williams R E O 1972 Taxonomy of some human viridans streptococci. In: Wannamaker L W, Matsen J M (eds) Streptococci and streptococcal diseases. Academic Press, New York pp 281–299

Corbishley C M 1977 Microbial flora of the vagina and cervix. Journal of Clinical Pathology 30: 745–748

Coufalik E D, Taylor-Robinson D, Csonka G W 1979 Treatment of non-gonococcal urethritis with rifampicin as a means of defining the role of Ureaplasma urealyticum. British Journal of Venereal Diseases 55: 36–43

Criswell B S, Ladwig C I, Gardner H L 1969 Haemophilus vaginalis: vaginitis by inoculation from culture. Obstetrics and Gynecology 33: 195–199

Crociani F, Matteuzzi D, Ghazvintzadeh H 1973 Spezies des Genus Bifidobacterium in der Frau. Zentralblatt fur Bakteriologie (Originale A) 223: 298–302

Cruickshank R, Sharman A 1934 The biology of the vagina in the human subject. Journal of Obstetrics and Gynaecology of the British Commonwealth 41: 190–266

Curtis E M, Pine L 1981 Actinomyces in the vaginas of women with and without intrauterine contraceptive devices. American Journal of Obstetrics and Gynecology 140: 880–884

Davies M E, Pearl S A 1938 Biology of human vagina in pregnancy. American Journal of Obstetrics and Gynecology 35: 77–97

Davis J P, Osterholm M T, Helms C M et al 1982 Tri-state toxic shock syndrome study: II. Clinical and laboratory findings. Journal of Infectious Diseases 145: 441–448

Delaha E C, Curtin J A, Stevens G, Osborne H J 1964 Incidence and significance of Haemophilus vaginalis in non specific vaginitis. American Journal of Obstetrics and Gynecology 89: 996–999

De Louvois J, Hurley R, Stanley V C, Jones J B, Faulkes J E B 1975a Microbiology of the female lower genital tract during pregnancy. Postgraduate Medical Journal 51: 156–160

De Louvois J, Hurley R, Stanley V C 1975b Microbial flora of the lower genital tract during pregnancy: relationship to morbidity. Journal of Clinical Pathology 28: 731–735

De Louvois J, Stanley V C, Leask B G S, Hurley R 1975c Ecological studies of the microbial flora of the female lower genital tract. Proceedings of the Royal Society of Medicine 68: 269–270

Delwicha E A, Pestka O J, Tortorello M L 1985 The Veillonellae gram-negative cocci with a unique physiology. Annual Review of Microbiology 39: 175–194

Duerden B I 1980 The isolation and identification of Bacteroides spp. from the normal vaginal flora. Journal of Medical Micro-biology 13: 79–87

Duguid H L D, Parrott D, Traynor R 1980 Actinomycetes-like organisms in cervical smears from women using intrauterine contraceptive devices. British Medical Journal 281: 534–541

Duignan N M, Lowe P A 1975 Preoperative disinfection of the vagina. Journal of Antimicrobial Chemotherapy 1: 117–120

Dunkelberg W E 1965 Diagnosis of Haemophilus vaginalis vaginitis by gram-stained smears. American Journal of Obstetrics and Gynecology 91: 998–1000

Dunkelberg W E, Hefner J D, Patow W E, Wyman F J, Orup H I 1962 Haemophilus vaginalis among asymptomatic women. Obstetrics and Gynecology 20: 629–632

Durfee M A, Forsyth P S, Hale J A, Holmes K K 1979 Ineffectiveness of erythromycin for treatment of Haemophilus vaginalis-associated vaginitis: possible relationship to acidity of vaginal secretions. Antimicrobial Agents and Chemotherapy 16: 635–637

Easmon C S F, Hastings M J, Clare A J et al 1981 Nosocomial transmission of Group B streptococci. British Medical Journal 283: 459–461

Easmon C S F, Hastings M J, Bloxham B, Clare A J, Marwood R, Rivers R P A 1982 Group-B streptococcal colonisation in mothers and babies. In: Holm S E, Christiansen P P (eds) Basic concepts of streptococci and streptococcus diseases. Reedbooks UK, Chertsey, Surrey, pp 295–296

Edmunds P N 1959 Haemophilus vaginalis: its association with puerperal pyrexia and leucorrhoea. Journal of Obstetrics and Gynaecology of the British Empire 66: 917–926

Elliot S D, Alexander T J L, Thomas J H 1966 Streptococcal infections in young pigs II. Epidemiology and experimental production of the disease. Journal of Hygiene (Cambridge) 64: 213–220

Eschenbach D A, Gravett M G, Chen K C S, Hoyne V B, Holmes K K 1984 Bacterial vaginosis during pregnancy. An association with prematurity and postpartum complications. In: Mardh P A, Taylor Robinson D (eds) Bacterial vaginosis. Almquist & Wiksell, Stockholm, pp 213–221

Eschenbach D A, Rosene K, Tompkins L S, Watkins H, Gravett M G 1986 Endometrial cultures obtained by a triple method from afebrile and febrile postpartum women. Journal of Infectious Diseases 153: 1038–45

Ezaki T, Yamamoto N, Ninomiya K, Suzuki S, Yabauchi E 1983 Transfer of Peptococcus indolicus, Peptococcus asaccharolyticus, Peptococcus prevoti and Peptococcus magnus to the genus Peptostreptococcus and proposal of Peptostreptococcus tetradius sp. nov. International Journal of Systemic Bacteriology 33: 683–698

Facklam P R 1977 Physiological differentiation of viridans streptococci. Journal of Clinical Microbiology 5: 184–201

Facklam R R, Rutledge L 1985 Physiologic and in vitro virulence differences among four beta-haemolytic group C streptococcus species. In: Kimura Y, Kotami S, Shiokawa Y (eds) Recent advances in streptococci and streptococcal diseases. Reedbooks UK, Chertsey, Surrey, pp 64–66

Fallon R J 1974 The rapid recognition of Lancefield Group B haemolytic streptococci. Journal of Clinical Pathology 27: 902–905

Falls F H 1933 Endometritis and pyometra due to Welch bacillus. American Journal of Obstetrics and Gynecology 25: 280–288

Feigin R D 1976 The perinatal Group B streptococcal problem: the questions and the answers. New England Journal of Medicine 294: 106–107

Fenton L J, Harper M H 1979 Evaluation of colistin and nalidi-

xic acid in Todd-Hewitt broth for selective isolation of Group B streptococci. Journal of Clinical Microbiology 9: 167–169

Ferreiri P, Cleary P P, Seeds A E 1977 Epidemiology of Group B streptococcal carriage in pregnant women and newborn infants. Journal of Medical Microbiology 10: 103–114

Fienberg R, Cohen R B 1967 Enzymes of glycogen metabolism in the squamous epithelium of the cervix: histochemical study. Obstetrics and Gynecology 31: 608

Fox A, Phillips I. 1984 Two curved rods in non-specific vaginitis. In: Mardh P A, Taylor Robinson D (eds) Bacterial vaginosis. Almquist & Wiksell, Stockholm, pp 93–96

Foy H M, Kenny G E, Levinsohn E M, Grayston J T 1970 Acquisition of mycoplasma and T-strains during infancy. Journal of Infectious Diseases 121: 579–587

Foy H, Kenny G, Bor E, Hammar S, Hickman R 1975 Prevalence of Mycoplasma hominis and Ureaplasma urealyticum (T-strains) in urine of adolescents. Journal of Clinical Microbiology 2: 226–230

Frampton J, Lee Y 1964 Is Haemophilus vaginalis a pathogen in the female genital tract? Journal of Obstetrics and Gynaecology of the British Commonwealth 71: 436–444

Freundt E A 1953 The occurrence of micromyces (pleuropneumonia-like organisms) in the female genital tract. Relation to the pH and general flora of the vagina. Acta Pathologica et Microbiologica Scandinavica B 32: 468–480

Fry R M 1938 Fatal infections by haemolytic streptococci Group B. Lancet i: 199–201

Gardner H L 1980 Haemophilus vaginalis vaginitis after twenty five years. American Journal of Obstetrics and Gynecology 137: 385–391

Gardner H L, Dukes C D 1955 Haemophilus vaginalis vaginitis. American Journal of Obstetrics and Gynecology 69: 962–976

George W L, Kirby B D, Sutter V L, Citron D M, Finegold S M 1981 Gram-negative anaerobic bacilli, their role in infection and patterns of susceptibility to antimicrobial agents. 11. Little known Fusobacterium species and miscellaneous genera. Review of Infectious Diseases 3: 599–625

Gibbs R S, Blanco J D, Castaneda Y S, St Clair P J 1980 Therapy of obstetrical infections with moxalactam. Antimicrobial Agents and Chemotherapy 17: 1004–1007

Gibbs R S, Blanco J D, St Clair P J, Castaneda Y S 1982 Quantitative bacteriology of amniotic fluid from women with clinical intraamniotic infection at term. Journal of Infectious Diseases 145: 1–9

Gillespie W A, Sellin M A, Gill P et al 1978 Urinary infection in young women with special reference to Staphylococcus saprophyticus. Journal of Clinical Pathology 31: 348–350

Golberg R L, Washington J A III 1976 Comparison of isolation of Haemophilus vaginalis (Corynebacterium vaginale) from peptone-starch-dextrose agar and Columbia colistin-nalidixic acid agar. Journal of Clinical Microbiology 4: 245–247

Goldacre M J, Watt B, Loudon N, Milne L J R, Loudon J D O, Vessey M P 1979 Vaginal microbial flora in normal young women. British Medical Journal 1: 1450–1453

Goldacre M J, Milne L J R, Watt B, Loudon N, Vessey M P 1981 Prevalence of yeast and fungi other than Candida albicans in the vagina of normal young women. British Journal of Obstetrics and Gynaecology 88: 596–600

Goplerud C P, Ohm M J, Galask R P 1976 Aerobic and anaerobic flora of the cervix during pregnancy and the puerperium. American Journal of Obstetrics and Gynecology 126: 858–865

Gorbach S L, Tabaqchali S 1969 Bacteria, bile and the small bowel. Gut 10: 963–972

Gorbach S L, Menda K B, Thadepalli H, Keith L 1973 Anaerobic microflora of the cervix in healthy women. American Journal of Obstetrics and Gynecology 117: 1053–1055

Greenwood J R, Pickett M J 1979 Salient features of Haemophilus vaginalis. Journal of Clinical Microbiology 9: 200–204

Greenwood J R, Pickett M J 1980 Transfer of Haemophilus vaginalis (Gardner and Dukes) to a new genus Gardnerella: G. vaginalis (Gardner and Dukes). International Journal of Systemic Bacteriology 30: 170–178

Greenwood J R, Pickett M J, Martin W J, Mack E G 1977 Haemophilus vaginalis (Corynebacterium vaginale): method for isolation and rapid biochemical identification. Health Laboratory Science 14: 102–106

Gregoire A T, Rankin J, Johnson W D, Rakoff A E, Adams A 1967 Alpha-amylase content in cervical mucus of females receiving sequential, non-sequential, or no contraceptive therapy. Fertility and Sterility 18: 836–839

Grice G C, Hafiz S 1983 Actinomyces in the female genital tract. A preliminary report. British Journal of Venereal Diseases 59: 317–319

Grossman J H III, Adams R L 1979 Vaginal flora in women undergoing hysterectomy with antibiotic prophylaxis. Obstetrics and Gynecology 53: 23–26

Guinan M E, Dan B B, Guidotti R J et al 1982 Vaginal colonisation with Staphylococcus aureus in healthy women: a review of four studies. Annals of Internal Medicine 96: 944–947

Gupta P K, Woodruff J D 1982 Actinomyces in vaginal smears. Journal of the American Medical Association 247: 1175–1176

Haffar A N, Fuselier P A, Baker C J 1983 Species distribution of non-group D alpha-haemolytic streptococci in maternal genital and neonatal blood cultures. Journal of Clinical Microbiology 18: 101–103

Hafiz S, McEntegart M G, Morton R S, Waitkins S A 1975 Clostridium difficile in the urogenital tract of males and females. Lancet i: 420–421

Hammann R 1982 A reassessment of the microbial flora of the female genital tract with special reference to the occurrence of Bacteroides species. Journal of Medical Microbiology 15: 293–302

Hammerschlag M R, Alpert S, Onderdonk A B et al 1978a Anaerobic microflora of the vagina in children. American Journal of Obstetrics and Gynecology 131: 853–856

Hammerschlag M R, Alpert S, Rosnerl et al 1978b Microbiology of the vagina in children: normal and potentially pathogenic organisms. Pediatrics 62: 57–62

Hartley C L, Clements H M, Linton K B 1977 Escherichia coli in the faecal flora of man. Journal of Applied Bacteriology 43: 261–269

Hedges A J, Howe K, Linton A H 1977 Statistical considerations in the sampling of Escherichia coli from intestinal sources for serotyping. Journal of Applied Bacteriology 43: 271–288

Hill A M 1964 Why be morbid? Paths of progress in the control of obstetric infections. Medical Journal of Australia 1: 101–111

Hill G B, Ayers O M 1985 Antimicrobial susceptibilities of anaerobic bacteria isolated from female genital tract infections. Antimicrobial Agents and Chemotherapy 27: 324–331

Holst E, Hofmann H, Mardh P A 1984a Anaerobic curved rods in genital samples of women. In: Mardh P A, Taylor Robinson D (eds) Bacterial vaginosis. Almquist & Wiksell, Stockholm, pp 117–124

Holst E, Svensson H, Skorm A, Westrom L, Mardh P A 1984b Vaginal colonisation with Gardnerella vaginalis and anaerobic curved rods. In: Mardh P A, Taylor Robinson D (eds) Bacterial vaginosis. Almquist & Wiksell, Stockholm, pp 147–152

Huang J C C, Diena B B 1982 Serotype distribution of group B streptococci isolated from human and animal sources in Canada. In: Holm S E, Christensen P (eds) Basic concepts of streptococcal diseases. Reedbooks UK, Chertsey, Surrey, pp 46–47

Hurley R, Stanley V C, Leask B G S, De Louvois J 1974 The microflora of the vagina during pregnancy. In: The normal microflora of man. Skinner F A, Carr J G (eds) Academic Press, London, pp 155–185

Islam A K M S 1981 Primary carrier sites of Group B streptococci in pregnant women correlated with serotype distributions and maternal parity. Journal of Clinical Pathology 34: 78–81

Islam A, Thomas E 1980 Faecal carriage of Group B streptococci. Journal of Clinical Pathology 33: 1006–1008

Jacob A E, Douglas G J, Hobss S J 1975 Self transferrable plasmid determining the haemolysin and bacteriocin of Streptococcus faecalis var. zymogenes. Journal of Bacteriology 121: 863–872

Jensen N E, Berg B 1982 Sewage and aquatic biotypes as potential reservoir of Group B streptococci. In: Holm S E, Christensen P (eds) Basic concepts of streptococcal diseases. Reedbooks UK, Chertsey, Surrey, pp 107–108

Jones D E, Friedl E M, Kanarek K S, Williams J K, Lim D V 1983a Rapid identification of pregnant women heavily colonised with Group B streptococci. Journal of Clinical Microbiology 18: 558–560

Jones J B, Kaplan W, Brown J M, White W 1983b Studies of cervicovaginal smears for the presence of actinomycetes. Mycopathologia 83: 53–55

Kallenius G, Wimberg J 1978 Bacterial adherence to periurethral epithelial cells in girls prone to urinary tract infection. Lancet ii: 540–562

Karnaky K J 1959 Comparisons of battery pH reading and electronic pH recordings of the vagina in Trichomonas vaginalis infestation. American Journal of Obstetrics and Gynecology 77: 149–154

Kirby B D, George W L, Sutter V L, Citron D M, Finegold S M 1980 Gram-negative anaerobic bacilli: their role in infections and patterns of susceptibility to antimicrobial agents. 1 Little known Bacteroides species. Review of Infectious Diseases 2: 914–951

Klein J O, Buckland D, Finland M 1969 Colonisation of newborn infants by mycoplasmas. New England Journal of Medicine 280: 1025–1030

Knuppel R A, Scerbo J C, Dzink J, Mitchell G W, Cetrulo C L, Bartlett J 1981 Quantitative transcervical uterine cultures with a new device. Obstetrics and Gynecology 57: 243–248

Kummel J 1963 Klinische und bakteriologische Untersuchungen über die unspezifische Scheidenzundung. Archiv fur Gynaekologie 199: 5–42

Lamont R J, Postlethwaite R 1986 Carriage of lysteria monocytogenes and related species in pregnant and non-pregnant women in Aberdeen, Scotland. Journal of Infection 13: 187–194

Lapage S P 1961 Haemophilus vaginalis and its role in vaginitis. Acta Pathologica et Microbiologica Scandinavica B 52: 34–54

Larsen B, Galask R P 1980 Vaginal microbial flora: practical and theoretic relevance. Obstetrics and Gynecology 55: 100–113

Larsen B, Galask R P 1982 Vaginal microbial flora: composition and influences of host physiology. Annals of Internal Medicine 96: 926–930

Laughton N 1950 Vaginal corynebacteria. Journal of Hygiene (Cambridge) 48: 346–356

Lee Y H, McCormack W M, Marcy S M, Klein J O 1974 The genital mycoplasmas: their role in disorders of reproduction and in paediatric infections. Pediatric Clinics of North America 21: 457–466

Levison M E, Corman L C, Carrington E R, Kaye D 1977 Quantitative microflora of the vagina. American Journal of Obstetrics and Gynecology 127: 80–85

Levison M E, Trestman I, Quach R, Sladowski C, Floro C N 1979 Quantitative bacteriology of the vaginal flora in vaginitis. American Journal of Obstetrics and Gynecology 133: 139–144

Lim D V, Kanarek K S, Peterson M E 1982 Magnitude of colonisation and sepsis by Group B streptococci in newborn infants. Current Developments in Microbiology 7: 99–101

Lindner J G E M, Plantema F H F, Hoogkamp-Korstanje J A A 1978 Quantitative studies of the vaginal flora of health women and of obstetric and gynaecological patients. Journal of Medical Microbiology 11: 233–241

Linneman C C, Stareck J L, Hornsten S et al 1982 The epidemiology of genital colonization with Staphylococcus aureus. Annals of Internal Medicine 96: 940–944

McCormack W M, Rankins J S, Lee Y H 1973a Localisation of genital mycoplasmas in women. American Journal of Obstetrics and Gynecology 112: 920–923

McCormack W M, Rosner B, Lee Y H 1973b Colonisation with genital mycoplasmas in women. American Journal of Epidemiology 97: 240–245

McCormack W M, Hayes C H, Rosner B et al 1977 Vaginal colonization with Corynebacterium vaginale. Journal of Infectious Diseases 156: 740–745

McEntegart M G, Hafiz S, Kinghorn G R 1982 Haemophilus ducreyi infections—time for reappraisal. Journal of Hygiene (Cambridge) 89: 467–478

McLauchlin J, Audurier A, Taylor A G 1986 Aspects of the epidemiology of human listeria monocytogenes infection in Britain 1967–1984; the use of sero typing and phoge typing. Journal of Medical Microbiology 22: 367–377

Mardh P A, Soltesz L V 1983 In vitro interactions between Lactobacilli and other micro organisms occurring in the vaginal flora. Scandinavian Journal of Infectious Diseases Supplement 40: 47–51

Mardh P A, Holst E, Moller B R 1984 The grivet monkey as a model for study of vaginitis. Challenge with anaerobic curved rods and Gardnerella vaginalis. Scandinavian Journal of Urology and Nephrology Supplement 86: 201

Mead P B 1978 Cervical vaginal flora of women with invasive cervical cancer. Obstetrics and Gynecology 52: 601–604

Meers P D 1974 The bacteriological examination of urine: a computer-aided study. Journal of Hygiene (Cambridge) 72: 229–244

Meleney F L 1931 Bacterial synergism in disease processes. Annals of Surgery 94: 961–981

Mhalu F S 1977 Reservoir of Group B streptococci in women in labour. British Medical Journal 1: 812

Michell D R, Bell J H, Good R G, Moyer D L 1966 The intrauterine device: a bacteriologic study of the endometrial cavity. American Journal of Obstetrics and Gynecology 96: 119–126

Mitchell R G 1968 Classification of Staphylococcus albus strains isolated from the urinary tract. Journal of Clinical Pathology 21: 93–96

Mitchell R G, Crow M R 1984 Actinomyces odontolyticus isolated from the female genital tract. Journal of Clinical Pathology 37: 1379–1383

Moberg P, Eneroth P, Harlin J, Ljung-Wadstrom A, Nord C E 1978 Cervical bacterial flora in infertile and pregnant women. Medical Microbiology and Immunology 165: 139–145

Moellering R C, Korzeniowski O M, Sande M A, Wennersten

C B 1979 Species specific resistance to antimicrobial synergism in Streptococcus faecium and Streptococcus faecalis. Journal of Infectious Diseases 140: 203–208

Moi H, Danielsson D, Schoenknecht F 1984 An in vitro study of the attachment to vaginal epithelial cells of anaerobic curved rods, Bacteroides bivius and Bacteroides disiens. In: Mardh P A, Taylor-Robinson D (eds) Bacterial vaginosis. Almquist & Wiksell, Stockholm, pp 185–190

Morris C A, Morris D F 1967 Normal vaginal microbiology of women of childbearing age in relation to the use of oral contraceptions and vaginal tampons. Journal of Clinical Pathology 20: 636–640

Nakkash A F Y, Jones D 1982 Studies on Group B streptococci. In: Holme S E, Christensen P (eds) Basic concepts of streptococcal diseases. Reedbooks UK, Chertsey, Surrey, pp 44–45

Neary M P, Allen J, Okubadejo O A, Payne D J H 1973 Preoperative vaginal bacteria and postoperative infections in gynaecological patients. Lancet ii: 1291–1294

Noble M A, Bent J M, West A B 1983 Detection and identification of group B streptococci by use of pigment production. Journal of Clinical Pathology 36: 350–352

O'Farrell S, Wilks M, Nash J Q, Tabaqchali S 1984 A selective enrichment broth for the isolation of Clostridium difficile. Journal of Clinical Pathology 37: 98–99

Ohm M J, Galask R P 1975 Bacterial flora of the cervix from 100 prehysterectomy patients. American Journal of Obstetrics and Gynecology 122: 683–687

Ohm M J, Galask R P 1976 The effect of antibiotic prophylaxis on patients undergoing total abdominal hysterectomy. II Alterations of microbial flora. American Journal of Obstetrics and Gynecology 125: 448–454

Onderdonk A B, Polk B F, Moon N E, Goren B, Bartlett J G 1977 Methods for quantitative vaginal flora studies. American Journal of Obstetrics and Gynecology 128: 777–781

Osborne N G, Wright R C 1977 Effect of pre-operative scrub on the bacterial flora of the endocervix and vagina. Obstetrics and Gynecology 50: 148–151

Osborne N G, Wright R C, Grubin L 1979 Genital bacteriology: a comparative study of premenopausal women with postmenopausal women. American Journal of Obstetrics and Gynecology 135: 195–197

Osterholm M T, Davis J P, Gibson R W et al 1982 Tri-state toxic shock syndrome study. I Epidemiologic findings. Journal of Infectious Diseases 145: 431–440

Pattman R S 1984 The significance of finding curved rods in the vaginal secretion of patients attending a genito-urinary medical clinic. In: Mardh P A, Taylor-Robinson D (eds) Bacterial vaginosis. Almquist & Wiksell, Stockholm, pp 143–146

Pead H, Crump J, Maskell R 1977 Staphylococci as urinary pathogens. Journal of Clinical Pathology 30: 427–431

Percival-Smith R, Bartlett K H, Chow A W 1983 Vaginal colonisation of Escherichia coli and its relation to contraceptive methods. Contraception 27: 497–504

Peterson D R 1982 Epidemiologic comparisons of toxic shock syndrome. Annals of Internal Medicine 96: 891–892

Pezzlo M T, Hesser J W, Morgan T, Valter P J, Thrupp P D 1979 Improved laboratory efficiency and diagnostic accuracy with new double-masked swab for endometrial specimens. Journal of Clinical Microbiology 9: 56–59

Pheifer T A, Forsyth P S, Durfee M A, Pollock H M, Holmes K K 1978 Role of Haemophilus vaginalis and treatment with metronidazole. New England Journal of Medicine 298: 1429–1434

Pine L, Malcolm G B, Curtis E M, Brown J M 1981 Demonstration of Actinomyces and Arachnia species in cervicovaginal smears by direct staining with species specific fluorescent-antibody conjugate. Journal of Clinical Microbiology 13: 15–21

Piot P, Van Dyck E, Goodfellow M, Falkow S 1980 A taxonomic study of Gardnerella vaginalis (Haemophilus vaginalis) Gardner and Dukes 1955. Journal of General Microbiology 119: 373–376

Piot P, Van Dyck E, Totten P A, Holmes K K 1982 Identification of Gardnerella (Haemophilus) vaginalis. Journal of Clinical Microbiology 15: 19–24

Rabinowitz M, Toaff R, Krochik N 1963 The possible role of Listeria monocytogenes in habitual abortion. In: Gray M L (ed) 2nd Symposium on Listeric Infection. Bozeman Montana State College, pp 309–314

Rappaport F, Rabinowitz M, Toaff R, Krochik N 1960 Genital listeriosis as a cause of repeated abortion. Lancet i: 1273–1275

Redmond D L, Kotcher E 1963 Comparison of cultural and immunoflorescent processes for identification of Haemophilus vaginalis. Journal of General Microbiology 33: 89–94

Ridley M 1959 Perineal carriage of Staphylococcus aureus. British Medical Journal 1: 270–273

Rogosa M, Sharpe M E 1960 Species differentiation of human vaginal lactobacilli. Journal of General Microbiology 23: 197–209

Romano N, Romano F 1968 Reperto e significato di Micoplasmi nelle infezioni infiammatorie del tratto vaginale. Giornale di Malattie Infettive e Parassitarie 20: 585–591

Ross P W, Cumming C G 1982 Association of Group B streptococci with symptoms and signs of venereal infection in women. In: Holm S E, Christensen P (eds) Basic concepts of streptococci and streptococcal diseases. Reedbooks UK, Chertsey, Surrey, pp 103–104

Ross J M, Needham J R 1980 Genital flora during pregnancy and colonization of the newborn. Journal of Royal Society of Medicine 73: 105–110

Salm R 1944 The occurrence and significance of Clostridium welchii in the female genital tract. Journal of Obstetrics and Gynecology 51: 121–126

Sanderson P J, Ross J, Stringer J 1981 Source of Group B streptococii in the female genital tract. Journal of Clinical Pathology 34: 84–86

Sautter R L, Brown W J 1980 Sequential vaginal cultures from normal young women. Journal of Clinical Microbiology 11: 479–484

Schaeffer A J, Stamey T A 1977 Studies of introital colonisation in women with recurrent urinary tract infection IX: Role of antimicrobial therapy. Journal of Urology 118: 221–224

Schaeffer A J, Jones J M, Dunn J K 1981 Association of in vitro Escherichia coli adherence to vaginal and buccal epithelial cells with susceptibility of women to recurrent urinary tract infections. New England Journal of Medicine 304: 1062–1066

Schlievert P M, Osterholm M T, Kelly J A, Nishimura R D 1982 Toxin and enzyme characterisation of Staphylococcus aureus isolates from patients with and without toxic shock syndrome. Annals of Internal Medicine 96: 937–940

Sellin M, Cooke D I, Gillespie W A, Sylvester D G H, Anderson J D 1975 Micrococcal urinary-track infections in young women. Lancet ii: 570–572

Smith L D S 1975 The pathogenic anerobic bacteria. C C Thomas, Springfield, Illinois

Sparks R A, Purrier B G A, Watt P J, Elstein M 1977 The bacteriology of the cervix and uterus. British Journal of Obstetrics and Gynaecology 84: 701–707

Spencer R C, Nanayakarra C S, Coup A J 1982 Fulminant neonatal sepsis due to Streptococcus milleri. Journal of Infection 4: 88–89

Spiegel C A, Roberts M 1984 Mobiluncus geni nov, Mobiluncus curtisii subsp. curtisii sp. nov, Mobiluncus curtisii subsp. holmesii subsp. nov. and Mobiluncus mulieris sp. nov; curved rods from the human vagina. International Journal of Systemic Bacteriology 34: 117–184

Spiegel C A, Amsel R, Eschenbach D, Schoenknecht F, Holmes K K 1980 Anaerobic bacteria in non-specific vaginitis. New England Journal of Medicine 303: 601–606

Stamey T A, Condy M 1975 The diffusion and concentration of trimethoprim in human vaginal fluid. Journal of Infectious Diseases 131: 261–266

Stamey T A, Sexton C C 1975 The role of vaginal colonization with Enterobacteriaceae in recurrent urinary infections. Journal of Urology 113: 214–216

Stamey T A, Condy M, Mihora G 1977 Prophylactic efficacy of nitrofurantoin macrocrystals and trimethoprim-sulphamethoxazole in urinary infections. Biological effects on the vaginal and rectal flora. New England Journal of Medicine 296: 780–783

Stark P L, Lee A 1982 The microbial ecology of the large bowel of breast-fed and formula-fed infants during the first year of life. Journal of Medical Microbiology 15: 189–203

Stringer J 1982 Bacteriophages of Lancefield Group B streptococci. In: Holm S E, Christensen P (eds) Basic concepts of streptococci and streptococcal diseases. Reedbooks UK, Chertsey, Surrey, pp 51–53

Sutter V L, Citron D M, Finegold S M 1980 Wadsworth anaerobic bacteriology manual. 3rd edn. C V Mosby, London.

Swenson R M, Michaelson T C, Daly M J, Spaulding E H 1973 Anaerobic bacterial infections of the female genital tract. Obstetrics and Gynecology 42: 538–541

Tarlinton M N, D'Abrera V St E 1974 Haemophilus vaginalis—further investigations into its identity. Journal of Medical Microbiology 7: 537–541

Tashjian J H, Coulam C B, Washington J A II 1976 Vaginal flora in asymptomatic women. Mayo Clinic Proceedings 51: 557–561

Taylor E, Blackwell A L, Barlow D, Phillips I 1982 Gardnerella vaginalis, anaerobes, and vaginal discharge. Lancet i: 1376–1379.

Teare E L, Bakhtiar M, Rogers T R, Oates J K 1981 Non specific vaginitis: its diagnosis and treatment. Journal of Antimicrobial Chemotherapy 8: 496–497

Thadepalli H, Gorbach S L, Keith L 1973 Anaerobic infections of the female genital tract: bacteriologic and therapeutic aspects. American Journal of Obstetrics and Gynecology 117: 1034–1040

Toaff R, Krochik N, Rabinowitz M 1962 Genital listeriosis in the male. Lancet ii: 482–483

Totten P A, Amsel R, Hale R, Piot P, Holmes K K 1982 Selective differential human blood bilayer media for isolation of Gardnerella (Haemophilus) vaginalis. Journal of Clinical Microbiology 15: 141–147

Traynor R M, Parrett D, Duguid H L D, Duncan I D 1981 Isolation of actinomyces from cervical specimens. Journal of Clinical Pathology 34: 914–916

Ursi J P, Van Dyck E, Ballard R C, Jacob W, Piot P, Meheus A Z 1982 Characterisation of an unusual bacterium from genital ulcers. Journal of Medical Microbiology 15: 97–103

Valicenti J F, Pappos A A, Gruber C D, Williams H O, Wills H F 1982 Detection and prevalence of IUD associated Actinomyces colonisation and related morbidity. Journal of the American Medical Association 247: 1149–1152

Van der Waaij D, Berghuis J M, Lekkerkerk J E C 1972 Colonisation resistance of the digestive tract of mice during systemic antibiotic treatment. Journal of Hygiene (Cambridge) 70: 605–610

Vergeront J M, Stolz S J, Cross B A, Nelson D B, Davis J P, Bergdoll M S 1983 Prevalance of serum antibody to staphylococcal enterotoxin F among Wisconsin residents: implications for toxic-shock syndrome. Journal of Infectious Diseases 148: 692–698

Wallace R J Jr, Baker C J, Quinones F J, Hollis D G, Weaver R E, Wiss K 1983 Nontypeable Haemophilus influenzae (biotype 4) as a neonatal, maternal and genital pathogen. Review of Infectious Diseases 5: 123–136

Watt B, Goldacre M J, Loudon N, Annat D J, Harris R I, Vessey M P 1981 Prevalence of bacteria in the vagina of normal young women. British Journal of Obstetrics and Gynaecology 88: 588–595

Werner H, Lang N, Kraseman C, Tolmitt T G, Feddern R 1978 Epidemiology of anaerobic infections of the female genitourinary tract and preliminary results of therapy with erythromycin. Current Medical Research Opinions 5 (Supplement 2): 52–55

Wiegersma N, Jansen G, Van der Waaij D 1982 Effect of twelve antimicrobial drugs on the colonization resistance of the digestive tract of mice and on endogenous potentially pathogenic bacteria. Journal of Hygiene (Cambridge) 88: 221–230

Wilks M, Thin R N, Tabaqchali S 1982 Quantitative methods of studies on vaginal flora. Journal of Medical Microbiology 15: 141–147

Wimberley N, Faling L J, Bartlett J G 1979 A fibreoptic bronchoscopy technique to obtain noncontaminated lower airway secretions for bacterial culture. American Review of Respiratory Diseases 119: 337–343

Windsor R S, Elliot S D 1975 Streptococcal infection in young pigs. IV An outbreak of streptococcal meningitis in weaned pigs. Journal of Hygiene (Cambridge) 75: 69–78

Wren M W D 1980 Prolonged primary incubation in the isolation of anaerobic bacteria from clinical specimens. Journal of Medical Microbiology 13: 257–263

Wren M W D, Eldon C P, Dakin G H 1977 Novobiocin and the differentiation of peptococci and peptostreptococci. Journal of Clinical Pathology 30: 620–622

Wylie J G, Henderson A 1969 Identification and glycogen-fermenting ability of lactobacilli isolated from the vagina of pregnant women. Journal of Medical Microbiology 2: 363–365

Yong D C T, Thompson J S 1982 Rapid microbiochemical method for identification of Gardnerella (Haemophilus) vaginalis. Journal of Clinical Microbiology 16: 30–33

Cytology of the female genital tract: cytological and histopathological recognition of infection
P Cooper

HISTOLOGY AND CYTOLOGY OF THE FEMALE GENITAL TRACT

Three types of epithelium are present in the uterus and vagina. Squamous epithelium lines the labia minora, vagina and ectocervix. The endocervical canal and endometrium are lined by a single layer of columnar epithelium. These epithelia are under hormonal influence. The following description is based on their appearances during the child-bearing years when hormonal influences are at their peak. Subsequently the epithelial and cytologic changes which occur during the menstrual cycle and in prepubertal and postmenopausal women will be described.

Stratified squamous epithelium

When fully mature three zones are observed within the epithelium: the basal layer, the midzone or prickle cell layer, which constitutes the bulk of the epithelium, and the superficial zone (Fig. 3.1). The basal layer is composed of a single layer of small cells with active nuclei and indistinct cytoplasm. Under normal circumstances the process of epithelial regeneration is confined to the basal layer and occasional mitoses are seen.

The midzone is composed of maturing squamous cells. The smaller cells adjacent to the basal layer are called parabasal cells. The larger cells adjacent to the surface layers are called intermediate cells and as the cells mature towards the surface the volume of cytoplasm increases whereas the nuclear size remains fairly constant.

The superficial zone is composed of several layers of cells which are larger than intermediate cells. The nuclei are pyknotic. The most super-

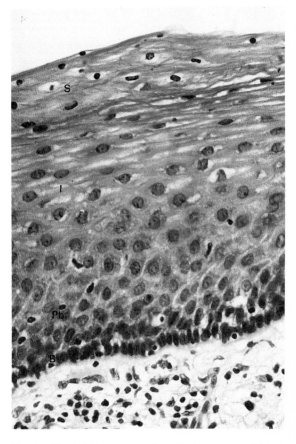

Fig. 3.1 Cervical biopsy: normal stratified squamous epithelium. B = basal cells; Pb = parabasal cells; I = intermediate cells; S = superficial cells. ×350. Haematoxylin and eosin.

ficial cells are cast off by a mechanism known as desquamation or exfoliation. Squamous cells throughout the intermediate and superficial zones are tightly bound to each other by well developed intercellular bridges. These bonds are split and ex-

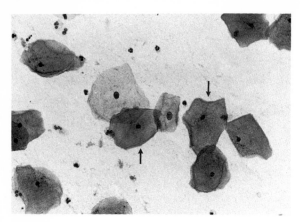

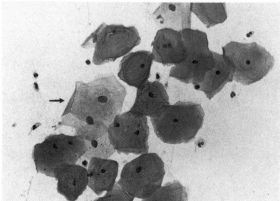

Fig. 3.2 Cervical smear: superficial squamous cells (arrows). ×250. Papanicolaou.

Fig. 3.3 Cervical smear: intermediate squamous cells (arrow). ×250. Papanicolaou.

foliation occurs, but the mechanism for this is unknown.

The squamous epithelium of the cervix and vagina is rich in glycogen. Precursors of keratin are present in the cytoplasm of the most superficial cells, but full development of keratin only occurs under abnormal circumstances, for example prolapse.

The epithelium is supported by a basement membrane and a connective tissue stroma.

Cytological characteristics of cells shed from the normal squamous epithelium of cervix and vagina

Superficial squamous cells (Fig. 3.2)

These are large polygonal-shaped cells with a small pyknotic nucleus, 5 μm diameter, and delicate transparent cytoplasm. The cell shape reflects the rigidity of the cytoplasm which is due to the presence of numerous tonofibrils. The majority of superficial cells stain pink in a Papanicolaou stained smear. These cells predominate in a smear taken at the peak of oestrogenic activity.

Intermediate squamous cells (Fig. 3.3)

Squamous cells of this type which are adjacent to the superficial zone are of the same size as superficial cells but their cytoplasm is delicate and basophilic. The cytoplasm at the edge of the cell often exhibits folding. In the deeper layers of the intermediate zone the cells are smaller and have rather dense cytoplasm. The main difference be-

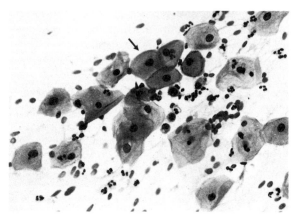

Fig. 3.4 Cervical smear: navicular cells (arrow). ×250. Papanicolaou.

tween intermediate cells and superficial cells lies in the structure of the nucleus. The nucleus of the intermediate cells is round or oval, 8 μm diameter with a well defined nuclear membrane and a delicate chromatin pattern. Chromocentres and sex chromatin may be seen within the nucleus.

Navicular cells (Fig. 3.4)

Navicular cells are a frequent variant of intermediate cells. They are seen in smears during pregnancy and after the menopause. Navicular cells are boat-shaped and the cytoplasm characteristically contains abundant glycogen. In a variety of pathological and physiological conditions the squamous

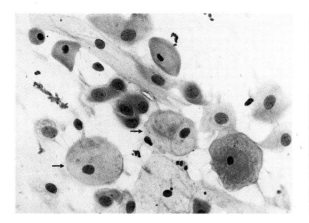

Fig. 3.5 Cervical smear: parabasal cells (arrows). ×320. Papanicolaou.

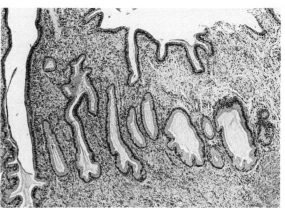

Fig. 3.6 Columnar cell epithelium of the endocervical canal. ×40. Haematoxylin and eosin.

epithelium of the genital tract may fail to reach full maturation and under these circumstances intermediate cells will predominate in the smear.

Parabasal cells (Fig. 3.5)

Parabasal cells are the least common type of squamous cell seen in cervical or vaginal smears taken during the reproductive years. Under normal physiological conditions they appear before puberty, after the menopause and during lactation. The cells are round or oval and have dense basophilic cytoplasm. The nuclei are similar to those of intermediate cells and appear larger only because they occupy a larger proportion of the total cell volume.

Basal cells

These are rarely seen in smears. Their presence indicates that the upper layers of the squamous epithelium have been severely damaged. Basal cells appear as very small oval cells. Their nuclei are large and occasionally contain small nucleoli.

Endocervical epithelium

The endocervical canal and the endocervical glands are lined by a single layer of mucus-secreting epithelium composed of tall columnar cells with basal nuclei (Fig. 3.6). Ciliated columnar cells are also found within this epithelium.

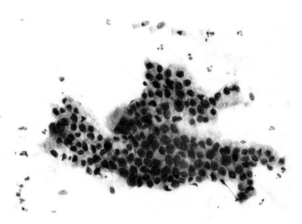

Fig. 3.7 Cervical smear. Endocervical cells show a 'honeycomb' pattern. Mucus-secreting cells predominate. ×390. Papanicolaou.

Endocervical cells

These are often well preserved in cervical smears and may occur in tight clusters. If the cluster is 'on end' the cells assume a very characteristic honeycomb appearance (Fig. 3.7). If in rows, their columnar appearance is well displayed and mucus-secreting and ciliated cells can be readily identified (Fig. 3.8). The nuclei of endocervical cells are finely granular and frequently contain one or two small nucleoli. The nuclei are approximately the same size as those of intermediate squamous cells. 'Stripped' nuclei are often seen when the delicate cytoplasm of the columnar cells disintegrates (Fig. 3.9). The endocervical cells secrete mucus during

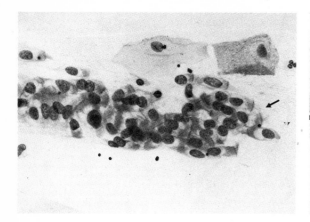

Fig. 3.8 Cervical smear. Ciliated cells predominate (arrow). ×390. Papanicolaou.

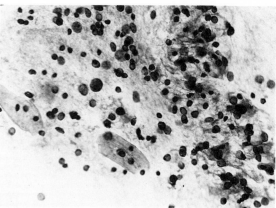

Fig. 3.9 Cervical smear. Numerous 'stripped' endocervical cell nuclei are seen. ×200. Papanicolaou.

the reproductive years. The alkaline mucus is abundant and of low viscosity during the oestrogenic phase of the cycle. After ovulation the mucus becomes viscous, under the influence of progesterone.

Endometrium

The endometrium is composed of tubular glands surrounded by densely packed stromal cells (Fig. 3.10). The appearance of the glands and the stroma changes with the phase of the menstrual cycle.

Endometrial cells may be seen in smears from the onset of the menstrual flow until the 12th day of the cycle. The appearance of endometrial cells in cervicovaginal smears after the 12th day of the cycle must be considered abnormal. Although endometrial glandular cells and endometrial stromal cells are readily distinguished in histological sections, identification of these two types in cervical or vaginal smears is often difficult. Well preserved cells originating from endometrial glands are usually seen in clusters with overlapping nuclei (Fig. 3.11) whereas stromal cells are arranged in flat sheets or single files. The epithelial cells from the endometrium are distinguished from endocervical cells by their scanty cytoplasm and smaller nuclei. The nuclei are round or oval and have evenly dispersed but coarsely granular chromatin.

· Stromal cells have very indistinct cytoplasm and elongated nuclei.

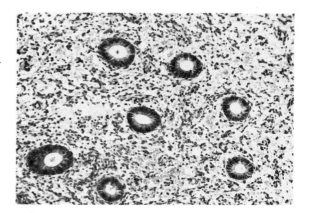

Fig. 3.10 Endometrial curettings: proliferative phase of the endometrium. ×200. Haematoxylin and eosin.

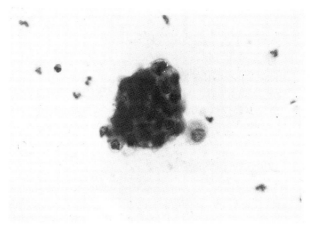

Fig. 3.11 Cervical smear: a tight cluster of endometrial glandular cells. ×390. Papanicolaou.

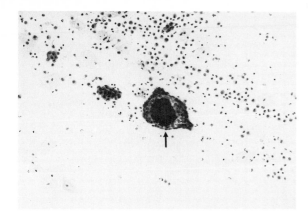

Fig. 3.12 Cervical smear: menstrual exodus. A large cluster of endometrial cells (arrow). Stromal cells form the core of these cellular balls. ×25. Papanicolaou.

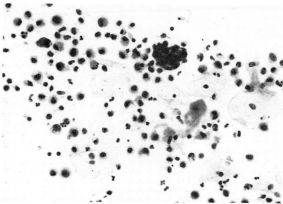

Fig. 3.13 Cervical smear: the menstrual exodus. Clusters of endometrial cells are surrounded by granulocytes and histiocytes. ×250. Papanicolaou.

The exodus

From the fifth to the sixth day of menstruation clusters of glandular cells and stromal cells accompanied by histiocytes are present in the smear (Figs 3.12–3.14). This particular pattern is known as the exodus. Single endometrial cells are extremely difficult to identify in smears.

Non-epithelial components of a normal smear

These include leucocytes, histiocytes, spermatozoa and the normal vaginal flora.

Physiological changes in the genital tract

In the prepubertal child the squamous epithelium of the cervix and vagina is thin and matures only to parabasal or intermediate cell level (Fig. 3.15). This epithelium is more susceptible to infection than the fully mature epithelium present during the reproductive years. Smears taken during childhood reflect this lack of maturation and the predominant cells are of parabasal or intermediate cell type.

During the reproductive years the smear pattern reflects the hormonal changes of the menstrual cycle. In the first half of the cycle, as the level of oestrogen rises, the number of fully mature squamous cells increases until at midcycle the predominant cells are of superficial and large intermediate cell type (Fig. 3.16) and these lie separately in a clean background. As the level of progesterone increases

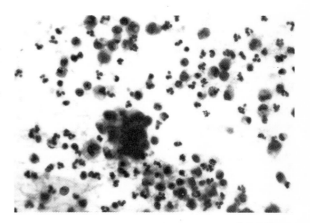

Fig. 3.14 Cervical smear: the menstrual exodus. A group of endometrial cells is readily identified, but the single cells are easily confused with histiocytes. ×390. Papanicolaou.

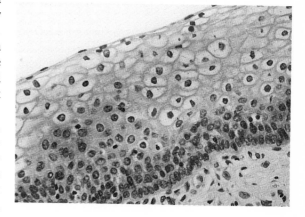

Fig. 3.15 Cervical biopsy: prepubertal stratified squamous epithelium. ×250. Haematoxylin and eosin.

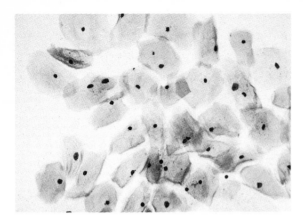

Fig. 3.16 Cervical smear taken at midcycle. Numerous superficial cells are seen. ×250. Papanicolaou.

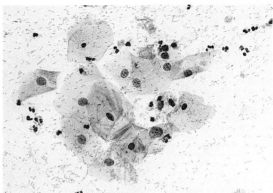

Fig. 3.17 Postovulatory cervical smear. Intermediate cells predominate. Döderlein bacilli are numerous. ×350. Papanicolaou.

in the postovulatory half of the cycle, the maturation of the smear decreases and intermediate cells lie in clumps with folded cytoplasmic borders (Fig. 3.17). The bacterial population increases, particularly Döderlein bacilli, and these feed upon the glycogen of the squamous cell cytoplasm which results in cytolysis. Polymorphonuclear leucocytes become more numerous and towards the end of the secretory phase cytolytic squamous cells and bare nuclei are seen against a background of polymorphs and bacteria (Fig. 3.18). When assessing a smear the stage of the menstrual cycle should be taken into account. Many reports erroneously suggest inflammation when in reality only physiological changes are present.

During menstruation red blood cells, endometrial cells and histiocytes are superimposed on this 'dirty' background.

After the menopause the smear pattern becomes atrophic, but this may take several years. Small intermediate cells and parabasal cells predominate (Fig. 3.19). This mimics the childhood state and again this epithelium is susceptible to infection.

Pregnancy

In the first trimester of pregnancy the female sex hormones are secreted by the corpus luteum and later by the placenta. Oestrogenic activity gradually decreases and progesterone predominates. These hormonal changes are reflected in the smear pattern. Cyclical changes cease and the smear contains

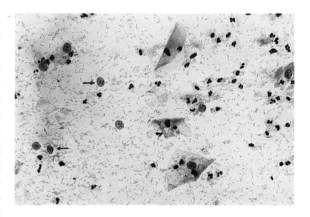

Fig. 3.18 Cervical smear showing marked cytolysis and a number of naked nuclei (arrows). ×320. Papanicolaou.

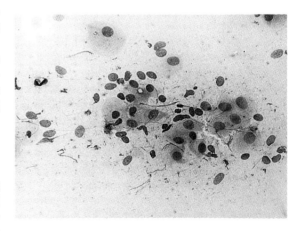

Fig. 3.19 Cervical smear: Atrophic postmenopausal pattern with parabasal cells and many 'naked' nuclei. ×210. Papanicolaou.

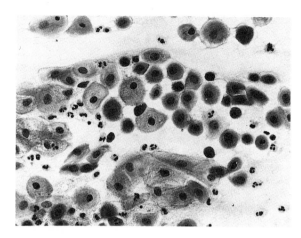

Fig. 3.20 Cervical smear. Postpartum pattern. Numerous very small parabasal cells, some with pyknotic nuclei. ×250. Papanicolaou.

clusters of glycogen-rich intermediate cells with folded cytoplasmic borders, so-called navicular cells. However, not all pregnant women show this characteristic smear pattern. The poor epithelial maturation during pregnancy and the abundant glycogen available may result in a very cytolytic smear pattern. These features also predispose the epithelium to infection. Superficial cells may be present in small numbers but a smear in which they predominate may indicate placental insufficiency.

In the initial postpartum period the cytological picture is characterised by the presence of inflammatory cells, but after about 10 days 'postpartum' cells predominate. These are parabasal cells with thickened cytoplasmic borders, abundant glycogen and pyknotic nuclei (Fig. 3.20). This atrophic smear pattern tends to persist until normal cyclical activity is re-established. Similar changes are seen in smears after the menopause and in other conditions of low oestrogen or high progesterone activity, so that no cytological picture can be said to be truly diagnostic of pregnancy.

Oral contraception

Today many of the smears routinely screened are from patients taking oral contraceptive drugs. The normal cyclical pattern is abolished. The smear pattern will reflect the type and balance of hormones given but usually shows a progesterone effect, hence the appearance of the smear is essen-

tially similar to one taken in the second half of a normal cycle. Clumps of intermediate cells with folded cytoplasmic borders predominate. Cytolysis is often marked in a background of bacteria, numerous Döderlein bacilli and polymorphonuclear leucocytes.

Squamous metaplasia

The cervix and vagina are covered by non-keratinised stratified squamous epithelium. The endocervical canal and crypts are lined by delicate columnar epithelium composed of a single layer of mucus-secreting and ciliated cells. In an ideal state the point of contact of these two epithelia, i.e. the squamocolumnar junction, lies at the external cervical os. At certain times of life, particularly late fetal life, adolescence and pregnancy, the position of the squamocolumnar junction changes. At these times, under the influence of increased hormonal stimulation, particularly by oestradiol, there is a change in cervical volume and in the shape of the cervical lips. The cervix everts and mucus-secreting columnar epithelium comes to lie exposed on the cervical portio forming the so-called endocervical ectropion. The everted endocervical mucosa forms a red granular zone which contrasts sharply with the smooth pale pink surface of the adjacent squamous epithelium. This zone is often referred to as an 'erosion'. This is incorrect, because there is no loss of epithelium and the redness merely reflects blood vessels which are more clearly visible through the transparent endocervical epithelium than through multilayered squamous epithelium. Histologically an ectropion consists of endocervical epithelium which may be thrown into villi or papillary folds. The stroma often contains an inflammatory cell infiltrate (Fig. 3.21).

After the menopause the cervical lips retract and the squamocolumnar junction is usually situated within the endocervical canal.

The normal environment for endocervical cells within the endocervical canal is at an alkaline pH. Exposure to an acid vaginal pH is thought to interfere with the buffering action of the mucus covering the endocervical cells (Singer & Jordan 1976). This in turn results in damage to the endocervical cell nucleus and cytoplasm. As a result subcolumnar reserve cells in the damaged area are stimulated.

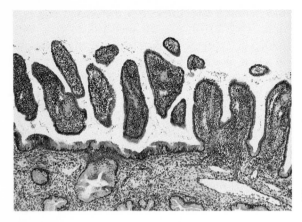

Fig. 3.21 A cervical ectropion. ×10. Haematoxylin and eosin.

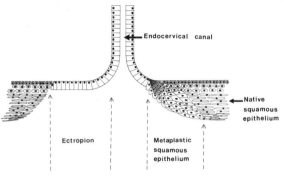

Fig. 3.22 The process of squamous metaplasia.

These rapidly proliferate and differentiate towards squamous cells. This is the process of *squamous metaplasia*, and the area undergoing squamous metaplasia is known as the *transformation zone* (Figs. 3.22–3.25). When fully mature this metaplastic squamous epithelium is virtually indistinguishable from native squamous epithelium, but unlike the latter, metaplastic epithelium overlies the endocervical crypts, which are to some extent also involved in the metaplastic process. The mouths of endocervical crypts sometimes become blocked by proliferating squamous epithelium. Mucus secretion continues and this eventually leads to cystic dilatation of the glands and the formation of Nabothian follicles. Identification of the endocervical crypts and Nabothian follicles on the ectocervix is of help in defining the limits of the transformation zone. Squamous metaplasia proceeds in a random fashion and small islands of metaplastic epithelium eventually fuse. The final outcome of squamous metaplasia is replacement of columnar epithelium exposed on the ectocervix by a multilayered squamous epithelium, which is more suited to the environment.

The main stimulus for squamous metaplasia to occur is the exposure of columnar epithelium to an acid vaginal pH. However, inflammatory processes, chronic physical or chemical irritation may possibly have a role to play. The origin of subcolumnar reserve cells is still debated but recent work suggests that they are derived from subepithelial stromal cells (Lawrence & Shingleton 1980). Identification of the squamocolumnar junction and

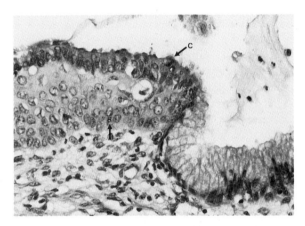

Fig. 3.23 A cervical biopsy showing reserve cell hyperplasia (R). These proliferating cells are covered by a row of degenerate endocervical columnar cells (C). ×250. Haematoxylin and eosin.

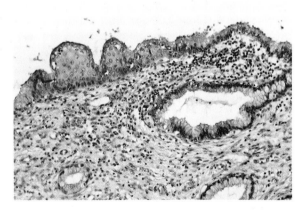

Fig. 3.24 A cervical biopsy showing small islands of immature metaplastic squamous epithelium replacing columnar epithelium. ×100. Haematoxylin and eosin.

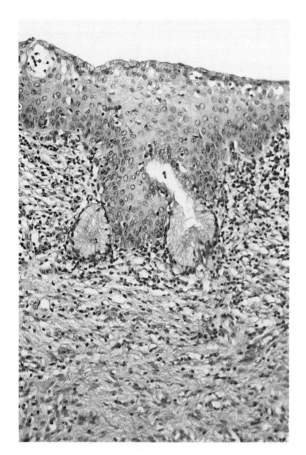

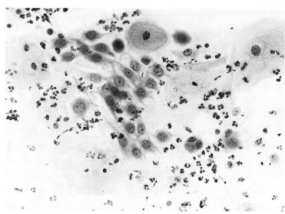

Fig. 3.26 Cervical smear: metaplastic squamous cells. Intercellular bridges are conspicuous. ×250. Papanicolaou.

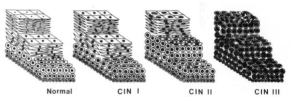

Fig. 3.27 Epithelial changes in intraepithelial neoplasia.

Fig. 3.25 Cervical biopsy. Metaplastic squamous epithelium is replacing the columnar epithelium of the endocervical crypts. ×140. Haematoxylin and eosin.

transformation zone is important because virtually all cervical intraepithelial neoplasia is confined to this zone.

Metaplastic cells often appear in cervical smears. Usually they are seen as sheets of angular cells, sometimes with finely vacuolated cytoplasm. Intercellular bridges are often conspicuous, hence the term 'spider cells' (Fig. 3.26). The nuclei are oval with delicate chromatin and sometimes prominent nucleoli. The cells not infrequently contain ingested polymorphonuclear neutrophil leucocytes. The presence of metaplastic squamous cells in a cervical smear confirms the transformation zone has been sampled and therefore provides a reliable indication that an adequate cervical smear has been taken.

Cervical intraepithelial neoplasia

Richart (1973) defined cervical intraepithelial neoplasia (CIN) as a spectrum of intraepithelial change which begins as a generally well differentiated intraepithelial neoplasm, which has traditionally been classified as very mild dysplasia, and ends with invasive carcinoma.

The histological changes of CIN are characterised by an abnormal epithelium in which cellular organisation, polarity and maturation are disturbed. The squamous cells show nuclear abnormalities consistent with malignancy. These include nuclear irregularity, hyperchromasia and a coarse granular chromatin pattern. Mitoses are frequent and many are abnormal. These nuclear abnormalities are found at all levels of the epithelium regardless of the degree of cytoplasmic maturation, but the nuclear abnormalities increase with increasing severity of the lesion. The epithelial changes which characterise CIN have been divided into three categories (Fig. 3.27).

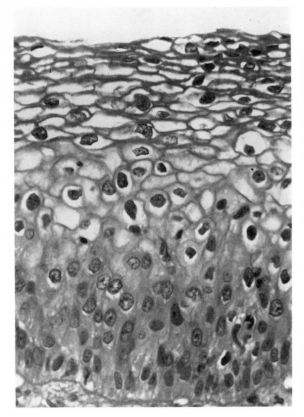

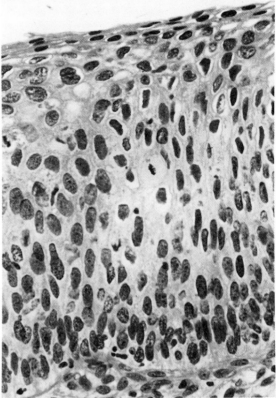

Fig. 3.28 Cervical intraepithelial neoplasia Grade I. ×290. Haematoxylin and eosin.

Fig. 3.29 Cervical intraepithelial neoplasia Grade II. ×290. Haematoxylin and eosin.

CIN Grade I (Fig. 3.28) Squamous cells in the upper two-thirds of the epithelium show evidence of cytoplasmic maturation, but marked nuclear abnormalities are seen (as described above).

CIN Grade II (Fig. 3.29) Up to two-thirds of the epithelium is replaced by undifferentiated cells. Cytoplasmic membranes are indistinct and the nuclear-cytoplasmic ratio is in favour of the nucleus. Some attempt at cytoplasmic maturation is seen only in the upper layers of the epithelium.

CIN Grade III The epithelium is completely replaced by undifferentiated cells. Mitotic figures are seen at all levels in the epithelium. With increasing atypia there is loss of intracytoplasmic glycogen. Cell cohesion is diminished, cell turnover is increased and this explains why smears from patients with severe atypias frequently contain numerous abnormal cells. Lesions of Grade III CIN are some-

times further subdivided into three histological types:

Small-cell carcinoma in situ (Fig. 3.30)

Large-cell keratinising carcinoma in situ (Fig. 3.31)

Large-cell non-keratinising carcinoma in situ (Fig. 3.32)

The small-cell variety is usually situated close to the external os or within the endocervical canal. The large-cell keratinising form is found on the exposed part of the cervix away from the external os. The commonest type is the large-cell non-keratinising form which occurs in the transformation zone.

It is now generally agreed that virtually all CIN arises in the transformation zone with one edge of the lesion at the squamocolumnar junction. The border between normal and neoplastic squamous

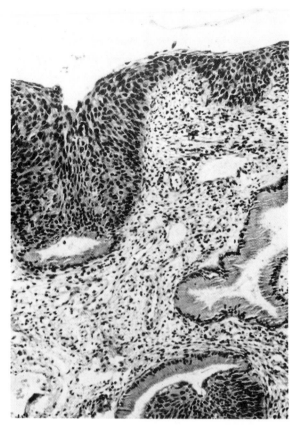

Fig. 3.30 Small-cell carcinoma in situ showing involvement of endocervical crypts. ×8. Haematoxylin and eosin.

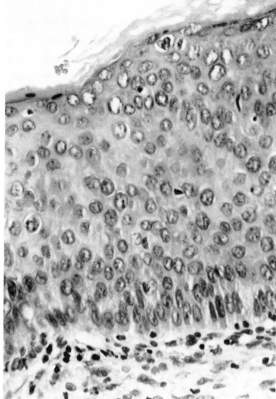

Fig. 3.31 Large-cell keratinising carcinoma in situ. ×280. Haematoxylin and eosin.

epithelium is always sharply defined (Figs. 3.33, 3.34). The process of normal squamous metaplasia is interrupted at a very early stage by carcinogenic agents which divert cell differentiation along a path which may eventually lead to CIN or invasive squamous cell carcinoma. The factors associated with a high risk of cervical cancer are related to sexual intercourse and cervical cancer is regarded as a venereally transmitted disease. The causative agent(s) have yet to be finally established, but herpes simplex virus, basic proteins in sperm heads and viral envelopes (Singer et al 1976) and human papilloma virus are all proposed as possible agents.

The cytological recognition of CIN is based upon the epithelial cells scraped from the surface layers of the lesion. The term *dyskaryosis* is used to describe these cells and a dyskaryotic cell is best de-

fined as a cell with an abnormal nucleus, but with well differentiated cytoplasm.

Histological diagnosis	Cytological diagnosis
CIN I	Mild dyskaryosis—dyskaryotic squamous cells of superficial and large intermediate cell type (Fig. 3.35)
CIN II	Moderate dyskaryosis—dyskaryotic squamous cells of small intermediate cell type (Fig. 3.36)
CIN III	Severe dyskaryosis—dyskaryotic squamous cells of parabasal type (Fig. 3.37)

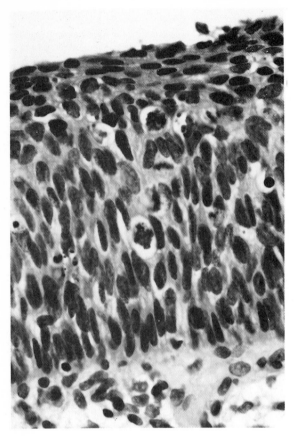

Fig. 3.32 Large-cell non-keratinising carcinoma in situ. ×550. Haematoxylin and eosin.

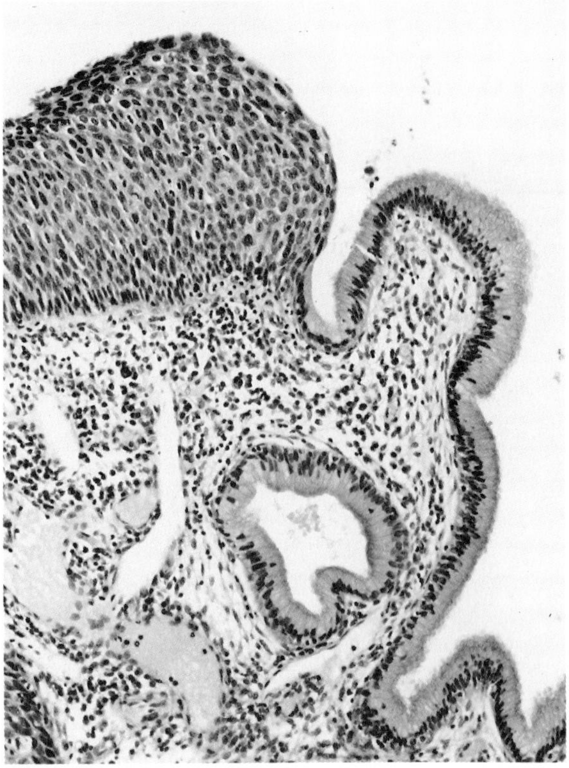

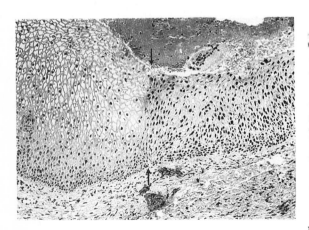

Fig. 3.33 Small-cell carcinoma in situ arising at the squamocolumnar junction. ×125. Haematoxylin and eosin.

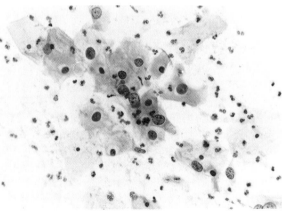

Fig. 3.34 Cervical biopsy. The border between normal and neoplastic epithelium is clearly demarcated (arrows). ×80. Haematoxylin and eosin.

Fig. 3.35 Cervical smear: mild squamous cell dyskaryosis. Cells with large hyperchromatic nuclei in the centre of the field. Compare with normal superficial cells at the periphery of the group. ×250. Papanicolaou.

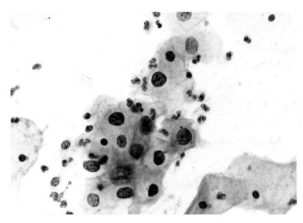

Fig. 3.36 Cervical smear: moderate squamous cell dyskaryosis. ×390. Papanicolaou.

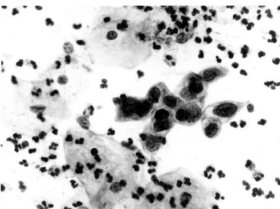

Fig. 3.37 Cervical smear: severe squamous cell dyskaryosis. ×380. Papanicolaou.

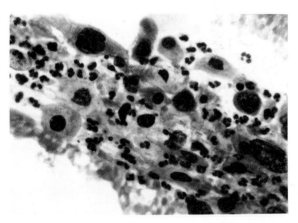

Fig. 3.38 Cervical smear: invasive squamous cell carcinoma characterised by conspicuous nuclear hyperchromasia and pleomorphism. ×320. Papanicolaou.

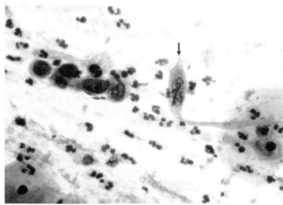

Fig. 3.39 Cervical smear: invasive squamous cell carcinoma. 'Tadpole'-shaped malignant cells may be seen (arrow). ×320. Papanicolaou.

Although lesions at the milder end of the CIN spectrum may regress, there is considerable evidence that CIN lesions of any grade may persist or progress to a more severe form (Richart & Barron 1969; Kinlen & Spriggs 1978; Spriggs & Boddington 1980). In the light of this evidence it is essential that all patients with dyskaryotic squamous cells in their smears are kept under frequent cytological review. If the dyskaryosis persists or progresses to a more severe form further investigation by colposcopy and biopsy should be advised.

In preinvasive disease diagnosis by cytology is the method of choice. If invasive disease is suspected, biopsy diagnosis is the correct procedure.

Invasive squamous cell carcinoma can be diagnosed cytologically (Figs. 3.38, 3.39) but false negatives do occur because of the presence of blood, necrotic debris and inflammatory cells. This slough may obscure any malignant cells present. Often in an ulcerated tumour viable malignant cells may not appear in the smear.

Inflammatory changes in the epithelia of the vagina and cervix

The stratified squamous epithelium of the cervix and the columnar epithelium of the endocervical canal may be damaged by infection, trauma and by

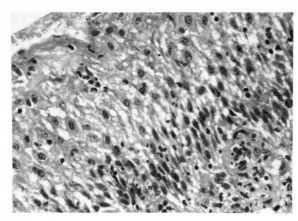

Fig. 3.40 Cervical biopsy: acute cervicitis. ×320. Haematoxylin and eosin.

physical and chemical agents. Sometimes the responsible agent can be identifed by characteristic changes in the histology or cytology. In many cases, however, the stimulus produces a non-specific inflammatory response. The importance of recognising this non-specific picture in tissue sections and in cervicovaginal smears is to avoid confusion between the so-called 'benign atypias' and premalignant disorders.

Changes in squamous epithelium

In the early stages there is increased vascularity and oedema. The epithelium may be infiltrated with polymorphonuclear leucocytes and the upper layers of the epithelium may be shed (Fig. 3.40). Loss of the superficial layers of the epithelium makes it

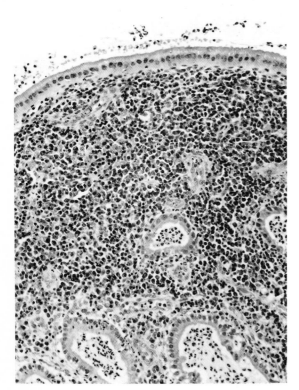

Fig. 3.41 Cervical biopsy showing acute inflammation of endocervical tissue. Note the intense stromal inflammation and the inflammatory exudate within crypts. ×140. Haematoxylin and eosin.

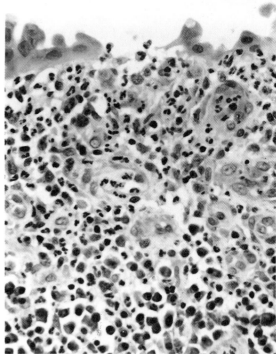

Fig. 3.42 Cervical biopsy: acute endocervicitis with partial loss of surface epithelium. The remaining columnar cells show loss of mucus secretion. ×550. Haematoxylin and eosin.

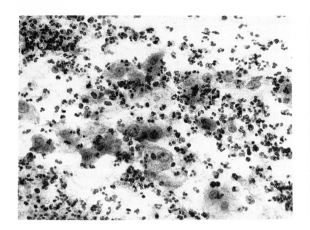

Fig. 3.43 Cervical smear. Squamous cells have enlarged nuclei and ragged cytoplasmic membranes. Polymorphonuclear neutrophil granulocytes are numerous. ×310. Papanicolaou.

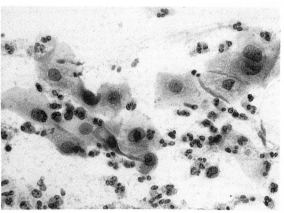

Fig. 3.44 Cervical smear. Nuclear enlargement, hyperchromasia and binucleation are seen in this inflammatory smear pattern. ×320. Papanicolaou.

vulnerable to further damage. In severe inflammation there may be epithelial ulceration and necrosis. The stromal involvement may be mild, but in severe inflammation the stroma usually contains a dense inflammatory cell infiltrate.

Changes in endocervical columnar epithelium

The epithelial surface is often covered by a thin purulent exudate, but the most intense inflammatory reaction often occurs in the crypts. The columnar epithelium may show loss of mucus secretion, there may be ulceration and usually there is an intense inflammatory cell infiltrate in the stroma (Figs. 3.41, 3.42).

Changes in the smear pattern

Inflammation may alter the proportions of parabasal, intermediate and superficial cells in a smear. Under normal circumstances a postmenopausal smear will contain exclusively or predominantly parabasal cells, but when inflammation occurs superficial and intermediate cells may appear in the smear. This increase in maturation may be due to increased vascularity of the inflamed tissue.

Conversely the smear of a woman during childbearing years contains predominantly superficial and intermediate cells, but an inflammatory smear may contain many parabasal cells. This is a con-

sequence both of exposure of the deeper layers of the epithelium during inflammation and of the presence of immature squamous epithelium during the process of repair.

Because of the marked cellular changes which may occur as a result of inflammation, hormonal assessment should not be undertaken on an inflammatory smear.

Changes within epithelial cells

Significant inflammation of the cervix or vagina will result in the presence of a large number of polymorphonuclear leucocytes, histiocytes and cellular debris in the smear. Should the epithelial cells be obscured by the inflammatory exudate a second smear should be requested when the inflammation has cleared.

Squamous cells. Changes occur in both the nucleus and the cytoplasm. Nuclear changes include nuclear pyknosis, karyorrhexis and condensation of chromatin at the periphery of the nucleus. Karyolysis, or nuclear enlargement and binucleation, may also occur (Figs. 3.43, 3.44). Cytoplasmic changes include an eosinophilic staining reaction, cytoplasmic vacuolation and a ragged cytoplasmic membrane.

Columnar cells. Nuclei may become greatly enlarged and multinucleate cells are not uncommon (Fig. 3.45). The chromatin pattern, however, remains uniform from cell to cell. The nuclei often

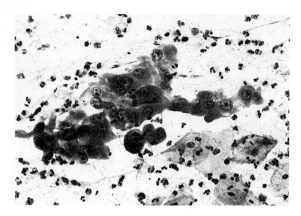

Fig. 3.45 Cervical smear. Inflammatory changes in endocervical cells. ×320. Papanicolaou.

contain a number of chromocentres and conspicuous nucleoli. Bare nuclei are common and may be a trap for the unwary. A comparison of the stripped nuclei with those of well preserved endocervical cells will facilitate correct identification.

Sometimes the cellular changes produced by inflammation or healing cannot be readily distinguished from those of dyskaryosis. Under these circumstances the patient should be followed with regular smears. In most cases the changes will improve, but where doubt remains a colposcopic examination and biopsy are indicated.

CYTOLOGICAL RECOGNITION OF INFECTIONS

Introduction

Strict criteria must be used in the cytological diagnosis of infections of the lower genital tract. A normal bacterial flora is always present and the number of organisms varies with the stage of the menstrual cycle. Inflammatory cells and histiocytes are a normal component of a cervical or vaginal smear and their presence alone does not indicate infection. The overall appearance of the smear, the age of the patient and the clinical details must be taken into account.

Cervical and vaginal squamous epithelium respond to oestrogen by proliferation and maturation of epithelial cells. At the peak of oestrogenic activity the epithelium reaches maximum height and superficial cells predominate in the smear. Progesterone

inhibits the maturation of squamous epithelium. Intermediate and parabasal cells predominate in the smear and the epithelium is rather thin. This atrophic epithelium is more susceptible to infection.

Lactobacillus vaginalis (Döderlein's bacillus), which is normally present in the vagina, metabolises glycogen to lactic acid, which maintains the vaginal pH at 4.5. This mechanism is said to be an effective barrier against colonisation by pathogenic flora, although this concept has been recently challenged (Larsen & Galask 1980).

It follows that natural protection of the epithelia of the cervix and vagina depends on the integrity of the squamous epithelium, possibly the low pH of the vagina, an equilibrium between micro-organisms, as well as the general health of the individual. Disturbance of one or more of these factors may result in invasion by pathogenic bacteria or the overgrowth of a commensal.

Senile vaginitis

As the level of oestrogen falls after the menopause, the maturation of vaginal and cervical epithelium also decreases. The atrophic epithelium which results is more susceptible to infection than fully mature epithelium. A postmenopausal smear contains squamous cells of small intermediate and parabasal type. Many of the parabasal cells have pyknotic or fragmented nuclei and sheets of atrophic cells and naked nuclei are seen (Fig. 3.46). Polymorphonuc-

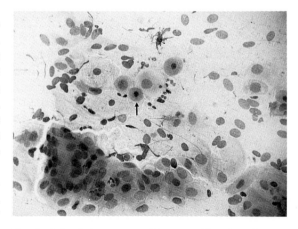

Fig. 3.46 Cervical smear: atrophic pattern. Note the pyknotic nuclei (arrow) and the many naked nuclei. ×200. Papanicolaou.

lear leucocytes may be numerous. Squamous cells may change their staining characteristics from blue to red, so-called 'red atrophy'. A variety of commensal organisms are probably responsible for the inflammatory reaction in senile vaginitis. The organisms are able to flourish in the changed hormonal environment. It may be difficult to interpret a postmenopausal smear pattern with pyknotic nuclei or large naked nuclei. The use of local or systemic oestrogen preparations will improve the maturation of the squamous epithelium and any true cellular abnormalities can then be recognised.

'Non-specific' vaginitis

This is a common condition characterised by an increased vaginal discharge often foul smelling, which is not attributable to *Trichomonas* or *Candida* infection. In the past confusion has reigned over the organism(s) causing this condition but it now appears that *Gardnerella vaginalis* plays a significant role, possibly with anaerobic bacteria (Taylor et al 1982). The confusion has been further increased because *G. vaginalis* was previously known as *Haemophilus vaginalis* and then as *Corynebacterium vaginale*. The organism is a Gram-negative or Gram-variable bacillus or coccobacillus which is transmitted by sexual intercourse. Isolation of *G. vaginalis* in a routine laboratory can be difficult and often the diagnosis is made in the outpatient clinic from wet preparations and Gram-stained smears. Some workers report a poor correlation between the isolation rates and microscopic diagnoses and suggest that a considerable number of cases are missed when the diagnosis is based on microscopy alone (Ison et al 1982); other workers disagree (Jones 1983).

The diagnosis in wet preparations and fixed cytological smears is based on the presence of the characteristic bacilli and 'clue cells' (Fig. 3.47) (Gardner & Dukes 1955). These are squamous cells covered with bacilli which adhere to the surface of the cell. The epithelial cells often stain purple and appear rather hazy. Not all cells are involved. The organism does not penetrate the mucosa nor invoke a significant inflammatory cell reaction and the smears contain few inflammatory cells and sections of the mucosa appear normal (Dawson & Harris 1983). However, the

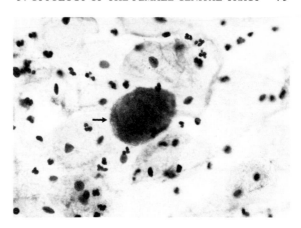

Fig. 3.47 Cervical smear. 'Clue cell' (arrow). ×390. Papanicolaou.

specificity of 'clue cells' as a hallmark of this infection remains an issue for debate.

Trichomonas vaginalis

This protozoan is a common cause of an offensive vaginal discharge. From 20–30% of women harbour the organism but it is pathogenic in a much smaller percentage. In the female infection is usually limited to the vulva, vagina and cervix. The mucosal surfaces may be tender, ulcerated and covered by a frothy cream-coloured discharge. In the male the prostate, seminal vesicles and urethra may be infected and approximately 10% of infected males have a thin white urethral discharge. The infection is venereally transmitted.

Trichomonas vaginalis is an actively motile, unicellular pear-shaped protozoan, 8–30 μm long, with four anterior flagella and one posterior flagellum. It is phagocytic and can ingest other microorganisms (Street et al 1984). A pH of 5.5 to 6.0 is preferred and the organism cannot survive for long in normal acid vaginal secretions, nor at the neutral vaginal pH found in young girls and elderly women.

The protozoan attacks the stratified squamous epithelium of the cervix and vagina. Biopsies are not usually taken in this condition, but when they are the squamous epithelium shows oedema, vascular dilatation, superficial ulceration and focal small haemorrhages. Both the epithelium and stroma contain an inflammatory cell infiltrate of leucocytes

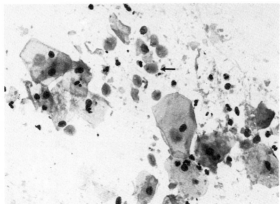

Fig. 3.48 Cervical smear: *Trichomonas vaginalis* (arrow). ×390. Papanicolaou.

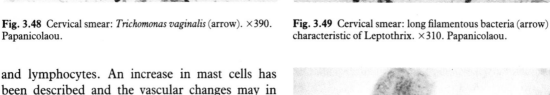

Fig. 3.49 Cervical smear: long filamentous bacteria (arrow) characteristic of Leptothrix. ×310. Papanicolaou.

and lymphocytes. An increase in mast cells has been described and the vascular changes may in part be due to the release of mast cell products (Kobayashi et al 1983).

Positive identification of *T. vaginalis* in cervical smears may be difficult and wet preparations and cultures are more reliable. The protozoa usually appear as hazy greyish-green round or oval bodies with a small eccentric nucleus. Small eosinophilic granules may be identified in the cytoplasm. Flagella are rarely seen (Fig. 3.48). Identification of the nucleus is essential to avoid confusion with cell fragments and mucus. *Leptothrix* is often found in smears in association with *Trichomonas* (Fig. 3.49) but the reason for this association is not known.

A clue that *T. vaginalis* is present may be afforded by the overall appearance of the smear which shows a diffuse eosinophilic staining of the epithelial cells. Cytolysis is marked and there may be an increase in the number of parabasal cells as a result of destruction of cervical and vaginal epithelium. Leucocytes are numerous. Squamous cells may show nuclear enlargement, binucleation, hyperchromasia, chromatin clumping and nuclear pyknosis or karyorrhexis. A characteristic cytoplasmic change is the presence of perinuclear haloes (Fig. 3.50). These should not be confused with the changes of koilocytotic atypia (see section on Papilloma Virus).

The nuclear and cytoplasmic appearances produced by *T. vaginalis* are probably the result of degenerative changes within the cells.

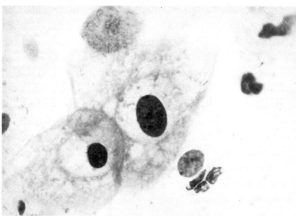

Fig. 3.50 Cervical smear: *Trichomonas vaginalis* infection. Squamous cells show nuclear enlargement and perinuclear haloes. ×390. Papanicolaou.

Some interest has been shown in the possible relationship of *T. vaginalis* to cervical carcinogenesis (Koss & Wolinska 1959). The organism does produce some epithelial atypia, but in most cases this regresses after treatment. There is insufficient evidence to link this infection with true CIN. A cytological diagnosis of a significant degree of CIN should not be withheld because of a coexisting *Trichomonas* infection, but at the mild end of the CIN spectrum treatment of the infection is advisable before a final cytological grading is given.

The incidence of *T. vaginalis* infection in patients with carcinoma in situ is higher than in the general population. However, the same is true for

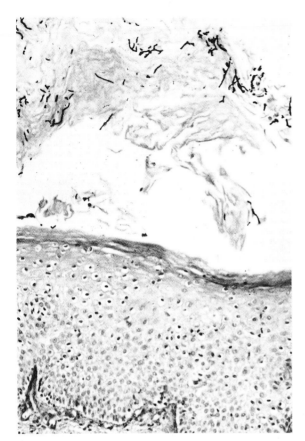

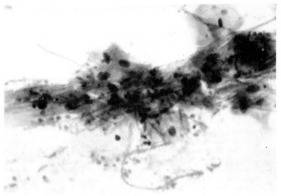

Fig. 3.52 Cervical smear: *Candida albicans*. A tangled mass of yeasts and hyphae. ×200. Papanicolaou.

Fig. 3.51 Cervical biopsy: *Candida albicans* in surface keratin. ×120. Periodic acid Schiff.

other gynaecological disorders and it is probably due to an associated epithelial injury which favours the growth of *Trichomonas*.

Candida albicans

This fungus forms part of the normal flora of the mucous membranes of the female genital tract. As such it may be identified in cervical and vaginal smears without any associated inflammatory cell reaction. Under certain circumstances, however, it may gain dominance and cause inflammation of the cervix, vagina and vulva. Clinically the infection is characterised by intense itching, irritation and a white discharge which forms plaques. These adhere to the mucous membranes, but are easily wiped away. Predisposing conditions are: diabetes mellitus, disturbance of the bacterial equilibrium,

by the use of broad spectrum antibiotics, high levels of progesterone—during pregnancy or with oral contraceptives—and immunosuppression. However, it should be stressed that in many women with this common vulvovaginal infection no predisposing factors can be identified (Sobel 1984).

The fungus is an oval budding yeast 2–3 × 4–6 μm which produces a pseudomycelium. Usually it does not penetrate the mucosa, but when associated with inflammation it can be identified within the mucosa together with cellular debris and polymorphonuclear neutrophil leucocytes (Fig. 3.51). The submucosa shows mild oedema and an inflammatory cell infiltrate of lymphocytes, plasma cells and neutrophil leucocytes.

In Papanicolaou stained cervical smears long eosinophilic hyphae and yeast spores are recognised. These protrude from clumps of folded intermediate cells (Fig. 3.52) Squamous cells may show some nuclear swelling and hyperchromasia.

Herpes simplex virus

The precise incidence of herpes genitalis infection is unknown because a large number of patients exhibit only mild symptoms or are asymptomatic. Primary infection occurs in a host without antibodies. In many cases the virus assumes a latent stage in neurones within the sensory ganglia of the host (Galloway et al 1979). Recurrent infection in the presence of antibody is common.

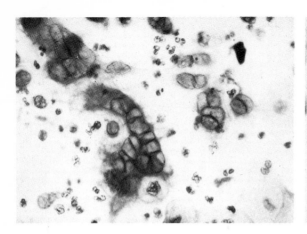

Fig. 3.53 Cervical smear. Infected cells show the syncytial arrangement, nuclear moulding and multinucleation characteristic of herpes virus infection. ×250. Papanicolaou.

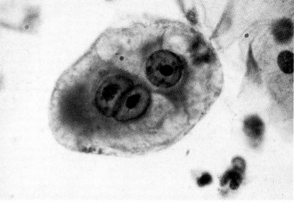

Fig. 3.54 Cervical smear: herpes simplex Type A intranuclear inclusions. ×20. Papanicolaou.

Herpes simplex virus (HSV) is a double-stranded DNA virus. The complete virus particle measures 150–200 nm diameter. There are two types:

HSV Type I causes aphthous stomatitis and herpes labialis (cold sores).

HSV Type II causes genital herpetic infection with vesicular eruptions on the penis, cervix, vulva, vagina and perineum. Some cases are also caused by HSV Type I.

Type I infection occurs in childhood. Type II infections are venereally transmitted or may be acquired during passage through the birth canal.

Primary genital herpetic infections produce symptoms 3–7 days after exposure. When clinically apparent there may be severe vulvar pain, tenderness, dysuria and a watery vaginal discharge. Symptoms in recurrent attacks are often less severe. Stimuli which precipitate an attack of Type I or Type II infection include exposure to sunlight, fever, menstruation and emotional stress.

Mutiple vesicles appear which later form shallow ulcers. A mass of ulcerated and secondarily infected vesicles on the cervix may be mistaken for cervical carcinoma.

A biopsy taken in the vesicular stage shows suprabasal vesicles filled with serum, degenerate epidermal cells and cells with the characteristic nuclear inclusions. Subsequently the infected cells undergo karyorrhexis and lysis and a biopsy or smear taken in the later ulcerative phase may show no specific diagnostic features.

A Papanicolaou stained smear taken from lesions in the vesicular stage shows characteristic cellular changes. The abnormalities produced make it difficult to identify the cell type with certainty, but most are squamous cells and a few are endocervical cells. When HSV enters the host cell nucleus normal cell DNA and protein synthesis cease and virus replication begins.

On a morphological basis three stages of development have been described (Patten 1978):

Stage I. Nuclear enlargement. The cells may be mononuclear or multinucleate. There is increased granularity and clumping of chromatin.

Stage II. Margination of chromatin beneath the nuclear membrane. The nuclei have a smudged 'ground-glass' appearance with moulding of adjacent nuclei. At this stage the nuclei are basophilic and Feulgen-positive. Cytoplasmic volume increases and the large multinucleate cells have a syncytial appearance. Multinucleation and syncytial formation may be the result of cell aggregation and fusion (Fig. 3.53).

Stage III. Virus particles lose their content of nuclear protein, shrink from the nuclear membrane and appear as an eosinophilic mass surrounded by a halo in a nucleus with marginated chromatin. This is the classic Type A inclusion of Cowdry (Fig. 3.54).

Virus particles can be observed in single cells removed from cervical smear preparations using a transmission electron microscopy (TEM) technique described by Coleman et al (1977; Fig. 3.55). Except for the multinucleate giant cells seen in a

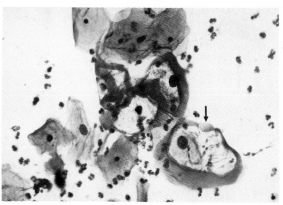

Fig. 3.59 Koilocytes (arrow) in a cervical smear. ×250. Papanicolaou.

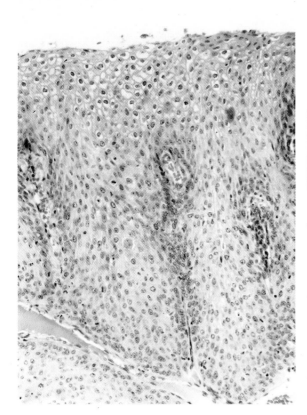

Fig. 3.58 Cervical biopsy. An inverted condyloma in which the surface is flat, but the epithelium shows pronounced acanthosis. ×110. Haematoxylin and eosin.

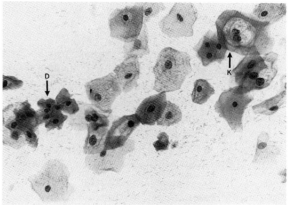

Fig. 3.60 Cervical smear: a binucleate koilocyte (K) and a group of small dyskeratotic squamous cells (D). ×240. Papanicolaou.

Recently considerable interest has centred on the possible role of human papilloma virus (HPV) in cervical carcinogenesis. This group of viruses is known to be implicated in the development of malignant skin tumours in the human disease of epidermodysplasia verruciformis (Orth et al 1980) and in causing some malignant alimentary tumours in cattle (Jarrett 1981). The presence of HPV DNA has been demonstrated in the tumour cells using DNA and RNA hybridisation techniques.

Although the majority of condylomatous lesions on the cervix do show some nuclear pleomorphism a small percentage show very marked cytological and histological atypia (Meisels et al 1981). The term 'atypical condylomata' has been used to describe these lesions.

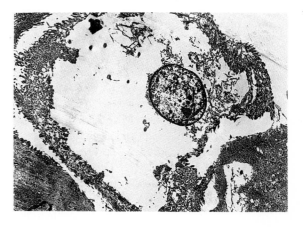

Fig. 3.61 Transmission electron microscopy of a koilocyte taken from a cervical smear. ×4000.

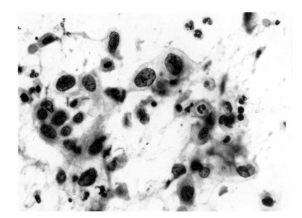

Fig. 3.62 Cervical smear. Dyskaryotic squamous cells are present in addition to small dyskeratotic and binucleate abnormal cells which suggest origin from an atypical condyloma. ×390. Papanicolaou.

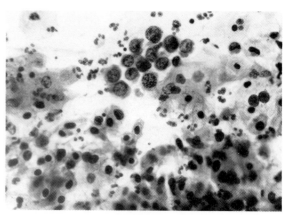

Fig. 3.63 Cervical smear: cells from an atypical condyloma. Note the smudged nuclear chromatin in many cells, although one severely dyskaryotic group does show a well preserved abnormal chromatin pattern. ×320. Papanicolaou.

Smears from atypical condylomata usually contain few, if any, of the characteristic 'balloon cells' or dyskeratotic cells. More often the smear contains groups of parabasal cells with large irregular hyperchromatic nuclei and amphophilic cytoplasm (Fig. 3.62). Even more worrying is a pattern consisting of very pleomorphic mature squamous cells. These may be single or lie in thick sheets on the smear. The nuclei are large, very hyperchromatic and irregular in shape. The cytoplasm is often strikingly orangophilic and at first sight these may be mistaken for cells shed from an invasive keratinising squamous cell carcinoma, but there is no tumour diathesis (Fig. 3.63). Karyorrhexis and smudging of nuclear chromatin are features often seen in condylomatous lesions and these features may provide a clue to the aetiology of the lesion.

Histologically the atypical condylomata are usually flat but a mild degree of papillomatosis may be seen. In mild atypia the basal layers of the epithelium are often relatively normal. Koilocytes are seen in the middle layers and large, often multinucleate cells with a smudged chromatin pattern are seen in the surface layers. Dyskeratotic cells may be present on the surface. In more severe degrees of atypia enlarged darkly staining irregular nuclei can be seen in all layers of the epithelium. Occasional koilocytes may be found and often a few almost normal cells are scattered through the

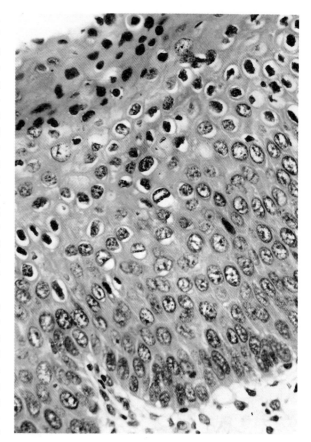

Fig. 3.64 Cervical biopsy: atypical condyloma, flat type. ×350. Haematoxylin and eosin.

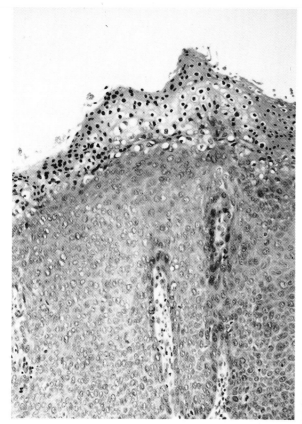

Fig. 3.65 Cervical biopsy: atypical condyloma, papillary type. ×110. Haematoxylin and eosin.

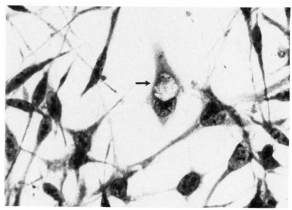

Fig. 3.66 McCoy cell culture infected with *Chlamydia trachomatis*. Intracytoplasmic inclusion (arrowed). ×380. May-Grünwald-Giemsa.

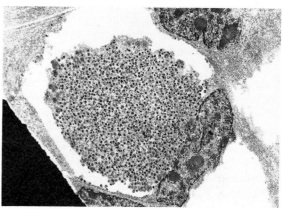

Fig. 3.67 McCoy cell culture. Transmission electron microscopy of a single infected cell. The intracytoplasmic inclusion contains numerous elementary bodies. ×2200.

epithelium (Figs. 3.64, 3.65). We have seen biopsies where the epithelial changes in adjacent fields progress from a typical condyloma through dysplasia to very severe epithelial changes, indistinguishable from carcinoma in situ. There is no doubt that in some patients condylomatous lesions progress to more severe forms of CIN and possibly to squamous cell carcinoma (Syrjanen 1980). All patients with cervical condylomata, even of the classical type, should have regular cytological examinations, followed by colposcopy and biopsy when required.

Chlamydia trachomatis

These organisms are classified as Gram-negative bacteria. They lack some important mechanisms for generating energy, hence they are obligate intracellular parasites. The host cells supply the deficient energy needs.

Chlamydia are divided into two species: *C. psittaci* and *C. trachomatis*. All chlamydia have similar morphological features and multiply in the host cytoplasm by a distinctive developmental cycle (Taylor-Robinson & Thomas 1980). In cell culture characteristic intracytoplasmic inclusions are seen which are filled with elementary bodies (Figs. 3.66–3.68). The infected cells are enlarged and may show nuclear enlargement and multinucleation (Fig. 3.69).

C. trachomatis is the agent implicated in a variety of genital tract and associated infections. It is sexually transmitted and is probably the most common pathogen causing non-gonococcal genital infections

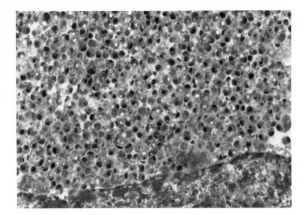

Fig. 3.68 McCoy cell culture. Numerous elementary bodies. ×6300.

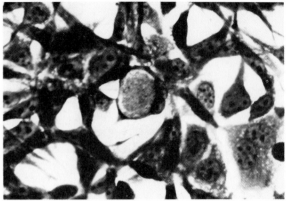

Fig. 3.69 McCoy cell culture. Binucleate infected cells. ×390. May-Grünwald-Giemsa.

in both sexes (Schachter 1978). The infection may be asymptomatic, but the organism may cause urethritis in the male and cervicitis, salpingitis and pelvic inflammatory disease in the female (Oriel & Ridgeway 1983, Weström & Mardh, 1983). Chlamydial infection has been implicated as a cause of the Curtis-Fitz-Hugh syndrome: perihepatitis associated with genital tract infection (Bolton & Darougar 1983). It causes inclusion conjunctivitis in the newborn and follicular conjunctivitis in adults. Some cases of neonatal pneumonia are attributable to this organism (Hammerschlag 1978; Hobson et al 1983). It is the agent of lymphogranuloma venereum. The organism grows in the urethral epithelium of the male and in the columnar and metaplastic squamous epithelium in the cervix of the female.

In the acute stage of infection with *C. trachomatis* there is an acute inflammatory reaction in the infected tissues and a purulent discharge. Cellular inclusions are rarely identified. Chronic infection with this organism, particularly in the eye, results in a chronic follicular inflammatory reaction characterised by the presence of lymphoid follicles in the affected tissues (Dunlop et al 1964).

Recently the entity of chronic follicular cervicitis has been linked with chlamydial infection of the cervix (Dunlop et al 1964; Hare et al 1981). In this condition the cervical stroma contains an intense lymphocytic and plasma cell infiltrate. Lymphoid follicles, often with germinal centres, are seen in many cases. The follicles always lie beneath columnar epithelium or metaplastic squamous epithelium

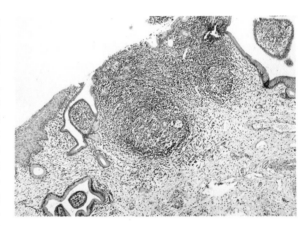

Fig. 3.70 Cervical biopsy. Lymphoid follicles beneath endocervical columnar epithelium. ×40. Haematoxylin and eosin.

(Fig. 3.70). Intracytoplasmic inclusions are rarely seen but their light microscopic and TEM appearances have been described in cervical biopsies by Swanson et al (1975). The infected cells contain intracytoplasmic vesicles. The vesicles are often large and occupy almost the entire volume of the cell. Numerous small spherical bodies, approximately 1 μm in diameter, are visible within the vesicles. The organisms are most easily identified in endocervical columnar cells.

Chronic follicular cervicitis can be diagnosed readily from cervical smears. Ulceration of the epithelium or firm scraping of the cervix will result in cells from the lymphoid follicles appearing in the smear. These include lymphocytes, reticulum cells, phagocytic cells and plasma cells. Mitoses are seen.

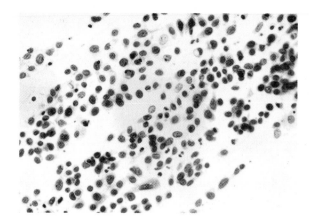

Fig. 3.71 Cervical smear. Streaks of lymphocytes and histiocytic cells are characteristic of follicular cervicitis. ×100. Papanicolaou.

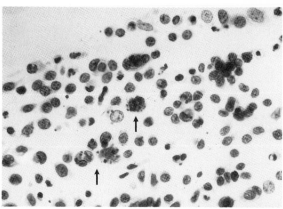

Fig. 3.72 Cervical smear: follicular cervicitis. 'Tingible-body' macrophages (arrows) can be identified. ×250. Papanicolaou.

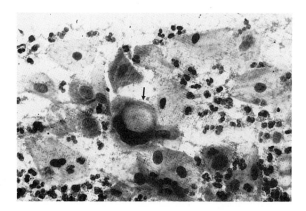

Fig. 3.73a Cervical smear: chronic follicular cervicitis. A single epithelial cell contains a large intracytoplasmic inclusion (arrow). ×320. Papanicolaou.

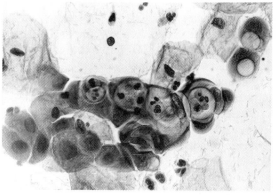

Fig. 3.73b Cervical smear: inflammatory changes in metaplastic squamous cells. Intracytoplasmic vacuolation is common and should not be confused with the changes of a chlamydial infection. ×320. Papanicolaou.

Characteristically single cells form streaks across the smear and there is no cellular aggregation (Fig. 3.71). These cells may be easily mistaken for small undifferentiated malignant cells, or a leukaemic or lymphomatous infiltrate. However, the cells lack the monotony of the cell population usually associated with leukaemia or lymphoma. In our experience the recognition of debris-laden macrophages is a useful indicator of the true diagnosis (Fig. 3.72). If the follicles are lying deep within the stroma or beneath mature metaplastic squamous epithelium they are unlikely to be represented in the smear.

In the absence of follicular cells in the smear there are no other easily identifiable criteria of this infection. Gupta et al (1979) described detailed morphological changes in metaplastic squamous cells and endocervical cells infected with *C. trachomatis*. We have examined a series of cervical smears, stained by the Papanicolaou and May-Grünwald-Giemsa techniques, from a group of women who had positive cultures for *C. trachomatis*. Some had histological or cytological evidence of follicular cervicitis. However, very few smears contained recognisably infected cells. When present the cells showed nuclear enlargement or multinucleation and had abundant vacuolated cytoplasm (Fig. 3.73a). Small coccoid structures were sometimes identified within the cytoplasmic vacuoles, but caution should be exercised in diagnosing a chlamydial infection from smears. Vacuolated

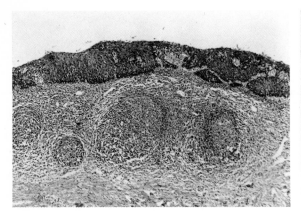

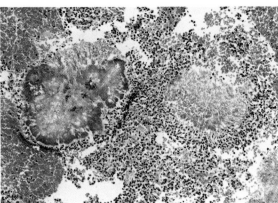

Fig. 3.74 Cervical biopsy. Several lymphoid follicles lie beneath dysplastic squamous epithelium. ×40. Haematoxylin and eosin.

Fig. 3.75 Curettings from the endocervix. Colonies of *Actinomyces* organisms surrounded by a purulent exudate. ×100. Haematoxylin and eosin.

metaplastic cells are common, particularly in inflammatory smears and these changes should not be misinterpreted (Fig. 3.73b). At the end of our study we concluded that the diagnosis of chlamydial infections using cervical cytology alone was both unreliable and impractical for a busy routine screening laboratory.

It is unlikely that all cases of chronic follicular cervicitis are due to an associated chlamydial infection and Roberts & Ng (1975) found this entity to be more common in postmenopausal women.

A number of authors have suggested a possible association between *C. trachomatis* and CIN (Schachter et al 1975, 1982; Paavonen et al 1979; Hare et al 1982). The organism has been isolated from the cervices of some women who showed CIN and in some cases well developed lymphoid follicles were seen beneath the dysplastic epithelium (Fig. 3.74). It has been suggested that CIN in these cases may be reversible if the infection is adequately treated (Carr et al 1979).

Actinomyces

Actinomyces are Gram-positive filamentous bacteria which superficially resemble fungi. The characteristic growth pattern is one of a *branched* mycelium which tends to fragment into bacteria-like pieces. Free-living forms are found mostly in the soil. Anaerobic species form part of the normal flora of the mouth, genital and gastrointestinal

tracts. Actinomycosis of the female genital tract is usually caused by *A. israelii* and results from surgical instrumentation, surgical abortion or by direct extension from lesions in the appendix or anus.

Recently considerable interest has been shown in these organisms because they have been identified in the female genital tract in association with the intrauterine contraceptive device (IUCD) (Eschenbach et al 1977; Hager et al 1979; Kaufman et al 1980).

Actinomyces do not usually invade mucosal surfaces, but the presence of an IUCD with the associated tissue injury and decreased oxygenation favours colonisation with *Actinomyces* and other anaerobic organisms. *Actinomyces* probably form part of a polymicrobial anaerobic infestation developing in the presence of a foreign body (Duguid et al 1982). The result may be a chronic endocervicitis, endometritis or a tubovarian abscess.

Biopsies of tissues infected with *Actinomyces* show abscesses, fibrosis and sinus formation. The organism can be identified in the tissues as a colony of Gram-positive mycelial filaments surrounded by eosinophilic 'clubs' (Figs. 3.75, 3.76). The latter may be antigen-antibody complexes. This colony may be recognised macroscopically in pus as a yellow granule, hence the name 'sulphur granule'.

Colonies of *Actinomyces* can be identified in routine cervical smears (Gupta et al 1976; Gupta 1982) where they appear as cotton wool-like balls

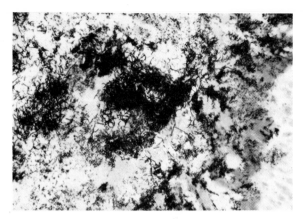

Fig. 3.76 Curettings from the endocervix. Colonies of filamentous branching bacteria characteristic of *Actinomyces*. ×390. Gram.

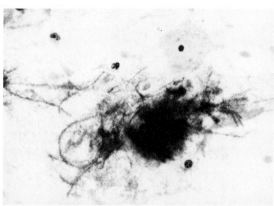

Fig. 3.77 Cervical smear: *Actinomyces* organisms may be difficult to identify in a routine smear. ×390. Papanicolaou.

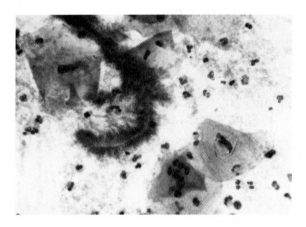

Fig. 3.78 Cervical smear: *Actinomyces* organisms may show a characteristic feathered appearance which is a helpful diagnostic feature. ×320. Papanicolaou.

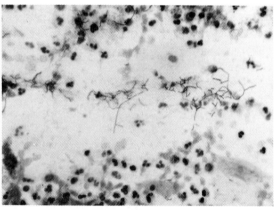

Fig. 3.79 Cervical smear: *Actinomyces* organisms. Branching filaments are clearly seen. ×320. Gram.

with projecting radiating filaments (Figs. 3.77, 3.78). Often the colonies are fragmented and many bacteria-like pieces are seen. The filaments may have a beaded appearance. Care must be taken to make a positive identification of the organism by the recognition of *branching* filaments (Fig. 3.79). The cervical smears of IUCD users often contain large 'fluffy' aggregates of bacteria which at first glance may be mistaken for *Actinomyces*. When in doubt a Gram stain of the smear will resolve the problem. Identification of the organism should be confirmed, whenever possible, by culture of material from an endocervical swab. Direct immunofluorescence using fluorescein isothiocyanate

labelled antisera against *A. israelii* is the most sensitive and specific test, but it is not widely used (Valicenti et al 1982).

Amoebae have been recognised in association with *Actinomyces* in the cervical smears of IUCD users (McNeill & de Moraes-Ruehsen 1978).

The prevalence of *Actinomyces* in IUCD users is still debated. Any type of IUCD may predispose the patient to colonisation with *Actinomyces*, although some authors claim a much lower incidence in women using copper devices (Duguid et al 1980, 1982). This may be due to the weak antibacterial and antifungal action of the copper salts. Another possibility is that the lower incidence

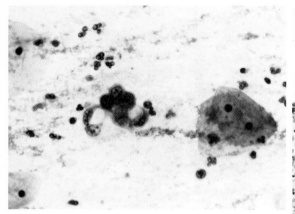

Fig. 3.80 Cervical smear: vacuolated endometrial cells in the smear of an IUCD user. ×390. Papanicolaou.

merely reflects the fact that copper devices are changed more frequently than their plastic counterparts. Prolonged usage of an IUCD seems to favour colonisation of the genital tract by *Actinomyces*-like organisms (Keebler et al 1983; Petitti et al 1983). The recognition of *Actinomyces* in IUCD users is important because several studies have shown that pelvic inflammatory disease is more likely to develop among IUCD users than among non-users (Nilsson et al 1981; Burman et al 1982; Duguid et al 1982; Valicenti et al 1982), but it is a rare complication. One study has shown that the presence of *Actinomyces* in a cervical smear is quite a sensitive indicator of the prevalence of the organism in the genital tract, but careful culture techniques have proved to be more sensitive indicators (Duguid et al 1982).

In addition to infections the presence of an IUCD poses other problems for the cytopathologist. Endometrial cells may be present in a smear at any time of the menstrual cycle. The cells may show marked nuclear enlargement and cytoplasmic vacuolation and an erroneous diagnosis of endometrial carcinoma may be made (Fig. 3.80). These abnormalities create particular difficulty in the smear of an older woman when the presence of endometrial hyperplasia or carcinoma is a real possibility.

Endocervical cells too may show nuclear enlargement, prominent nucleoli and mitotic activity. Large papillary clusters may be shed.

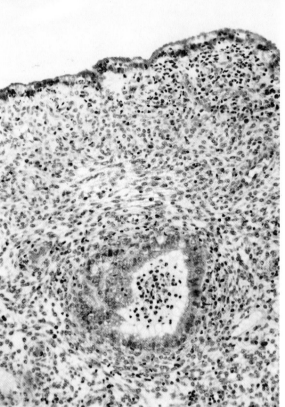

Fig. 3.81 Endometrial curettings: an acute focal endometritis. Inflammatory cells are present beneath the surface epithelium and within glands. ×110. Haematoxylin and eosin.

Fragments of an IUCD, in the form of amorphous brown staining material, may be present in a cervical smear. These fragments may be associated with aggregates of *Actinomyces* and are thought to be the foreign bodies necessary for the growth of this organism (Duguid et al 1980). The fragments are often encrusted with calcium or iron and occasionally psammoma bodies are seen in the tissues and in cervical smears.

Atypical and dyskaryotic squamous cells have been reported in cervical smears in association with an IUCD and in the presence of *Actinomyces* (Sykes & Shelley 1981).

Endometrial curettings from IUCD users show the features of a focal acute and chronic endometritis (Moyer & Michell 1971) with leucocytes, lymphocytes, plasma cells, macrophages and rarely foreign body giant cells (Fig. 3.81). Squamous metaplasia of the endometrium sometimes occurs. There may be a premature predecidual reaction, focal fibrosis and pressure atrophy of the endometrium beneath the device.

The above pattern is usually seen with plastic devices. Copper-containing IUCDs cause a less florid reaction with leucocytes confined to gland lumens and forming a surface exudate. Progesterone impregnated devices cause a marked decidual reaction in the endometrial stroma, which may be localised or diffuse (Martinez-Manautou et al 1975).

Gonococcus

Neisseria gonorrhoeae is a Gram-negative diplococcus which is an intracellular parasite. The individual cocci are kidney-shaped and are arranged in pairs with concave sides adjacent.

N. gonorrhoeae is the causative organism of acute and chronic gonorrhoea, the most common venereal disease. Gonococci attack the mucous membranes of the genitourinary tract in both sexes. Infection in the male is usually symptomatic and causes an acute purulent urethritis. The prostate gland, epididymis or rectum may be involved. Healing with fibrosis may result in urethral or rectal strictures.

In the female, infection causes an acute urethritis and cervicitis with a purulent discharge; it may however be asymptomatic. Spread of the gonococcus to the fallopian tubes may cause pelvic inflammatory disease with the possible long-term sequelae of fibrosis, obliteration of the fallopian tubes and sterility.

The vaginal mucosa in the adult is usually resistant to penetration by the gonococcus, but vaginitis does occur in children and adolescents because the vaginal mucosa is thin and less vascular.

Gonococcal conjunctivitis of the newborn (ophthalmia neonatorum) is a serious condition which may result in blindness.

Gonococcal infection does not result in immunity and reinfection is common (Johnson 1981).

A presumptive diagnosis of gonococcal infection can be made when polymorphonuclear leucocytes containing intracellular diplococci are identified in the discharge. The cytological and histological changes of acute gonococcal cervicitis are nonspecific.

The organisms can be identified in routine Papanicolaou stained smears in the cytoplasm of polymorphonuclear leucocytes and attached to or within the cytoplasm of squamous cells. However, the morphological separation of *N. gonorrhoeae* from other species of *Neisseria* and from other organisms is not possible in cervical smears (Johnson 1983) and it is advisable to confirm the diagnosis by culture.

Techniques of cytological sampling and slide preparation

The quality of a cytological diagnosis depends to a great extent on the techniques used to obtain the cellular samples. Specimens which contain too few cells or are heavily contaminated with blood or inflammatory cells, or which are poorly spread, fixed or stained may result in false negative reports. Accurate sampling of the area or lesion is, of course, essential.

The cervical smear

The main purpose of taking a cervical smear is to exclude the presence of CIN. This lesion arises in the transformation zone and in taking a cervical smear this area must be thoroughly sampled. The usual method of taking a smear is to place the shaped end of an Ayre's spatula into the external os and to rotate the spatula through 360 degrees. This technique is adequate when the whole transformation zone is covered by the spatula (Fig. 3.82a). In many cases, however, the transformation zone extends beyond the normal sweep of the spatula. It is then necessary to take a second sample from the area not covered by the original sweep (Fig. 3.82b). The cells obtained may be put on to one slide or a second slide made if preferred. An adequate cervical smear should include mature squamous cells, metaplastic squamous cells and endocervical cells.

Endocervical swab/brush sample

The squamocolumnar junction is not always visible and in older women it may retreat into the endocer-

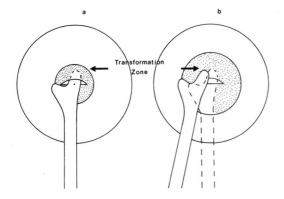

Fig. 3.82 Taking a cervical smear.

vical canal. In this situation, in addition to taking a smear with an Ayre's spatula, as in Fig. 3.82, an endocervical sample should be obtained. The tip of a cotton wool swab moistened with physiologic saline is rotated in the endocervical canal and the cellular sample obtained is smeared on to a glass slide by rolling the cotton wool swab across the slide. The technique is similar for an endocervical brush, which can be used dry.

Vaginal smear

Some laboratories routinely request both cervical and vaginal smears on all patients. Many laboratories, however, issue all routine reports on a cervical smear alone. In certain clinical situations, however, a vaginal sample increases the chance of an accurate cytological diagnosis; most important is the diagnosis of endometrial carcinoma. Diagnostic cells may not always be present at the moment a cervical smear is taken, but these cells tend to collect in the posterior vaginal fornix. A smear taken from this site should be included when endometrial carcinoma is suspected. The material can be aspirated using a glass pipette with a suction bulb or collected with the smooth end of an Ayre's spatula.

The vaginal smear should be taken as the first step in the gynaecological examination. The speculum should not be lubricated as lubricant may contaminate a smear taken from the cervix or vagina and produce a basophilic background which obscures cellular detail. Neither cervical nor vaginal smears are a sufficiently reliable diagnostic tool

for the detection of endometrial carcinoma and if the smears are negative endometrial samples should be obtained by direct aspiration or curettage of the endometrial cavity.

A vaginal sample alone is a poor method for the detection of cervical lesions.

Smear from the upper third of the lateral wall of the vagina. Cells are obtained by scraping with a spatula. Avoid contamination with squamous cells from the vulva or skin which make the hormonal determination unreliable.

Purpose of specific sampling techniques

Cervical smear. Detection of CIN, invasive squamous cell carcinoma and endocervical adenocarcinoma.

Endocervical smear. Detection of CIN and squamous cell carcinoma higher in the endocervical canal, endocervical and endometrial carcinoma.

Posterior fornix smear. Detection of endometrial carcinoma, ovarian or tubal carcinoma.

Lateral vaginal wall smear. Hormonal evaluation.

Most infections of the genital tract detected during routine screening are diagnosed from a cervical smear.

Slide preparation

Many smears are inadequate because correct preparation of the smear has been neglected. When the cellular sample is collected it should be thinly, evenly and rapidly spread on to a slide which has already been labelled with the relevant patient details. Thick smears with numerous overlapping cells are impossible to interpret. Rapid fixation is very important and an air-drying artefact is all too common. The smear must be fixed immediately after spreading. Immersion in 95% ethyl alcohol in a Coplin jar, or the use of a coating fixative, either sprayed or dropped on to the slide, are the methods most commonly used. The smears must remain immersed in 95% ethyl alcohol for a minimum of 15 minutes. Prolonged fixation however will not materially alter the appearance of the smear. Coating fixatives should be allowed to dry on the smear. This usually takes 5–10 minutes. The smears are then stained by the Papanicolaou method.

REFERENCES

Bolton J P, Darougar S 1983 Perihepatitis. British Medical Bulletin 39(2): 159–62

Burman R, Schlesselman S, McCaffrey L, Gupta P K, Spence M 1982 The relationship of genital tract Actinomyces and the development of pelvic inflammatory disease. American Journal of Obstetrics & Gynecology 143: 585–589

Cabral G A, Fry D, Marciano-Cabral F, Lumpkin C, Mercer L, Goplerud 1983 A herpes virus antigen in human premalignant and malignant cervical biopsies and explants. American Journal of Obstetrics & Gynecology 145: 79–86

Carr M C, Hanna L, Jawetz E 1979 Chlamydiae, cervicitis and abnormal Papanicolaou smears. Obstetrics & Gynecology 53: 27–30

Coleman D V, Russell W J I, Hodgson J, Tun Pe, Mowbray J F 1977 Human papovavirus in Papanicolaou smears of urinary sediment detected by transmission electron microscopy. Journal of Clinical Pathology 30: 1015–1020

Dawson S G, Harris J R W 1983 Venereal disease, Gardnerella vaginalis and non-specific vaginitis. British Journal of Hospital Medicine 29(1): 28–37

Duguid H L D, Parratt D, Traynor R 1980 Actinomyces-like organisms in cervical smears from women using intrauterine contraceptive devices. British Medical Journal 281: 534–537

Duguid H L D, Parratt D, Traynor R, Taylor D, Duncan I D, Elias-Jones J 1982 Studies on uterine tract infections and the intrauterine contraceptive device with special reference to actinomyces. British Journal of Obstetrics & Gynaecology 89 (Suppl 4): 32–39

Dunlop E M C, Jones B R, al-Hussaini M K 1964 Genital infection in association with TRIC virus infection of the eye. British Journal of Venereal Diseases 40: 33–42

Eschenbach D A, Harnisch J P, Holmes K K 1977 Pathogenesis of acute pelvic inflammatory disease: role of contraception and other risk factors. American Journal of Obstetrics & Gynecology 128: 838–850

Galloway D A, Fenoglio C, Shevchuck M, McDougall J K 1979 Detection of herpes simplex RNA in human sensory ganglia. Virology 95: 265–268

Gardner H L, Dukes C D 1955 Haemophilus vaginalis vaginitis. American Journal of Obstetrics & Gynecology 69: 962–976

Gilman S C, Docherty J J, Clarke A, Rawls W E 1980 Reaction patterns of herpes simplex virus type 1 and type 2 proteins with sera of patients with uterine cervical carcinoma and matched controls. Cancer Research 40: 4640–4647

Gissmann L, Boshart M, Durst M, Ikenberg H, Wagner D, Zur Hausen H 1984 Presence of human papillomavirus in genital tumours. Journal of Investigative Dermatology 83: 26s–28s

Gupta P K 1982 Intrauterine contraceptive devices. Vaginal cytology, pathologic changes and clinical implications. Acta Cytologica 26: 571–613

Gupta P K, Hollander D H, Frost J K 1976 Actinomyces in cervico-vaginal smears: an association with intrauterine contraceptive device usage. Acta Cytologica 20: 295–297

Gupta P K, Lee E F, Erozan Y S, Frost J K, Geddes S T, Donovan P A 1979 Cytologic investigations in chlamydia infection. Acta Cytologica 23: 315–320

Hager W D, Douglas B, Majmuder B et al 1979 Pelvic colonisation with Actinomyces in women using intrauterine contraceptive devices. American Journal of Obstetrics & Gynecology 135: 680–684

Hammerschlag M R 1978 Chlamydial pneumonia in infants. New England Journal of Medicine 298: 1083–1084

Hare M J, Toone E, Taylor-Robinson D et al 1981 Follicular cervicitis—colposcopic appearances and association with chlamydia trachomatis. British Journal of Obstetrics & Gynaecology 88: 174–180

Hare M J, Taylor-Robinson D, Cooper P 1982 Evidence for an association between Chlamydia trachomatis and cervical intraepithelial neoplasia. British Journal of Obstetrics & Gynaecology 89: 489–492

Heise E R, Kucera L S, Raben M, Homesley H 1979 Serological response patterns to herpes virus type 2 early and late antigens in cervical carcinoma patients. Cancer Research 39: 4022–4026

Hobson D, Rees E, Visuralingam N D 1983 Chlamydial infections in neonates and older children. British Medical Bulletin 39(2): 128–132

Ison C A, Dawson S G, Hilton J, Csonka G W, Easmon C S F 1982 Comparison of culture and microscopy in the diagnosis of Gardnerella vaginalis infection. Journal of Clinical Pathology 35: 550–554

Jarrett W F H 1981 Papilloma viruses and cancer. In: Anthony P P, MacSween R N M (eds) Recent advances in histopathology 11. Churchill Livingstone, Edinburgh, 35–48

Johnson A P 1981 The pathogenesis of gonorrhoea. Journal of Infection 3(4): 299–308

Johnson A P 1983 The pathogenic potential of commensal species of Neisseria. Journal of Clinical Pathology 36: 213–223

Jones B M 1983 Gardnerella vaginalis-associated vaginitis—a 'new' sexually transmitted disease. Medical Laboratory Science 40(1): 53–57

Kaufman D W, Shapiro S, Rosenberg L et al 1980 Intrauterine contraceptive device use and pelvic inflammatory disease. American Journal of Obstetrics & Gynecology 136: 159–162

Keebler C, Chatwani A, Schwartz R 1983 Actinomycosis infection associated with intrauterine contraceptive devices. American Journal of Obstetrics & Gynecology 145(5): 596–599

Kinlen L J, Spriggs A I 1978 Women with positive cervical smears, but without surgical intervention. A follow-up study. Lancet ii: 463–465

Kobayashi T K, Fujimoto T, Okamoto H, Yuasa M, Sawaragi I 1983 Association of mast cells with vaginal Trichomoniasis in endocervical smears. Acta Cytologica (Baltimore) Mar–Apr 27(2): 133–137

Koss L G, 1968 Diagnostic cytology and its histopathologic basis. 2nd ed. J B Lippincott Company, London

Koss L G, Wolinska W H 1959 Trichomonas vaginalis cervicitis and its relationship to cervical cancer. Cancer 12(ii): 1171–1193

Kurman R J, Shah K H, Lancaster W D, Jenson A B 1981 Immunoperoxidase localisation of papilloma virus antigens in cervical dysplasia and vulvar condylomas. American Journal of Obstetrics & Gynecology 140: 931–935

Larsen B, Galask R P 1980 Vaginal microbial flora: practical and theoretic relevance. Obstetrics and Gynecology 55 (Supp 5): 100S–113S

Lawrence W D, Shingleton H M 1980 Early physiologic squamous metaplasia of the cervix: light and electron microscopic observations. American Journal of Obstetrics & Gynecology 137: 661–671

McDougall J K, Galloway D A, Fenoglio C M 1980 Cervical carcinoma: detection of herpes simplex virus RNA in cells undergoing neoplastic change. International Journal of Cancer 25: 1–8

McNeill R E, de Moraes-Ruehsen M 1978 Amoeba trophozoites in cervicovaginal smear of a patient using an intrauterine device: a case report. Acta Cytologica 22: 91

Martinez-Manautou J, Maqueo M, Aznar R, Pharriss B B, Zaffaroni A 1975 Endometrial morphology in women exposed to uterine systems releasing progesterone. American Journal of Obstetrics & Gynecology 121: 175–179

Meisels A, Fortin R 1976 Condylomatous lesions of the cervix and vagina, I. Cytologic patterns. Acta Cytologica 20: 505–509

Meisels A, Roy M, Fortier M et al 1981 Human papilloma virus infection of the cervix: the atypical condyloma. Acta Cytologica 25: 7–16

Moyer D L, Michell D R 1971 Reactions of human endometrium to the intrauterine foreign body: II. Long term effects on the endometrial histology and cytology. American Journal of Obstetrics & Gynecology III: 66–80

Naib Z M, Nahmias J A, Josey W E, Kramer J H 1969 Genital herpetic infection. Association with cervical dysplasia and carcinoma. Cancer 23: 940–945

Nilsson C G, Vartiainen E, Widholm O 1981 Bacterial cultures from intrauterine devices removed from patients with pelvic inflammatory disease. Acta Obstetrica et Gynecologica Scandinavica 60: 563–566

Oriel J D, Ridgeway G L 1983 Genital infections in men. British Medical Bulletin 39(2): 133–137

Orth G, Jablonska S, Favre M et al 1980 Epidermodysplasia verruciformis: a model for the role of papilloma viruses and human cancer. In: Essex M, Todaro G, Zur Hansen H (eds) Viruses in naturally occurring cancers. Cold Spring Harbour Laboratory, New York, pp 1043–1428

Paavonen J, Vesterinen E, Meyer B et al. 1979 Genital Chlamydia trachomatis infections in patients with cervical atypia. Obstetrics & Gynecology 54: 289–291

Papanicolaou G N 1960 Atlas of exfoliative cytology supplement 2. Harvard University Press, Cambridge, Mass.

Patten S F Jr 1978 Diagnostic cytopathology of the uterine cervix. In: Wied G L (ed) Monographs in clinical cytology, 2nd edn, vol 3, S Karger, Basel pp 88–91

Petitti D B, Yamamoto D, Morgenstern N 1983 Factors associated with Actinomyces-like organisms on Papanicolaou smears in users of intrauterine contraceptive devices. American Journal of Obstetrics & Gynecology 145(3): 338–341

Richart R M 1973 Cervical intraepithelial neoplasia. In: Somers S C (ed) Pathology annual. Appleton-Century-Crofts, New York, pp 301–328

Richart R M, Barron B A 1969 A follow-up study of patients with cervical dysplasia. American Journal of Obstetrics & Gynecology 105: 386–393

Roberts T H, Ng A B P 1975 Chronic lymphocytic cervicitis: cytologic and histopathologic manifestations. Acta Cytologica 19: 235–243

Schachter J 1978 Chlamydial infections: first of three parts. New England Journal of Medicine 298: 428–435

Schachter J, Hill E C, King E B, Coleman V R, Jones P, Meyer K F 1975 Chlamydial infection in women with cervical dysplasia. American Journal of Obstetrics & Gynecology 123: 753–757

Schachter J, Hill E C, King E B et al 1982 Chlamydia trachomatis and cervical neoplasia. Journal of the American Medical Association 248: 2134–2138

Singer A, Jordan J A (eds) 1976 The anatomy of the cervix. In: The cervix. W B Saunders, London, 13–36

Singer A, Reid B, Coppleston M 1976 A hypothesis; the role of the high risk male in the aetiology of cervical cancer. American Journal of Obstetrics & Gynecology 126: 110–115

Sobel J D 1984 Vulvovaginal candidiasis—what we do and do not know. Annals of Internal Medicine 101(3): 390–392

Spriggs A I, Boddington M M 1980 Progression and regression of cervical lesions. Journal of Clinical Pathology 33: 517–522

Street D A, Wells C, Taylor-Robinson D, Ackers J P 1984 Interaction between Trichomonas vaginalis and other pathogenic microorganisms of the human genital tract. British Journal of Venereal Diseases 60(1): 31–38

Swanson J, Eschenbach D A, Alexander E R, Holmes K K 1975 Light and electron microscopic study of Chlamydia trachomatis infection of the uterine cervix. Journal of Infectious Diseases 131: 678–687

Sykes G S, Shelley G 1981 Actinomyces-like structures and their association with intrauterine contraceptive devices, pelvic infection and abnormal cervical cytology. British Journal of Obstetrics & Gynaecology 88: 934–937

Syrjanen K J 1980 Current views on the condylomatous lesions in uterine cervix and their possible relationship to cervical squamous cell carcinoma. Obstetrical & Gynecological Survey 35: 685–694

Taylor E, Barlow D, Blackwell A L, Phillips I 1982 Gardnerella vaginalis, anaerobes and vaginal discharge. Lancet i: 1376–1379

Taylor-Robinson D, Thomas B J 1980 The role of Chlamydia trachomatis in genital tract and associated diseases. Journal of Clinical Pathology 33: 205–233

Thomas D B, Rawls W E 1978 Relationship of herpes simplex virus type-2 antibodies and squamous dysplasia to cervical carcinoma in situ. Cancer 42: 2716–2725

Valicenti J F Jr, Pappas A A, Graber C D, Williamson H O, Willis N F 1982 Detection and prevalence of intrauterine contraceptive device-associated Actinomyces colonisation and related morbidity. Journal of the American Medical Association 247: 1149–1152

Weström L, Mardh P-A 1983 Chlamydial salpingitis. British Medical Bulletin 39(2): 145–150

Woodruff J D, Braun L, Cavalieri R, Gupta P, Pass F, Shah K V 1980 Immunologic identification of papilloma virus antigen in condyloma tissues from the female genital tract. Obstetrics & Gynaecology 56: 727–732

Epidemiological aspects of genital tract infection in the female
M W Adler and A Mindel

GONORRHOEA

Size of the problem

Even though gonorrhoea is a large and increasing problem the actual numerical size of this is not really known. Approximately 200 million new cases of gonorrhoea per year are notified to the World Health Organization (WHO). However, this figure is an underestimate because some countries do not report to the WHO and others that do have different notification and health care systems which often lead to underestimates of the actual amount of disease in any one country and mean that comparisons between countries have to be treated with caution.

Some of the developing countries provide examples, both of countries not notifying to the WHO, and also of those with no centrally organised control programme for the sexually transmitted diseases (STDs). In this situation it is only possible to obtain limited information, as a result of specially conducted screening surveys. For example in Africa anything from 3% (antenatal; Osoba and Onifade 1973) to 17% of women (family planning clinics; Hopcroft et al 1973) are found to have gonorrhoea on screening; non-hospital based population surveys indicate that 18% of women and 9% of men suffer from gonorrhoea (Arya et al 1973). Naturally, such high rates carry with them a high incidence of complications, and in particular of salpingitis and infertility. It has been pointed out that gonorrhoea is so common in certain parts of Nigeria that its presence is viewed as evidence of adolescence and sexual potency (Osoba 1981b). It is, however, salutary that the complication of infertility immediately alters a woman's social standing and marriage prospects.

Table 4.1 Age-specific rates per 100 000 population (women) for postpubertal gonorrhoea in the United Kingdom and United States in 1984

Age group (years)	United Kingdom	United States
15–19	304	1376
20–24	349	1340
25+	69	128

In developing countries the figures tend to be more complete and representative of what is occurring. Even so the standards vary and countries such as the United Kingdom with a network of STD clinics and routine notification have more accurate figures than the United States, where the majority of patients are treated outside clinics, by private physicians who do not report cases (Fleming et al 1970). In 1984 (latest available figures) there were 53 802 cases of gonorrhoea (male 33 734; female 20 068) in the UK. This is thought to be a fairly accurate picture compared to the USA where the reported cases for 1984 were 878 556 (male 508 725; female 369 831) but was estimated to be nearer 1.6–2.0 million cases. In the UK the age-specific rates for women range from 69 per 100 000 population (age group 25+ years) to 349 per 100 000 (20–24 years). In the USA the highest rate in females is found in those aged 15–19 years, namely 1376 per 100 000 (Table 4.1). This fourfold difference in rates between British and American women is most probably a reflection of a less adequate control programme in the latter country rather than an inadequate notification system in the former. These differences are on the basis of reported rates but, as indicated, these are an underestimate in the USA and therefore the difference between that country and the UK is even greater.

Table 4.2 Number of cases of gonorrhoea and percentage increase (base year 1955) in the United Kingdom

Year	Male		Female	
	Number	% Increase	Number	% Increase
1955	16 232	–	4 158	–
1977	41 542	156	24 421	487
1980	38 226	135	22 598	443
1984	33 734	108	20 068	383

Trends

As indicated, gonorrhoea constitutes a major health problem and one that is increasing in size. Even though there has been a flattening off or slight decrease in the number of cases, this short-term trend should be put into the context of what has occurred over the last few decades. In the United Kingdom the number of cases of gonorrhoea in females was particularly low in 1955 (4158 cases) and this increased to a peak in 1977 (24 421) with a decrease over the next 7 years (Table 4.2). Despite this drop the increase from the mid 1950s to early 1980s is over 400%. This contrasts with men where the increase is a third greater. A similar situation is also found in the United States.

The age-specific rates over time give an idea of those at greatest risk. The largest rise since 1965 has been in the group of women aged less than 20 years, the 1975 rate being nearly $3\frac{1}{2}$ times the 1965 rate, although this has declined slightly since. Similar but less marked changes have occurred in the 20–24 years age group and, as indicated earlier, they have the highest age-specific rates.

There are two major problems associated with all the figures described so far which affect the total epidemiological picture of gonorrhoea. These are that the figures only related to:
1. patients seeking care for disease and/or
2. special case-finding studies.

Illustrations of these two problems can be found within the UK. The only notification of STDs is from the physicians working in the 230 specialised clinics. Thus, there is no notification of patients treated in general or private practice and in antenatal and gynaecological clinics. Additionally there is no routine way of calculating the number of symptomless patients who may never attend clinics. Case-finding studies in special clinical situations can help to quantify those treated in alterna-

tive agencies and the asymptomatic. Table 4.3 summarises the findings of some recent surveys carried out in the UK. These attempted to estimate the proportion of women with gonorrhoea in gynaecological, obstetric and family planning clinics. Unfortunately, this ad hoc approach means that the results are limited to specific age groups and to patients who have opted to seek medical care, often for an unrelated condition. To some extent the varying rates of reported gonorrhoea (0.16–2.9%) in these types of studies reflect these demographic and consulting differences and not 'true' differences in disease prevalence. Additionally, since these studies refer to only one part of the total population 'at risk' of contracting or suffering from an STD, and therefore do not refer to a defined population, they lack a denominator and cannot be used to estimate incidence and/or prevalence rates. These problems can only be overcome by population based studies that attempt to identify asymptomatic and symptomatic subjects and those seeking care as well as those not doing so. Such an approach has shown that the proportion of women with gonococcal infections not receiving care in the UK is low (Adler et al 1981).

CHLAMYDIA

Eleven of the 15 serotypes of *Chlamydia trachomatis* may cause genital infection. Types D to K are associated with non-gonococcal and postgonococcal urethritis in males and a variety of clinical syndromes in females including cervicitis, urethritis, bartholinitis and pelvic inflammatory disease (PID). Serotypes L1, L2 and L3 cause lymphogranuloma venereum (LGV).

LGV is common in many tropical and subtropical countries (Osoba 1981a). In contrast, only a

Table 4.3 Screening surveys for gonorrhoea in the United Kingdom

Series	Type of clinic	% of patients with disease
Hughes & Davis 1971	Gyn.	0.3
Silverstone et al 1974	Gyn.	0.3
Adler et al 1981	Gyn.	0.5
Driscoll et al 1970	Gyn.	2.9
Sparks et al 1975	Obs.	0.16
Cassie & Stevenson 1973	Obs.	0.2
Adler et al 1981	Obs.	0.3
Rees & Hamlett 1972	Obs.	0.6
Nabarro et al 1978	FPC	0.4

Gyn. = gynaecological; Obs. = obstetric; FPC = family planning clinic.

handful of cases occur in each European country each year (Willcox 1975) and almost all of these are acquired abroad. In the UK only 43 cases were reported from STD clinics in 1983.

Infection with serotypes D to K appears to be very common throughout the world. However, as most infections in women are asymptomatic the true incidence of this infection has not been determined.

C. trachomatis can be isolated from 12–31% of female STD clinic attenders (Wentworth et al 1973; Hilton et al 1974; Oriel et al 1974; Macdonald-Burns et al 1975; Nayyar et al 1976; Ridgway & Orien 1977). The isolation rate from females attending family planning clinics or who are gynaecological outpatients is considerably lower (Hilton et al 1974; McCormack et al 1979).

Most female chlamydial isolates come from contacts with non-gonoccal urethritis (NGU) or gonorrhoea. In female contacts of males with chlamydia-positive NGU the isolation rate varies from 45–68%, compared with only 4–18% in chlamydia-negative NGU contacts (Oriel et al 1972a; Holmes et al 1975; Alani et al 1977; Terho 1978). In women with gonorrhoea, chlamydia may be isolated in 27–63% of cases (Hilton et al 1974; Oriel et al 1974; Nayyar et al 1976; Davies et al 1978).

C. trachomatis has also been implicated as a major cause of PID. In Sweden, Mardh (1977) found that 19 of 53 women with salpingitis had chlamydial infection of the cervix and of those who had laparoscopy 6 of 7 grew *C. trachomatis* from the fallopian tubes. Other studies using serological tests have also suggested a strong association between PID and chlamydia (Eschenbach 1975; Simmons et al 1979; Treharne et al 1979). A treatment study by

Rees (1980) further supports the role of chlamydia in salpingitis. In this study 343 women with gonorrhoea were randomly treated with either penicillin or tetracycline. A significantly greater proportion of the women receiving penicillin developed PID and many but not all, had chlamydia isolated from the cervix.

C. trachomatis infection in the newborn usually occur as a result of delivery through an infected birth canal.

Of infants born to mothers with positive cervical cultures, 44–67% will themselves have culture-proven *C. trachomatis* infection. However, only 35–50% of the infected infants will develop conjunctivitis and 11–20% pneumonia (Schachter et al 1979; Frommell et al 1979; Hammerschlag et al 1979).

Harrison & Alexander (1984) have calculated the incidence of chlamydial conjunctivitis in the USA, considering an estimated 5% prevalence of cervical infection in pregnancy, to be 18–25 cases per 1000 live births and of chlamydial pneumonia 5–10 cases per 1000 live births.

PELVIC INFLAMMATORY DISEASE

It is no longer reasonable to regard the STDs only as acute infectious diseases. The chronic morbidity associated with some of the diseases, such as PID and carcinoma of the cervix, make them expensive and fatal.

The incidence and prevalence of PID varies throughout the world but in most developed and developing countries is rapidly increasing. The factors associated with PID are the STDs, use of intrauterine contraceptive devices (IUCDs), post-abortion and puerperal infections. The relative importance of these various factors and aetiological agents differs in different parts of the world.

In developed countries the increased use of IUCDs and a rise in non-gonococcal infections are now important factors. In Sweden and the USA the risk of PID has been calculated as being 7–9 times greater among nulliparous IUCD users than among those without IUCDs (Weström et al 1976; Eschenbach et al 1977). Other studies also show a risk, but which is lower in both nulliparous and parous women (Targum & Wright 1974; Kaufman et al 1980; Burkman et al 1981). It is suggested that IUCDs are replacing gonorrhoea as a major factor in the incidence of PID in Sweden.

In England and Wales the number of cases of acute PID admitted to hospital has doubled in the last 20 years. The number of hospitalised cases in 1981 (latest available figures) reached 14 690. These figures only related to hospitalised patients. Physicians in genitourinary medicine and gynaecologists are the two major groups seeing and treating women with PID. Certainly, many of the patients with PID diagnosed in STD clinics are managed on an outpatient basis.

The age-specific rates for PID are similar to those described previously for gonorrhoea, with the major increases occurring in the 15–19 and 20–24 year age group. In the USA PID is a major and costly health problem. It has been estimated that over 850 000 episodes of PID occur annually and that these account for 212 000 hospital admissions, 115 000 surgical procedures and 2 500 000 physician visits (Curran 1980). The direct cost alone of these is calculated at 645 million dollars. Enormous as this is, it does not take account of direct costs of ectopic pregnancy or the indirect costs associated with PID.

PID also represents a major health and social problem in developing countries but the data are sparse. It is suggested that pelvic infection is the commonest gynaecological disease in African women (Lithgow & Rubin 1972). In Uganda and Zimbabwe the proportion of gynaecological admissions due to this condition are 30 and 44% respectively (Grech et al 1972; Brown & Cruickshank 1976).

These figures of the annual numbers of acute cases and projected costs only give part of the picture and it is reasonable to suppose that in association with the increase in acute disease, there is also an increase in long-term complications and morbidity. The most disastrous consequence of salpingitis is sterility. Weström (1975) has reported tubal occlusion in 13% of Swedish women with one attack of salpingitis, rising to 75% with three or more attacks. Holtz (1930) followed up patients for 4 years after acute salpingitis and found 17% to be involuntarily sterile; Hedberg & Speyz (1958) reported a 40% sterility, also after a 4-year follow-up. Even if women with PID are able to conceive eventually their chances of suffering an ectopic pregnancy are high. Weström (1980) has reported a seven- to 10-fold increased risk of ectopic pregnancy in women who had suffered PID compared to those who had not had PID.

In Africa the consequence of infertility, subfertility and ectopic pregnancy is also substantial. Arya & Taber (1975) found an association between gonorrhoea, PID and subsequent infertility in rural Uganda. This work was based on population surveys, which will tend to give a clearer picture than case-finding studies in specific clinical settings. By necessity, most other African studies have been of the latter type. Amongst hospitalised patients with PID in Uganda, one-third were suffering from a gonococcal infection and 25% of all the patients were infertile (Grech et al 1972). A high rate of pregnancy wastage (29% of all pregnancies) was also reported. It has been reported from Zambia that 46% of hospitalised patients with PID had gonococcal infections, all confirmed microbiologically (Ratnam et al 1980). Studies carried out in the Western Pacific have shown combined primary and secondary infertility rates of 40%, and in certain tribes 74% of married couples were infertile (Scragg 1957).

Even though infertility and ectopic pregnancy are the most dramatic sequelae of PID, others exist. Chronic abdominal pain can create long-term morbidity for both the patient and attending doctor. Weström (1975) has reported that 18% of patients had pain lasting longer than 6 months causing them to seek medical advice, while Falk (1965) reported a similar figure. Another prospective controlled study reported higher figures; thus, over a 2-year follow-up period 74% of patients had com-

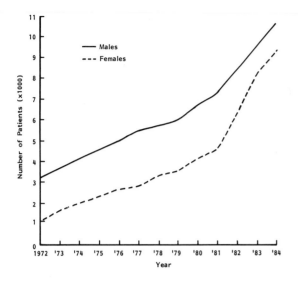

Fig. 4.1 Reported cases of genital herpes in the United Kingdom for the period 1972–1984

plained of abdominal pain, and even though this decreased over time, 20% still reported this 2 years after the initial attack of PID (Adler et al 1982). A proportion of patients with persistent pain require readmission to hospital and laparoscopy. Persistent pain of a nature requiring hospitalisation presents a substantial problem. Over 10 000 women have laparoscopic examination for abdominal pain in England and Wales per year (Working Party of the Confidential Enquiry into Gynaecological Laparoscopy 1978).

Pain can also be experienced during menstruation and sexual intercourse. Adler (1982) showed that by the end of a 2-year follow-up of PID 80% of patients had noticed some change in their periods, in that they tended to be longer and more painful. Also, 40% of patients had experienced dyspareunia over the 2 years. Other features of PID and its long-term morbidity were reported in relation to increased contact with general practitioners and alteration of normal daily routine.

GENITAL HERPES

Since the human being is the only host of the herpes simplex viruses (HSV) the infected person is the sole reservoir. Infection occurs when susceptible individuals come into contact with infected secretions during close personal contact and as these viruses are very unstable this appears to be the only important method of transmission. The incubation period is 2–14 days for both viruses with initial infection occurring at the site of inoculation (Rawls & Campione-Piccardo 1981). Latency is a particular property of these viruses with periodic reactivation at the site originally infected. Virus excretion associated with such reactivations constitutes the major source of infection.

Most oral infections are caused by HSV-1; however, genital infection may be caused by either viral type.

Genital infections caused by HSV-2 are spread by sexual intercourse with a partner who has genital sores at the time, whereas HSV-1 genital infections are usually contracted by oral genital contact with a person who has active cold sores. Of genital isolates, 13–60% are due to HSV-1 (Wolontis & Jeansson 1977; Corey et al 1981; Barton et al 1982; Peutherer et al 1982).

Trends

Genital herpes was first reported from STD clinics in the UK in 1972 when 4501 cases were reported. The number of cases has increased each year and by 1984 the number of cases reported was 19 869 (Communicable Disease Surveillance Centre 1985), an increase of 340%. Just under half the cases occur in females (Fig. 4.1). The percentage changes for the other important STDs are shown in Table 4.4, Genital herpes shows the largest percentage increase and is now the fifth commonest diagnosis in STD clinics.

The trends in genital herpes may have been due in part to increased publicity (both medical and non-medical) about the disease and current antiviral treatments, the inclusion of both primary and recurrent cases in clinic returns (Hindley & Adler 1985) and the increased use of viral culture for diagnosis. The size of the increase, however, suggests that a considerable part of it is real.

The size of the problem in other countries is less clear. In the USA no accurate national data are available; however, herpes is said to be one of the most common STDs. Estimates in the popular

Table 4.4 Percentage changes in the six commonest diseases seen in STD clinics in 1972–1983

	1972	1983	% Change
Non-specific genital infection	83 558	155 075	+86
Gonorrhoea	60 241	53 802	−11
Candidiasis	30 423	64 173	+110
Trichomoniasis	19 514	17 921	−8
Warts	16 311	49 884	+206
Genital herpes	4 501	19 869	+341

press in the USA put the number of herpes sufferers between 2 and 20 million. The Centers for Disease Control have estimated that there are between 300 000 and 500 000 new cases of herpes each year in the USA, based on a survey of 10 STD clinics. However, the validity of this figure is questionable as the majority of patients attending such clinics are of lower socioeconomic status and do not represent a reasonable cross section of the population (MMWR 1982).

In Scandinavia herpes is also common. A survey in a Swedish STD clinic found that herpes could be isolated from 8.4% of the cervices of all female attenders (Jeansson & Molin 1974) and the situation in other western countries appears to be similar.

In the Third World very little information is available. However, in these countries tropical infections, in particular chancroid, appear to be the commonest cause of genital ulceration.

Herpes in pregnancy and the epidemiology of neonatal herpes

One of the areas of greatest concern to women with herpes is the risk of transmitting the infection to the neonate. Neonatal herpes is a devastating disease with 60% mortality and a high morbidity (Nahmias et al 1970). Both congenital and intrapartum infection have been described (Nahmias et al 1970; Florman et al 1973). Congenital infection appears to be rare whereas neonatal infection is an increasing problem.

In addition to the risk of neonatal infection mothers with primary genital herpes before 20 weeks' gestation have an increased risk of spontaneous abortion and those after 23 weeks' have an increased risk of having a premature infant (Nahmias et al 1971).

Estimates of the incidence of neonatal herpes in the USA vary from 5-33/100 000 live births (Nahmias 1974). However, as the reporting system is only voluntary this is only a rough estimate. The incidence of neonatal HSV in the USA does however appear to be rising (MMWR 1982; Sullivan-Bolyai et al 1983).

There are very few cases of neonatal infection seen in the UK. In 1981 11 cases of neonatal herpes were reported to the Communicable Disease Surveillance Centre (Public Health Laboratory Service—unpublished data).

Information about the risk of neonatal infection following delivery through an infected birth canal is scarce. Nahmias and co-workers (1971) found that 3 of 6 females (50%) with primary herpes and only 1 of 23 women (4%) with recurrent herpes at delivery gave birth to an infected infant. The relevance of these data has been questioned as most of the women were young indigenous Blacks with inadequate antenatal care.

In addition to the patients with obvious clinical herpes or a history of herpes there are several other possible sources of neonatal herpes. Asymptomatic viral shedding has been reported from both the cervix and vulva in pregnant women with recurrent herpes (Vontver et al 1982). Other documented sources of neonatal infection include father to baby (Douglas et al 1983; Yaeger et al 1983) and baby to baby transmission (Francis et al 1975; Linneman et al 1975). It has also been suggested that contact with other adults, including hospital personnel, may be implicated (Light 1979).

The association of HSV with carcinoma of the cervix

The data linking HSV-2 with carcinoma of the cervix come from three sources:

1. Seroepidemiological studies;
2. Virus-specific antigens in cervical cancer tissue;
3. Virus-specific RNA and DNA in cancer tissue.

Seroepidemiological studies

Several studies have shown that the presence of HSV-2 is more common in women with cervical dysplasia, carcinoma in situ and invasive carcinoma than in controls, and that there is a graded effect (Rawls et al 1969; Nahmias et al 1970; Catalano & Johnson 1971). Thus positive antibodies are common in women with cervical carcinoma, less so in patients with carcinoma in situ and least common in those with dysplasia.

Interpretation of the results of seroepidemiological studies is complicated by two important limitations. The first is that the methods used for HSV-2 assay vary and there is considerable cross-reactivity between HSV-1 and HSV-2. Secondly, controlling for other sexual attributes possibly associated with carcinoma of the cervix (e.g. age at first sexual intercourse, number of sexual parters, marital status, previous STDs) has proved difficult.

Virus-specific antigens in cervical cancer tissue

Studies reporting on the detection of HSV-2-specific antigens from exfoliated cervical cells have shown that such antigens are present in the majority of patients with invasive carcinoma, in fewer patients with dysplasia and in almost none of the controls. In addition, when the tumour is successfully treated HSV antigens are no longer detected in cervical cells (Aurelian et al 1973; Pacsa et al 1975).

Virus-specific RNA and DNA in cancer tissue

In situ hybridisation techniques have shown that HSV-specific RNA can be detected in CIN, as well as preinvasive and invasive cervical carcinoma (McDougall et al 1980).

These studies suggest that there is some HSV RNA in cervical neoplastic cells; however, the absence of DNA, except in one study (Frenkel et al 1972), suggests that HSV is unlikely to be the cause of the tumour. A recent postulate is that HSV may be a cofactor in the causation of carcinoma of the cervix together with human papilloma virus (Zur Hausen 1982).

CYTOMEGALOVIRUS

Infection with cytomegalovirus (CMV) in adults may be asymptomatic or may cause a disease which is clinically indistinguishable from infectious mononucleosis. The virus has been recovered from virtually all body fluids including saliva, vaginal and cervical secretions and semen, and transmission occurs with close interpersonal contact.

CMV infection is widespread, but the age at which infection is acquired varies from one country to another. Antibody studies have shown that in many poorer parts of the world the infection is acquired very early in childhood, and that 95–100% of children are infected by 3–5 years old (Krech 1973). In the United Kingdom, most of western Europe and the USA, 50–60% of the population will eventually acquire the infection: about one-third during childhood and the rest between 15–35 years (Stern & Elek 1965).

The evidence for the sexual spread of CMV is circumstantial. Jordan et al (1973) reported that CMV was isolated in 13% of 120 women with suspected venereal infection compared with none in 76 having routine gynaecological examinations. Chretein et al (1977) reported two cases of CMV mononucleosis which was apparently sexually transmitted from the same female.

Whether the source of the infection is sexual or not, transplacental spread from the cervix of the pregnant mother to the fetus can result in a spectrum of illness, including hepatosplenomegaly, neonatal jaundice, microcephaly, choroidoretinitis, polycystic kidneys, mental retardation and deafness.

The neonate may acquire the virus in two ways. The most serious neonatal infections usually result from a primary infection in the mother during pregnancy and up to 3% of infants born to such mothers will have the infection, although only a small percentage of these will have severe manifestations (Griffiths et al 1980). It is evident that the level of immunity to CMV in mothers during

Table 4.5 Diagnoses made concurrently with trichomoniasis and candidosis in STD clinics (England and Wales, 1978)

Diagnosis	Trichomoniasis (%)	Candidosis (%)
Gonorrhoea	19.4	7.1
Non-specific genital infection	4.5	9.2
Trichomoniasis	–	5.6
Candidosis	9.4	–
Genital herpes	1.4	1.0
Genital warts	3.7	6.1
Other conditions requiring treatment	2.0	3.1
Other	1.9	3.2
All diagnoses	35.8	30.9

From Belsey & Adler 1981.

the child-bearing years has a direct relationship to the number of infants born with disseminated neonatal CMV infections. Neonates may also be 'infected' from mothers having a recrudescence of the infection during pregnancy. Virus may be isolated in a small percentage of such infants; however none of the serious manifestations associated with disseminated neonatal CMV infectious have been described.

In 1982, 32 cases of neonatal CMV infection were reported to PHLS for England and Wales (PHLS—unpublished data). In the USA, CMV is suggested as the leading congenital viral infection involving 2-22/1000 live births (Stagno et al 1983). Only 10% of the estimated 33 000 infants born each year in the USA are symptomatic at birth. These infants have severe disease with a 20–30% mortality. Those that survive often develop late sequelae, including mental retardation, seizures, learning difficulties, choroidoretinitis and optic atrophy (Pass et al 1980; Stagno et al 1983).

Of the 90% of infants with no clinical manifestations at birth about 10% develop clinical manifestations by 2 years. The single most important late sequela in this group is sensorineural hearing loss (Kumar et al 1984).

TRICHOMONIASIS

Even though trichomoniasis is usually considered to be sexually acquired, the association has been hard to prove. This arises from the difficulty in isolating *Trichomonas vaginalis* from males who have undoubtedly been exposed to the infection. This

may be because the infection is of a short duration in the male, with spontaneous cure, or because the conventional examination of urethral material is not the most appropriate technique for identification. Other approaches such as examining semen, prostatic fluid and urine deposits, and urine cultures have been used (Watt & Jennison 1960; Shapira 1965; Summers & Ford 1972). Isolation rates with these techniques, in male contacts of women with proven trichomoniasis, gave positive results in anything from 28–71% of the men. Catterall & Nicol (1960) looked at the problem in reverse by examining the female contacts of 56 men with trichomoniasis and found the parasite in all of them.

Additional strength is given to the contention that trichomoniasis is usually sexually transmitted by the finding that the condition is often seen in association with another sexually transmitted agent. A recent study examined all cases of female trichomoniasis isolated in women in STD clinics in England and Wales and found that in 19% of instances the infection was associated with gonorrhoea (Belsey & Adler 1981; Table 4.5).

Other modes of spread, apart from sexual intercourse, have been suggested to account for the rare infections in neonates, virgins and those fervently denying the possibility of sexual spread. The role of infected towels, lavatory seats and speculae have been investigated (Whittington 1957).

As with any of the other infections discussed in this chapter the true incidence and prevalence of the condition is difficult to assess and figures usually relate to STD clinic attenders or those screened in antenatal and gynaecology clinics. The number

Table 4.6 Screening surveys for trichomoniasis in the United Kingdom

Series	Type of clinic	% of patients with disease
Hughes & Davis 1971	Gyn.	3.5
Adler et al 1981	Gyn.	6.3
Driscoll et al 1970	Gyn.	23.5
Adler et al 1981	Obs.	3.6
Rees & Hamlet 1972	Obs.	4.0
Thin & Michael 1970	Obs.	8.9

Gyn. = gynaecological; Obs. = obstetric.

of cases attending STD clinics in the UK has remained fairly constant: between 18 000–21 000 over the last 5 years. The latest available figures (1984) show a total of 17 921 cases (female 16 632; male 1289). Screening in antenatal and gynaecology clinics shows rates of isolation varying from 3.5–23.5% (Table 4.6). The prevalence of trichomoniasis in a defined population varies between clinical settings and has been found to range from 32–70 per 1000 (Adler et al 1981).

CANDIDOSIS

Vaginal candidiasis is usually caused by *Candida albicans*, but other pathogenic species can be isolated (*Torulopsis glabrata*, *C. stellatoidea* and *C. tropicalis*). Screening of women attending an STD clinic has shown that 81% of those with a yeast infection had *C. albicans* present, 16% had *T. glabrata* and other yeasts were present in 3% (Oriel et al 1972a).

Opinions differ as to whether the presence of *C. albicans* in the vagina necessarily signifies disease. Carroll et al (1973) correlated macroscopic vaginitis with the presence of *C. albicans* and concluded that the organism is always pathogenic. This view has since been supported by some workers, whereas others have suggested that *C. albicans* is only pathogenic if associated with symptoms, and in the absence of these symptoms it should be regarded as a commensal and remain untreated. This controversy is further complicated by the poor predictive value of genital symptoms and signs. Controlled observations show that women with vaginal candidosis, compared to those without, complain of vaginal and/or vulval irritation and dysuria significantly more frequently and are found to have a

thick white discharge with plaques and inflammation of the vulva and vagina more often. However, the frequency with which these symptoms and signs occur in the non-diseased women make them of little diagnostic value (Adler & Belsey 1984).

Data on the incidence and prevalence of vaginal candidosis are invariably confined to special groups and those seeking care. Screening surveys in antenatal and gynaecology clinics show that the proportion of women with candidosis ranges from 15–71% (Thin & Michael 1970; Hughes & Davies 1971). The number of patients attending STD clinics in the UK with candidosis has steadily increased and in 1984 reached 64 173. Most cases occurred in women (49 649) and constituted the commonest diagnoses amongst women seen in STD clinics.

The figures relating to the proportion of antenatal and gynaecology patients with candidosis and the numbers seen in STD clinics give a limited view of the epidemiology of this condition, since they are confined only to hospital attenders. Vaginal discharge is an important reason for consultation in general practice and vaginal candidosis is frequently treated in this non-hospital situation (Wright & Palmer 1978). Even though these data are community based, they are still confined to those seeking care. The true incidence and prevalence of vaginal candidosis is only to be found by examining those attending general practice and hospital as well as those who do not seek any form of medical care. Such epidemiological work shows that the prevalence is higher in women not consulting than in antenatal, gynaecology and family planning clinics (Adler & Belsey 1981).

There are various predisposing factors associated with candidosis. Pregnancy has been shown to be stongly associated with the development of the condition. Antibiotics, and in particular, tetracycline, have been shown to predispose to infection (Oriel & Waterworth 1975). Even though the oral contraceptive pill has been implicated in the past (Catterall 1966), this has not been substantitated in recent epidemiological studies (Goldacre et al 1979). This change or difference could well be associated with the introduction of low oestrogen-containing pills.

Traditionally it is maintained that candidosis in women is rarely sexually transmitted, but that it is invariably so in men (Davidson 1977). However, this is probably changing and it has been reported that yeast infection was sexually acquired in women more frequently than men (Thin et al 1977). Candidosis, even if sexually acquired, has always been regarded as innocuous; again, this is no longer true if one bears in mind the fact that concurrent infections can exist in the same patient. For example, in STD clinics one-third of cases of female candidosis are associated with one or more additional conditions (Belsey & Adler 1981). Table 4.5 shows the concurrent diagnoses associated with candidosis; thus, in 9% of instances non-specific genital infection was diagnosed and in 7% gonorrhoea. These recent observations concerning sexual transmission and association with other sexually transmitted agents requiring treatment must change the approach to the management of such a disease outside STD clinics.

SYPHILIS

As with virtually all the STDs, the current magnitude of the problem represented by syphilis in any one country and comparisons with others is difficult to ascertain. This is not a new problem: for example, in 1910 the Registrar General in England and Wales reported 1639 deaths due to syphilis in adults and 1200 in infants (Adler 1980). Osler was of the view that this was a considerable underestimate and calculated that adult deaths were probably nearer 60 000.

The advent of penicillin made a dramatic and rapid impact on the incidence of early infectious syphilis throughout the world in the 1950s. Unfortunately, this effect has not been maintained in all countries.

Table 4.7 Reported new cases of congenital syphilis

Year	UK (<2 years)	USA (0–1 year)
1970	13	345
1971	18	451
1972	16	383
1973	9	314
1974	15	270
1975	10	180
1976	12	167
1977	17	144
1978	9	107
1979	16	130
1980	8	–

In the United Kingdom a decline in syphilis has been witnessed and virtually maintained. There has been an increase in all forms of syphilis amongst males during the last decade, whereas the number of cases in females has continued to fall. This disparity is explained by the fact that most primary and secondary syphilis (58%) occurs amongs homosexuals (British Co-operative Clinical Group, 1980). The age-specific rates indicate that the greatest increase in males was in those aged 20–24 years.

Particularly encouraging is the fall in congenital syphilis in developed countries (Table 4.7). This is largely due to widescale antenatal screening. Happily, in association with this fall infant mortality due to this condition is negligible. In the UK in 1980 there were no such cases and in the USA in 1979 there were a total of four instances of infant mortality due to syphilis. Unfortunately, congenital syphilis still represents a major health problem in many developing countries.

ANAEROBIC VAGINOSIS

Non-specific vaginitis or bacterial vaginosis is now a recognised clinical entity consisting of malodorous vaginal discharge, the discharge being grey, homogenous and adherent to the vaginal walls, and a vaginal pH above 5.0 and where *Trichomonas vaginalis* or other organisms are not isolated.

The role of *Gardnerella vaginalis* in this syndrome has been disputed (Dunkelburg 1977). The organism was originally implicated in 1955 by Gardner & Dukes as the cause of this distinct clinical entity. However, more recent studies have suggested that anaerobic bacteria may act in sym-biosis with *Gardnerella* to cause the infection. The presence of anaerobes has a higher correlation with the clinical syndrome than the presence of *Gardnerella* (Taylor et al 1982).

Since there is a lack of unanimity concerning the causative organism or the criteria for diagnosing non-specific vaginitis, it is almost impossible to determine how common the infection is, its pathogenesis, its mode of spread and whether patients with the condition suffer any long-term morbidity.

The evidence for sexual transmission is circum-stantial. Firstly, studies have shown that *G. vaginalis* of the same biotype may be isolated from the urethra of males who are contacts of vaginally in-fected females (Gardner & Dukes 1955; Pheifer et al 1978). Secondly, *Gardnerella* is often associated with other STDs (Josey & Lambe 1976), and final-ly, treatment of the male contact has resulted in clearance of recurrent infection in females (Malouf et al 1981).

In 1977 Dunkelburg estimated that 15% of women of child-bearing age in the USA were in-fected with *G. vaginalis*. He calculated that there were 7.5 million infected at that time in the USA.

Until such time as there are more exact diagnos-tic criteria for non-specific vaginitis and until the role of *G. vaginalis* in this condition has been fully elucidated there will be no way of verifying such figures or indeed of conducting any meaningful epidemiological surveys.

GROUP B STREPTOCOCCI

Patients with colonisation of the genital tract with Group B streptococci are usually asymptomatic. Several studies suggest that the infection may be spread by sexual intercourse. Baker (1980) showed that the colonisation rate of the genital tract was higher in sexually active females than in virgins, and women attending STD clinics were more likely to be colonised than those attending other out-patient departments. Secondly, Franciosi and co-workers (1973) reported that Group B streptococci could be isolated from 45% of husbands whose wives were vaginally infected and when both part-ners were treated the wives remained persistent-ly negative. Finally, Christensen and colleagues (1974) reported that colonisation with Group B streptococci was associated with gonococcal infec-tion.

Although the infection is asymptomatic in adults, neonatal infection is often severe, with a 30% mortality. Virtually all infants born to mothers with Group B streptococci in their genital tracts be-come colonised with the bacteria; however, overt infection resulting in respiratory distress, mening-itis, septicaemia, cellulitis, arthritis or osteomyeli-tis only occurs in about 1% of these infants (Horn et al 1974).

The number of neonates who have Group B streptococcal infection per year is unknown. Hill (1984) has estimated that the annual incidence in the USA was 3.5–4.2/1000 live births. In the UK there were 138 cases reported to the Communicable Disease Surveillance Centre in 1980 (PHLS, un-published data). The size of the problem in the Third World remains unknown.

THE ACQUIRED IMMUNE DEFICIENCY SYNDROME

Five cases of *Pneumocystis carinii* pneumonia and 26 of Kaposi's sarcoma were reported in homosexual men in Los Angeles, New York and California in mid-1981 (Friedman-Kien et al 1981, 1982; Got-tlieb et al 1981a, 1981b; Hymes et al 1981). This phenomenon subsequently became known as the acquired immune deficiency syndrome (Aids). The Centre for Disease Control (CDC) in Atlanta sub-sequently defined this as a person

1. with a reliably diagnosed disease that is at least moderately indicative of an underlying cellular immune deficiency; for example, Kaposi's sarcoma in a patient aged less than 60 years, or opportunistic infection;
2. who has no known underlying cause of cellu-lar immune deficiency or any other cause of reduced resistance reported to be associated with the disease.

This definition was accepted for surveillance purposes by most other countries and was the one used within the UK. The definition has sub-sequently been slightly modified in June 1985 in the light of laboratory tests to detect HIV antibody and includes additional serious conditions.

Following the initial reports the spectrum of the syndrome has increased to include other tumours, such as lymphomas (Ziegler et al 1982) and other opportunistic infections caused by virus, bacteria, fungi and protozoa. It is now also appreciated that groups other than homosexual men are at risk of Aids. These include heterosexual intravenous drug abusers (Moll et al 1982; Wormser et al 1983), haemophiliacs (Centers for Disease Control 1982a) and Haitian immigrants (Centers for Disease Control 1982b, 1985; Viesa et al 1983).

There are currently (March 1987) 31 526 cases in the USA, 4500 in Europe (Centers for Disease Control 1987) and 724 in the UK. In the UK proportionately more homosexuals are involved than in the USA; 87% of cases compared with 73%. The overall and eventual mortality are 46 and 100% respectively. Median survival after diagnosis varies with the manifestation of the disease and is approximately 9 months for a patient with an opportunistic infection and 31 months for those suffering from Kaposi's sarcoma.

Recently, HIV has been strongly implicated in the aetiology of Aids. (Barre-Sinoussi et al 1983; Gallo et al 1983). In Britain, 2000 persons were examined serologically for antibodies to HIV (Cheingsong-Popov et al 1984). Of Aids patients, 97% had antibodies; 89% with PGL and 42% of the sexual contacts of the two groups. Equally worrying was the fact that 17% of healthy homosexual men attending STD clinics had presence of antibodies. Recent work shows that the prevalence in the Department of Genitourinary Medicine at the Middlesex Hospital has increased from 3.7% of British homosexual men attending in March 1982 to 21% in July 1984 (Carne et al 1985). Even though it is thought that only the minority of those infected with the virus will develop Aids it would be prudent to assume that they are infectious.

Females, unless they belong to the risk groups of intravenous drug abusers or haemophiliacs, are not at high risk of acquiring Aids in Europe or the USA. At the end of December 1986, 3.6% of Aids occurred in females in the UK, while in the USA 6.5% were in females. However, only 14% of these American women had contracted Aids through heterosexual contact and the largest group (53%) were intravenous drug users. The fact that heterosexual spread can occur, and in Africa is apparently more common than in Europe and the USA, is of concern since this is probably the only way that HIV infection could break out of the (so far) well defined high risk groups (Piot et al 1984; Van de Perre et al 1984).

Prostitutes

If heterosexual transmission of HIV can occur to women from bisexual men and then back to males, it is likely that female prostitutes with multiple partners would act as an important source of infection and transmission. It is suggested that some of the cases in the USA that do not belong to any risk group may have contracted Aids through heterosexual contact with infected prostitutes (Chamberland et al 1984). By November 1984, 263 (3.8%) of Aids cases in the USA belonged to the 'non-characteristic' group (Centers for Disease Control 1984). Detailed investigations of 65 of the males in this group indicated that 17 admitted sexual intercourse with female prostitutes. One of the 9 women belonging to the non-characteristic group was a former prostitute. Another study has shown that of 36 male Aids cases without known risk factors in New York, 11 reported one or more episodes of intercourse with female prostitutes in the 5 years prior to the onset of the disease and two further men had experienced intercourse with intravenous drug-abusing women (Abkin et al 1985). Contact with prostitutes is also cited as a mode of transmission in another study in army personnel (Redfield et al 1985); however, the strict penalties against homo-sexuality in the army cannot rule out homosexual, as opposed to prostitute, contact as the risk factor.

Some women engaging in prostitution do so to finance their drug addiction and thus also belong to a high risk group for Aids. In the USA approximately a third of women who had sought treatment for their drug addiction had practised prostitution to obtain money for drugs (Grizburg et al, in press).

The heterosexual transmission of HIV infection to women is of particular concern because of the possibilities of ensuing vertical transmission. Aids has now been reported (March 1987) in 456 children (under 13 years old) in the USA. Most of the mothers had Aids, were sexual contacts of bisexual men or were themselves intravenous drug addicts. It is thought that transmission of the virus can occur transplacentally, during delivery and through breast milk.

REFERENCES

Abkin R R, Lekatsas A, Walker J 1985 Acquired immunodeficiency syndrome in heterosexual males associated with sexual contacts. Paper presented at International Conference on Acquired Immunodeficiency Syndrome (AIDS) April 14–17 1985, Atlanta

Adler M W 1980 The terrible peril: a historical perspective on the venereal diseases. British Medical Journal 281: 206–211

Adler M W, Belsey E M 1984 The value of genital symptoms and signs in women. The British Journal of Family Planning 10: 84–88

Adler M W, Belsey E M, Rogers J S 1981 Sexually transmitted diseases in a defined population of women. British Medical Journal 283: 29–32

Adler M W, Belsey E M, O'Connor B H 1982 Morbidity associated with pelvic inflammatory disease. British Journal of Venereal Diseases 58: 151–157

Alani M D, Darougar S, MacDonald-Burns D C, Thin R N, Dunn H 1977 Isolation of chlamydia trachomatis from the male urethra. British Journal of Venereal Diseases 53: 88–92

Arya O P, Taber J R 1975 Correlates of venereal diseases and fertility in rural Uganda. WHO/VDT/Res 75,339 World Health Organisation, Geneva

Arya O P, Nsamzumahire H, Taber S R 1973 Clinical, cultural and demographic aspects of gonorrhoea in a rural community in Uganda. Bulletin of the World Health Organization 49: 587–595

Aurelian L, Schumann B, Marcus R L, Davis H J 1973 Antibody to HSV 2 induced tumour specific antigens in serum from patients with cervical carcinoma. Science 181: 161–164

Baker C J 1980 Group B streptococcal infections. Advances in Internal Medicine 25: 475–501

Barre-Sinoussi F, Chermann J C, Rey F et al 1983 Isolation of T lymphotropic etrovirus for a patient at risk of acquired immune deficiency syndrome (AIDS). Science 220: 868–870

Barton I G, Kinghorn G R, Najem S, Al-Omar L S, Potter C W 1982 Incidence of herpes simplex virus types 1 and 2 isolated in patients with herpes genitalis in Sheffield. British Journal of Venereal Diseases 58: 44–47

Belsey E M, Adler M W 1981 Study of STD clinic attenders in England and Wales, 1978. 2: Patterns of diagnosis. British Journal of Venereal Diseases 57: 290–294

British Co-operative Clinical Group 1980 Homosexuality and venereal disease. In the United Kingdom: a secondary study. British Journal of Venereal Diseases 56: 6–11

Brown I McL, Cruickshank J G 1976 Aetiological factors in pelvic inflammatory disease in urban Blacks in Rhodesia. South African Medical Journal 50: 1342

Burkman R T et al 1981 Association between intrauterine device and pelvic inflammatory disease. Obstetrics and Gynecology 57: 269–275

Carne C, Weller I V D, Sutherland S et al 1985 Rising prevalence of human T lymphotropic virus type III (HTLV III) infection in homosexual men in London. Lancet i: 1261–1262

Carroll C J, Stanley V C, Hurley R 1973 Criteria for the diagnosis of candida vulvovaginitis in pregnant women. Journal of Obstetrics and Gynaecology of the British Commonwealth 80: 258–263

Cassie R, Stevenson A 1973 Screening for gonorrhoea, trichomoniasis, moniliasis and syphilis in pregnancy. Journal of Obstetrics and Gynaecology of the British Commonwealth 80: 48–51

Catalano L W, Johnson L D 1971 Herpes virus antibody and carcinoma in situ of the cervix. Journal of the American Medical Association 217: 447–450

Catterall R D 1966 Candida albicans and the contraceptive pill. Lancet ii: 830–831

Catterall R D, Nicol C S 1960 Is trichomonas infestation a venereal disease? British Medical Journal 1: 1177–1179

Centers for Disease Control 1982a Opportunistic infections and Kaposi's sarcoma among Haitians in the United States. Morbidity and Mortality Weekly Report 31: 353–361

Centers for Disease Control 1982b Update on acquired immune deficiency syndrome (AIDS) among patients with haemophilia A. Morbidity and Mortality Weekly Report 31: 644–652

Centers for Disease Control 1984 Update: acquired immunodeficiency syndrome (AIDS)—United States. Morbidity and Mortality Weekly Report 33: 661–664

Centers for Disease Control 1985 Update: acquired immunodeficiency syndrome—United States. Morbidity and Mortality Weekly Report 34: 245–248

Chamberland M E, Castro K G, Haverkos H W et al 1984 Acquired immunodeficiency syndrome in the United States: an analysis of cases outside high incidence groups. Annals of Internal Medicine 101: 617–623

Cheingsong-Popov R, Weiss R A, Dalgleish A et al 1984 Prevalence of antibody to human T lymphotropic virus type III in AIDS and AIDS risk patients in Britain. Lancet ii: 477–480

Chretein J H, McGinnis C G, Muller A 1977 Venereal causes of cytomegalovirus mononucleosis. Journal of the American Medical Association 238: 1644–1645

Christensen K K, Christensen P, Flamholg L, Ripa T 1974 Frequencies of streptococci of groups A, B, C, D, and G in urethra and cervix swab specimens from patients with suspected gonococcal infection. Acta Pathologica Microbiologica Scandinavica (B) 82: 470–474

Communicable Disease Surveillance Centre and the Academic Department of Genito Urinary Medicine 1985 Sexually transmitted diseases 1983. British Medical Journal 291: 528–530

Corey L, Holmes K K, Benedetti J, Critchlow C 1981 Clinical course of genital herpes: implications for therapeutic trials. In: Nahmias A J, Dowdle W R, Schinazi F (eds) The human herpes virus. Elsevier, New York, pp. 496–502

Curran J W 1980 Economic consequences of pelvic inflammatory disease in the United States. American Journal of Obstetrics and Gynecology 132, 2: 848–851

Davidson F 1977 Yeasts and circumcision in the male. British Journal of Venereal Diseases 53: 121–123

Davies J A, Rees K, Hobson D, Karayiannis P 1978 Isolation of chlamydia trachomatis from Bartholin's ducts. British Journal of Venereal Diseases 54: 409–413

Douglas J, Schmidt O, Corey L 1983 Acquisition of neonatal HSV 1 infection from a paternal source contact. Journal of Pediatrics 103(6): 908–910

Driscoll A M, Mccoy D R, Nicol C S, Barrow J 1970 Sexually

transmitted disease in gynaecological out-patients with vaginal discharge. British Journal of Venereal Diseases 46: 125

Dunkelburg W E 1977 Corynebacterium vaginale. Sexually Transmitted Diseases 1: 69–75

Eschenbach D A 1975 Polymicrobial etiology of acute pelvic inflammatory diseases. New England Journal of Medicine 293: 166–171

Eschenbach D A, Harrish J P, Holmes K K 1977 Pathogenesis of acute pelvic inflammatory disease: role of contraception and other risk factors. American Journal of Obstetrics and Gynecology 128: 838

Falk V 1965 Treatment of acute non-tuberculous salpingitis with antibiotics alone and in combination with glucocorticoids. A prospective double blind controlled study of the clinical course and prognosis. Acta Obstetrica Gynecologica Scandinavica 44 (Suppl 6): 3

Fleming W L, Brown W S, Donohue J F, Branigin P W 1970 National survey of venereal disease treated by physicians in 1968. Journal of the American Medical Association 211: 1827

Florman A L, Gershon A A, Blackett P R, Nahmias A J 1973 Intrauterine infection with herpes simplex virus. Resultant congenital malformations. Journal of the American Medical Association 225: 129–132

Franciosi R A, Knostman J D, Zimmerman R A 1973 Group B streptococcal neonatal and infant infection. Journal of Pediatrics 82: 707

Francis D P, Herrman K L, MacMahon J R, Chavigny J R, Sanderlin K C 1975 Nosocomial and maternally acquired herpesvirus hominis infections. A report of four cases in neonates. American Journal of Diseases in Children 129: 889–893

Frenkel N, Roizman B, Cassai E, Nahmias A 1972 A DNA fragment of herpes simplex 2 and its transcription in human cervical cancer tissue. Proceedings of the National Academy of Science USA 69: 3734–3789

Friedman-Kien A, Laubenstein L, Marmor M et al 1981 Kaposi's sarcoma and pneumocystis among homosexual men— New York City and California. Morbidity and Mortality Weekly Report 30: 305–308

Friedman-Kien A, Laubenstein L J, Rubinstein P et al 1982 Disseminated Kaposi's sarcoma in homosexual men. Annals of Internal Medicine 96: 693–700

Frommell G T, Rothenberg R, Wang S-P, McIntosh K 1979 Chlamydial infection of mothers and their infants. Journal of Pediatrics 95: 28–32

Gallo R C, Savin P S, Gelman E P et al 1983 Isolation of human T cell leukaemia virus in acquired immune deficiency syndrome (AIDS). Science 220: 865–867

Gardner H L, Dukes C D 1955 Haemophilus vaginalis vaginitis. American Journal of Obstetrics and Gynecology 69: 962–976

Goldacre M J, Watt B, Loudon N, Milne L S R, Loudon J D O, Vessey M P 1979 Vaginal microbial flora in normal young women. British Medical Journal 2: 1450–1453

Gottlieb M S, Schanker H M, Fan P T, Saxon A, Weisman J D, Pzalski I 1981a Pneumocystis pneumonia—Los Angeles. Morbidity and Mortality Weekly Reports 30: 250–252

Gottlieb M S, Schroff R, Schanker H M et al 1981b Pneumocystis carinii pneumonia and mucosal candidiasis in previously healthy homosexual men: evidence of a new acquired cellular immunodeficiency. New England Journal of Medicine 305: 1425–1431

Grech E S, Everett J V, Mukasa F 1972 Epidemiological aspects of acute pelvic inflammatory disease in Uganda. Tropical Doctor 3: 123–127

Griffiths P D, Campbell-Benzie A, Heath R B 1980 A prospective study of primary cytomegalovirus infection in pregnant women. British Journal of Obstetrics and Gynaecology 87: 308–314

Grizburg H M, Weiss S H, MacDonald et al HTLV III exposure among drug users. Cancer Research (in press)

Hammerschlag M R, Anderka M, Semine D Z, McComb D, McCormack W M 1979 Prospective study of maternal and infantile infection with C trachomatis. Pediatrics 64: 142–148

Harrison H R, Alexander E R 1984 Chlamydia trachomatis infection of the infant. In: Holmes K K, Mardh P A, Sparling P T, Weisner P J (eds) Sexually transmitted diseases. McGraw Hill, New York, pp. 207–280

Hedberg E, Speyz S O 1958 Acute salpingitis. Views on prognosis and treatment. Acta Obstetrica Gynecologica Scandinavica 37: 131

Hill H R 1984 Group B streptococcal infections. In: Holmes K K, Mardh P A, Sparling P F, Weisner P J (eds) Sexually transmitted diseases. McGraw-Hill Book, New York, pp 397–407

Hilton A L, Richmond S J, Milne J D, Hindley F, Clark S K R 1974 Chlamydia A in the female genital tract. British Journal of Venereal Diseases 50: 1–9

Hindley D J, Adler M W 1985 Genital herpes: an increasing problem? Genitourinary Medicine 61: 56–58

Holmes K K, Handsfield H H, Wang S P et al 1975 Etiology of non-gonococcal urethritis. New England Journal of Medicine 292: 1199–1206

Holtz F 1930 Klinische Studien über die nicht tuberkulose Salpingoophritis. Acta Obstetrica Gynecologica Scandinavica 10 (Suppl 1)

Hopcroft M, Verhagen A R, Ngigi S, Haya A C A 1973 Genital infections in developing countries: experience in a family planning clinic. Bulletin of the World Health Organization 48: 581–586

Horn K A, Zimmerman R A, Knostman J D, Meyer W T 1974 Neurological sequelae of group B streptococcal neonatal infections. Pediatrics 53: 501

Hughes W H, Davies J M 1971 Better specimens from the female genital tract. British Medical Journal 4: 424–425

Hymes K B, Cheung T, Greene J B 1981 Kaposi's sarcoma in homosexual men—a report of eight cases. Lancet ii: 598–600

Jeansson S, Molin L 1974 On the occurrence of genital herpes simplex virus infection. Acta Dermatologica 54: 479–485

Jordan C M, Rousseau W E, Noble G R, Stewart J A, Chin T D Y 1973 Association of cervical cytomegaloviruses with venereal disease. New England Journal of Medicine 288: 932–934

Josey W E, Lambe D W 1976 Epidemiological characteristics of women infected with corynebacterium vaginale. Journal of the American Venereal Disease Association 3: 9–13

Kaufman D W, Watson, Rosenburg L et al 1980 Intrauterine contraceptive device use and pelvic inflammatory disease. American Journal of Obstetrics and Gynecology 136: 159–162

Krech U 1973 Complement fixing antibodies against cytomegalovirus in different parts of the world. Bulletin of the World Health Organization 49: 103

Kumar M L, Nankervis G A, Jacobs I B et al 1984 Congenital and post natally acquired cytomegalovirus infection: long term follow up. Journal of Pediatrics 104: 674–679

Light I J 1979 Postnatal acquisition of HSV by the newborn infant: a review of the literature. Pediatrics 63: 480–482

Linneman C C Jr, Buchman T G, Light I J, Ballard J L, Roizman B 1975 Transmission of herpes simplex type I in a nursery for new born. Identification of viral isolates from DNA 'finger printing'. Lancet i: 964–966

Lithgow D M, Rubin A 1972 Gynaecology in Southern Africa.

Witwatersrand University Press, Johannesburg

McCormack W M, Alpert S, McComb D E, Nichols R L, Semine Z, Zinner S H 1979 Fifteen month follow-up study of women infected with C trachomatis. New England Journal of Medicine 300: 123–125

Macdonald Burns D C, Darougar S, Thin R N, Lothian L, Nicol C S 1975 Isolation of chlamydia from women attending a clinic for sexually transmitted diseases. British Journal of Venereal Diseases 51: 314–318

McDougall J K, Galloway D A, Fenoglio C M. 1980 Cervical carcinoma: detection of herpes simplex virus RNA in cells undergoing neoplastic change. International Journal of Cancer 25: 1–8

Malouf M, Fortier M, Moran G, Dube J -L 1981 Treatment of Haemophilus vaginalis vaginitis. Obstetrics and Gynecology 57: 711–714

Mardh P A 1977 Chlamydia trachomatis infection in patients with acute salpingitis. New England Journal of Medicine 296: 1377–1379

Moll B, Emeson E E, Small C B et al 1982 Inverted ratios of inducer to suppressor and lymphocyte subsets in drug abusers with opportunistic infections. Clinical Immunology and Immuno Pathology 25(3): 417–423

MMWR 1982 Genital herpes infection United States 1966–1979 31: 137–139

Nabarro J M, Grant A M, Simon R, Beral V, Catterall R D 1978 Screening for gonorrhoea in a central London family planning clinic. Fertility and Contraception 2: 1–4

Nahmias A J 1974 The Torch syndrome of perinatal infections. Hospital Practice 9: 65

Nahmias A J, Alford C A, Korones S B 1970 Infection of the newborn with herpes virus hominis. Advances in Pediatrics 17: 185–226

Nahmias A J, Josey W E, Naib Z M et al 1971 Perinatal risk associated with maternal genital herpes simplex virus infection. American Journal of Obstetrics and Gynaecology 110: 825–837

Nayyar K C, O'Neill J J, Hambling M H, Waugh M A 1976 Isolation of Chlamydia trachomatis from women attending a clinic for sexually transmitted diseases. British Journal of Venereal Diseases 52: 396–398

Oriel J D, Partridge B M, Denny M S, Coleman J C 1972a Genital yeast infection. British Medical Journal 4: 761–764

Oriel J D, Reeve P, Powis P A, Miller A, Nicol C S 1972b Chlamydial infection: isolation of chlamydia from patients with non-specific genital infection. British Journal of Venereal Diseases 48: 429–436

Oriel J D, Pouris P A, Reeve P, Miller A, Nicol C S 1974 Chlamydia infections of the cervix. British Journal of Venereal Diseases 50: 11–16

Oriel J D, Waterworth P M 1975 Effect of minocycline and tetracycline on the vaginal yeast flora. Journal of Clinical Pathology 28: 403–406

Osler W 1917 The campaign against venereal disease. British Medical Journal i: 694–696

Osoba A O 1981a Lymphogranuloma venereum In: Harris J R W (ed) Recent advances in sexually transmitted disease 2. Churchhill Livingstone, London

Osoba A O 1981b Sexually transmitted diseases in tropical Africa: a review of the present situation. British Journal of Venereal Diseases 57: 89–94

Osoba A O, Onifade A 1973 Venereal diseases among women in Ibadan. West African Medical Journal 22: 23–25

Pacsa A S, Kummaerlander L, Pejtsik B, Pali K 1975 Herpesvirus antibodies and antigen in patients with cervical anaplasia

and in controls. Journal of the National Cancer Institute 55: 775

Pass R F, Stagno S, Myers G J, Alford C A 1980 Outcome of symptomatic congenital cytomegalovirus infection; results of long-term longitudinal follow-up. Pediatrics 66: 658–662

Peutherer J F, Smith I W, Robertson D H H 1982 Genital infection with herpes simplex virus type 1. Journal of Infection 4: 33–35

Pheifer T A, Forsyth P, Durfree M A, Pollock H M, Holmes K K 1978 Non-specific vaginitis role of Haemophilus vaginalis and treatment with metronidazole. New England Journal of Medicine 298: 1429–1434

Piot P, Quinn T C, Taelman H et al 1984 Acquired immunodeficiency syndrome in a heterosexual population in Zaire. Lancet ii: 65–69

Ratnam A V, Din S N, Chatterjee T K 1980 Gonococcal infection in women with pelvic inflammatory disease in Lusaka, Zambia. American Journal of Obstetrics and Gynecology 138: 965–968

Rawls W E, Campione-Piccardo J 1981 Epidemiology of herpes simplex virus type 1 and type 2 infections. In: Nahmias A J, Dowdle W R, Schinazi F (eds) The human herpesviruses. Elsevier, New York

Rawls W E, Tompkins W A F, Melnick J L 1969 The association of herpesvirus type 2 and carcinoma of the uterine cervix. American Journal of Epidemiology 89: 547–554

Redfield R R, Rhkam P D, Salahuddin J Z 1985 Heterosexual promiscuity: an emerging risk factor for HTLV III disease? Paper presented at International Conference on Acquired Immunodeficiency Syndrome (AIDS) April 14–17 1985, Atlanta

Rees E 1980 The treatment of pelvic inflammatory disease. Annals of Obstetrics and Gynecology 138: 1042–1047

Rees D A, Hamlett J D 1972 Screening for gonorrhoea in pregnancy. Journal of Obstetrics and Gynaecology of the British Commonwealth 79: 344–347

Ridgway G L, Oriel J D 1977 Interrelationship of C trachomatis and other pathogens in the female genital tract. Journal of Clinical Pathology 30: 933–936

Schachter J, Grossman M, Holt J, Sweet R, Goodner E, Mills J 1979 Prospective study of chlamydial infection in neonates. Lancet ii: 377–379

Scragg R F R 1957 Depopulation in New Ireland: a study of demography and fertility. Administration of Papua and New Guinea

Shapira H E 1965 Studies on metronidazole (flagyl) in the therapy of urogenital trichomoniasis in the male patient. Journal of Urology 93: 303–306

Silverstone P I, Snodgrass C A, Wigfield A S 1974 Value of screening for gonorrhoea in obstetrics and gynaecology. British Journal of Venereal Diseases 50: 53–56

Simmons P D, Forsey T, Thin R N et al 1979 Antichlamydia antibodies in pelvic inflammatory disease. British Journal of Venereal Diseases 55: 419–424

Sparks R A, Williams O L, Boyce J M H, Fitzgerald T C, Shelley G 1975 Antenatal screening for candidiasis, trichomoniasis and gonorrhoea. British Journal of Venereal Diseases 61: 110–115

Stagno S, Pass R F, Dworsky M E, Alford C A 1983 Congenital and perinatal cytomegalovirus infection. Seminars Perinatal 7: 31–42

Stern H, Elek S D 1965 The evidence of infection with cytomegalovirus in a normal population. A serological study in Greater London. Journal of London 65: 79–87

Sullivan-Bolyai J, Hull H F, Wilson C, Corey L 1983 Neonatal herpes simplex virus infection in King County, Washington.

Increasing incidence and epidemiologic correlates. Journal of American Medical Association 250: 3059–3062

Summers J L, Ford M L 1972 The Papanicolaou smear as a diagnostic tool in male trichomoniasis. Journal of Urology 107: 840–842

Targum S D, Wright N H 1974 Association of the intrauterine device and pelvic inflammatory disease: a retrospective pilot study. American Journal of Epidemiology 100: 262–271

Taylor E, Blackwell A L, Barlow D, Phillips I 1982 Gardnerella vaginalis, anaerobes and vaginal discharge. Lancet i: 1376–1379

Terho P 1978 Chlamydia trachomatis in non-specific urethritis. British Journal of Venereal Diseases 54: 251–256

Thin R N, Michael A N 1970 Sexually transmitted disease in antenatal patients. British Journal of Venereal Diseases 46: 126–128

Thin R N, Leighton M, Dixon M J 1977 How often is genital yeast infection sexually transmitted? British Medical Journal 2: 93–94

Treharne J D, Ripa K T, Mardh P A, Svensson L, Weström L, Darougar S 1979 Antibodies to C trachomatis in acute salpingitis. British Journal of Venereal Diseases 55: 26–29

Van de Perre P, Rouvroy D, LePage P et al 1984 Acquired immunodeficiency syndrome in Rwanda. Lancet ii: 62–65

Viesa J, Frank E, Spira T J, Landesman S H 1983 Acquired immune deficiency in Haitians: opportunistic infections in previously healthy Haitian immigrants. New England Journal of Medicine 308: 124–129

Vontver L A, Hickok D E, Brown Z, Reid L, Corey L 1982 Recurrent genital herpes virus infection in pregnancy: infant outcome and frequency of asymptomatic recurrences. American Journal of Obstetrics and Gynaecology 143: 75–84

Watt L, Jennison R F 1960 Incidence of trichomonas vaginalis in marital partners. British Journal of Venereal Diseases 36: 163–166

Wentworth B B, Bonin P, Holmes K K, Gutman L, Wiesnar P, Alexander E R 1973 Isolation of viruses, bacteria and other organisms from venereal disease clinics and patients: methodology and problems associated with multiple isolation. Health Laboratory Sciences 10: 75–81

Weström L 1975 Effect of acute pelvic inflammatory disease on fertility. American Journal of Obstetrics and Gynecology 121: 707–713

Weström L 1980 Incidence, prevalence and trends of pelvic inflammatory disease and its consequences in industrialised countries. American Journal of Obstetrics and Gynaecology 138: 880

Weström L, Bengtsson L P, Mardh P A 1976 The risk of pelvic inflammatory disease in women using intrauterine contraceptive devices as compared to non-users. Lancet 2: 221

Whittington M J 1957 Epidemiology of infections with trichomonas vaginalis in the light of improved diagnostic methods. British Journal of Venereal Diseases 33: 80–91

Willcox R R 1975 Importance of the so called 'other' sexually transmitted disease. British Journal of Disease 51: 221–226

Wolontis S, Jeansson S 1977 Correlations of herpes simplex virus type 1 and 2 with clinical features of infection. Journal of Infectious Diseases 135: 28–33

Working Party of the Confidential Enquiry into Gynaecological Laparoscopy 1978 Gynaecological laparoscopy. British Journal of Obstetrics and Gynaecology 85: 401.

Wormser G P, Krupp L B, Hanrahan J P et al 1983 Acquired immunodeficiency syndrome in male prisoners. Annals of Internal Medicine 98: 297–303

Wright H J, Palmer A 1978 The prevalence and clinical diagnosis of vaginal candidosis in non-pregnant patients with vaginal discharge and pruritis vulvae. Journal of the Royal College of General Practitioners 28: 719–723

Yaeger A S, Ashley R L, Corey L 1983 Transmission of herpes simplex from father to neonate. Journal of Pediatrics 103(6): 905–907

Zeigler J L, Daw W I, Miler R C 1982 Outbreak of Burkitt's like lymphoma in homosexual men. Lancet ii: 631–633

Zur Hausen H 1982 Human genital cancer: synergism between two virus infections or synergism between a virus infection and initiating events? Lancet ii: 1370–1372

PART II

The investigation of infection in the female genital tract

The diagnosis of lower genital tract infection
M J Hare

THE NORMAL FEMALE LOWER GENITAL TRACT AND ITS EXAMINATION

Techniques of examination

In the examination of the female genital tract two factors are of paramount importance: good exposure and good lighting. The former is sometimes very difficult to achieve, particularly when modesty, fear or cultural background lead to reluctance to be examined, especially by a male doctor. Under such circumstances female staff should, whenever possible, conduct the examination and gently coax the woman into the best available position. The advice following in this chapter represents the ideal situation.

Position for examination

Although British and some European doctors have in the past favoured either the left lateral or Sims' semiprone position for gynaecological examination, this has little to recommend it when the possible diagnosis is genital tract infection. The dorsal position is to be preferred, and the examination couch should be designed specifically for such examination. The woman to be examined rests on it in a semisitting position; the back of the couch should be adjustable to her comfort. Her legs are supported either by knee crutches or projecting ankle stirrups, whichever she prefers; and these are both adjustable to height and length. The examining doctor or nurse sits between her legs with a light source from over his shoulder, or he may prefer to use a headlamp. The couch should be adjustable for height and also for head-town tilt; this latter is most important for examination of the cervix when the uterus is acutely retroflexed or retroverted,

when the vagina is angled more toward the ventral surface of the body and the cervix points upwards. A tray positioned under the buttocks can be used to receive used instruments and soiled swabs, and also catch spilt fluid if the vagina is washed out with diagnostic solutions such as acetic acid.

Instruments

Clean instruments should be laid up on a trolley beside the examining doctor or nurse. These should comprise the following:

Vaginal specula. There are three basic patterns of vaginal specula available for diagnostic uses: the single-bladed (or Sims') pattern, the double-bladed adjustable self-retaining pattern (sometimes referred to as the duckbill or Cusco speculum) and the cylindrical (or Ferguson) pattern. For most aspects of the examination for genital tract infection the Cusco instrument is the best. In its closed form it is easy to pass into the vagina, and on opening the instrument the cervix comes readily into view. With the blade locked open by the screw the instrument is self-retaining, freeing both the examiner's hands. The view of the cervix is good but somewhat distorted, especially if the woman is parous or the external os is broad, for the canal will gape open giving the impression that the columnar cell tissue spreading on to the cervix (the cervical 'erosion') is larger than it actually is. The vagina is seen less well with the Cusco speculum, and special care must be taken not to miss lesions in the anterior and posterior fornices.

If the vagina needs to be examined in more detail than is possible with the Cusco instrument then the single-bladed Sims' speculum will provide a better view of the walls. In the highly parous woman the vagina may be very loose and lax, and additional specula and even side wall retractors such as those used in gynaecological surgery may be needed.

Cleaning materials. Once initial tests have been taken on any vaginal discharge that is present this should be wiped away to allow detailed inspection of the epithelial surfaces, and the taking of uncontaminated specimens from the more localised secretions. This can be done with gauze swabs held on the end of a sponge-holding forceps (Rampleys pattern). Cotton wool balls can be used as an alternative to gauze, but these sometimes leave fluffy threads behind on the area cleaned. A third option is to use 'Rocket' pattern disposable swabs which will absorb up to 3 ml fluid; these are an ideal shape and size.

Endocervical speculum. It is sometimes necessary to examine the inside of the endocervical canal, especially when looking for warts or polyps. This is best done with an endocervical speculum of the Kogan pattern.

Biopsy instruments and curettes. With the recent acknowledgement of the importance of wart virus infection in the genital tract even those who regard themselves as purely physicians may feel that they need to take tissue biopsies under certain circumstances. There are many patterns of small biopsy forceps available for this use but probably the best are the Eppendorfer pattern. It is essential that the forceps take a clean bite from the tissue to be sampled, and do not crush either the specimen for examination or the remaining area.

Lesions just inside the endocervical canal can sometimes be removed best using an endocervical curette rather than a biopsy forceps. The Kevorkian pattern is well designed, but should contain a basket behind its blade to receive the specimen— otherwise it is very easily lost on removal.

Tissue-holding forceps. Not infrequently on passage of the bivalve speculum the cervix is found to be angled to a degree that makes it impossible to see clearly the whole of the area surrounding the external os. Under these circumstances it is sometimes necessary to grasp the cervix and gently pull it forward into view. The traditional instrument for this purpose is the vulsellum, which is effectively fastened on to the cervix with three teeth. This often causes bleeding from that organ and its application can be painful; it is better not used in the conscious patient. The single-toothed variant (or tentenaculum) is kinder but less efficient, and the author's preference is to use a tissue-holding forceps for the purpose. Allis' pattern are gentle but probably not stout enough for the purpose: Littlewood's pattern are probably the best overall.

Sequence of genital tract examination

Relevant general examination

The examining doctor or nurse must decide on the detail to which a general examination should be performed in each case. When genital tract infection is a possible diagnosis a brief comment should be made on the general state of the woman: fitness, build, nutrition etc. The state of the hair, skin and mucous membranes should be noted, and palpation carried out for generalised lymph node enlargement. Many would also suggest that clinical examination for whatever reason gives an opportunity for preventative screening health measures, such as the recording of arterial blood pressure and breast palpation.

Superficial inspection

The vulva and perianal area should be inspected first. The inguinal lymph nodes are palpated for enlargement or tenderness, and the pubic hair examined for lice. The general condition of the vulva and surrounding skin is noted, including that of the anal margin. As well as obvious lesions such as condylomata the quality of the vulval skin is important, with the possibility of hypoplastic or hyperplastic change. Ulceration, both painful and painfree, should be sought and self-inflicted damage due to scratching. The sites of Bartholin's glands should be palpated for cystic swelling and tenderness.

Passage of the vaginal speculum

At this point a bivalve vaginal speculum is passed into the vagina to expose the cervix, having been previously warmed to body temperature. If the woman is in the position for examination already described and is well relaxed the passage of the speculum should require no force and cause no pain. Usually the instrument is positioned with the handle downwards, and if the labia are parted prior to its insertion it will slide in without being turned. This is preferable to the older technique of inserting it through the closed labia at right angles to its final position and turning it as it is pushed it. Once the instrument is in the vagina to its full depth the blades are separated to expose the cervix. Normally this will appear in a satisfactory 'end-on' view but further movement of the instrument may be necessary if the view obtained is unsatisfactory. Once an adequate view has been obtained the instrument is locked in the open position by a screw or a ratchet mechanism.

If the woman is in her reproductive years and the vagina is healthy, the normal secretions will be enough to provide lubrication for a smooth metal speculum and no added lubrication will be needed. However, if the vagina is inflamed or atrophic or the woman being examined is tense or poorly relaxed, then additional lubrication helps. This is also a help if she is menstruating, and especially if she has been using an internal tampon. Plastic specula are often more difficult to insert than the metal instruments, and more often need added lubrication. Tap water may be an adequate lubricant in some cases, but proprietary lubricants such as KY jelly are better. The jelly must *not* contain any antimicrobial preservative and should be used very sparingly so as not to dilute the material taken for culture or cytological investigation.

Inspection of the upper vagina and cervix

Although the bivalve speculum will hide the anterior and posterior walls of the vagina, at this point the lateral walls can be inspected for signs of infection, ulceration and warty growth. A sample of vaginal discharge is taken with a spatula or wire loop from the vaginal side wall or the pool of discharge in the posterior vaginal fornix, and this is emulsified in a drop of normal saline. Microscopic examination of this emulsion will reveal the presence of *Trichomonas vaginalis*, *Candida albicans* and other yeasts, 'clue' cells suggestive of *Gardnerella vaginalis* infection, polymorphonuclear leucocytes and a range of epithelial cells. Vaginal secretion can also be smeared directly on to a microscope slide and heat fixed for staining by

Gram's method. A general bacterial picture can be obtained from a culture swab either plated directly or stored in transport medium such as Stuart's or Amies'. Specialised cultures for *C. albicans*, *T. vaginalis* and mycoplasmas may be taken at this point.

The cervix is now inspected for evidence of inflammation, ulceration and warty growth. The normal appearance of the cervix is fully described in the section on colposcopy and reference should be made to that section for details of normal variation. The diagnosis of 'cervicitis' is especially difficult to make. Next a cervical scrape is taken with a wooden spatula and the material obtained smeared thinly on a microscope slide. This is immediately treated with a chemical fixative for staining by Papanicolaou's method; examination of this may reveal evidence of premalignant disease, and evidence of infection with herpes virus, wart virus, *T. vaginalis*, *C. albicans* and various other pathogens.

The cervix is next cleaned free of discharge and blood, to allow specimens to be taken from the endocervical canal without contamination. These may be taken with a wire loop, a conventional bacterial swab or a fine swab on a thin wire. Smears can be made for staining by Gram's method and by special techniques such as immunofluorescence for chlamydia. Cultures for the gonococcus may be plated immediately or placed in transport medium; specialised media are available for other organisms such as chlamydia. Should any areas of the cervix present a suspicious appearance (including warty growth) colposcopy and biopsy are essential.

Inspection of the lower vagina and urethral orifice

The vaginal speculum is now slowly withdrawn, allowing inspection of the previously concealed partition of the vaginal wall. This also 'milks' the urethra downwards towards its orifice, and any discharge which has collected in it presents there. This discharge can be sampled by smear and culture as previously described. The urethral introitus should be carefully inspected for inflammation, and in the elderly for prolapse and the presence of a caruncle, Skene's glands may be enlarged, and pressure on them may result in the discharge of pus.

Bimanual examination

Having completed the inspection and microbiological sampling of the lower genital tract, bimanual examination should be performed. For this the woman should have an empty bladder, whilst for the examination so far the bladder should *not* have been recently emptied as this would have washed away discharge, especially from the urethra. At this point, therefore, the woman should be asked to pass urine. This specimen should be tested for protein, ketones and sugar; and if the symptoms suggest a possible urinary tract infection a midstream specimen should be obtained for bacterial culture.

With the woman in the dorsal position the right-handed examiner should slip the gloved and lubricated middle and index fingers of his right hand into the vagina, whilst his left hand is placed on the abdomen immediately above the pubic symphysis. With the examining fingers in the *anterior* fornix of the vagina, the uterus in a normal position of *anteflexion* and *anteversion* will be between the examiner's two hands. It can be felt as a firm cylindrical mass some 10 cm long and 5 cm in diameter, broader at the top and tapering to the cervix. It should move freely on pressure, and although its palpation may be uncomfortable it should not be painful.

If the examiner now moves his left hand to the right and left of the uterus in turn, and his fingers in the vagina to the right and left fornices, he will be palpating the area containing the fallopian tube and ovary on each side. In the slim and well-relaxed subject the ovaries are certainly palpable, but this will not always be so in the normal subject. Generally speaking a palpable mass in the area of the fallopian tube or ovary should raise the question of an abnormal swelling. Similarly tenderness or pain experienced by the woman on bimanual palpation suggests disease, with the possible exception of tenderness in one ovary elicited around midcycle at the time of ovulation, which can be due to a tense developing follicle about to rupture at ovulation.

If no mass is felt anteriorly when the examiner's fingers are in the anterior fornix of the vagina, it should be concluded that the uterus is not anteflexed and anteverted in position. The examiner's fingers should next be placed in the posterior fornix when the uterus may be felt in an axial position (that is, in a line with the axis of the vagina) or in a retroverted position. The position of the cervix will give a guide to this: in anteversion it will point backwards, in retroversion it will point forwards towards the pubic symphysis and in the axial position it will be between these two. In full retroversion the body of the uterus will not be felt between the hands on bimanual examination as it is tucked away in the curve of the sacrum; under these circumstances the only way to palpate uterus, tubes and ovaries bimanually is with one finger in the anorectal canal.

It must be stressed that retroversion of itself is not a pathological condition. Up to a third of adult women will be found on examination to have a retroverted uterus, especially if they have borne children. Most of these will have a freely mobile pelvis, and if they are examined in a forward leaning position such as Sim's semiprone, the uterus will be found to have fallen forwards. As long as the uterus is freely mobile there should be no clinical problems. If the uterus is fixed in retroversion, perhaps by adhesions due to past pelvic inflammatory disease or endometriotic scarring, then clinical symptoms may occur. However the fixed retroverted uterus that is not causing symptoms can generally be left alone.

Examination of the anorectal canal

It is generally taught that no examination for genital tract infection in women is complete without examination of the anorectal canal, and certainly a number of patients will have obvious proctitis from which *Neisseria gonorrhoeae*, *Chlamydia trachomatis* and other organisms may be isolated. Nevertheless the practice of routine proctoscopy is physically uncomfortable for patient and mentally so for their attendants; one group reported frankly that, in a series of cases: 'The taking of anal specimens was discontinued primarily because of the reticence of both patients and examining physicians'. However in cases where the woman is thought likely to be suffering from sexually transmitted disease it is probably worth suggesting to the woman that the test is worthwhile. In earlier reports on gonorrhoea in women the anorectal canal was the only site of identification of the organism in up to 9% of cases: more recently, probably due to improved methods of detection at all sites, the proportion has dropped to 2% (Kinghorn & Rashid 1979); in my own series where direct and indirect immunofluorescence was used as well as conventional smears and cultures the proportion of cases where gonococcal proctitis was diagnosed without coexisting genital gonorrhoea was only 1.5% (Hare 1971) (see Plate 41).

Regarding *C. trachomatis*, Dunlop and others (1970) reported that of 28 women who presented because of signs of chlamydial disease in themselves, their sexual partners or their newborn children and for whom *C. trachomatis* was isolated, 13 produced rectal isolates and in one of these cases the rectum was the only site of isolation (see Plate 42). Vaughan-Jackson and others (1972) reported rectal isolates from 11 of 21 women who presented because of proven chlamydial eye disease, but in that series all were accompanied by cervical isolates as well. The rectal canal may also be infected by viral disease such as *Condylomata accuminata* and herpetic eruptions. The author is not aware of any data on the incidence of asymptomatic infection of the rectum by these organisms in the absence of genital site involvement.

If one accepts that routine proctoscopy is an unpleasant and distasteful procedure, and may have an adverse effect on future attendance by the patient and her acquaintants, it is necessary to justify the procedure before adopting it as routine. This would need to be on one or more of the following grounds:

1. That isolated infection of the rectum by particular pathogens in the absence of coexisting genital infection was a reasonably frequent occurrence.

2. That such an infection presented a threat to the health of the woman concerned, especially in relation to long-term consequences.

3. That the treatment of rectal infections required a different or higher dosage regime than the treatment of uncomplicated genital infection.

4. That isolated untreated rectal infection in women represents a potential source of reinfection to their sexual partners.

The answer to point 1 would seem to be equivocal, and depend very much on the sensitivity of diagnostic methods. Regarding point 2, gonorrhoeal and chlamydial proctitis in women appear to cause minimal symptoms. Although in the past symptoms of Neisserial proctorrhoea such as rectal bleeding, soreness, tenesmus, diarrhoea, painful defaecation and anorectal discharge were reported and said by one author to occur in over 30% of his patients (Martin 1935), such reports seem to have been associated with the preantibiotic era, and have dwindled markedly since the availability of effective treatment. Thus Dunlop (1963) reported that only 3% of women treated by him for gonorrhoea mentioned rectal symptoms. In a series of 343 women with bacteriologically proven genital gonorrhoea only 59 complained of rectal symptoms, although the gonococcus was identified in the rectum in two-thirds (Hare 1971). In 13 of the 59 cases it was thought that the symptoms were due to coexisting haemorrhoids. Of 308 women in whom the rectal mucosa was examined using a proctoscope 165 (54%) had a normal appearance, 79 (26%) doubtful changes and only 64 (20%) moderate or severe proctitis. Even in the small group of 27 women with clinically severe proctitis over half were asymptomatic. It must be concluded therefore that proctitis in women due to gonorrhoea is a mild and usually asymptomatic condition.

In the same way chlamydial proctitis in women appears to be predominantly asymptomatic. Munday et al (1985) reported that although chlamydial proctitis is more than twice as common as gonococcal proctitis amongst homosexual men, the condition is usually asymptomatic and important only because of the reservoir of infection thus created. Schuch et al (1984) described a case of chlamydial proctitis in a woman which presented as a vaginal mass and was diagnosed on biopsy, but they do not make it clear if the organism involved was of an oculogenital or lymphogranuloma subgroup. In contrast Jacobs (1976) reviewed 16 cases of proctitis due to *Herpes virus hominis* of whom 2 were women and reported symptoms in all. Perianal and anal warts also appear to cause identifiable symptoms.

Regarding the long-term consequences of anorectal infection, the main hazard reported prior to the antibiotic era was that of stricture. In 1923 Sir Charters Symonds gave his Presidential Address to the subsection of Proctology of the Royal Society of Medicine in London on the subject of gonorrhoeal stricture of the rectum, making the claim that the museums of five London teaching hospitals and that of the Royal College of Surgeons of London contained specimens illustrating this condition but wrongly labelled as syphilitic. Hayes (1929) stated that rectal stricture formation was 'fairly frequent' after gonorrhoea, and much more common in negroid rather than white women. This fact he attributed to a greater propensity to keloid scar formation. Since the advent of antibiotic therapy no further reports have appeared.

No long-term consequences appear to have been reported in association with anorectal infection by oculogenital chlamydia, herpes virus or wart virus, although the suggested associations between each of these organisms and lower genital tract cancer in women must pose a question regarding their long-term effects on the lower bowel.

In answer to point 3, some reports from the early years of penicillin treatment, when the single dose used was often under a million units, it was suggested that rectal gonorrhoea required higher doses for adequate treatment than uncomplicated genital infection. However with the routine use of high doses, this was accepted as not so, and for any organism of given sensitivity, an antibiotic schedule adequate to cure genital gonorrhoea may be assumed to be adequate for the rectal involvement (see Chapter 8). There has been no suggestion that chlamydial proctitis requires any different treatment schedule than chlamydial lower genital infection. Warts within the anorectal canal may require local management.

Concerning the fourth point, it has long been a matter of debate as to whether in women anorectal involvement with sexually transmitted organisms is predominantly due to direct inoculation by penoanal intercourse, as it is in men, or due normally to contamination of the anal margins by infected discharges and menstrual loss. This is obviously a significant matter, as if the first proposition is true infection of the male partners will occur from this practice, whilst if the second is the usual avenue of infection, infection of partners is unlikely.

In the past authorities have been divided on their conclusions concerning gonococcal proctitis in women. Most regarded soiling of the anal margins with contaminated vaginal discharge to be the main pathway of infection; their views are summarised by Hayes (1929) and supported by Kinghorn & Rashid (1979). A minority, however, thought heterosexual sodomy to be the usual method of

transfer (see Jensen 1953). Dans (1975) however found no difference in the rate of admission of this practice between those who had rectal involvement and those who did not. No definite evidence is available to link the finding of chlamydial proctitis in women with the practice of penoanal coitus, nor is this so for warty lesions. The reported number of cases of herpetic proctitis in women is too small for a definite conclusion to be made, although Jacobs (1976) has no doubt that the fiery and forthright views expressed by Astric (1736) are correct!

The answer to this question would appear to depend to a degree on the frequency of the practice of heterosexual penoanal coitus, a subject the discussion of which is still apparently taboo in our 'liberated' society. Kinsey et al (1948, 1953) felt unable to question their subjects concerning this, although they did ask about a variety of other sexual practices which are almost universally regarded as deviant. Goldberg & Sutherland (1963) reported that about one-third of men attending a clinic for venereal diseases in Kingston, Jamaica admitted to this practice when asked. The delicacy of the question meant that the present author (Hare 1971) felt able to ask only 125 (36%) of 343 women with gonorrhoea about this practice; 47 (38%) of these answered in the affirmative. Reasons given for the practice included experimentation, partner's request, mechanical difficulty of conventional coitus during pregnancy; a small number mentioned it as a measure to prevent the spread of genital infection. The recent publicity given in the United Kingdom to the risk of transfer of the agent of Aids by various sexual practices has led to further enquiry; Cumberbatch and Debney (1987) report that more than one in ten of a sample of female university students between 18 and 21 years of age had experienced anal intercourse. Interestingly, although penoanal coitus is usually considered a male homosexual practice, Masters & Johnson (1979) reported that this practice leads to frequent sexual orgasm in women, but not in men who adopt the passive role.

In summary, it would seem appropriate that proctoscopy continue as part of the routine examination of women being investigated as possibly infected with sexually transmitted organisms of major importance, such as *Neisseria gonorrhoeae*, *Trepomera pallidum*, *Chlamydia trachomatis*, herpes virus and wart virus. However, due regard must always be paid to the sensitivities and feelings of the women concerned, and the procedure should never be insisted upon, especially in inappropriate cases. If it is undertaken, relevant smears and cultures should be taken. A full discussion of proctitis related to sexually transmitted disease and sexual practice has been compiled by Goldmeier (1985). In his opinion the full range of parasites causing the condition in men need not be sought in women.

Serological tests

Blood can be taken for a variety of serological tests for micro-organisms that could be causing genital disease, and the examinations performed will depend on local interest and availability. Tests for syphilis (see Chapter 7) are routine in venereal disease clinics, antenatal clinics and, in some countries, for premarital screening, and in experienced hands their interpretation is accurate. However serological tests for other agents such as *C. trachomatis*, *N. gonorrhoeae*, and herpes virus are much less useful. Some additional information can be gained by dividing the antibodies detected into IgG and IgM fractions, but generally serial specimens at reasonable intervals are needed for definitive conclusions to be reached.

THE USE OF THE COLPOSCOPE FOR THE EXAMINATION OF THE LOWER GENITAL TRACT

Introduction

Even with good light and good exposure clinical inspection of the lower genital tract with the unaided eye leaves much undetected. In the course of his work on early cervical carcinoma, Hinselman in 1924 designed a low power microscope with which he expected to see early 'mini cancers' not visible to the naked eye. This hope proved unfounded, but he was able to describe definitive patterns indicating premalignant disease and his work laid the foundations for the understanding of the development of cervical carcinoma. It is now accepted that in all aspects of lower genital tract disease the colposcope can be a valuable aid to diagnosis and investigation.

The modern colposcope (see Frontispiece) is a binocular instrument which is either free-standing or attached by an arm to the examination couch. The overall combination of lenses should allow a range of magnification between $\times 6$ and $\times 40$, with a step or zoom progression between them. The basic light source, situated either behind the lens or relayed by glass fibres from a distant source, should be white, but a green filter should be available for the inspection of vascular patterns. A light source of variable intensity is an advantage, as is the means for photography. The working distance from the objective to the cervix should be at least 20 cm, and in the author's opinion ideally 30 cm, to allow room for instruments for manipulating the cervix and the taking of smears, biopsies and cultures to be used in front of the lens.

Although the term 'colposcope' implies that the instrument is for the inspection of the vagina, it is the examination of the uterine cervix which is the most enhanced. It is no exaggeration to say that a 'new world' is opened up in the cervical diagnosis by the use of this instrument. However to take advantage of this the examiner must fully understand the normal development of the cervix, and the semimicroscopic appearances of different tissues, both normal and abnormal.

Techniques involved in colposcopy

The basic colposcopic examination described in this section, follows the method used for the investigation of an abnormal cervical (Pap) smear. If the investigation is being undertaken because of suspected infection rather than premalignant change, then the procedures described earlier in this chapter should be included.

Firstly, having passed the bivalve speculum into the vagina and exposed the cervix, this organ is inspected at low and high magnification. If excessive discharge is present on its surface this should be wiped off with a swab which may be dry or soaked in saline. Features to be noted are the distribution on the cervix of different types of epithelium (columnar and squamous), and the presence of abnormal areas such as warts and polyps. Keratin may be seen in plaques which can be scraped off the cervix revealing the underlying epithelium; keratin may also be associated with warty or premalignant change. Rarely, an area of frank carcinoma may be seen as proliferative or ulcerative disease and this often bleeds profusely when touched. Precancerous change, referred to as cervical intraepithelial neoplasia or CIN, may be identifiable by abnormal vascular patterns, typically mosaicism and punctation. These are due to blood vessels persisting in the superficial layers of the epithelium, when normally they would be absent. Cervicitis and vaginitis may also be identified by an intense vascular pattern, the most typical being the 'strawberry' appearance said to typify trichomonal disease but also present in severe inflammation by other organisms. Vascular patterns are made more striking by the use of a green filter. If needed, a cervical smear should be taken at this point.

Secondly, the cervix is now gently washed with dilute (3–5%) acetic acid. This solution can be applied to the cervix on a swab or as a fine jet directed from a wash bottle. The effect of this solution is to render abnormal tissues opaque, whereas normal tissues remain semitranslucent and hence appear pink. No fully satisfactory explanation has been given for this change, but it seems that the acetic acid acts briefly on the nuclei of individual cells, rendering them opaque, but not on the cytoplasm. Thus the greater the nuclear–cytoplasmic ratio, the more opaque the appearance. These changes fade after a few minutes. As a rule of thumb the more abnormal the cell, the greater the nuclear–cytoplasmic ratio, and hence the more densely opaque the tissues become.

However, premalignant change is not the only reason for an increased nuclear–cytoplasmic ratio. Immaturity of the tissue, due to the presence of active or recent squamous metaplasia, will also give this effect, as will infection due to various agents. Specifically, warty areas can be identified by this technique, whether or not they are associated with CIN.

Thirdly, at this point the examining physician must try to define the positions of the original and present squamocolumnar junctions. The present junction is the easier to identify, being the border between the grape-like projections of columnar epithelium and the flat advancing tongues of squamous metaplasia. In the older woman especially the present squamocolumnar junction may be out of sight within the endocervical canal, and re-

vealed only when the external cervical os is opened using a Kogan intracervical speculum. The original squamocolumnar junction is harder to find; there may be a subtle change in the reaction of the tissues to acetic acid but the most reliable factor is the outer limit of the cervical glands, identified by gland openings or Nabothian follicles (retention cysts). In a minority of cases this border may be beyond the limits of the cervix and actually on the vagina.

Fourthly, an additional technique that is sometimes used is the application of Schiller's or Lugol's iodine solution to the cervix. Healthy mature squamous epithelium contains glycogen, and hence stains deep brown on reaction with iodine. Premalignant squamous epithelium does not, and remains unstained. However, columnar epithelium and immature but otherwise normal squamous epithelium also fail to take up iodine, and infected tissue may not react either. For this reason the iodine test (Schiller's test) is of limited use, and certainly of much less value than the acetic acid test.

Finally, appropriate tests for bacteria, protozoa, mycoplasmas, viruses, chlamydia and treponemes may have been taken at any stage of the examination, bearing in mind the possible antimicrobial effect of acetic acid and the lethal effect of iodine on micro-organisms. At the end of the colposcopic examination biopsies may be taken from atypical areas of the cervix with appearances suggestive of premalignant or malignant change, warts, chlamydial cervicitis, herpetic cervicitis and from any area where the appearance is not understood.

The crater left behind in the cervix after biopsy may bleed. Such bleeding may be controlled by the application of a styptic compound such as Monsell's solution (ferric subsulphate), but in most cases this needs to be combined with a fair degree of pressure exerted through a swab. This pressure may need to be continued for several minutes. In extreme cases such pressure may not be adequate and the cervix may need to be sutured or the vagina tightly packed with a gauze roll; equipment for both of these procedures should be available in the colposcopy clinic. When biopsy has been performed and haemostasis secured, a tampon may be pushed high in the vagina against the cervix to continue pressure; the women should be advised to remove this in 3 to 4 hours. She should be told to avoid coitus and expect 'spotting' for a few days after biopsy.

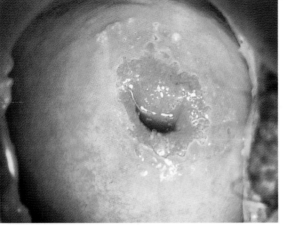

Plate 1

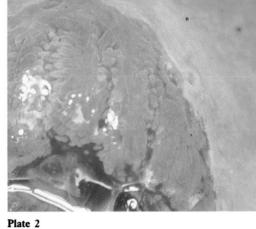

Plate 2

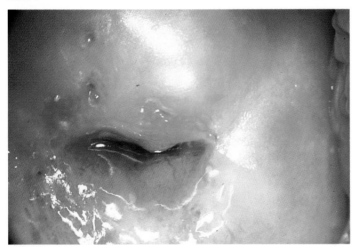

Plate 3

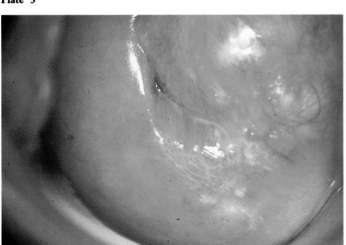

Plate 4

Plate 1 Healthy cervix, showing columnar cell ectopy of cervical 'erosion'.

Plate 2 Magnified view of the squamocolumnar junction. The grape-like projections of columnar epithelium are clearly seen, with crypts and clefts between them. Metaplastic squamous epithelium is encroaching columnar epithelium at the squamocolumnar junction.

Plate 3 Immature squamous metaplasia. The squamocolumnar junction is at the external os. 'Gland' openings are seen in the metaplastic area.

Plate 4 Mature squamous metaplasia. The squamocolumnar junction is out of sight in the endocervical canal. The 'gland' openings have been covered, by squamous epithelium, and the trapped secretory epithelium has produced mucus cysts or Nabothian follicles.

Plate 5 The cervix as seen by the naked eye. The diagnosis of thrush is easy, but who would suspect active herpes or cervical intraepithelial neoplasia?

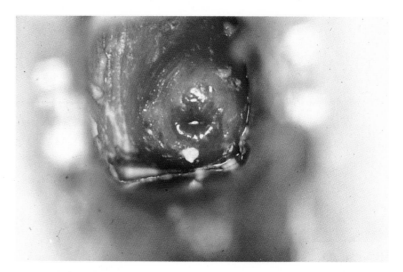

Plate 6 Normal columnar cell erosion. Difficult to assess with the naked eye or colposcope, but made much clearer after treatment with acetic acid.

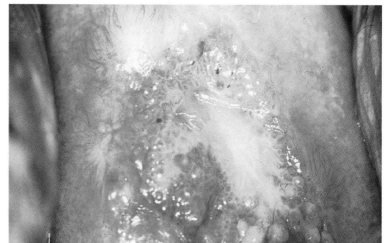

Plate 7 Plate 6 after treatment with acetic acid. Now the pattern of columnar cell ectopy is much clearer.

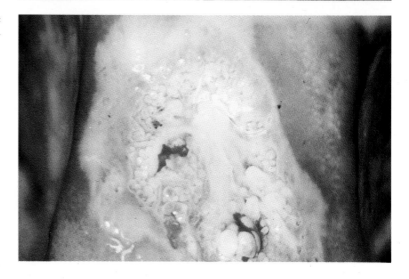

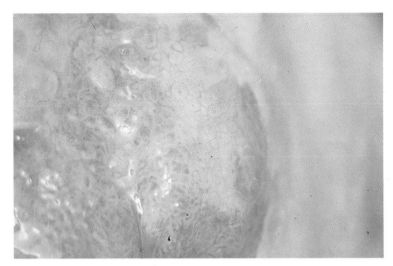

Plate 8 An area of cervical intraepithelial neoplasia grade 3 (CIN 3) showing a mosaic pattern, bounded by columnar epithelium.

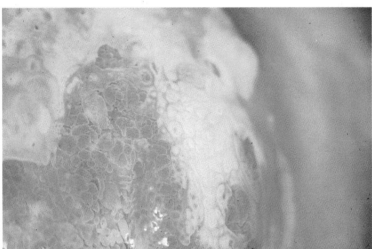

Plate 9 The same area as in Plate 8 after application of acetic acid. The abnormal area has become densely white.

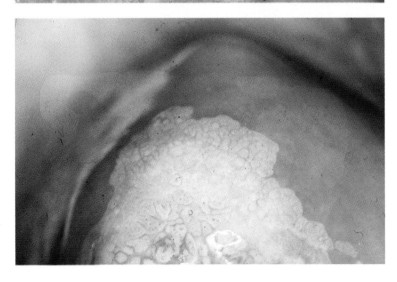

Plate 10 Grade 3 cervical intraepithelial neoplasia. A pronounced pattern of mosaic visible after treatment with acetic acid. Notice the clear-cut boundary between normal and abnormal tissue.

Plate 11 Mosaic pattern seen under high power colposcopy (CIN 3).

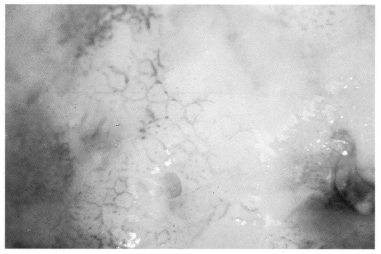

Plate 11

Plate 12 Schiller's test. Weak iodine solution is applied to the cervix. Normal tissue stains brown; abnormal and immature tissue does not take up the colour.

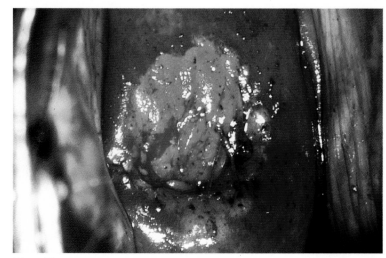

Plate 13 A very small area of CIN 3 in an otherwise normal cervix. To judge the size of the lesion, compare with the string of the intrauterine contraceptive device in the bottom left corner.

Plate 14 High power view of abnormal area showing coarse punctation. Suggestive of microinvasive carcinoma.

Plate 12

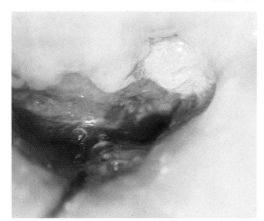

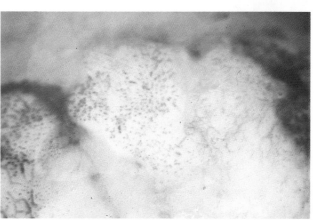

Plate 13

Plate 14

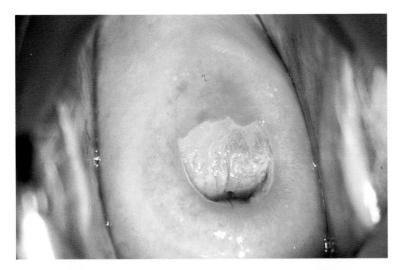

Plate 15 Small area of CIN 2 reaching into the endocervical canal.

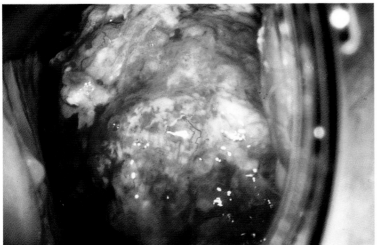

Plate 16 Invasive squamous cell carcinoma of the cervix. A fungating necrotic mass at the top of the vagina.

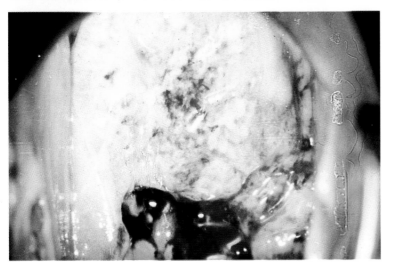

Plate 17 Necrotic, ulcerated cervix due to squamous cell carcinoma.

Plate 18, Plate 19 Cervical carcinoma, removed surgically. This stage I lesion has reached the border between the cervix and the body of the uterus, but not extended outwards.

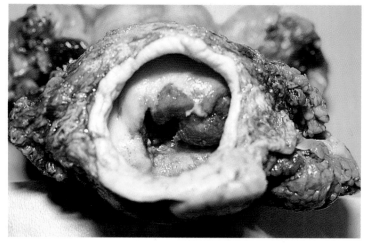

Plate 18

Plate 20 The use of the cervical speculum to allow inspection of the lower part of the endocervical canal.

Plate 21 Histology provides the definitive diagnosis of cervical lesions. Biopsy is easy on the conscious patient, and is seen here using Eppendorfer forceps.

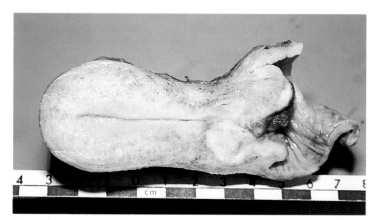

Plate 19

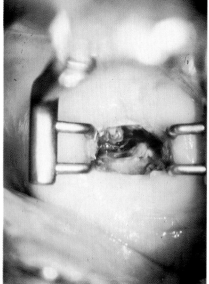

Plate 20

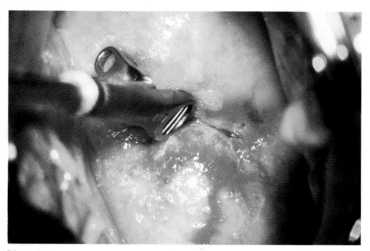

Plate 21

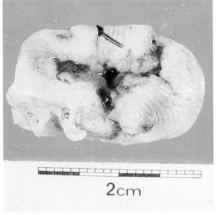

Plate 22

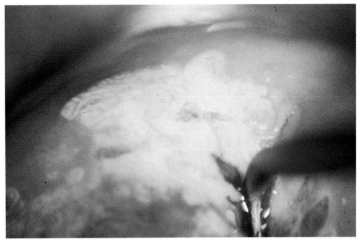

Plate 23

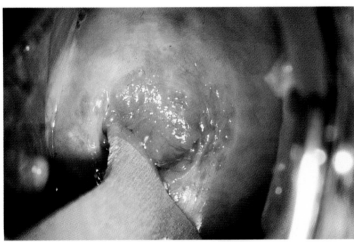

Plate 24

Plate 22 Cone biopsy is needed when the full extent of the lesion is not visible on colposcopy, or where invasive disease is suspected. A cone or cylindrical shaped piece of cervix is removed: the marker suture allows the pathologist to orientate the specimen.

Plate 23 A very dense acetowhite area well away from the endocervical canal. Biopsy showed microinvasive carcinoma.

Plate 24 Cervical smear taking. The spatula must fully scrape the whole of the 'transformation zone' of metaplastic squamous epithelium.

Plate 25 'Non-specific' cervicitis: inflamed columnar epithelium with yellow purulent discharge.

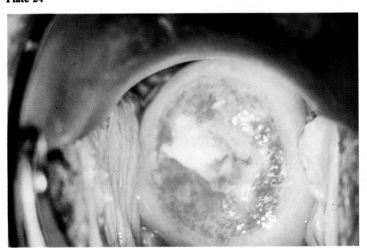

Plate 25

Plate 26 and **Plate 27** Follicular cervicitis related to *Chlamydia trachomatis* infection: general view and close-up of follicles.

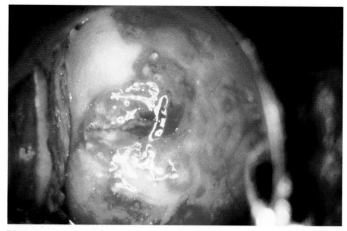

Plate 26

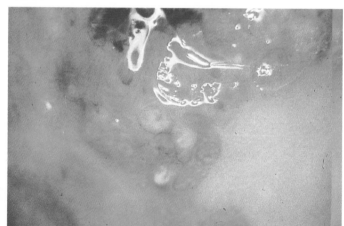

Plate 27

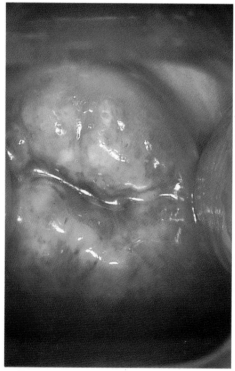

Plate 28 Herpetic cervicitis—also known as necrotic cervicitis.

Plate 28

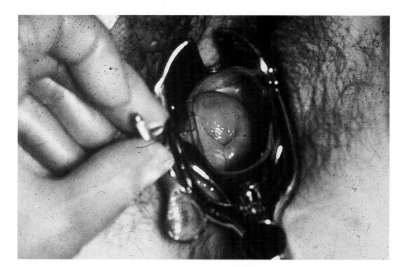

Plate 29 Primary chancre of the uterine cervix

Plate 30, Plate 31 Condylomatous wart on cervix showing showing typical vascular patterns: before and after application of acetic acid.

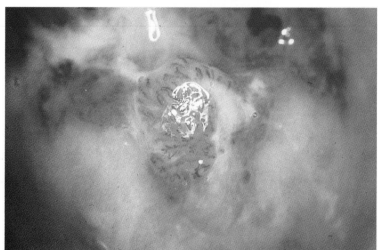

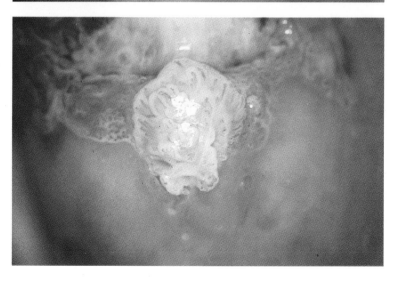

Plate 32 Heavily keratinised cervical wart: confusion could arise with cervical carcinoma.

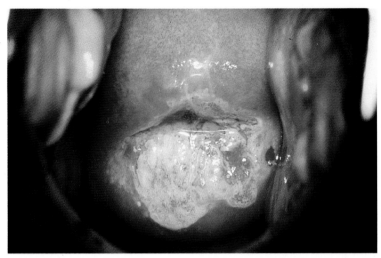

Plate 32

Plate 33 General view of cervical warts of both the condylomatous and flat kind. On colposcopy the finger-like projections of the condylomata are seen, together with the mosaic of the flat warts, which were associated with grade 2 CIN.

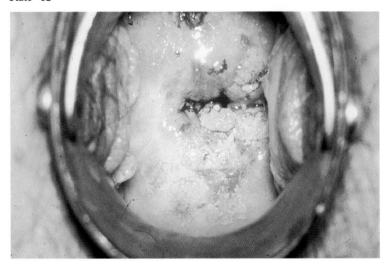

Plate 33

Plate 34, Plate 35 Treatment of the cervix by cryotherapy. Gas released under pressure into a shaped probe causes freezing. If this probe is placed against the cervix an ice-ball forms in the tissues.

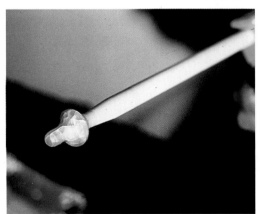

Plate 34

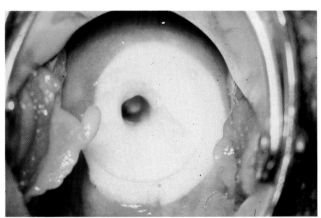

Plate 35

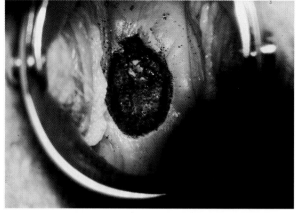

Plate 36

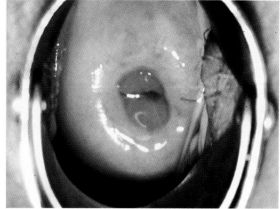

Plate 37

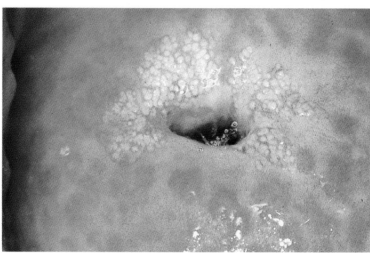

Plate 38

Plate 36 Crater in cervix caused by laser therapy; with this method abnormal tissue can be removed with least damage to normal. Electrodiathermy can produce a similar picture.

Plate 37 Healed cervix after laser treatment. The organ is anatomically and physiologically well recovered.

Plate 38 'Strawberry' vaginitis, seen on the ectocervix. This pattern is often associated with trichomonal infection, but can occur with others. Note that mosaicism is also present.

Plate 39 Severe vaginitis with purulent discharge, due to an overwhelming streptococcal infection.

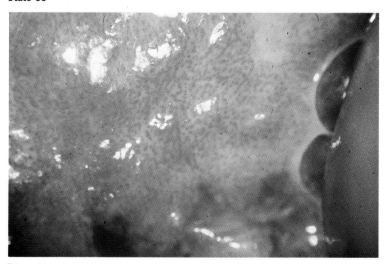

Plate 39

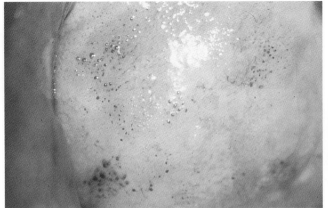

Plate 40

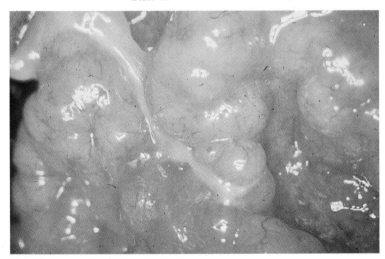

Plate 41

Plate 40 Atrophic vaginitis due to oestrogen lack.

Plate 41 Proctitis, with inflamed mucosa and mucopurulent discharge. This case was due to gonorrhoea.

Plate 42 Chlamydial proctitis, with follicles and mucopurulent discharge.

Plate 43 View of the cilial border of fallopian tubes in organ culture. Monitoring of the degree of activity can be used to assess tissue viability.

Plate 42

Plate 44 Primary chancre on the vulva

Plate 45 Condylomata of secondary syphilis

Plate 46 Florid growth of vulval warts.

Plate 47 Typical coalescing vesicles and ulcers due to herpetic infection.

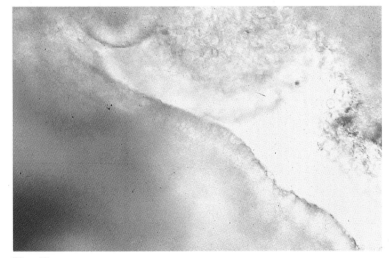

Plate 43

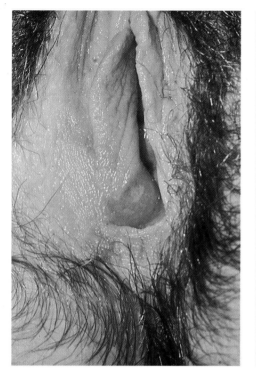

Plate 44

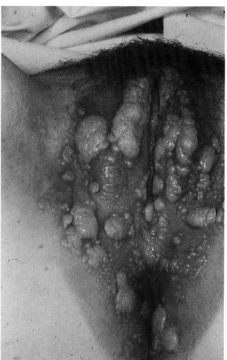

Plate 45

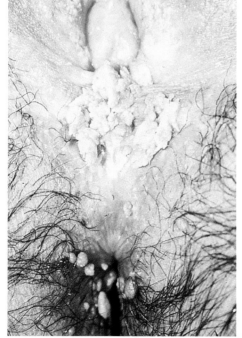

Plate 46

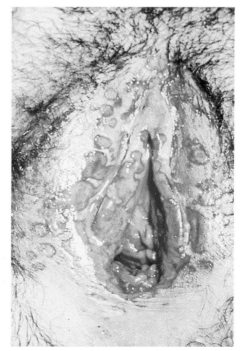

Plate 47

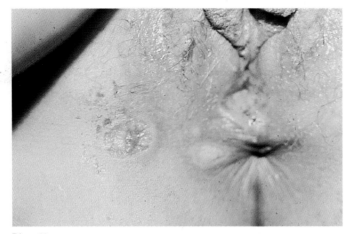

Plate 48

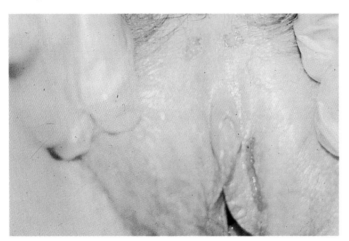

Plate 49

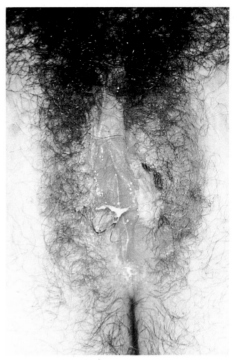

Plate 50

Plate 48 Twin syphilitic chancres at the anus, with a coexisting herpetic ulcer.

Plate 49 Asymptomatic herpetic ulcers.

Plate 50, Plate 51 Vulval ulcers due to Behçet's disease.

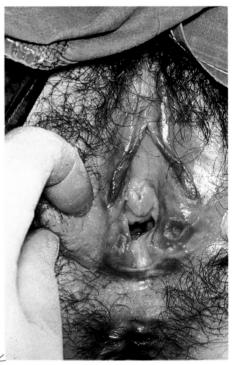

Plate 51

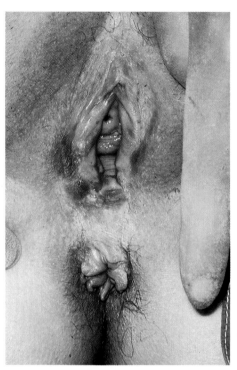

Plate 52 Atrophic vulval change with fissures. Areas such as this should undergo biopsy prior to treatment.

Plate 53 Perigenital scabies with nodular lesions.

Plate 54 Pediculosis pubis—lice (thick arrows) and nits (thin arrows).

Plate 55 Tick in umbilical fold.

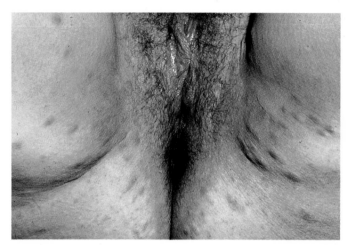

Plate 52

Plate 53

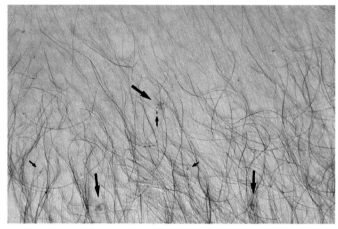

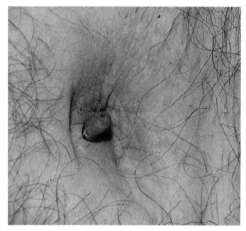

Plate 54

Plate 55

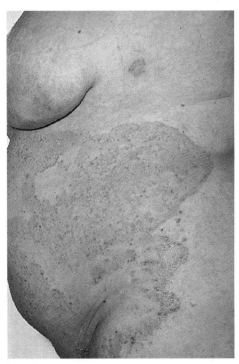

Plate 56   Tinea cruris with widespread involvement of the trunk.

Plate 57   *Candida intertrigo* with characteristic scaly fringe.

Plate 58   Furunculosis of groin.

Plate 59   Erysipelas of abdominal skin fold and erythrasma of the groin in an obese diabetic.

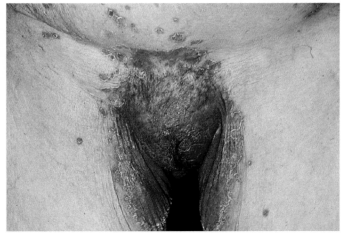

Plate 56

Plate 57

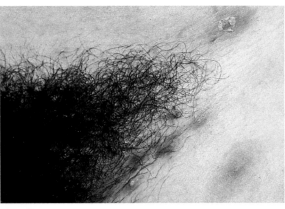

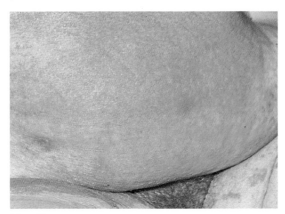

Plate 58

Plate 59

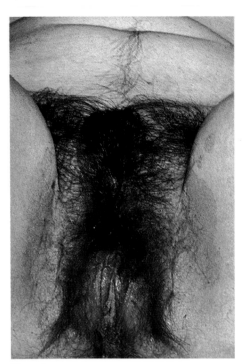

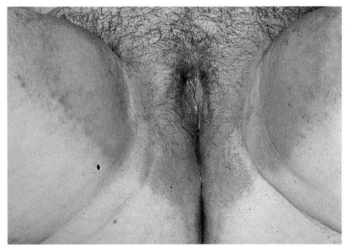

Plate 60

Plate 61

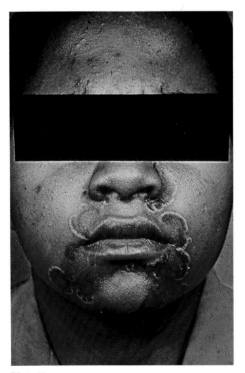

Plate 62

Normal colposcopic appearances

There is much confusion about the normal appearances of the cervix, and many that have exhibited what are completely normal variants have been subjected to medical, surgical and destructive assault through lack of understanding of their owners' medical advisers. It is essential for any physician or surgeon in any specialty involving the lower genital tract to understand its development and normal changes. Professor Kaufman has described these in greater detail in Chapter 1. In this section the description will confine itself to the colposcopic appearances normally seen in the sexually active woman (Plates 1–7, 12, 20 and 24).

Three types of epithelium are normally seen on the cervix: columnar epithelium, original squamous epithelium and metaplastic squamous epithelium. (In early development and intrauterine life there is a time at which the two different original epithelial layers, squamous and columnar, join together at the original squamocolumnar junction.) If a significant area of columnar epithelium is seen exposed on the cervix with its typical red appearance the area is commonly referred to as an 'erosion'. This term, first coined in the last century, is an obvious misnomer, as it implies an ulcer or tissue deficit. Colposcopic examination reveals the true nature of 'erosions', with the grape-like projections, clefts and crypts of columnar epithelium presenting a typical pattern. On application of acetic acid these become lightly outlined in white opacity. In early intrauterine development the columnar epithelium joins directly with the original squamous epithelium to form the original squamocolumnar junction, but this, however, is an appearance that will never be seen at colposcopy; squamous metaplasia will always have taken place.

Even before birth the process of squamous metaplasia will have started. It involves the columnar epithelium being overgrown by a sheet of metaplastic squamous epithelium, creating a new squamocolumnar junction which is ever moving inwards towards the endocervical canal. Initially tongues of squamous epithelium advance across the tops of the crypts of columnar epithelium; these then coalesce to form a flat plane with isolated gaps revealing columnar epithelium underneath; and these apertures then narrow, leaving only the gland openings which become ringed in faint whiteness on application of acetic acid and through which the secretions of the underlying columnar epithelium can be seen to be discharged. Eventually these will close over and the dammed up secretions behind them will form retention cysts or Nabothian follicles. These can become very large, and the cervix which contains many of them can resemble a small bunch of grapes (1 Kings 21, 1–10). On colposcopic examination the cystic nature of these areas is very obvious, and usually blood vessels can be seen tightly stretched over their surface. These are physiological not pathological features; it is very rare indeed for them to cause symptoms; they do not normally need to be treated or destroyed.

It is not fully known what causes squamous metaplasia to occur. The process appears to take place throughout the woman's life, from before birth up until death. It appears to be progressing most rapidly at times of greatest hormonal change, for example at birth, at the menarche, during pregnancy and at the climacteric. The rate of change seems also to be related to the area of columnar epithelium exposed in the vagina. As the pH in the vagina is less than that in the cervix, especially during the reproductive years, it has been postulated that acidity is one of the factors that stimulates squamous metaplasia. The greater the area exposed to the lower vaginal pH, the greater the area likely to undergo change.

The change in rate of squamous metaplasia at different times of life may lead to different appearances being visible on the cervix. Immature squamous cell tissue, because of its relatively high nuclear–cytoplasmic ratio, becomes moderately opaque on application of weak acetic acid. As this epithelium matures this change becomes fainter, and at the original squamocolumnar junction mature metaplastic squamous epithelium may blend imperceptibly with original squamous epithelium. Only the presence of gland openings, faintly ringed in white because of less mature metaplastic layers lining the canal, and of retention cysts, identify what is original and what is metaplastic tissue. If there has been a series of rapid changes in the rate of metaplasia during the woman's life two or three distinct zones may be visible, almost akin to the rings on a tree trunk.

During the life of a woman the overall movement

of the site of the squamocolumnar junction over the tissue is inwards towards the endocervical canal. However other factors may produce an apparent outward movement, due to pouting or extroversion of the cervix. These factors include trauma, such as abortion and particularly childbirth, when lateral splits often occur and the anterior lips of the cervix roll outwards. In the past such an appearance has been referred to as an ectropion to distinguish it from an erosion, but in practice the underlying tissue is the same; exposed endocervical columnar epithelium. Hormonal changes can have similar effects; the unstimulated cervix between birth and the menarche and after the climacteric tends to be shrunken with the canal inverted and the cervix during the reproductive years more turgid and extroverted. Constant progesterone stimulation as in pregnant women and those using hormonal contraception seems to lead to considerable extroversion and 'erosions' are common in such groups. As previously mentioned the use of the bivalve speculum exaggerates this appearance at examination.

It can be anticipated, therefore, that in the early reproductive years and in association with pregnancy a sizeable area of ectopy will be seen. This will gradually shrink in size with advancing age; and after the menopause usually only squamous epithelium will be visible. However there is marked individual variation in this pattern, but the examining physician must be prepared to note and investigate atypical findings.

Abnormal colposcopic findings

Premalignant change (Plates 8–11, 13–15 and 21–23)

When subjected to a variety of external stimuli related to sexual intercourse, columnar epithelium undergoes dysplastic rather than metaplastic change, and instead of healthy metaplastic squamous epithelium, dysplastic epithelium or CIN is formed. Professor Wilbanks in Chapter 20 describes the evidence for the possible relationships between CIN and invasive cancer and infection with various micro-organisms. As well as infection these changes have been linked with the following features:

Sexual intercourse. This correlation was first suggested by Rigoni-Stern in 1842, and it has been confirmed by many authors that celibate women do not develop cervical squamous cell precancer or cancer. Most authors would regard this relationship as absolute. This does not apply, however, to the development of cervical adenocarcinoma.

It is debatable as to whether spermatozoa act as a carcinogen or a cocarcinogen. Coppleston & Reid (1967) have demonstrated the ability of spermatozoa to penetrate immature cervical metaplastic squamous epithelium, and shown in contrast that they are not able to penetrate either mature squamous epithelium or columnar epithelium. Singer (1982) has reported a relationship between the histone content of man's sperm and the likelihood of his female sexual partners developing premalignant or malignant cervical change. This has led to the concept of the 'high risk male', but it is still not possible to say that such men are not also infected with and passing on sexually transmitted organisms. However vasectomy does appear to decrease the risk to the man's partner.

Vulnerability of the cervix. At times of rapid squamous metaplasia, and especially when large areas of columnar cell epithelium are undergoing this change, the cervix seems particularly likely to develop cellular atypia. This appears to be particularly likely at the menarche and during the first pregnancy. This probably explains the widespread observation that the earlier the age when a girl first has sexual intercourse, the more likely she is to develop premalignant and malignant cervical change.

In addition some women appear by inherited traits to be at greater risk than others from the development of premalignant and malignant change. This group appear to have an inherited deficiency in the synthesis of alpha$_1$ anti-trypsin, the enzyme concerned with the scavenging and clearance of the breakdown products of sperm, blood and micro-organisms from the cervix. The lack of this enzyme also leads to disease in other parts of the body, most obviously in the bronchial tree, with bronchitis and chronic obstructive airways disease (Singer 1982).

Promiscuity. The greater the number of the woman's sexual partners, and the greater the number of her partners' sexual partners, the greater is the likelihood that she will develop cervical carcinoma or one of its precursors. The former observation can be ascribed to an increased chance of meeting a 'high risk' or an infected male, the latter to a higher risk of the male partner becoming infected himself. It could also be postulated that genetically determined 'high risk' males might be promiscuous by nature!

Mineral and tar products. In the past coal tar products were implicated in the development of cervical cancer, and more recently textile workers have been shown to be at particular risk, perhaps because they work with oily machinery. Vulval carcinoma has also been shown to be related to this group in the past, possibly related to direct contamination of that area with mineral oil (Robinson 1982). The more recently proven association between cigarette smoking and cervical carcinoma may be due to systemic factors, or perhaps due to genital contact with tar-stained fingers.

Cervical intraepithelial neoplasia is found in the transformation zone between the original and present squamocolumnar junctions. It is identified by two features:

Firstly, the appearance of mosaicism or punctation on the epithelium prior to the application of acetic acid. In mosaicism the epithelium is crisscrossed by fine capillaries running parallel to the surface of the tissue, forming a delicate mosaic tracery. Punctation is due to the appearance of such vessels end-on, producing fine dots on the epithelial tissue. Generally speaking, fine and delicate patterns appear early in the progress of the disease, and the coarser the pattern the more advanced the lesion. The use of a green filter will enhance this appearance.

Secondly, whiteness on application of acetic acid. When this solution is sprayed on the cervix or applied with a swab CIN becomes opaque and white in appearance. There is usually a clear outline produced between normal and abnormal areas, and the appearance of any areas of mosaic and punctation may be enhanced. As a generalisation the more dense the white reaction on application of acetic acid, the more abnormal the epithelium.

However definite the picture gained by cytology and colposcopy abnormal areas should *always* be biopsied, and a definitive histological diagnosis obtained. Most lesions can be adequately biopsied by taking small samples from the areas with the most abnormal looking epithelium as seen in colpo-

scopy. However, if the lesion or the area of normal metaplastic epithelium goes into the endocervical canal and the top of it (the present squamocolumnar junction) cannot be seen, or if there is any doubt concerning its extent, cone biopsy is necessary. In the past the degree of abnormality was described from normality through mild, moderate and severe degrees of dysplasia, to carcinoma in situ, and to microinvasive and frankly invasive squamous cell cervical carcinoma. This classification had its drawbacks in that it implied a boundary between dysplasia and carcinoma in situ that did not exist; in fact many pathologists would regard carcinoma in situ and severe dysplasia as one and the same condition. The terminology that now meets more general approval is to regard all variations of change between normality and invasive carcinoma as intraepithelial neoplasia (IN). Thus premalignant change on the cervix is referred to as cervical intraepithelial neoplasia (CIN); if it occurs on the vulva it is vulval intraepithelial neoplasia (VIN); and in the vagina it is vaginal intraepithelial neoplasia (VaIN).

Infection with wart virus (Plates 30–33 and 46, Fig. 5.1)

Infection with human papilloma virus (HPV) is probably the commonest specific cervical infection, more common, even, than infection with *Chlamydia trachomatis* or *Neisseria gonorrhoeae*. Meisels et

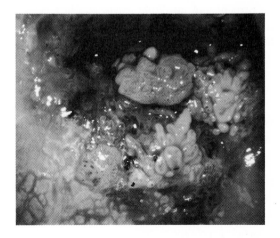

Fig. 5.1 Close-up view of cervical warts of both the condylomatous and flat kind.

al (1977), examining women who presented with cervical smears suggestive of wart virus infection of the cervix, reported that there were two distinct clinical patterns that might be identified on colposcopy. The first was the typical proliferative condylomatous lesion on the surface of the cervix, with finger-like projections outwards (kondylos = knuckle). The surface may be heavily keratinised, and if it is not, the whole area will usually become densely white on application of acetic acid. Once the acetic acid has worn off the blood supply can be seen to be in the form of regular single capillary loops, one in each projection. The differential diagnosis is with invasive cervical cancer; this generally has a much more 'broken down' and irregular appearance, and the vessels are much more irregular in their pattern. Invasive cervical carcinoma also is usually more friable and bleeds to touch. Nevertheless diagnostic confusion can occur between these lesions, and biopsy should always be performed. In the early stages these lesions may simply look like a roughening of the epithelial surface. If heavy surface deposits of keratin hide the diagnostic picture these can be scraped off prior to diagnosis.

The second appearance is that of the 'flat condyloma', a term which is self-contradicting but has come to be accepted. These are in individual appearance no different from CIN, with vessels forming mosaic and punctation patterns and the whole area becoming white on application of acetic acid. Features suggestive of wart virus infection are the presence of multiple small satellite lesions, most unusual in CIN, and the presence of lesions outside the transformation zone, as true CIN arises only in that area. These lesions are often seen together, and on biopsy CIN may contain signs of warty change. Flat condylomas are more commonly associated with CIN than the condylomatous, but either can be. Biopsy of the most abnormal looking areas prior to treatment is mandatory.

Infection with Herpes virus hominis (Plates 28, 47–49)

Herpetic cervicitis may present with one of three abnormal appearances, although in many cases the cervix that is infected and actively secreting the virus is completely normal to the naked eye and on colposcopy (Rattray et al 1978; Barton et al 1986). In the early stages of the infection one may see vesicles and small ulcers on the cervix, similar in all ways to typical lesions on the vulva and vagina (Kaufman et al 1973). However when these progress and coalesce the whole cervix often becomes involved in a very severe cervicitis to which the term 'necrotic' has been applied (Willcox 1968). The organ is tender, swollen and oedematous, and on its surface develops a thick yellow slough. Attempts to prise this off may cause bleeding or the release of a thick, mucopulent discharge. The whole is secondarily infected with bacteria. If the slough has separated an ulcer may result. The differential diagnosis is between herpes, cervical carcinoma and syphilis, and adequate tests for differentiation should be carried out. The third appearance is of 'non-specific' inflammation; mildly oedematous tissue with faint patterns of vascular abnormality and a weak white reaction on application of acetic acid.

Diagnosis is by identification of the causative organism. This may be by culture, by identification of herpetic inclusions in cytological or histological material taken from suspicious lesions, or by identification of the herpes antigen in such specimens by immunological techniques such as immunofluorescence or immunoperoxidase.

Infection with Chlamydia trachomatis (Plates 26, 27 and 42)

Many of the descriptions that have been applied in the past to *Chlamydia trachomatis* cervicitis have relied on naked eye observations, and have used terminology that does not correlate well with colposcopic, cytological and histological findings. Thus, terms such as 'hypertrophic erosion' and 'erythema' have no specific meaning, and although the non-specific picture of inflammation may indeed be most common when the cervix is infected with *C. trachomatis* these changes cannot be regarded as specific. On colposcopy, however, one typical feature can be found. Lymphoid follicles, identical in structure with those found in the eye in trachoma and related disorders, can be seen in a significant proportion of cases (Hare et al 1981), and on biopsy these are found to have a typical structure of a peripheral ring of small lymphocytes surrounding a pale germinal centre composed of large lymphocytes, reticular cells and macrophages. Sometimes the picture is not fully formed, and dense lymphocytic invasion only can be observed. Dunlop et al (1964) first linked this appearance to chlamydial infection, and Hare et al (1981) found it in 13 of 34 women who were the sexual partners of men with 'non-specific' urethritis (presumably chlamydial in many cases). Follicles were identified in 5 of 11 cases where *C. trachomatis* was isolated, compared with 1 of 15 cases where the organism was not isolated.

Paavonen et al (1980) described a more acute pattern of disease, with formation of microabscesses. No other workers have reported this, and the pattern may be non-specific.

Syphilis (Plates 29, 44–48)

Syphilitic chancres on the cervix are most uncommon; one newly retired genitourinary physician who had worked all his life in busy clinics in the United Kingdom stated recently that he had seen four in his professional career, all of whom had declined to be photographed! Suspicion should be raised by the woman's sexual history, and by the appearance of an atypical ulcer placed on the cervix, not following its normal contours. Specific diagnostic techniques for syphilis should be used.

Tropical infections

These are covered in Chapter 17.

Cervical polyps

Polypoid growths presenting at the uterine cervix are common. They may be one of the following:

Ectocervical. These are usually obvious outgrowths of metaplastic squamous epithelium. They cause no symptoms, and can be safely disregarded.

Endocervical. These present at the external os emerging from the endocervical canal, although their bases may be seen if an endocervical speculum is used. Exposed endocervical tissue in the vagina often becomes secondarily infected, leading to discharge and intermenstrual and postcoital bleeding and spotting. For this reason they are probably best

removed, and this can usually be done using a colposcopic biopsy forceps. Neither ectocervical or endocervical polyps have any greater tendency than their parent tissues to develop premalignant or malignant change, but it is a wise precaution to have a histological examination of all tissues removed.

Endometrial. Usually in the later years of a woman's reproductive life irregular shedding of the endometrium can lead to polyp formation, and these can become long and attenuated and present at the external os of the cervix. Like endocervical tissue, endometrium is not resistant to infection by vaginal organisms, and similar symptoms occur with the occasional addition of a cramp-like pain which may be caused by uterine contractions. Such polyps are best removed at a formal dilatation and curettage, as they are often multiple and the condition of the endometrium predisposes to further polyp formation if left. Although malignant change is unlikely, polyps and curettings should be examined histologically.

Fibroid. Leiomyomatous or fibroid polyps may form from outgrowths of the myometrium into the uterine cavity, and these often reach a diameter of several centimetres. They may be extruded through the cervical os and considerably distort the endocervical canal, and in extreme cases the condition may mimic uterovaginal prolapse. Removal of these larger lesions may require a major surgical procedure, and if the reproductive function is no longer required, hysterectomy may be appropriate. Sarcomatous change in association with fibroids is very rare.

Invasive cervical carcinoma (Plates 16–19 and 23)

Most cervical carcinomas are of the squamous cell type, only 1–10% being adenocarcinoma. Squamous cell tumours can mimic any appearance from an exaggerated CIN to ulceration and proliferative growth. As the lesion grows the top of the vagina may become involved. Except in the very early stages of microinvasive and occult invasive carcinoma the lesion is symptomatic, with vaginal discharge and postcoital bleeding being the commonest presenting feature. Unfortunately delay in diagnosis often occurs when the woman presents with a vaginal discharge and her physician attempts to treat this on microbiological grounds, without recognising that the tissue that has become infected is itself abnormal. Before treating a lower genital tract infection the whole area must be thoroughly inspected, and if treatment fails to eradicate the infection in the predicted time the whole genital tract must be inspected again.

If cervical carcinoma is suspected multiple biopsies must be taken, preferably under colposcopic control. Cytological investigation is *not* enough; the presence of blood, pus or necrotic debris can obscure the detail in a specimen and lead to an inconclusive or even false negative result. If doubt remains the matter must be pursued, if needs be by examination under anaesthesia.

In contrast to squamous cell carcinoma, in its early stages at least, columnar cell carcinoma of the cervix can present with an exaggerated but acceptable appearance of columnar cell ectopy, and cause no symptoms. At this stage it will be detected as the result of cervical cytology. Even at colposcopy the lesion may be difficult to identify, and good representative biopsies may be difficult to obtain. Under these circumstances cone biopsy and fractional endometrial and endocervical curettage will be necessary.

THE DEFINITION OF PATHOLOGICAL INFLAMMATORY CHANGE IN THE LOWER GENITAL TRACT

What is cervicitis? (Plate 25)

If cervicitis is taken to be an abnormal degree of polymorphonuclear response on the cervix, then the following factors must be taken into account when making the diagnosis:

Normal menstrual changes. In the first half of the menstrual cycle there is normally no pus on the cervix. However in the second half, where dominance is by progesterone rather than oestrogen, some pus is normal, and this can be diagnosed by the change of the mucus from clear to cloudy and confirmed by stained smears.

Oral contraception. Oral contraception relies for its effect on progesterone rather than oestrogen dominance; hence pus is a usual feature at all times in smears from these women (Jordan & Singer 1976).

Rapid squamous metaplasia. At times when the turnover of metaplastic cells on the cervix is very rapid pus forms as part of the scavenging response to the death of columnar cells. This is most commonly observed at the menarche, and during pregnancy.

Response to coitus. Especially early on in the reproductive years or in response to a new sexual partner the cervix reacts to the foreign presence of sperm and seminal fluid by a polymorphonuclear response. This must be regarded as the normal response to intercourse. When a relationship has lasted for a considerable time the cervix appears to become more tolerant of the partner's sperm, and the response become less marked.

Response to parturition. However smoothly delivery (or miscarriage) appears to progress trauma is almost inevitable (Wilbanks & Richart 1967). There will be a response of polymorphonuclear leucocytes to this trauma.

In summary, the presence of polymorphonuclear leucocytes on the cervix is a response to normal life events on many occasions. Fluhmann (1961) found such evidence of cervicitis in cervical secretions from 108 of 113 adult non-pregnant women, 34 of 35 pregnant women and 15 of 19 postmenopausal women.

Despite this evidence Brunham et al (1984) felt able to diagnose mucopurulent cervicitis on clinical and cytological findings. They state that the presence of yellow mucopus standing out against a white swab or the presence of 10 or more polymorphonuclear leucocytes per high power ($\times$ 1000) field in a gram-stained smear constitutes cervicitis, and correlates with infection with *C. trachomatis* but, most interestingly, not with gonococcal infection. However the population studied for this work comprised all young women attending a clinic for sexually transmitted disease, who had had on average a large number of sexual partners. It seems doubtful that these findings would have been the same in, for example, an antenatal clinic or a well woman cytology clinic. The advice put forward that such women and their sexual partners should be treated presumptively as cases of chlamydial infection may well be apposite in groups where chlamydial infection is common, but could lead to much worry and embarrassment and would not be correct in groups where such infection is rare and unlikely.

McCormack and others (1979) followed seven female college students with active chlamydial infection of the cervix for between 15 and 25 months. Only one complained of a discharge; on examination six of the seven were reported as remaining 'normal' for the whole period. Harrison et al (1985) reported on a group of university students attending a gynaecology clinic. They analysed a variety of symptoms and signs, both singly and in groups. When factors such as abdominal pain, gonorrhoea and a history of gonococcal or non-gonococcal urethritis in a recent partner are excluded the only useful symptom was a request for an 'oral contraception recheck' (42.9% incidence of chlamydial infection—a figure most unlikely to be found in most contraception clinics). On examination a green discharge was associated in 50% of cases with chlamydial infection, but a 'purulent' discharge in only 23.5% of cases, a yellow discharge in 12.5% of cases and a mucoid discharge in 7.5% of cases. They suggested a 'cervicitis score' with one point each for erythema, ectopy, friability and discharge. If discharge was present one point was added if it was thick and one point if it was yellow or green. Finally one point was added if 1–4 polymorphonuclear leucocytes were seen per $450 \times$ field, and two points if 5 or more were seen. All women with cervical chlamydial isolations had scores of 4 to 8, but so did 42% of those who did not have chlamydia isolated; only 19% of those with this score had chlamydial isolates. They concluded that the main relationship between the various factors discussed was that oral contraception predisposed to columnar cell ectopy, which predisposed to chlamydial infection, which predisposed to cervicitis.

A screen of the greatest number and widest spectrum of the population can be obtained by the examination of routinely taken cervical smears (Papanicolaou or Pap smears) for the presence of pus. Such 'inflammatory smears' are often reported by cytologists, and make a clear definition of the degree of dyskaryosis impossible. Oriel and others (1974), Simmonds & Vosmik (1974) and Paavonen et al (1978) all suggest that an inflammatory pattern in the cervical smear may point to chlamydial cervicitis. Burns et al (1975) found inflammatory changes in 72 of 80 women who were the sexual partners of men with non-specific urethritis, but also in 19 of 40 control subjects. All these studies are based on high risk populations, and the prediction value of an inflammatory smear in a low risk population is unknown.

In summary, symptoms, signs and cytological features of 'cervicitis' would seem to have a useful predictive value in high risk populations, such as promiscuous groups and those attending clinics for sexually transmitted disease. In the population as a whole the value is probably much less, and due weight must be given to the effect of pregnancy, childbirth, miscarriage, coitus and contraception.

What is vaginitis? (Plates 5, 38–40)

In Chapter 2 it has been shown that the vagina is usually colonised by a wide variety of organisms, and that the finding of micro-organisms in the vagina does not imply a disease state. Host defences that prevent such organisms causing clinical inflammatory change (Cohen et al 1984) include mucus (which has the ability to prevent bacterial adherence), the vaginal pH, lysozyme, and the presence in secretions of lactoferrin, which competes with the organism for the iron necessary for its metabolism. These authors have also noted high levels of zinc and fibronectin in vaginal fluid, although the significance of these is uncertain. There is also local antibody secretion.

Infections of the vagina can be roughly divided into five groups:

Vaginitis, due to specific pathogens such as Candida albicans and Trichomonas vaginalis. These may produce a typical pattern of inflammation. Symptoms are present and, on examination, reddened tissues are seen that may bleed to touch. Pus is present in the vaginal secretions. The colposcopic picture of trichomonal vaginitis (the so-called strawberry vagina) is not specific, and can be seen in acute infections by other organisms. A similar picture may be seen in atrophic vaginitis due to the relatively low levels of hormone stimulation present in the premenarchial and postmenopausal years. This subject has been fully covered by Professor Douglas in Chapter 16.

The accepted teaching is that *Neisseria gonorrhoeae* and *Chlamydia trachomatis* do not invade the vagina in the reproductive years, although each can cause vaginitis in the premenarche and after the menopause. However Barton et al (1985) did report the isolation of *C. trachomatis* from the vaginal vault in the cases of four women who had undergone hysterectomy. Whether this was due to contamination from urethritis, or because residual columnar epithelium was present at the top of the vagina, or a true colonisation of vaginal epithelium, remains unclear.

Non-specific vaginitis or vaginosis. In the past this has usually been associated with infection due to *Gardnerella vaginalis*, although now other organisms and possibly synergism between organisms have been implicated. Infections in this group are different in character from those of the first group specified; Eschenbach and others (1984) suggest that the diagnostic criteria should include three of the following:

A homogenous, thin appearance of the discharge;

A pH value of more than 4.5;

The presence of clue cells (see Chapter 15);

A fishy, amine odour, made more apparent when a few drops of 10% potassium hydroxide are mixed with discharge on a glass slide.

Paavonen et al (1984) stress that bacterial vaginosis may be associated with other micro-organisms as well as *G. vaginalis*, and these include mycoplasmas and many anaerobic bacteria including the newly reported anaerobic curved rods (with the proposed genus name *Mobiluncus*; Owen et al 1984).

Amsel et al (1983) stress that if non-specific vaginitis is diagnosed using criteria similar to those listed above, most of the women in whom the diagnosis is made will be asymptomatic. In their series, composed of college students, about half of whom presented because of untoward symptoms and half of whom came for routine gynaecological examination (usually for oral contraceptive prescription), symptoms of abnormal discharge, vaginal malodour or vulvar irritation were present in 32 (46%) of 69 women with non-specific vaginitis, and 77 (32%) of 242 'normal' women. These authors also report the usefulness of gas liquid chromatography for the detection of various fatty acids produced in non-sepcific vaginitis. An increased succinate to lactate ratio was found in 19 of 22 women with non-specific vaginitis but only one of 60 normal women. Propionate and/or butyrate were detected in 11 of 21 women with non-

specific vaginitis, and in none of 54 normal women. The absence of lactate in vaginal secretions from these women emphasises that non-specific vaginitis or vaginosis involves the displacement of the normal lactate producing organisms from the vagina by those with other metabolic pathways. In a previous communication (Spiegel et al 1980) they had identified *G. vaginalis* as the acetate producer, *Bacteroides* as the succinate producer and *Peptococcus* as producing butyrate and acetate. In their later paper they stressed the association between symptoms of vaginitis, the presence of anaerobic organisms and the wearing of an intrauterine contraceptive device, an association that has also been noted by other workers. One reported side-effect of trichomonal and non-specific vaginitis that might be of interest to patients is the effect it has on the sex-ratio of fetuses conceived during an attack. Minkoff et al (1985) report a definite bias towards females in this condition, suggesting that the X-bearing spermatozoa are more resistant than the Y-bearing ones to the hostile vaginal environment.

Vaginitis due to virus organisms specifically invading the vaginal epithelium. The two most common of these organisms are herpes virus and wart virus. Infection by each is dealt with fully in the relevant chapters, but it should be stressed that, particularly in the case of wart virus infection, the diagnosis is often missed. The vagina needs to be carefully inspected with the colposcope and Rylander et al (1984) have described the typical appearances: warty plaques on the vaginal walls with either keratinised surface layers giving a rough, white pattern prior to the application of acetic acid, or areas with abnormal vascular patterns which whiten with this agent. These warts may be condylomatous or flat. Chronic long-term infection of the cervix, vagina and vulva with wart virus infection is commonly seen in women taking long-term steroid or immunosuppressive therapy, for example after transplant procedures. In all patients, but especially in this group, such lesions may show premalignant change (vaginal intraepithelial neoplasia or VaIN), and biopsy should be used freely.

Behçet's disease, Stevens-Johnson syndrome and polyarteritis. These conditions are not due to an infective agent, though secondary infection of the lesions produced may occur. In all of them the basic lesion is an underlying perivasculitis leading to obstruction of the blood supply to the area and hence tissue necrosis, breaking down into ulceration. In all of the conditions lesions can appear elsewhere in the body, and Behçet's disease has an especially wide range, including the buccal mucosa, eye, bony joints, gastrointestinal tract and pericardium. For a full review of the pathological findings see Slavin (1976).

Atrophic vaginitis due to hormone insufficiency. This is dealt with in Chapter 16.

In dealing with the problem of vaginal discharge as a symptom it is essential to ascertain the source of the discharge. Thus it may be due to a reaction in the vagina, secretion from the endocervix or from the endometrial cavity. The treatment of each condition is usually different.

What is vulvitis? (Plates 44–52)

The epithelium of the vulva is of the full thickness squamous type, and is subject to dermatological infections that involve the skin elsewhere (see Chapter 18). It is also invaded by viral pathogens such as herpes virus and wart virus, fungal infections such as that due to *Candida albicans*, and bacterial infections especially outside the reproductive years. Infection with fungal and bacterial agents is particularly common in cases of uncontrolled diabetes mellitus, and has often been the presenting feature in these cases. Vulval ulcers may be due also to syphilis, Behçet's and Stevens-Johnson syndrome. They may be self-inflicted by scratching and rubbing the irritating areas. In the older woman malignant ulcers due to carcinoma must be considered.

There remains a large group of women who present with symptoms of vulvitis (soreness, irritation, itching, ulceration, sometimes with a discharge) or without symptoms, but in whom the vulval appearance is abnormal. Such cases are often due to vulval dystrophy, which may be atrophic or hypertrophic in type, and may be associated with premalignant change (vulval intraepithelial neoplasia or VIN). The description and diagnostic features of such lesions are outside the range of the volume, but it must be emphasised that, should any doubt remain about the nature of the lesions, multiple biopsies involving the clinically worst areas are mandatory.

THE TREATMENT OF LOWER GENITAL TRACT INFECTION

Introduction

The treatment of specific conditions due to known or suspected pathogens is described in each individual chapter, and will not be pursued here. There will remain, however, a large body of women with distressing symptoms which cannot be attributed to disease caused by a known pathogen. Although by presenting at a clinic for sexually transmitted diseases the women herself may imply that her symptoms are due to a sexually acquired condition this must not be assumed uncritically, and certainly it is most damaging to make such implications in women presenting under different circumstances. The possibility of a psychological overlay must also be considered.

For those women with genuine symptoms and signs with no evidence of specific infection, empirical treatment may be indicated. This may be with one or more of the following groups of agents:

Antibiotics, either systemic or local;

Sulphonamides;

Antiseptics;

Acid preparations.

An attempt may also be made to change the environment by hormonal preparations.

Antibiotics

The two conditions most commonly treated by antibiotics are non-specific cervicitis and non-specific vaginitis. Brunham et al (1984) support the recommendation of the Center for Disease Control (Atlanta) that non-gonococcal mucopurulent cervicitis (as previously defined) should be treated with an antichlamydial regime, for example the equivalent of 500 mg tetracycline hydrochloride by mouth four times a day for a minimum of 7 days. They recommend that the sexual partners of these women should be treated in the same way. Similar regimes can be given to clear the 'inflammatory' cervical smear, in which the inflammatory pattern obscures the cytological detail and makes a proper diagnosis impossible.

Non-specific vaginitis or vaginosis may respond to the nitroimidazole group of drugs. Paavonen et al (1984) recommend metronidazole or an equivalent at the dose of 500 mg twice daily for 5 to 7 days (this would need to be 400 mg three times daily in countries where the 250 mg preparation is not available). The value of treatment of sexual partners is not proven.

Local preparations are of unproven value. Metronidazole is available in 1 g or 500 mg rectal suppositories, but no proper evidence is available concerning their value as vaginal pessaries. Neomycin, natamycin and (in the past) chloromycetin pessaries are available, but again no real evidence has been produced for their usefulness: they are probably best avoided.

Sulphonamides

Local triple sulphonamide preparations have traditionally been used in gynaecology, especially for application to tissues healing after surgery and electrodiathermy. This preparation is available as a pessary or in the form of a cream, and contains sulphathiazole, sulphacetamide and sulphabenzamide. Despite their long and hallowed use very little has been published concerning their effectiveness. Hodge & Murdoch (1963) reported a trial (not double-blind) in which triple sulphonamide pessaries were compared with control pessaries in the treatment of vaginal discharge. Thirty-four of 50 women were improved after triple-sulpha, but only 19 of 50 after control treatment. However the microbiological investigations of the patients in this series left much to be desired, and there will be no general agreement with the author's contention that 'It is doubtful whether bacteriological investigations of the sort usually undertaken as routine are useful or necessary in the treatment of this complaint'. Jones et al (1982) found various *Bacteroides* species to be susceptible in vitro to the constituents of the triple sulphonamide preparation, although *Gardnerella vaginalis* was not. The acid pH of this preparation has also been considered an advantage. However, Paavonen et al (1984) report that triple sulphonamide was not as effective as nitroimidazoles in the treatment of bacterial vaginosis.

Antiseptics

In the past preparations containing arsenic (acetarsol) and mercury (hydrargaphen) have been used for the treatment of vaginitis with claimed success; however, the potential risks of absorption of these metals by the woman or her sexual partner have led to the withdrawal of arsenic preparations and will probably result in the withdrawal of mercurials in the near future. In recent years iodine preparations have gained some acceptance in the management of this condition. Monif et al (1980) reported that povidine–iodine solutions produced a dramatic fall in the total numbers of aerobes and anaerobes recoverable from the posterior vaginal pool in the first 10 minutes following administration, but from 30 minutes afterwards the organisms re-established themselves. When the vehicle for the administration of the preparations was changed to polyethylene glycol an antibacterial effect was observed over a 3-hour period. No properly controlled therapeutic trials have been conducted although Ahmed (1982) reported that povidine iodine was better than hydrargaphen. Mayhew (1981) and Beaton et al (1984) report enthusiastically on the use of povidine iodine preparations, which come as pessaries, gel and douche. However the statement of the latter group that treatment may be applied before laboratory examination is to be deprecated. Organic dyes such as gentian violet, and mixtures such as Bonney's blue, were introduced into gynaecological practice long before controlled trials were deemed appropriate: they have their devotees in practice but little written evidence in their favour. Eusol solution is also commonly used, especially in postoperative cases.

Acid preparations

To attempt to alter the pH of the vagina by acid preparations begs the whole question of cause and effect in vaginitis. Undoubtedly the acid vagina is generally in a better state of health than the neutral or alkaline vagina; but does acidity lead to a healthy environment or is it a byproduct of this? Lactic acid pessaries and acetic jelly have both been used in the vagina, but no real evidence exists as to their value. Slater (1950) showed some benefits from both lactic acid jelly and acetic acid pessaries during vaginal healing, and this may indicate a use for these preparations in postoperative cases and as adjuncts to other therapy.

The idea that colonisation of the vagina with the yoghurt yeast leads to easing the symptoms of intractable vaginitis is attractive to those who prefer a more natural approach to medicine, and certainly anecdotal reports of its value abound. The author is unable, however, to find a controlled account of its use in the medical literature.

Change in hormonal environment

In the premenarchial and postmenopausal years declining oestrogen levels may lead to the development of vaginitis, and this has been dealt with by Professor Douglas in Chapter 16. Variations in the hormonal environment also occur in response to pregnancy and oral contraception, and in both of these situations the vaginal pH moves towards neutrality and the resistance of the vaginal wall to infection, as measured by the fall in the karyopyknotic index (KPI). This is due to relative progesterone dominance. For more women this has no notable effect, but for some it leads to repeated vaginal infections. If this is in response to pregnancy not much can be done about it, but attempts can be made to vary the contents of oral contraceptive preparations to avoid such side-effects. As a group, however, oral contraceptives have a progestogenic effect, and change to a different form of contraception may be the only answer.

Immunotherapy

A recent introduction into the field of treatment for non-specific vaginitis is the use of a vaccine prepared against 'aberrant' lactobacilli. Whilst agreeing that the full mode of action is obscure, Harris (1984) reports cure of non-specific vaginitis in 74 of 77 cases followed for 6 months. Litschgi (1984) reported almost equally good results; most of his cases were related to infection with *Gardnerella vaginalis*. This is a new method, insufficiently assessed and explained; but if future work confirms the initial findings it may become very important in the future.

Surgical treatment of infection

Removal of foreign bodies

Part of the basic investigation of vaginal discharge is a thorough visual and digital examination of the vagina and cervix, and the removal of impacted foreign bodies in the vagina is undertaken then. The commonest of these will be the forgotten or lost vaginal tampon, and the clinical picture of toxic shock syndrome has been described by Dr Warren in Chapter 2. Also commonly found objects are male and female contraceptives and objects designed or adapted as adjuncts or stimulants to sexual enjoyment. In addition to these a large variety of objects have been recovered from the vagina; lost, stolen or strayed, or perhaps placed there on purpose. The late R R Willcox of St Mary's Hospital, London, reported the finding of a fine specimen of *Allium cepua*, a condition not reported before or since in the medical literature but no doubt observed by others (Willcox 1961).

The need to remove the intrauterine contraceptive device of a woman who presents with pelvic inflammatory disease is discussed in Chapter 21, but it may also be desirable to remove it because of lower genital tract infection. Amsel et al (1983) report that 18.8% of women with bacterial vaginosis in that study were intrauterine contraceptive device users, compared with only 5.4% intrauterine contraceptive device users amongst normal controls. In their study population half of the intrauterine contraceptive device users had non-specific vaginitis. Paavonen et al (1984) recommend the removal of intrauterine contraceptive devices from women with recurrent bacterial vaginosis. Care must be taken in the interpretation of such advice; whilst recognising the undesirability of intrauterine contraceptive decive usage in these circumstances, unwanted pregnancy may be an even worse alternative for the woman. It must always be remembered that removal of an intrauterine contraceptive device around or just after the midpoint of the menstrual cycle can result in pregnancy if coitus occurred in the few preceding days.

Surgical treatment of infected glands

The greater vestibular glands of Bartholin commonly become infected, and if a fluctuant abscess develops in the area surgical drainage is indicated. Chronic blockage of the duct can lead to a cyst of Bartholin's duct, when the gland area is again palpable and fluctuant but none of the other traditional signs of inflammation are present. The infecting organisms may be sexually transmitted or commensal, and the bias of published series to one type usually reflects the interest of the author and the populations from which his series is taken. Thus in gynaecological practice the organisms isolated from Bartholin's gland tend to be non-sexually transmitted, whilst in series from clinics for sexually transmitted disease the organisms isolated tend to be in the sexually transmitted group.

The treatment of acute bartholinitis follows the old surgical maxim that if pus is present it should be released. If the swelling is not fluctuant then appropriate antibiotic therapy is given. If it is fluctuant, then surgical drainage is appropriate. Aspiration even with the broadest gauge needle is probably not enough, and the piercing of the abscess with a broad-bladed knife under general anaesthesia is needed, followed by digital exploration to make sure that loculus formation has not resulted in incomplete drainage. The site of incision should be just exterior to the hymeneal remnants. The abscess cavity can then be packed with ribbon gauze soaked in antiseptic to encourage further drainage.

If the tissues are not too inflamed and friable continued drainage can be ensured by the technique of marsupialisation. After incision of the cavity the edges are sutured with fine absorbable material to the skin edges, leaving a drainage aperture with a maximum diameter of about 1 cm. Over the following weeks this aperture will shrink down, and if drainage ceases it will close over.

The non-tender, non-inflamed swelling of Bartholin's gland may be an old abscess, probably sterile, or a cyst due to a failure of drainage through the duct. Treatment of this may be by marsupialisation, or, especially if the lesion has recurred, by total excision under general anaesthesia. Excision of Bartholin's gland is not, however, to be taken on lightly, since the surrounding area is very vascular with ill defined tissue planes, and heavy bleeding can occur which may be difficult to control.

Inflammation of Skene's gland at the urethral meatus is usually part of the picture of urethritis, and settles with appropriate antibiotic treatment. Occasionally the glands become chronically blocked and cause dysuria and dyspareunia. They should then be drained and destroyed; electrodiathermy is the most appropriate surgical modality.

Also at the urethral meatus chronic inflammation can lead to the development of a urethral caruncle. This is a polypoid projection, usually less than a centimetre at its maximum length, and almost always occurs in postmenopausal women. Symptoms caused include bleeding and dysuria. Treatment is to destroy the lesion, either by electrodiathermy or laser, and local oestrogen therapy to help prevent a recurrence. Care should be taken to differentiate this condition from urethral prolapse, which is common in the same group. In this condition a sleeve of urethral lining is visible coming through the meatus, and needs to be excised.

Surgical treatment of the chronic infected 'erosion' (Plates 34–37)

Exposed columnar epithelium on the uterine cervix (columnar cell ectopy or cervical erosion) is a variant of normal, and the tradition from the past that it must be treated 'because it is there' must be resisted strongly. Nevertheless there will be a small number of women who repeatedly claim vaginal discharge from which no specific pathogen can be isolated, and on examination are found to have large areas of columnar cell ectopy producing an obvious mucoid secretion. The area may also be friable, and bleed to touch and on intercourse. Providing that malignant and premalignant change in the area has been discounted, at least by a negative cervical smear and preferably by colposcopy as well, an attempt may be made to reduce the area of exposed columnar epithelium by surgical means. The principle behind most techniques is to induce the columnar epithelium to undergo squamous metaplasia either by treating its surface or by destroying it to full thickness. Such techniques include:

The application of silver nitrate as a solid chemical. This is a traditional method, and no recent evidence is available as to its usefulness.

Cryotherapy. Destruction of columnar cell ectopy by freezing it to very low temperatures from which it will not recover causes only minor discomfort, and can easily be undertaken in the consulting room or outpatient clinic. The apparatus for this is comparatively inexpensive, and may depend on one of two principles:

1. Liquid nitrogen may be passed into a hollow

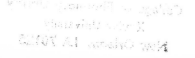

probe, and its evaporation lead to the freezing of the surrounding areas;

2. More commonly, gas under high pressure (nitrous oxide) is released inside the probe. The rapid fall in pressure that occurs leads to a dramatic fall in the temperature of the probe, and hence the freezing of the surrounding areas (Joule-Thompson effect).

Freezing of the tissue leads to cell death by alteration of the concentrations of the vital solutes and by damage to the cell membranes. Maximum damage is achieved during a rapid freeze but also during a slow thaw, and hence a popular technique is to freeze the cervix for 2 minutes, allow a partial thaw and then refreeze it for a further period. Repeated applications may be necessary.

Electrodiathermy. This technique has largely replaced that of cautery, where heat generated or contained in the cautery instrument is used to destroy the area of columnar epithelium. The application of an electric current across the tissues generates heat within them, and hence achieves destruction. Diathermy, especially of the bipolar kind, creates particular safety hazards, and if the instruments used are not fully insulated the slightest touch of the live probe on to a speculum or holding forceps can lead to a burn in the surrounding tissues. There is also the risk of fire or explosion if inflammable spirit-based sterilising fluid has been used. Often in the past diathermy has been inadequately performed and hence led to poor results and incomplete destruction of the target areas. To be fully effective, diathermy destruction must be to the same standards and level as laser destruction.

Laser. Light Amplification by Stimulated Emission of Radiation allows a powerful beam of energy with a wavelength just outside the range of visible light to be concentrated so that power of up to 40 watts can be focused on an area of 1 mm or less in diameter. Such immensely concentrated energy has enormous destructive power, and tissues subjected to it will disintegrate forcefully due to vaporisation of their contents. The carbon dioxide laser can be used to deliver a beam with a wavelength of 10.6 μm that destroys tissue irrespective of its colour and with a minimum of heat permeation into the surrounding tissues. Hence the operator can see fully what he is destroying, and be confident that there is no hidden destruction deeper than he can see.

Laser destruction of columnar epithelium should be to a depth of 7 mm, the normal limit of depth of the crypts and retention cysts of the cervix. In most women this can be done without anaesthesia, although for some the pain is intense. Laser surgery is usually bloodless because the beam has the effect of sealing all but the largest vessels. It is probably also the treatment of choice for warty lesions. Obviously the high price of the instrument would probably preclude its purchase solely for use in a clinic of genitourinary medicine, but if physicians in this field have the option of sharing a laser with another department they should consider it carefully.

Conisation and trachelorrhaphy. If all else fails and the physician is certain that the woman's discharge is due to columnar epithelium on her cervix, surgery may be considered. Conisation or cone biopsy involves the excision of a cone shaped area of tissue from the cervix, with sutures being placed in the remaining tissues to secure haemostasis. This technique has the advantage that the whole of the excised area can be examined in great detail by a histopathologist. Trachelorrhaphy is used if the exposure of columnar epithelium on the cervix is due to lateral splitting; the exposed area is not excised but inverted into the cervix by repairing the splits.

Granulation tissue

Following any surgery to the lower genital tract there is a risk of the formation of granulation tissue in the suture lines, probably as the result of a reaction to the suture material. The commonest sites for this to be found are at the vault of the vagina following hysterectomy, and along the suture lines marking the site of repair of an episiotomy or tear following childbirth. This tissue is red and friable, bleeds to touch and often becomes infected producing a foul discharge. Providing there is no doubt about the diagnosis it should be destroyed, preferably by laser, cryotherapy or diathermy. Surgery is inappropriate, as the placing of sutures to repair the tissue after excision of granulation tissue will open the risk of new granulation appearing round the new suture.

REFERENCES

Ahmed M Y 1982 A comparison of treatment of vaginitis. Practitioner 226: 353

Amsel R, Totten P A, Spiegel C A, Chen K C S, Eschenbach D, Holmes K K 1983 Non-specific vaginitis. Diagnostic criteria and microbial and epidermiologic associations. American Journal of Medicine 74: 14–22

Barton S E, Thomas B J, Taylor-Robinson D, Goldmeier D 1985 Detection of C. trachomatis in the vaginal vault of women who have had hysterectomies. British Medical Journal 291: 250

Barton S E, Wright L K, Link C M, Munday P E 1986 Screening to detect asymptomatic shedding of HSV in women with recurrent HSV infection. Genitourinary Medicine 62: 181–185

Beaton J H, Gibson F, Roland M 1984 Short-term use of a medicated douche preparation in symptomatic treatment of minor vaginal irritation, in some cases associated with infertility. International Journal of Infertility 29: 109–112

Brunham R C, Paavonen J, Stevens C E 1984 Mucopurulent cervicitis. The ignored counterpart in women of urethritis in men. New England Journal of Medicine 311: 1–6

Burns D C McD, Darougar S, Thin R N, Lothian L, Nicol C S 1975 Isolation of chlamydia from women attending a clinic for sexually transmitted disease. British Journal of Venereal Diseases 51: 314–318

Cohen M S, Black J R, Procter R A, Sparling P F 1984 Host defences and the vaginal mucosa: a re-evaluation. In: Mardh P-A, Taylor-Robinson D (eds) Bacterial vaginosis. Almqvist and Wiksell International, Stockholm, pp 13–22

Coppleston M, Reid B 1967 The search for mutagens, mutagenesis and carrier. In: Preclinical carcinoma of the cervix uteri. Pergamon Press, Oxford, p 254–282

Cumberbatch G, Debney L 1987 Unpublished data presented at the British Association in August 1987 and reported in The Guardian 28 August 1987

Dans P E 1975 Gonococcal anogenital infection. Clinical Obstetrics and Gynaecology 18: 103–119

Dunlop E M C 1963 British Journal of Venereal Disease 39: 109

Dunlop E M C, Jones B R, Al-Hussaini M K 1964 Genital infection in association with TRIC virus infection of the eye. British Journal of Venereal Diseases 42: 77–87

Dunlop E M C, Hare M J, Darougar S, Jones B R 1970 Chlamydial isolates from the rectum in association with chlamydial infection with the eye or genital tract. In: Nichols R L (ed) Trachoma and related disorders Excerpta Medica International Congress Series No 223, pp 507–512

Eschenbach D A, Bekassy S, Blackwell A, Ekgren J, Hallen A, Wathne B 1984 The diagnosis of bacterial vaginosis. In: Mardh P-A, Taylor-Robinson D (eds) Bacterial vaginosis Almqvist and Wiksell International, Stockholm, pp 260–261

Fluhmann C F 1961 The cervix uteri and its disease. W B Saunders, Philadelphia, pp 30–102

Goldberg J, Sutherland E S 1963 Studies on gonorrhoeae: some social and sexual parameters of male patients in Kingston, Jamaica. West Indian Medical Journal 12: 228–246

Goldmeier D 1985 Proctitis. In: Taylor-Robinson D (ed) Clinical problems in sexually transmitted diseases. Martinus Nijhoff, Dordrecht, pp 237–283

Hare M J 1971 Gonococcal proctitis in women. MD thesis, University of London.

Hare M J, Toone E, Taylor-Robinson D, Evans R T, Furr P M, Oates J K 1981 Follicular cervicitis: colposcopic appearances and association with C. trachomatis. British Journal of Obstetrics and Gynaecology 88: 174–180

Harris J R W 1984 Gynatrec solcovae in the treatment of non-specific vaginitis. Gynakologische Rundschau 24 (suppl 3): 50–57

Harrison H R, Costin M, Meder J B et al 1985 Cervical C trachomatis infection in university women: relationship to history, contraception, ectopy and cervicitis. American Journal of Obstetrics and Gynecology 153: 244–251

Hayes H T 1929 Gonorrhoea of the anus and rectum. Journal of the American Medical Association 93: 1878

Hodge C H, Murdoch C H 1963 Treatment of vaginal discharge by sulfonamide pessaries. American Journal of Obstetrics and Gynecology 86: 742–744

Jacobs E 1976 Anal infections caused by herpes simplex virus. Diseases of the Colon and Rectum 19: 151–157

Jensen T 1953 Rectal gonorrhoea in women. British Journal of Venereal Diseases 29: 222

Jones B M, Kinghorn G R, Geary I 1982 In vitro susceptibility of G. vaginalis and Bacteroides organisms associated with non-specific vaginitis to sulfonamide preparation. Antimicrobial Agents and Chemotherapy 21: 870–872

Jordan J A, Singer A 1976 Effect of oral contraceptive steroids upon epithelium and mucus. In: Jordan J A, Singer A (eds) The cervix W B Saunders, London, pp 192–208

Kaufman R H, Gardner H L, Rawls W E, Dixon R E, Young R L 1973 Clinical features of herpes genitalis. Cancer Research 33: 1446–1451

Kinghorn G R, Rashid S 1979 Prevalence of rectal and pharyngeal infection in women with gonorrhoea in Sheffield. British Journal of Venereal Diseases 55: 408–410

Kinsey A C, Pomeroy W B, Martin C E 1948 Sexual behaviour in the human male. W B Saunders, Philadelphia

Kinsey A C, Pomeroy W B, Martin C E, Gebhard P 1953 Sexual behaviour in the human female. W B Saunders, Philadelphia

Litschgi M 1984 Treatment of non-specific colpitis with gynatren/solco trichovac. Gynakologische Rundschau 24 (suppl 3): 58–62

McCormack W M, Alpert S, McComb D E, Nichols R L, Semine D Z, Zinner S H 1979 Fifteen-month follow-up study of women infected with C. trachomatis. New England Journal of Medicine 300: 123–125

Martin C L 1935 Rectal gonorrhoea in women. Journal of the American Medical Association 104: 192

Masters W M, Johnson V E 1979 Homosexuality in practice. Little, Brown, Boston

Mayhew S R 1981 Vaginitis: a study of the efficacy of povidine-iodine in unselected cases. Journal of International Medical Research 9: 157–159

Meisels A, Fortin R, Roy M 1977 Condylomatous lesions of the cervix: cytologic, colposcopic and histopathologic study. Acta Cytologica 21: 379–390

Minkoff H, Grunebaum A, McCormack W M, Schwarz H 1985 Relationship of vaginitis to the sex of conceptuses. American Journal of Obstetrics and Gynecology 66: 239–240

Monif G R G, Thompson J L, Stephens H D, Baer H 1980 Quantitative and qualitative effects of povidine-iodine liquid and gel on the aerobic and anaerobic flora of the female genital tract. American Journal of Obstetrics and Gynecology 137: 432–438

Munday P E, Cardner J M, Taylor-Robinson D 1985 Chlamydial proctitis? British Journal of Venereal Diseases 61: 376–378

Oriel J D, Powis P A, Reeve P, Miller A, Nicol C S 1974

Chlamydial infections of the cervix. British Journal of Venereal Diseases 50: 11–16

Owen R, Christiansen G, Hansen E et al 1984 Taxonomy of anaerobic curved rods. In: Mardh P-A, Taylor-Robinson D (eds) Bacterial vaginosis. Almqvist and Wiksell International, Stockholm, pp 264–265

Paavonen J, Saikku A, Vesterinen E, Meyer B, Vartiainen E, Saksela E 1978 Genital chlamydial infections in patients attending a gynaecological outpatient clinic. British Journal of Venereal Diseases 54: 257–261

Paavonen J, Meyer B, Vesterinen E, Saksela E 1980 Colposcopic and histological findings in cervical chlamydial infection. Lancet ii: 320

Paavonen J, Kallings I, Norling B et al 1984 Therapy of bacterial vaginosis. In: Mardh P-A, Taylor-Robinson D (eds) Bacterial vaginosis. Almqvist and Wiksell International, Stockholm, pp 265–266

Rattray M C, Corey L, Reeves W C, Vontver L A, Holmes K K 1978 Recurrent genital herpes amongst women: symptomatic v. asymptomatic viral shedding. British Journal of Venereal Diseases 54: 262–265

Robinson J 1982 Cancer of the cervix: occupational risks of husbands and wives and possible preventive strategies. In: Jordan J A, Sharp F, Singer A (eds) Pre-clinical neoplasia of the cervix. Royal College of Obstetricians and Gynaecologists, London

Rylander E, Eriksson A, von Schoultz B 1984 Wart virus infection of the cervix uteri and vagina in women with atypical cervical cytology. In: Mardh P-A, Taylor-Robinson D (eds) Bacterial vaginosis. Wiksell International, Stockholm, pp 223–226

Schuch R J, Musich J R, Nelson R L 1984 Chlamydial proctitis, unusual presentation as a symptomatic vaginal mass. Obstetrics and Gynecology 62: 132–134

Simmonds P D, Vosmik F 1974 Cervical cytology in non-specific genital infection: an aid to diagnosis. British Journal of Venereal Diseases 50: 313–314

Singer A 1982 What causes squamous carcinoma of the cervix? In: Jordan J A, Sharp F, Singer A (eds) Pre-clinical neoplasia of the cervix. Royal College of Obstetricians and Gynaecologists, London

Slater F 1950 The effect of vaginal pH on wound healing. American Journal of Obstetrics and Gynecology 59: 1089–1094

Slavin G 1976 The pathology of cervical inflammatory disease. In: Jordan J A, Singer A (eds) The cervix. W B Saunders, London, pp 251–269

Spiegel C A, Amsel R A, Eschenbach D, Schoeknecht F, Holmes K K 1980 Anaerobic bacteria in non-specific vaginitis. New England Journal of Medicine 303: 601–607

Vaughan-Jackson J D, Dunlop E M C, Darougar S, Dwyer R Sr C, Jones B R 1972 Results of tests for chlamydia in patients suffering from acute Reiters disease compared with results of tests of the genital tract and rectum in patients with ocular infection due to TRIC agent. British Journal of Venereal Diseases 48: 437–444

Wilbanks G D, Richart R M 1967 The puerperal cervix, injuries and healing: a colposcopic study. American Journal of Obstetrics and Gynecology 97: 1105–1110

Willcox R R 1961 An unusual case of vaginal tumour. British Journal of Venereal Diseases 37: 284

Willcox R R 1968 Necrotic cervicitis due to primary infection with the virus of herpes simplex. British Medical Journal i: 610–612

Pelvic inflammatory disease
M J Hare

INTRODUCTION AND DEFINITION

Pelvic inflammatory disease may be described as inflammation of the upper female genital tract, that is above the level of the uterine cervix. Such changes are almost always related to microbial infection, although in certain rare circumstances other stimuli such as chemical irritation may be responsible. Inflammatory changes may be confined to the endometrium (endometritis); or may have spread to the fallopian tubes (salpingitis); or may have spread further to involve the ovaries as well as the tubes (salpingo-oophoritis). Further spread may involve the peritoneal cavity (peritonitis) and localised abscess formation. Spread may occur along the paracolic gutter to the liver to cause perihepatitis (Fitz-Hugh Curtis syndrome).

Almost always spread is upward, with the endometrium first becoming infected followed by the tubes, the ovaries and then other structures. Adnexal involvement is usually bilateral although one side will often be at a more advanced stage than the other. Rarely pelvic inflammation is secondary to localised infection elsewhere in the body, for example from appendicitis, and in this case the spread is downwards and the condition usually unilateral. It may also occur as the consequence of a generalised infection such as tuberculosis.

Although taken literally the terms pelvic inflammatory disease and salpingitis (together with adnexitis, which is occasionally used) should have different meanings, in practice they tend to be used interchangeably in publications. In this chapter the term pelvic inflammatory disease will be used throughout except when reference is being made to published work when the author's preference will be followed.

PATHOGENESIS

Theories of development

The cavities of the uterus, tubes and peritoneum can be regarded as microbiologically sterile under normal, healthy circumstances, with the exception of the time of labour and immediately following delivery when the uterine cavity becomes colonised by micro-organisms, miscarriage, and in the woman who uses an intra-uterine contraceptive device (see Chapter 2). In contrast the cervix and vagina are normally colonised by a wide variety of micro-organisms. With the exception of the rare group of patients where tubal infection is a consequence of spread from a non-genital intra-abdominal focus of infection (less than 1% of all cases; see Weström 1980), and in cases of tuberculosis, a route must be postulated between the colonised lower and the sterile upper genital tracts. Two alternatives have classically been described (Keith et al 1984), these being:

1. Upward spread through the cavities of the cervix, uterine body and tubes, and
2. Through the lymphatic drainage of the cervix, bypassing the endometrial cavity.

This second option of lymphatic spread now seems to be involved hardly ever, if at all. Recent studies have shown endometritis to be present in virtually all cases of salpingitis (Heinonen et al 1985), and an earlier report by Falk (1946) demonstrated that cornual resection effectively prevents recurrent attacks of salpingitis, suggesting that there was no alternative route to the fallopian tubes.

The physiological barriers

The bar to the upward spread of infection appears to occur mainly at the uterine cervix, with a secondary barrier at the uterotubal junction. At the cervix ascent is blocked by mechanical, biochemical and immunological factors, and these vary between the non-pregnant and pregnant states. The mechanical factors include the small diameter of the pelvic canal, especially in the nulliparous state, and the downward flow of cervical mucus, enhanced by cilial activity. In established pregnancy this cervical barrier is made virtually absolute by the tight application of the amnion and chorion across the internal cervical os. Pelvic inflammatory disease in pregnancy, although not impossible, is an extreme rarity and the incidence decreases the further the pregnancy progresses (Acosta et al 1971). The biochemical barrier of the cervix is the production of lysozyme, an enzyme capable of hydrolysing the beta 1–4 peptidoglycan linkage of microorganisms, allowing osmotic lysis. The action of lysozyme may be enhanced by the presence of secretory IgA (Cohen et al 1984), which is also produced by the cervix (Rebello et al 1975).

Factors that will compromise the cervical barrier include childbirth and abortion, surgical instrumentation and the insertion of intrauterine contraceptive devices. After spontaneous or instrumental dilation the cervix is very slow to constrict down, and after the first delivery or miscarriage will never completely regain its prepregnancy state. Moreover at delivery especially some degree of splitting and distortion is inevitable. Around these events the upper genital tract is especially vulnerable to ascending infection, both by sexually transmitted organisms and those that normally inhabit the woman's own vagina and bowel, the risk gradually falling off as the uterus and cervix involute.

Surgical intervention is particularly likely to lead to pelvic infection if the woman is pregnant, and so procedures for pregnancy termination cause particular risk. Even with the best technique it is virtually impossible to sterilise the vagina and cervix preoperatively, and although women are at especial risk if they are infected with sexually transmitted organisms (Moller et al 1982), 'normal inhabitants' may also be the cause of pelvic inflammation following these events. It is now generally accepted that high risk events such as pregnancy termination should be covered by prophylactic antibiotics (Grimes et al 1984). The role of the intrauterine contraceptive device is discussed later.

However, pelvic inflammatory disease does occur in women who have experienced none of the compromising events detailed above; young women who have never had a child, miscarriage, curettage or any other procedure on the genital tract and who do not have an intrauterine contraceptive device; and a theory is needed to explain why in such otherwise healthy women the cervical barrier is broached and pelvic inflammatory disease develops. Such theories may be divided into those postulating transport of the causative microorganism by other motile organisms, and the physiological changes in the cervix and the uterus produced by the menstrual cycle and coitus.

Past and present authors have consistently affirmed that coitus is a prerequisite for the development of pelvic inflammatory disease, to the degree that if the condition occurs in a virgin it is assumed always to be due to spread of infection from elsewhere in the abdomen (Keith et al 1984). Whether this is true or not has not been tested by modern research, but the fact can probably be accepted. The organisms that cause pelvic inflammatory disease are not sufficiently mobile to progress upwards by their own efforts, but at intercourse both *Trichomonas vaginalis* and spermatozoa may be deposited, and the authors consider that each may provide transport for potential pathogens.

T. vaginalis can penetrate both the cervical and uterotubal barriers and has been found in both the fallopian tubes and the peritoneal cavity, although it has never been thought of as a causative agent (Mardh & Weström 1970). Trichomoniasis is also commonly found coexisting with pelvic inflammatory disease, and the organism has therefore been suggested as a vector for upper genital tract pathogens. Keith et al (1984) discussed the published evidence supporting this view, and themselves demonstrated in the laboratory attachment between *Escherichia coli* and *T. vaginalis*, apparently with harm to neither. However the same does not occur with sexually transmitted pathogens.

Francioli et al (1983) incubated strains of *Neisseria gonorrhoeae* with *T. vaginalis* and showed a rapid decline in the viability of the gonococci. This effect was enhanced by the presence of human serum, and for one strain was dependent on it. *T. vaginalis* was observed to phagocytose and then kill the gonococci; interestingly, when *N. gonorrhoeae* were incubated with the cattle parasite *Tritrichomonas fetus* neither effect was observed. Street et al (1984) confirmed this reaction between the gonococcus and *Trichomonas vaginalis* and reported similar results when *T. vaginalis* and *Mycoplasma hominis* were incubated together. This experiment, involving *T. vaginalis* and *Chlamydia trachomatis*, gave less clear results, and certainly the latter organism was not ingested by the former. These authors had designed their experiments partly to test the unpublished assertion of another investigator that trichomonads enhanced the survival of chlamydiae, a claim they could not confirm. It must be concluded, therefore, that although *T. vaginalis* cannot act as a vector for *N. gonorrhoeae* or *M. hominis* it may do so for other micro-organisms.

The evidence in favour of spermatozoa acting as vectors is much stronger. Amongst the organisms that can become attached to sperm and remain viable are *N. gonorrhoeae* (Gomez et al 1979), T-mycoplasmas (now classified as *Ureaplasma urealyticum*; Gnarpe & Friberg 1973), *C. trachomatis* (Wolner-Hanssen & Mardh 1984) and various aerobic and anaerobic micro-organisms (Toth et al 1982; Keith et al 1984). No investigator has reported harmful interactions between spermatozoa and these micro-organisms, and as sperm normally reach the fallopian tubes their role as vector seems very likely. Penetration of cervical mucus by sperm is reduced in women using hormonal contraception, and this may correlate with the apparent reduction of the incidence of gonococcal pelvic inflammatory disease in this group. However, the relationship between hormonal contraception and infection is complex, and will be examined in detail later.

The risk of developing gonococcal pelvic inflammatory disease seems to vary with the phase of the menstrual cycle with the highest rates being reported in the week after menstruation (Eschenbach et al 1977). This may be an effect specific to the gonococcal form of the infection, in that the discharge of menstrual blood and debris produces an environment most condusive to the growth of *N. gonorrhoeae*. Certainly pelvic inflammation due to *C. trachomatis* and other micro-organisms does not seem to be commonest at that time.

As has been previously noted the definite relationship between coitus and pelvic inflammatory disease has always been considered important if not axiomatic, and various work has been reported suggesting that female orgasmic uterine contractions may be responsible for drawing both sperm and micro-organisms through the cervical barrier. Fox et al (1970) report a very steep pressure gradient in the immediate postorgasmic period from the vagina (maximum +35 cm water) to the uterine cavity (minimum −26 cm water), and postulated that this would result in a postcoital 'insuck' of the vaginal contents including the ejaculate. Elgi & Newton (1961) demonstrated transport of carbon particles from the vagina to the fallopian tubes in women about to undergo hysterectomy and who had received oxytocin injections. They suggested that this was caused by the rhythmic contractions of the uterus produced by the drug and drew a parallel with the orgasmic response; however, their patients were under general anaesthesia and the possible effects of anaesthetics and muscle relaxants are not taken into account in their work. The women they studied were also highly parous. The 'pressure gradient' theory for the development of pelvic inflammatory disease may also help to explain anecdotal reports of the condition occurring following water-skiing, which can result in very high water pressure on the perineal region, and following anogenital coitus when air has been blown into the vagina. Previous infection also seems to compromise the defence mechanisms of the genital tract, and women who have had one attack are at significant risk of recurrence. This subject is dealt with fully by Professor Weström in Chapter 21.

There appears to be a secondary barrier to the upward spread of infection, and this has been described in an animal model by Chow et al (1980). It appears to depend on the small size of the tubal aperture and the downward flow of mucus. Certainly in the human endometritis is not always accompanied by salpingitis, although this may be because spread has not yet occurred rather than definitely arrested.

Once in the fallopian tubes infectious material can leak out into the pelvic peritoneal cavity, leading to oophoritis. Adhesions soon occur to limit the infection, and the ends of the tubes become clubbed and sealed off. Outside the pelvis the main area of spread is upwards along the right paracolic gutter to the liver and surrounding area, leading to the syndrome of perihepatitis named after the authors of two early descriptions, Fitz-Hugh (1934) and Curtis (1930). Until recently this was thought to be a specific manifestation of gonococcal disease, but recently chlamydial infection has also been implicated.

To summarise, therefore, almost all cases of non-tuberculous pelvic inflammatory disease spread upward from the lower genital tract. The cervix and the uterotubal junction usually provide an effective barrier against such spread, but this becomes less effective as a consequence of childbirth and miscarriage and various surgical and medical insults. Most lower genital infections remain confined, but in the sexually transmitted diseases such as gonorrhoea and chlamydial cervicitis, around 10% will develop into pelvic inflammatory disease. Possible ways in which the cervical barrier is overcome include transport upwards on vectors and the physiological pressure changes within the genital tract.

The role of contraception

Each of the common forms of artificial contraception has an effect on the acquisition and development of pelvic inflammatory disease, and with some methods the effect is complex with different factors causing sometimes contrary effects. In this section the methods will be considered in groups, viz.:

Barrier methods, male and female;
The intrauterine contraceptive device;
Hormonal methods;
Permanent methods.

Barrier methods

It is generally agreed that proper use of the condom will prevent the transfer of *Neisseria gonorrhoeae*, although its value in the prevention of chlamydial infections seems much more questionable (Barlow 1977). Kelaghan et al (1982) in a case control study claimed that the protective influence of barrier contraceptives extends to pelvic inflammatory disease, reducing the risk by almost a half. This extended to both primary and recurrent attacks, to both sheaths and diaphragms and, interestingly, to the use of spermicides alone. Spermicidal preparations are known to have a weak antimicrobial action (Singh et al 1972), and Kelaghan et al postulate that it is the antibacterial effect of the spermicide that is responsible for the success of the diaphragm in the prevention of pelvic inflammatory disease.

It is impossible to deduce from the evidence presented by Kelaghan and his colleagues, and other published work, what the reason is for their results. Is it simply that the transfer of sexually transmitted infections such as gonorrhoea is prevented by barrier contraception, but that if these women do acquire such an infection it is just as likely to progress to pelvic inflammatory disease in them as in others? Or is the mechanism of cervical bypass modified in this group? If so, this would seem to support the sperm vector theory, as amongst the temporary methods of contraception only in barrier method usage are sperm kept completely away from the uterine cervix.

The intrauterine contraceptive device

There is no doubt that the use of an intrauterine contraceptive device markedly increases for that woman the risk of developing pelvic inflammatory disease. Senanayake & Kramer (1980) reviewed a large number of reports on this relationship, and found the risk to be stated as up to a 10-fold increase over women using no contraception or other methods. Typical of such series was that of Targum & Wright (1974) in which 48% of women experiencing a first attack of pelvic inflammatory disease had an intrauterine contraceptive device in place, compared with 9% of matched controls. The authors stressed, however, that the condition was often mild and could be managed with the device in place. Vessey et al (1981) reported hospital admission rates in the United Kingdom with a diagnosis of acute pelvic inflammatory disease to be 1.51 per 1000 women for intrauterine device users, compared with 0.14/1000 for non-users. They found the Dalkon shield (now withdrawn) to be associated with the highest risk and copper-containing devices to be associated with the lowest risk. Smith & Soderstrom (1976) claimed an even higher instance of disease; they reported that tubal biopsies taken from women undergoing sterilisation procedure revealed inflammatory change in 47% of intrauterine contraceptive device users, compared with less than 1% in non-users.

A degree of endometritis is found in all intrauterine device users and indeed, this may be part of the mechanism of action as it produces an environment hostile to spermatozoa and the fertilised ovum. This reaction is normally associated with the presence in the uterine cavity of bacteria representative of the vaginal population if the device has a string or tail reaching through the cervix into the vagina, although when the device has no tail the cavity is often bacteriologically sterile (Sparkes et al 1981). Such colonisation may be irrelevant to the clinical state of the woman under normal conditions, but may flare up into clinical pelvic inflammation when potentially precipitating events occur. Thus Paavonen et al (1981) noted that in cases of both gonococcal and non-gonococcal pelvic inflammatory disease antibodies to two normal vaginal bacterial inhabitants (enteric bacteria and *Bacteroides fragilis*) were present more commonly in those who were intrauterine device users than in non-users.

Whether or not pelvic inflammatory disease in intrauterine contraceptive device users is more likely to lead to abscess formation remains uncertain. Edelman & Berger (1980) review the previous literature which contains conflicting reports and present their own series. In this a higher proportion of intrauterine device users had acute pelvic inflammatory disease, but a lower proportion of these women required surgical treatment than in a group of non-users. Niebyl et al (1978) interestingly report the association of unilateral ovarian (rather than tubo-ovarian) abscess with intrauterine device usage; they postulate that bacteria are shed continuously through the fallopian tubes resulting in infection of the corpus luteum which is a unilateral structure.

Despite the alarming incidence of pelvic inflammation in intrauterine device users, Targum & Wright (1974) feel that the risk to the total health of the woman must not be overstated. Overall they consider the risk of death through intrauterine contraceptive device usage to be much lower than that attributable to hormonal contraception.

Hormonal contraception

Hormonal contraceptives, usually in the form of the combined oestrogen–progesterone oral pill, are the commonest form of fertility control used in the age groups in which pelvic inflammatory disease is most prevalent. Epidemiological studies have been conducted in many centres on the possible relationship between these two factors, and almost all have concluded that the taking of oral contraceptives protects against the development of pelvic inflammatory disease. For example Rubin et al (1982) looked at 648 women hospitalised with a diagnosis of pelvic inflammatory disease and compared them with 2516 case controls. They concluded that women using oral contraceptives for more than one year had the risk of developing pelvic inflammatory disease reduced by one-third compared with those who used no contraception. This protective advantage was not demonstrable in those who had used oral contraceptives for a shorter time. However these authors consider than the use of oral contraceptives confers a greater benefit on the health of the American nation, preventing 12 500 hospital admissions for pelvic inflammatory disease that would otherwise be expected, and would use this as a relevant factor when advising young women about contraception.

Svensson et al (1984) came to similar conclusions about the 'protective' effect of oral contraception in salpingitis. They looked at 546 women experiencing their first attack of salpingitis; all underwent diagnostic laparoscopy and a significantly greater proportion of the women using oral contraception had mild rather than moderate or severe disease when compared with those using intrauterine devices and those not using oral contraceptives or intrauterine devices. They concluded that oral contraceptives diminished the inflammatory reaction in the fallopian tubes in acute salpingitis, and, as the degree of inflammation is correlated with the future fecundity of the woman, considered that women at risk of developing acute salpingitis should be advised to use oral contraceptives.

This view is not shared by Washington et al

(1985) in a carefully argued review article that merits full consideration. Whilst accepting that oral contraception may have a protective function against severe or acute pelvic inflammatory disease of the degree that requires hospital admission, they conclude that from studies already published no evidence exists for such protection against mild disease. They point out that:

1. All the studies commonly quoted showing a negative correlation between oral contraception and pelvic inflammatory disease are of the case control type and involve hospitalised patients: none of a smaller group of cross-sectional studies provide the same result and the only one based on outpatients shows a positive correlation with an increased risk of pelvic inflammatory disease for oral contraceptive users of 1.7 (Noonen & Adams 1974).

2. Almost all authors agree that oral contraceptive use increases the risk of chlamydial cervicitis. Of 14 papers quoted, 12 show an increased risk of up to fourfold and two show an equal risk when compared with non-users.

3. Although in animal studies progesterone is observed to suppress the growth of *Neisseria gonorrhoeae* (whereas oestrogen slightly enhances this), both oestrogen and progesterone enhance the growth, survival and ascension of genital chlamydial infection. In experiments with mice Taylor-Robinson et al (1982) reported that chlamydial infections lasted at least four times as long if the mice were pretreated with progesterone, and Rank & Barron (1982) reported similar findings with oestrogen.

It is also reported that chlamydial infection of the fallopian tubes often produces a markedly milder clinical picture than non-chlamydial salpingitis (Svensson et al 1984); indeed Henry-Suchet et al (1980) reported a 25.4% tubal isolation rate for *Chlamydia trachomatis* from women with obstructive infertility but without signs of pelvic inflammatory disease, compared with a 23.5% tubal isolate rate from women with acute pelvic inflammatory disease, and no such isolations from 36 control women. Interestingly, this control group was described as containing some women with ovarian causes for infertility, who probably had low levels of both oestrogen and progesterone, or high levels of oestrogen and low levels of progesterone. Obviously these women would not have been

current users of oral contraception, but could well have done so in the past. The evidence appears to suggest that undetected chlamydial pelvic inflammatory disease may well run a mild or even subclinical course, with the gradual progression of tubal damage. Theoretically, at least, oral contraceptive usage could encourage this pattern.

Permanent methods

For women, permanent contraception or sterilisation is most commonly achieved by blocking the fallopian tubes to prevent the union of the ovum with a spermatozoon, either by surgical division and ligation (Pomeroy's method) or by the application of a silastic band or self-locking clip under laparoscopic control. From many studies it is clear that such procedures reduce the likelihood of both primary and recurrent pelvic inflammatory disease developing, and probably prevent new infections completely. Falk (1946) reported on over 1000 cases of pelvic inflammatory disease treated by cornual resection and claimed 'in no instance have we seen or heard of a reinfection occurring'.

Male sterilisation techniques have not been investigated so well. Certainly if the sperm vector theory of development of pelvic inflammatory disease is valid it would be expected that the female sexual partners of men who had undergone vasectomy would be at lower risk of developing pelvic inflammatory disease than those of fertile men. No evidence on this has been published, but Toth et al (1982) report the clinical observation that salpingitis was a rare event in the wives of several hundred azoospermic males who came for infertility consultation.

THE CLINICAL FEATURES AND DIAGNOSIS OF PELVIC INFLAMMATORY DISEASE

Clinical features

The accurate diagnosis of the cause of lower abdominal pain in a young woman in her reproductive years is one of the most difficult of commonly occurring clinical situations. Jacobsen & Weström (1969) reported that, when made by trained gynaecologists, the diagnosis of pelvic inflammatory disease was accurate in only two-thirds of cases. General surgeons are just as inaccurate; Robinson & Burch (1984) report the diagnostic accuracy for acute appendicitis in young women to be as low or even lower. In routine clinical practice, when the results are not being prepared for publication or subjected to regular peer review, diagnostic accuracy is probably at least as bad, and many women with abdominal pain not obviously due to another cause will be labelled as suffering from pelvic inflammatory disease. Once such a diagnosis has been made it tends to stick for ever, and further episodes of pain are diagnosed as recurrent pelvic inflammatory disease without much consideration of alternatives.

If the diagnosis of pelvic inflammatory disease is to be made and relied upon clinical and basic laboratory findings, then very strict criteria must be used. Hager et al (1983) published such criteria on behalf of the Infectious Disease Society for Obstetrics and Gynecology of the USA. The recommendation is that for the diagnosis of pelvic inflammatory disease to be made the following three features should be present:

Abdominal direct tenderness, with or without rebound tenderness;
Tenderness with motion of the cervix and uterus;
Adnexal tenderness;

together with at least one of the following:

Gram-negative intracellular diplococci identified in endocervical secretions;
Body temperature greater than 38° Celsius;
Leucocytosis greater than 10 000 per mm³;
Purulent material obtained from peritoneal cavity by culdocentesis or laparoscopy;
Pelvic abscess or inflammatory complex on bimanual examination or by sonography.

(Given the present availability of the rapid immunofluorescent test for the identification of *Chlamydia trachomatis* using monoclonal antibodies, it would seem logical to include with these criteria the identification of this organism in the cervix, as an alternative to the gonococcus.)

This diagnostic method depends on signs rather than symptoms. In their paper previously quoted, Jacobsen & Weström (1969) had assessed the importance of symptoms, including low abdominal pain (almost always the presenting symptom), increased vaginal discharge, self-measured pyrexia or 'fever chills', irregular vaginal bleeding, urinary symptoms, vomiting and symptoms of proctitis. When they looked at these symptoms in women who had been diagnosed as suffering from pelvic inflammatory disease, and compared the incidence of each in the group who had the diagnosis confirmed on laparoscopy with the group whose pelvic findings were normal on laparoscopy, only symptoms of pyrexia or proctitis were significantly different in each group, both being commoner in the group of women who had the diagnosis confirmed. All the other symptoms were as common, and sometimes more common, in the 'normal' group. These authors also confirmed that signs were more reliable; tenderness on bimanual examination, the impression of a palpable mass or swelling in the pelvis, an observed abnormal vaginal discharge and a measured pyrexia were all significantly commoner in women with a confirmed diagnosis of pelvic inflammatory disease than in those with laparoscopically normal pelves. From the laboratory they regarded a raised erythrocyte sedimentation rate as significant. The best diagnostic combinations appeared to be pelvic pain, increased vaginal discharge, raised erythrocyte sedimentation rate with marked adnexal tenderness. The presence of a palpable mass made the diagnosis even more likely, but with all these features present 6 of 135 women did not have pelvic inflammatory disease. Of the diagnostic symptoms and signs mentioned more than seven had to be present together for complete diagnostic accuracy.

Hager et al (1983) also described a system for grading pelvic inflammatory disease by clinical features. They suggested:

Grade I. Uncomplicated (limited to tubes and/or ovaries);
with or without pelvic peritonitis.

Grade II. Complicated (inflammatory mass or abscess involving tubes or ovaries;
with or without pelvic peritonitis.

Grade III. Spread to structures beyond the pelvis, i.e. ruptured tubo-ovarian abscess.

The use of diagnostic and staging criteria is to be recommended. If these criteria were universally adopted they would not only act as a brake on thinly based diagnosis, but also form a basis for the comparison of work produced by different units.

The need for laparoscopy

Jacobsen & Weström (1969) stressed the inaccuracy of the clinical diagnosis of pelvic inflammatory disease, even when that diagnosis has been made by a specialist gynaecologist, an inaccuracy that is in keeping with the accuracy achieved by other specialists dealing with the other causes of lower abdominal pain in women. They performed a diagnostic laparoscopy on each of 814 women with a preoperative diagnosis of acute salpingitis. In 532 cases (65%) the diagnosis was confirmed; in 184 cases (23%) no pathological change could be seen (or came to light subsequently), and in 98 cases (12%) other pathological findings were present. These findings included acute appendicitis in 24 cases, endometriosis in 16 cases, bleeding from a ruptured corpus luteum in 12 cases, ectopic pregnancy in 11 cases and an ovarian tumour in 7 cases. Some of these conditions are life-threatening; none will respond to antibiotic therapy; and all require alternative medical or surgical management. Lundberg et al (1973) produce similar results, and especially highlight the unreliability of the clinical diagnosis of a pelvic mass in such cases. They cited 25 women with abdominal pain who were thought preoperatively to have a pelvic mass; the diagnosis was confirmed at laparoscopy in only eight. A pelvic mass was found at laparoscopy in 4 of 47 who were thought preoperativly not to have one.

Diagnostic laparoscopy would appear to be a safe and reliable way of confirming the diagnosis in these cases. In a large nationwide survey in the United Kingdom, Chamberlain & Carron-Brown (1978) found the mortality associated with diagnostic laparoscopy to be 4.9 per 100 000 cases, and that operative complications severe enough to warrant laparotomy occurred at the rate of 6.6 cases in every 1000. These risks would appear to be outweighed by the changes of severe blood loss from an undetected ectopic pregnancy or ruptured corpus luteum, or of neglect of a gangrenous appendix.

However it must be admitted that the majority of gynaecologists and genitourinary physicians both in the United Kingdom and abroad do not recognise the need for laparoscopy as part of the routine investigation of women with a presumptive diagnosis of pelvic inflammatory disease. If this attitude is held certain exceptions need to be made when laparoscopy becomes highly desirable if not obligatory. These would be:

—in severely ill women, especially if cardiovascular shock is present;
—in the older woman, when the alternative diagnosis of endometriosis and malignant disease is more likely;
—when a history of menstrual irregularity makes pregnancy a greater possibility;
—in women claiming no sexual experience;
—when diagnosis is in real doubt.

Otherwise, if the diagnosis is clear-cut according to the criteria already described, a trial of antibiotic therapy is acceptable by present day conventions. A positive response should be noted within 72 hours of the start of such treatment, and if this does not occur laparoscopy should be undertaken at that point.

The diagnostic features of pelvic inflammatory disease as seen down the laparoscope were described by Jacobsen & Weström (1969) as pronounced hyperanaemia of the tubal surface, oedema of the tubal wall, and a sticky exudate of the tubal surface and from the fimbrial ends when these are patent. Hager et al (1983) suggest the following grading on findings at laparoscopy or laparotomy:

Mild. Erythema, oedema, no spontaneous discharge of pus, tubes freely mobile.

Moderate. Grossly purulent material evident. More marked erythema and oedema. Tubes may not be freely mobile, and the fimbrial stoma may not be patent.

Severe. The presence of a pyosalpinx, inflammatory complex, or abscess.

Endometrial biopsy

On the assumption that the route of infection from the lower genital tract to the tubes and ovaries lies through the uterine cavity, it has recently been suggested that histological or cytological evidence of endometritis might strengthen the diagnosis of pelvic inflammatory disease sufficiently to make diagnostic laparoscopy unnecessary. Small endometrial biopsies are easy to obtain on a conscious patient with a 3 mm suction curette (Vabra curette, Ferrosan Co., Copenhagen, Denmark), and these can be quickly processed and examined for histological evidence of endometritis. Paavonen et al (1985a) compared the use of endometrial biopsy with diagnostic laparoscopy in 27 cases. Nineteen women had endometritis and 18 had typical changes of pelvic inflammatory disease at laparoscopy; three had endometritis without the laparoscopic appearance of salpingitis being present, and two had salpingitis without endometritis. Taking also into account the finding of evidence of inflammation in cytological smears from peritoneal fluid, these authors suggest that endometritis may be a more sensitive indicator of pelvic inflammatory disease than laparoscopic appearance. If this is so, and the incidence of endometritis associated with cervicitis is as high as 40%, as suggested by the same author (Paavonen et al 1985b), then the risk of developing pelvic inflammatory disease from cervicitis is considerably higher than is usually stated. At present the safety and usefulness of this technique have not been fully assessed, but it may be of considerable clinical use in the future.

Ultrasound and other imaging techniques

Over the past decade vast experience has been gained in the application of diagnostic ultrasound, and the female pelvis has been one of the areas most intensely studied. Landers & Sweet (1985) review recent reports on the use of this technique in the management of pelvic inflammatory disease, and conclude that it is highly accurate in the diagnosis of tubal abscess and related changes. Spirtos et al (1982) showed ultrasound to be more than twice as accurate as clinical assessment in the detection of pelvic masses, on a par with laparoscopy. One great advantage of ultrasound over almost any other method is that repeated examinations can be made with accurate measurements of the size of each abscess, and hence the response to treatment can be charted.

Other imaging techniques that have shown themselves to be of value are radionucleotide scanning (using gallium 67 or indium 111 marked white blood cells) and computed tomographic scans.

Both such techniques are highly accurate but both are much more expensive to perform than ultrasound, and so they have limited usefulness.

MICROBIOLOGICAL INVESTIGATIONS

Introduction

Laboratory investigations are performed in an attempt to identify the causative agent or agents in an attack of pelvic inflammatory disease, and hence to provide guidelines on suitable antibiotic therapy. The range of potentially pathogenic micro-organisms to be sought is vast, from the true viruses through chlamydia and mycoplasmas to aerobic and anaerobic bacteria, and even to protozoa. The sites that may be tested are also numerous. Inevitably, therefore, not every site can be tested or every specialised microbiological technique used; indeed some sites and tests are obviously of more value to research than as aids to the management of individual patients. A reasoned decision must be made in each case, therefore, as to what should or should not be done. This must be based to a degree on the probability of particular organisms being involved in that case, but allowance must be made for the possibility that this opinion is wrong!

The possible useful sites of microbiological investigation for pelvic inflammatory disease include:
The lower genital tract, the oropharynx and the rectum;
The endometrial cavity;
The peritoneal fluid present in the pouch of Douglas, removed by culdocentesis;
Pus, epithelial debris and minute biopsy material removed from the fallopian tubes under direct vision at laparoscopy, together with peritoneal fluid aspirated at the same time by a cannula inserted through the abdominal wall;
Blood for culture and antibody studies;
Material from the genital tract or oropharynx of the woman's sexual partner or partners.

Material from the lower genital tract, oropharynx and rectum

These should be taken under direct vision after the passage of a bivalve speculum, and full details will be found in Chapter 5. Material from the urethra and cervix should first be smeared on to a slide, heat fixed and stained by Gram's method for the presence of pus and gonococci. A 'wet' preparation (diluted in saline) should be examined immediately for *Trichomonas vaginalis* which, although not itself a cause of pelvic inflammatory disease, should be treated at the same time. Cultures are then taken from the vaginal walls, the cervix and the urethra and either plated directly or placed in transport medium: these are examined for gonococci and other bacteria. It is important that material from one of these sites—usually the vagina—is cultured for anaerobic organisms.

A swab is now revolved firmly around the walls of the endocervix, and the material so obtained is examined for the presence of *Chlamydia trachomatis*, either by culture or using immunofluorescence techniques to demonstrate the organism or antibody to it. Other tests that may be taken at this point include those for mycoplasmas, ureaplasmas and viruses. A cervical smear for Papanicolaou staining can also be taken at this point: this will not only reveal changes suggestive of premalignant disease but also indicate infection with agents such as wart virus, herpes virus, *T. vaginalis*, *Candida albicans* and *Actinomyces*.

Whether or not rectal and pharyngeal specimens are taken must be decided by the clinician managing the case. Certainly the taking of rectal specimens is distasteful to most women, and many will consider this an implication that they have participated in penoanal coitus. One way round this potential problem is to take the specimens under general anaesthesia prior to laparoscopy. It is, however, unlikely that any extra evidence will be obtained from rectal or pharyngeal specimens to help in the management of pelvic inflammatory disease.

The endometrial cavity

The vagina is not normally sterile; as Dr Warren has shown in Chapter 2 it can be colonised by a vast range of potentially pathogenic aerobic and anaerobic organisms and the results of lower genital tract culture may well not reveal the true nature of the organisms infecting the upper genital tract. In contrast, good correlation has been shown between cultures from the endometrial cavity and cultures from the fallopian tubes, with some evidence suggesting the endometrium is the more useful site to sample (Heinonen et al 1985). To take specimens from the endometrial cavity the cervix must be wiped thoroughly free of debris and a thin catheter passed through the endocervical canal into the body of the uterus. Material can then be obtained using suction or a rotary swab. Small biopsies can be obtained as described previously. A full range of relevant microbiological tests should be performed on these specimens.

Peritoneal fluid obtained by culdocentesis

Culdocentesis is the technique where the rectovaginal pouch of Douglas is entered by a sharp needle pushed through the posterior vaginal fornix, the cervix being deflected anteriorly to facilitate this. If during the procedure the woman is lying on her back in a semisupported position any free fluid in the peritoneal cavity will have run down and collected in this area and can be aspirated through the needle. At aspiration the nature of the fluid will be noted, and if it is frank blood or heavily blood-stained the possibility of an ectopic pregnancy or ruptured corpus luteum must be considered. Otherwise a portion of the aspirate should be centrifuged and examined under the microscope for the presence of pus. The remainder can be examined by various techniques for the presence of the microbial organisms already noted, although for the intracellular pathogens (viruses, chlamydia) culture of the centrifuged deposit will be more effective. Immunofluorescence techniques may show the presence of gonococci, chlamydia and some bacteria including the anaerobic group. The fluid may also be examined for the breakdown products of bacterial activity by gas liquid chromatography; volatile fatty acids (butyric, isobutyric, valeric and isovaleric) are not normally present but are produced by the metabolism of anaerobes. This technique is described more fully in Chapter 5.

On first appraisal, therefore, culdocentesis would seem to be an ideal investigative procedure: quick, easy to undertake, relatively painless for the patient concerned, with a wealth of information to come from the specimens obtained. Cunningham et al (1978) reviewed 344 cases of pelvic inflammatory disease; culdocentesis was attempted in 246 and fluid obtained in 133 cases. Bacteria were identified in 104 of these specimens. The gonococcus was isolated in peritoneal fluid in over half the cases where it had been isolated from the cervix, sometimes alone but more commonly with other organisms. Altogether 272 strains of micro-organisms were isolated from the 104 specimens. Cultures for chlamydia, mycoplasmas and urea-plasmas were not undertaken.

However the picture is less encouraging when control cases are taken into account. Peritoneal fluid was obtained by culdocentesis from 27 women prior to elective sterilisation; none had any evidence of pelvic inflammation at laparoscopy. Bacteria were grown from the specimens of peritoneal fluid obtained by culdocentesis from 8 of the 27. In another study (Sweet et al 1979) specimens were obtained in parallel, first by direct aspiration at laparoscopy and then by culdocentesis. Consistently higher isolation rates were obtained from the culdocentesis specimens, when compared with laparoscopy specimens, suggesting that material obtained by this way is very prone to contamination, probably from the vagina, and this seems to be the only way to explain these findings in control cases.

Specimens taken under direct vision at laparoscopy

If laparoscopy is undertaken to confirm the diagnosis of pelvic inflammatory disease, specimens can be taken under direct vision for laboratory examination. If the fallopian tubes are open and pus can be expelled from them by pressure with blunt instruments this can be sampled directly on to a swab or by aspiration. If the tubes are inflamed and oedematous but no obvious pus is visible, a thin swab or catheter may be introduced into the tubal astia to try to obtain cellular material. Blocked, swollen tubes may be punctured and the pus aspirated. Usually a fairly large volume of peritoneal fluid may be drawn out of the pouch of Douglas.

From this site, as elsewhere, *Chlamydia trachomatis* is far more likely to be identified if the specimen contains epithelial cells. Although a group of researchers from Sweden have described good culture results from microbiopsies taken from the fimbrial ends of the tubes and are sure that this technique carries no additional risk for the patient (Mardh et al 1977), this procedure would seem to be more appropriate to research studies than clinical management.

Blood culture and antibody studies

If the woman is febrile and it is thought septicaemia might be present blood cultures should be performed. Serological studies will give useful information about infection with certain organisms, conventionally by the demonstration of a significant rise in titre during the course of the disease in paired specimens taken some 7–10 days apart. For this reason serum antibody levels are of little value in the management of the acute phase of pelvic inflammatory disease, but can provide useful retrospective evidence for clinical audit and research. More detailed tests describing the balance between the various immunoglobulin fractions may, however, give diagnostic results from a single specimen.

Examination of sexual partners

The need to trace, interview and examine the sexual partners of women with pelvic inflammatory disease which may be due to sexually transmitted agents is fully recognised by genitourinary physicians and epidermologists but usually forgotten or disregarded by gynaecologists and general practitioners. That this is a very necessary part of the case management has been amply demonstrated. Gilstrap et al (1977) traced 161 male contacts of 100 women with gonococcal pelvic inflammation, and 69 male contacts of 46 women with non-gonococcal pelvic inflammation. Of the 161 contacts of women with gonococcal disease, 63 had gonorrhoea and 14 of these were asymptomatic and unaware of the condition. Of the 69 partners of women with a diagnosis of non-gonococcal pelvic inflammatory disease 10 had gonorrhoea, 3 being asymptomatic. This contact tracing was not only of benefit to the man concerned and his potential other sexual partners, but also may provide evidence leading to a reappraisal of the woman's condition. Osser & Persson (1982) produced similar figures relating to chlamydial disease. In their series 68% of the male partners of women with chlamydial salpingitis had chlamydial urethritis, as did 12% of the partners of women with salpingitis and from whom chlamydia was not isolated.

THE RANGE OF MICRO-ORGANISMS INVOLVED IN PELVIC INFLAMMATORY DISEASE

Introduction: single or multiple infecting organisms

When reviewed on a worldwide basis the published literature contains reference to a vast range of organisms implicated as causative agents of pelvic inflammatory disease, and these range in size from the viruses to the protozoa. No single hospital or laboratory will be able to test for all of these, and individual and local factors must be taken into account when planning investigations. These factors will also need to be borne in mind when planning treatment, which must usually be started before the full results of investigation are available.

There is also a deep division amongst authorities and research workers as to whether pelvic inflammatory disease is usually caused by a single infecting organism, or whether a number of agents may be relevant in one case. The 'single organism' school is mainly European in origin, and, for example, the group from Lund in Sweden rarely report multiple infection (Mardh & Westrom, 1970; Mardh et al 1977). In contrast most reports from the USA stress the polymicrobial nature of the condition. Eschenbach et al (1975) report that mixed infections were common in peritoneal specimens from women with pelvic inflammatory disease, whether or not gonococci were found. Monif et al (1976) claimed that in their series most gonococcal cases were superinfected with other agents, and Chow et al (1975) isolated a total of 80 strains of bacteria from 18 patients. In this latter series all specimens were obtained by culdocentesis and some organisms, for example *Candida* sp., were obviously contaminants. Cunningham et al (1978) also used culdocentesis and isolated 272 strains of bacteria from specimens from 104 women. Sweet et al (1979) compared specimens obtained at laparoscopy with those from culdocentesis: mixed infections were found in 5 of 15 positive laparoscopy

specimens and 10 of 21 positive culdocentesis specimens.

Paavonen et al (1981) reported that in a long-standing case of pelvic inflammatory disease antibodies to anaerobic and aerobic bacteria were more likely to be present than in cases of shorter duration, and this was irrespective of the presence of *Neisseria gonorrhoeae* or *Chlamydia trachomatis*, suggesting superinfection of the gonococcal or chlamydial condition with new invaders. Many authors feel that this and other evidence suggests that commonly gonococci and chlamydia initiate an infection, but are replaced by these later opportunistic invaders. This would partly explain the apparently different isolation rates for various organisms in different countries, for the stage of the disease at which women present varies markedly.

Gonococcal pelvic inflammatory disease

Neisseria gonorrhoeae provides the classical model of salpingitis and pelvic inflammatory disease, and medical literature for the past hundred years abounds with good accounts of this condition. What is described is a progressive condition which, unless rupture of an abscess causes an acute crisis, usually runs a course of 10–14 days, after which time the symptoms and signs of disease settle and the fallopian tubes actually become free of organisms (Curtis 1921). If a further 'flare-up' of gonococcal disease occurs it is due to reinfection from the lower genital tract rather than the persistence of the organism in the adnexal structures. These observations were based on salpingectomy specimens obtained in the preantibiotic era, and it is interesting to note that a similar duration is observed in laboratory experiments in which healthy tubes removed at hysterectomy are maintained in organ culture and inoculated with gonococci (Carney & Taylor-Robinson 1973; Hare & Barnes 1979).

Gonorrhoea should be suspected as a potential cause in all cases of pelvic inflammatory disease, but especially when the patient is young and likely to have been in contact with partners with sexually transmitted infection. However, over the past 20 years the proportion of pelvic inflammatory disease related to gonorrhoea appears to be falling in some countries of western Europe (Mardh 1980), although in other parts of the world it remains high. There is also the problem that in many cases gonococci may be present in cervical secretions in cases of pelvic inflammatory disease but cannot be found in the fallopian tubes. Thus, in a series of 50 patients, Mardh & Weström (1970) reported a 34% isolate rate from the lower genital tract, but only a 4% rate from the fallopian tubes during laparoscopy. Sweet et al (1979) reported somewhat better correlation, with 5 positives from the fallopian tubes from 13 cases where gonococci had been identified in the endocervix, and the number rose to 8 if culdocentesis specimens were used. Cunningham et al (1978) used only culdocentesis and reported the same correlation (54%) between cervix and peritoneal fluid, but Eschenbach et al (1975), using the same method, reported only 7 in 21. Chow et al (1975) could find only 1 culdocentesis specimen positive in 13 cases with positive endocervical cultures.

No satisfactory explanation for these differences has been advanced, and Mardh (1980) discusses the current theories. Lip & Burgoyne (1966) have shown that the earlier in the disease the test is done, the greater the chance of demonstrating gonococci in cul-de-sac cultures. Perhaps, therefore, the gonococci simply die out early in the course of the infection, as they do in organ culture, and the damaged tissue is infected by other organisms. Possibly other organisms colonise the infected areas and produce toxins to destroy the gonococci; such toxins are known to be produced by *Escherichia coli* (Simpson & Davis 1979). Alternatively in the tube and cul-de-sac negative cases the gonococcal infection may have always been confined to the cervix, and another organism, possibly sexually transmitted, possibly endogenous, may have ascended incidentally and caused the pelvic inflammatory disease. The author has also been confronted with a case of acute appendicitis and cervical gonorrhoea which gave rise, not unjustifiably, to the clinical diagnosis of gonococcal salpingitis. All these factors strengthen the case for routine laparoscopy in all cases of pelvic inflammatory disease.

Chlamydial pelvic inflammatory disease

Although on clinical grounds chlamydial pelvic inflammatory disease has been suggested for several years before the isolation of the organism from the upper genital tract, this was first reported by Eschenbach et al (1975) from culdocentesis fluid and by Eilard et al (1976) directly from the fallopian tubes at laparoscopy. Since then a major role has been postulated for this organism in the causation of pelvic inflammation. Mardh et al (1977) isolated the organism from the tubes of 30% of acute cases at laparoscopy; Henry-Suchet et al (1980) from 23.5% of cases; and Gjonnaes et al (1982) from 16.1% of cases. Evidence from endometrial cultures suggests an even greater rate of involvement, and from cervical cultures greater still; for example Wolner-Hanssen et al (1982) reported on 18 women with a tubal (laparoscopic) isolation from 1, endometrial isolations from 8 and cervical isolations from 13. All 18 had laparoscopic evidence of salpingitis, and 12 showed a significant rise in antichlamydial antibodies as the disease progressed.

The most dramatic evidence comes from antibody studies. Treharne et al (1979) reported on 143 cases; 62% had what they would consider diagnostically high serum antichlamydial IgG levels and 23% had IgM present in serum. Antichlamydial IgA was also present in pouch of Douglas fluid. Osser & Persson (1982) reported a fourfold rise in antichlamydial IgG or significant IgM, or both, in 51% of 72 cases of salpingitis. And although Sweet et al (1979) were unable to isolate *Chlamydia trachomatis* from the fallopian tubes in any of their cases, a subsequent report on the same series (Sweet et al 1980a) showed a fourfold rise of antichlamydial IgG and IgM in 23% of cases.

There is also experimental evidence supporting a causative role. Ripa et al (1979) induced salpingitis in grivat monkeys with inoculations of *C. trachomatis*, and Sweet et al (1980b) did the same in guinea pigs with *C. psittaci*. Both of these experiments appears to create a benign self-limiting condition, but the latter group reported later that some of the guinea-pigs in their studies had developed permanent tubal damage (Schachter et al 1982). Patton et al (1983) induced chlamydial salpingitis in four pig-tailed monkeys. A lymphocytic response was observed which reached its zenith on days 14–21 and had settled by day 35. By then extensive deciliation and epithelial degeneration had occurred.

The degree of pelvic inflammation produced by the 'pure' chlamydial infection remains a matter for debate. Svensson et al (1980) compared three groups of women with salpingitis, classified into chlamydial, gonococcal and non-gonococcal non-chlamydial. The main differences that emerged were that:

—Older women (30 years or more) were more likely to be in the non-chlamydial, non-gonococcal group than in either of the other two groups. Women aged 20–24 years were less likely to be in this group.

—Women with chlamydial salpingitis were less likely to present for help in the first 3 days of their illness than those in the other two groups. (It could be deduced from this that the symptoms are less severe).

—At laparoscopy non-chlamydial non-gonococcal cases are more likely to be classified as mild (rather than moderate or severe) than cases in the other two groups.

Henry-Suchet et al (1980) went further than this, claiming that a higher isolation rate of chlamydia from the fallopian tubes was obtained from women *with no sign of pelvic inflammatory disease* who were undergoing laparoscopy for infertility and were found to have occluded tubes. Despite the obvious implication of this finding for the management of infertility no other workers have confirmed these findings. There is, however, further evidence on serological grounds that chlamydial salpingitis may cause few or no symptoms. Punnonen et al (1979) showed that antibodies to *Chlamydia trachomatis* were present in infertile women to a degree about halfway between the high levels of women who were the sexual partners of men with non-gonococcal urethritis, and the low levels in healthy pregnant women. A quarter of this group had very high levels, and these included nine women with completely blocked fallopian tubes but no previous history suggestive of an attack of pelvic inflammatory disease. These findings from Finland have been confirmed in Italy by Cevenini et al (1982) and in the USA by Gump et al (1982). *C. trachomatis* can also be grown in fallopian tube organ culture, where it runs a much more benign course than *Neisseria gonorrhoeae*, producing far less cilial damage and leaving viable organs after 7–10 days (Hutchinson et al 1979).

There is, therefore, a body of evidence suggesting that chlamydial pelvic inflammatory disease may often run a benign course, causing minimal or even no discomfort to the woman concerned. Despite this lack of symptoms and signs the disease process can lead to permanent tubal damage and destruction, possibly over a long period of time. If these deductions are true and occur in a significant number of women—perhaps a third of more of those with untreated chlamydial cervicitis (Wölner-Hanssen et al 1982)—the need to seek out by contact-tracing or any other appropriate means all women with lower genital tract chlamydial infections and treat them adequately becomes imperative. McCormack et al (1979) followed 20 young women with chlamydial cervicitis for 15 months and none developed signs of pelvic inflammatory disease during that time; however it is possible that over that period a number sustained tubal damage from 'silent' tubal involvement. It is also important that all treatment regimes for pelvic inflammatory disease contain an antichlamydial agent; Sweet et al (1983) demonstrated persistence of *C. trachomatis* despite apparently adequate clinical cure of salpingitis with beta-lactam antibiotics.

Mycoplasmas and ureaplasmas

Only recently has an agreement been reached on the nomenclature for these organisms, and therefore even in the comparatively recent past a variety of names was used. In reports before the last decade one must expect mycoplasmas to be referred to also as pleuropneumonia-like organisms (PPLO) and L-forms, and ureaplasmas as tiny mycoplasmas (T-mycoplasmas). They were first isolated from pelvic abscess material in the 1940s, but the first proper series was that of Mardh & Weström (1970). These workers reported *Mycoplasma hominis* isolations from the fallopian tubes at laparoscopy from 8% of a series of women with pelvic inflammatory disease, and tubal isolation of *Ureaplasma urealyticum* of the same group. In patients with pelvic inflammatory disease associated with *M. hominis* infection a rise in antibody titre to the agent was observed during the progressive course of the disease. Other authors have reported isolations at about the same rate: Sweet et al (1979) reported an isolation of *U. urealyticum* from the fallopian tubes in only 1 of 26 cases of acute salpingitis, although culdocentesis specimens yielded 4 isolates of *U.*

urealyticum and one of *M. hominis*. Using culdocentesis Eschenbach et al (1975) obtained two
isolates of *M. hominis* and one of *U. urealyticum*
from 54 cases. Thompson et al (1980) have produced the highest figures; using culdocentesis they
reported a 20% isolation rate for *M. hominis* and a
17% isolation rate for *U. urealyticum* from cul-de-
sac fluid. Most of these isolations were as part of a
mixed infection.

As described in Chapter 12 both mycoplasmas
and ureaplasmas are very commonly present in the
genital tract of sexually active women, and it is not
tenable to regard them universally as pathogens. It
is certainly possible that on occasions either of
them may become a tubal pathogen, probably on
an opportunistic basis. They usually respond to the
same group of antibiotics that are used in the
treatment of chlamydial infection, and so will be
covered if that condition is managed adequately.

Endogenous aerobic and anaerobic bacteria
(Plate 43, Figs. 6.1 and 6.2)

The recent development of new technical skills for
the isolation of delicate bacteria, especially
anaerobes, has led to a plethora of publications in
the last decade reporting their isolation from cases
of pelvic inflammatory disease. Such studies include those of Cunningham et al (1978) who
obtained a total of 188 isolates of anaerobic bacteria
and 104 isolates of aerobic organisms from 104
peritoneal specimens. Almost all the anaerobic
specimens came from the species *Peptococcus* and
Bacteroides, with *P. prevotii*, *P. anaerobius* and *B.
fragilis* being the commonest. Aerobes were mainly
streptococci and coliforms, together with gonococci. Thadepalli et al (1973) looked at 33 women with
severe pelvic infection, including abscess formation
and puerperal infections. Anaerobes were recovered from the infected sites in all cases, and
aerobes in 20. *B. fragilis* was isolated from 26 of 32
cases, and a peptostreptococcus from 18. Other
anaerobes were much less common. Twelve of
these women had septicaemia, half due to *B. fragilis*. Of the aerobic organisms *Escherichia coli* were
the most commonly isolated. Chow et al (1975)
looked at 20 women with salpingitis; aerobic organisms were more commonly isolated in his series,
with streptococci bieng the commonest. No *Bacter-*

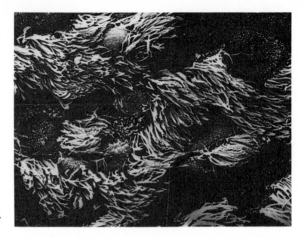

Fig. 6.1 Electron micrograph of fallopian tube cilia from
specimen prior to inoculation with *Bacteroides fragilis*.

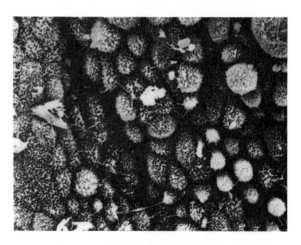

Fig. 6.2 Electron micrograph of tissue from same specimen as
Fig. 6.1 after 48 hours of *Bacteroides fragilis* infection. The
epithelium has been denuded of cilia.

oides sp. were found. Eschenbach et al (1975)
reported 94 isolates from 54 peritoneal specimens
from women with pelvic inflammatory disease;
amongst the anaerobes *B. fragilis* was the commonest organism with 14 isolates and haemolytic
streptococci were the commonest aerobes found.
Monif et al (1976) obtained a growth of *Neisseria
gonorrhoeae* from culdocentesis fluid in 11 of 17
women with gonococcal salpingitis. In 6 of these
11, and in the 6 remaining anaerobic and aerobic
bacteria were also grown. In 6 cases these were
Bacteroides sp. (usually *fragilis*); other common
organisms were streptococci and enterococci.

Thompson et al (1980) looked at 30 cases of acute pelvic inflammatory disease, 80% of which had cervical gonorrhoeae and 30% of which had the gonococcus isolated from their peritoneal fluid. Of this group, 63% had aerobes in the purulent material aspirated from the pouch of Douglas, and the organisms identified included 11 isolates of *Bacteroides* sp. (none *fragilis*), 11 *Peptococcus* sp. and 10 *Propionobacterium* sp. Amongst other anaerobes isolated were 7 isolates of streptococci and 5 of enterobacteriaceae.

Unfortunately the credibility of some of these reports is somewhat unsound because culdocentesis was used to obtain the specimens, rather than laparoscopy. Laparoscopically obtained results have also been obtained. Eilard et al (1976) reported 2 tubal isolates of *Bacteroides*, one with an anaerobic streptococcus. Sweet et al (1979) isolated only 4 anaerobes (other than gonococci) and 4 aerobes via the laparoscope in their series of 26 cases, though using culdocentesis in the same group 34 isolates were obtained. The anaerobes isolated at laparoscopy were all *Peptococcus* sp.. Heinonen et al (1985) reported tubal isolates of bacteria from 4 of 25 cases of salpingitis (coliforms, streptococci, *Bacteroides*) and isolates from 13 of the endometrial cavities of the same group. One isolate (of *Streptococcus faecalis*) was obtained from the tubes by laparoscopy in a control case.

A vital clue to the role of endogenous bacteria in pelvic inflammatory disease was provided by Paavonen et al (1981). They looked at serological evidence of infection with facultative enteric bacteria and *Bacteroides fragilis* in 101 women with pelvic inflammatory disease. Significant antibodies to each were found in about one-third of the patients, whether or not lower genital tract culture yielded *Neisseria gonorrhoeae* or *Chlamydia trachomatis*. The relevant factors were the duration of symptoms, the use of an intrauterine contraceptive device, and the presence of an adnexal mass.

The significance of these findings is of great importance. Anaerobic organisms run a very destructive course in tubal specimens maintained in organ culture (Hare & Barnes 1979), and the work of Thadepalli et al (1973) clearly shows that they are often associated with the most severe infections. The result of recent research would seem to lend itself to three possible interpretations:

1. Such organisms are almost always contaminants, and they can therefore be neglected;

2. They are tubal invaders either as primary pathogens or as secondary colonisers following a primary attack of pelvic inflammatory disease initiated by another organism;

3. Alternatively, they are released from the large bowel, possibly as a response of infection spreading to that organ from the upper genital tract. This might explain the commoner occurrence of such organisms in peritoneal fluid than in the tubes themselves, and suggest that colonisation of the peritoneal fluid occurs before invasion of the tubes.

If the second or third of these options is true, then treatment must include adequate cover for the very wide range of these organisms.

Pelvic inflammation due to true viruses

From first principles there would seem to be a possibility that viruses could act as upper genital tract infections, but reports on possible clinical cases are very scanty. Mardh & Weström (1970) reported virus isolations obtained at laparoscopy from 2 of 15 women with salpingitis, one a coxsackie B5 and one an echo B6. No comment is made concerning their possible role in the disease process. More recently Heinonen et al (1985) and Paavonen et al (1985c) have both reported the isolation of *Herpes virus hominis* type II from the fallopian tubes and from the endometrial cavity in cases of pelvic inflammatory disease. (These authors are from the same group and it is possible that the patients are the same.) Herpes virus is a virulent and common pathogen in the lower genital tract and certainly women with this condition often have symptoms and signs of upper genital tract infection, and so the role of this organism as a tubal pathogen seems very likely.

The original work on infection of fallopian tube organ cultures by micro-organism was performed with viruses. Barski et al (1959) described the original techniques for the maintenance of such organs in culture, and described a 'pathogenic' response after infection of rabbit oviducts with herpes or vaccinia, comparing this with the non-pathogenic response in human fallopian tubes after inoculation with poliovirus, adenovirus and encephalovirus. It is very tempting to speculate on the responses that might have been seen if the experiments had been the opposite way round. Mardh (1980) also mentions rhinoviruses in human fallopian tube culture.

With the possible exception of herpes virus this question remains academic. Certainly there is no reason to deny that virus could play a part in the pathogenesis of pelvic inflammatory disease; if so the clinical symptoms and signs might well be due to superinfection with other organisms rather than the virus disease itself.

Pelvic inflammatory disease due to oropharangeal organisms

Given the accepted high rates of orogenital sexual practices recorded in many sexual groups, it is not surprising that organisms commonly or usually found in the oropharynx play a part in the pathogenesis of pelvic inflammatory disease. The roles of anaerobic bacteria and herpes virus have already been discussed. *Haemophilus influenzae* was isolated from peritoneal fluid obtained by culdocentesis from 3 of 54 cases in the series of Eschenbach (1975), and at laparoscopy from 2 of 26 patients in the series of Sweet (1979). Heinonen et al (1985) reported the isolation of this organism at laparoscopy from 2 of 26 women; in both cases a pyosalpinx was present. Two further cases are reported by Paavonen et al (1985d), although as these authors are from the same group it is possible that they are the same cases.

It is possible also that some of the techniques used in orogenital sexual stimulation, such as the blowing of air into the vagina, might result in upward spread of organisms introduced from the partner's mouth. This might explain some attacks of pelvic inflammatory disease in homosexual women.

Pelvic inflammatory disease due to Actinomyces sp.

At the time of writing, there is no clear picture as to the significance or importance of the part played by *Actinomyces* in the pathogenesis of pelvic inflammatory disease. These organisms, long regarded as fungi, have recently been reclassified as gram-positive bacteria, are very difficult to culture, and the fact that they can be identified by their typical appearances on cervical smears has been recognised for less than a decade.

The common organism associated with human disease is *Actinomyces israelii*. It is reported to colonise the lower female genital tract in between 1 and 39% of women; reports differ as to whether or not intrauterine contraceptive device usage increases the incidence of such colonisation. Orogenital sexual stimulation may be the source of colonisation for some women. The risk of 'aggressive disease'—symptomatic pelvic inflammation—developing has been put as high as 25% by one group: however in this series the overall colonisation rate was the lowest report at 0.4%. In series reporting higher rates of colonisation, much lower rates are given for the development of pelvic inflammatory disease.

What does emerge from the literature, however, is that pelvic inflammation and abscess formation in relationship to *A. israelii* is much commoner if the woman is the wearer of an intrauterine contraceptive device. There remains, therefore, the problem of the advice to give to a woman who uses an intrauterine contraceptive device and in whom *A. israelii* is detected on routine cytological screening. There is a general consensus that treatment is necessary and the organism responds well to penicillin or tetracycline. What is controversial is whether or not the intrauterine contraceptive device should be left in place. In view of the inability of the experts in the field to agree over this it should depend to a major degree on the contraceptive needs of the woman. If alternative measures would be acceptable to her on medical and other grounds, the device should probably be removed, although if subsequent tests show the vagina and cervix to be free of the organism another may be inserted. If, however, removal of the device would be a great problem for the woman concerned, possibly laying her open to the risk of an unwanted pregnancy, then it is probably best to treat the organism with it in place.

No particular type of intrauterine contraceptive device has been particularly associated with actinomycotic sepius, and no difference is recorded between those devices which contain metal and those which do not.

Pelvic tuberculosis

The clinical picture of pelvic tuberculosis has changed markedly through the ages, and is still changing. At its orginal description 200 years ago the condition was a florid one, with symptoms and palpable pelvic masses. By the middle of this century this had changed, with infertility and abdominal pain being the most common reasons for presentation. More recent studies from developed countries (Falk et al 1980; Sutherland 1982) suggest that the age of presentation is becoming much older. Falk et al (1980) and Nogales-Ortiz et al (1979) both stress the dramatic fall in the incidence of this condition in developed countries over the past two decades.

Falk et al (1980) record that the majority of their patients are now postmenopausal on presentation, and that peri- or postmenopausal bleeding is the most common presenting symptom. Pain, including dysmenorrhoea, was the next common and infertility was the reason for presentation in only 1 in 8. Of the women presenting, 10% were asymptomatic, and 38% had had previously diagnosed tuberculosis at another extragenital site. On examination 46 patients—about a quarter—had palpable pelvic mass; 5 of these were adnexal cancer, 2 benign ovarian lesions and the rest inflammatory masses. In most cases the diagnosis was based on the appearance of the endometrium, and a bacteriological diagnosis was reached in only 29% of the cases. In 27% the diagnosis was reached after resection of the fallopian tubes.

This is the picture of tuberculosis in modern-day Sweden, a highly developed country with a good public health network. The accounts from Sutherland (1982) from Scotland and Nogales-Ortiz et al (1979) from Spain described a more traditional situation, with most women presenting during their reproductive years, with infertility as the main feature. Nogales-Ortiz et al (1979) stress particularly that the fallopian tubes were involved in all of the 1436 cases they report. The authors remark on the fact that the uterus is often small, almost infantile in such cases, and they regard the appearance at laparoscopy of such a uterus with bilateral inflamed tubes as suspicious of this condition. They report that serosal granulomes, frequently reported in past literature, are uncommon, and neither they nor Falk et al (1980) find hysterosalpingographic appearance as valuable as previously suggested.

Treatment is by antituberculous antibiotics, and because cases of pelvic tuberculosis are so comparatively rare the pattern for this is set by chest physicians. Sutherland (1982) reports good results from a combination of rifampicin, ethambutol and isoniazid;* Surgery is often needed, and all authors stress their great reluctance to 'tailor' this to preserve fertility, because of the high risk of ectopic pregnancy in this group. Total hysterectomy and bilateral salpingectomy is most appropriate, although if possible the ovaries should be conserved in the premenopausal woman.

Conclusions on the pathogenesis of pelvic inflammatory disease

From the work presented and discussed earlier in this chapter it is possible to construct a classification of pelvic inflammatory disease which will be of use in planning the suitability of investigations and treatment regimes. The traditional divisions would seem too simple for this purpose, and the following is suggested:

Primary pelvic inflammatory disease (First attack, no precipitating cause)

1. Due to exogenous sexually transmitted agents (common, especially in the younger woman).

2. Due to endogenous organisms (rare, usually in the older age group; beware of missed underlying cause).

Secondary pelvic inflammatory disease

1. Leading on from primary, when endogenous organisms replace exogenous organisms in an ongoing infection.

2. Secondary to a significant event such as the insertion of an intrauterine contraceptive device,

---

*Stark (personal communication) suggests that pyrazinamide should be added to this.

pregnancy termination, miscarriage, childbirth, surgical intervention. Endogenous or exogenous organisms.

3. Secondary to the wearing of an intrauterine contraceptive device, usually endogenous infection.

4. Secondary to a focus of infection elsewhere in the body. This may be intra-abdominal, e.g. an inflamed appendix, where endogenous organisms will be responsible, or anywhere for a tuberculous focus.

Recurrent pelvic inflammatory disease

1. Recurrence related to a further exposure to an exogenous source of sexually transmitted disease.

2. Recurrence involving endogenous organisms, due to reduced host defences to infection after the primary attack.

Although the classification will act as a guide to the types of organisms to be expected, in some cases it will not be definite. For example, women undergoing termination of pregnancy are at risk of subsequent pelvic inflammatory disease, not only from endogenous organisms that might be introduced into the traumatised endometrial cavity from the vagina, but also from sexually transmitted agents such as chlamydia which they may be harbouring in the cervix (Moller et al 1982).

IMMEDIATE AND SHORT-TERM COMPLICATIONS OF PELVIC INFLAMMATORY DISEASE

These mainly involved the development of abscesses and inflammatory masses; peritonitis and perihepatitis (Fitz-Hugh Curtis syndrome); and sacroiliitis.

Pelvic abscesses and inflammatory masses

Tubo-ovarian abscess is the commonest short-term complication of pelvic inflammatory disease, occurring perhaps in up to one-third of women needing hospital admission for this condition (Landers & Sweet 1985). It occurs most commonly in women in the age group 20–40 years: up to half are nulli-

parous: and, contrary to traditional statements, up to one-half of the women concerned will be undergoing their first attack of pelvic inflammatory disease.

The diagnosis is suspected from the sensation on bimanual examination that a palpable mass is present in the pelvis apart from the uterus, and this will need to be confirmed. In the past, this would have necessitated laparotomy and this may still be needed; however, now other methods are possible alternatives. Whatever method is used, its aim must be to distinguish between a tubo-ovarian abscess with the production of pus, an adhesive mass of bowel and pelvic organs without a purulent collection, and tubal oedema and tenderness without abscess formation.

Laparoscopy is often of use, and Adducci (1981) describes its application in 20 cases. All had a presumptive diagnosis of pelvic inflammatory disease with abscess formation. In 8 the diagnosis was entirely wrong: 6 had endometriosis and 2 appendicitis. Twelve had the diagnosis confirmed: only 2 needed laparotomy and the rest had pelvic drains inserted under laparoscopic control.

It is probable, however, that laparoscopy will not provide adequate information in a number of cases, and some operators may be wary of using it when large pelvic masses are present for fear of puncturing or damaging the delicate and friable inflamed tissues. In such cases the use of an imaging technique is certainly of value, and the methods available include ultrasound, radioisotope scanning and computerised tomography. Of these ultrasound is probably the cheapest and most widely available at the present time, and in skilled and practised hands has good diagnostic reliability (Spirtos et al 1982). If nuclear medicine diagnostic facilities are available then scanning may be used after injection of the patient with white cells labelled with gallium 67 or indium 111. These methods appear to be highly accurate in the localisation of abscesses elsewhere in the body, although detailed studies of their use in the pelvis are not available. In the same way computerised tomography would possibly appear to have great use in the future for the detection of pelvic abscesses, but again evidence concerning the sensitvity and specificity of this method is lacking at the present.

Whatever the cause of the initial attack of pelvic

inflammatory disease, when abscess formation occurs anaerobic organisms are almost invariably involved, often in conjunction with aerobes (Landers & Sweet 1985). This is in keeping with current theories on the development of intra-abdominal sepsis, where facultative aerobes such as *Escherichia coli* are associated with the early peritonitis–sepsis stage and anaerobes, especially *Bacteroides* sp., with the later abscess formation. The authors report the rarity of isolation of the gonococcus from such abscesses, and the absence in any reports in published literature of the isolation from an abscess of *Chlamydia trachomatis*. They also highlight the confused state of knowledge regarding *Actinomyces israelii*; in many large series it is not amongst the organisms isolated from tubo-ovarian abscesses, even in intrauterine contraceptive device users. However the difficulties in identifying the organism are also stressed.

Treatment of such cases also remains a matter of controversy. In the past it was always by surgery, following the old maxim 'if there is pus present, let it out'. If possible, drainage routes were extraperitoneal; through the posterior vaginal fornix, through the rectum and under the inguinal ligament. The problem with such approaches was that providing the diagnosis was correct and the abscess abutted directly against the drainage site all was well; however if the peritoneum or another structure intervened between the two then an attempt at drainage could make the matter far worse. For smaller defined abscesses surgical removal was possible, accompanied in many cases by hysterectomy and bilateral salpingo-oophorectomy.

More recently conservative treatment with vigorous antibiotic therapy has been attempted with some success. Most authors now agree that for a small or moderate size abscess (up to 8 cm maximum diameter) medical treatment is worth a trial (Ginsburg et al 1980). The details of the most appropriate antibiotic combination will be discussed in a later section, but it would appear that penicillin or another beta lactam antibiotic, aminoglycoside and an agent such as metronidazole, which is highly active against anaerobes, should all be used together. Careful monitoring of the clinical state of the patient is needed, including if possible ultrasonic assessment of the size of the abscess. If any worsening occurs, or if distinct im-

provement in her condition is not apparent within 48–72 hours of starting treatment, then surgical treatment is needed.

If surgical intervention is needed it must be tailored to the individual case, her clinical condition and her future need of fertility. All studies report a very poor fertility prognosis after antibiotic treatment for pelvic abscess complicating pelvic inflammatory disease, and Hager (1983) claims that if a unilateral abscess is present the fertility prognosis is better if a unilateral salpingo-oophorectomy is performed rather than an attempt made at conservative management. In all cases if the abscess is large or not responding to antibiotic therapy then operative intervention should occur. This will nowadays almost always be through an abdominal approach and full antibiotic cover should be given. If possible the unruptured abscess should be dissected free and removed intact: whether or not this should be accompanied by hysterectomy and removal of the other ovary and tube remains a matter for debate. Certainly in the past better long-term results have been obtained by this radical approach, but with the advent of improved microbiological techniques and an ever-widening range of antibiotics more conservative methods are being used (Landers & Sweet 1985). The next few years may show a dramatic swing in the approach to this condition. All authors agree that rupture of a pelvic abscess constitutes a surgical emergency, and requires immediate laparotomy under full antibiotic cover.

Peritonitis and perihepatitis (Fitz-Hugh Curtis syndrome)

This condition, which occurs in about 4% of cases of acute pelvic inflammatory disease (Wang et al 1980), is probably due to infected material from the pelvis running up the gutter present on the right side of the abdomen in the recumbent patient and directly infecting the liver. Inflammation of the liver capsule then develops, and is characterised by the formation of 'piano-string' adhesions between the liver and the surrounding structure and abdominal walls. The symptoms produced by the condition include upper abdominal tenderness and pleuritic pain. If the diagnosis of pelvic inflammatory disease is being confirmed by laparoscopy it is very easy indeed to turn the instrument round and inspect the upper part of the abdomen. Reddening and inflammation of the liver capsule is then seen, with the typical adhesions present in the longer-standing cases.

Classically this condition was thought to be a complication of gonococcal salpingitis, but more recently *Chlamydia trachomatis* appears to have been identified as a more common cause (Wang et al 1980). Whether the condition may arise when pelvic inflammatory disease is due to an organism other than these is uncertain. No special treatment seems necessary apart from adequate antibiotic treatment of the underlying pelvic inflammation, and there appear to be no long-term consequences of note.

MEDICAL TREATMENT OF PELVIC INFLAMMATORY DISEASE

Choice of antibiotic therapy

As has been seen in the previous sections, pelvic inflammatory disease may be due to a variety of organisms, and often more than one of these appears to be relevant to the disease process. Although evidence as to the nature of the infecting organism will come from the woman's age, social background and clinical state, and the results of rapid staining techniques, the diagnosis will be at the best tentative when antibiotic therapy is started. The physician in charge of the case, therefore, must often make what is an inspired guess as to the correct management, hoping to have his decision ratified later by good clinical progress and the results of microbiological tests.

Bell & James (1980) analysed by computer the isolation results of culdocentesis or laparoscopy specimens obtained in nine major studies of pelvic inflammatory disease, looking at the levels of 13 antibiotics needed to provide adequate treatment for the eradication of these organisms. They looked at the drugs singly, in pairs and in triple combinations, and for each calculated the percentage likelihood that adequate treatment would be provided by that regime. The organisms studied included aerobic and anaerobic bacteria, mycoplasmas, urea-plasmas and chlamydia, and drugs were assessed on levels obtained by both oral and intravenous routes. Their initial conclusion was that no single antibiotic therapy was adequate: the best drugs (carbenicillin or tetracycline given intravenously) gave only an 84% chance of cover and the best oral drug (tetracyline) only 74%. Double therapy is much more effective with a theoretical 96% effectiveness of gentamicin and clindamycin or carbenicillin, each given intravenously. The best oral pair were cotrimoxazole and tetracycline, theoretically 94% efficient. A large variety of triple regimes reached the highest level of efficiency at a theoretical 97% and some oral triple therapies reached 96%; interestingly, very few of them appear to have been used in practice. Where the combinations analysed in this work had been used in clinical practice, the reported results showed good agreement with the authors' predicted performances.

From this work and from clinical results it would seem unacceptable to treat pelvic inflammatory disease with a single antiobiotic. Double therapy is the least that should be offered and triple therapy may often be best.

Management of the patient in hospital

For most women acute pelvic inflammatory disease is best managed in hospital, to enable frequent observation to be made and parenteral drug therapy to be given. Individual cases may well need individual management, but for the moderately or seriously ill woman in the acute stage of the disease the following will be needed:

1. A general antibiotic, effective especially against gram-negative organisms. Gentamicin would seem one of the most appropriate.

2. An antibiotic with specific action against anaerobic organisms. In the United Kingdom metronidazole would be the first choice for this.

3. Antichlamydial cover. Sweet et al (1983) demonstrated that, if no appropriate antibiotic was used, *Chlamydia trachomatis* could persist in cases of pelvic inflammatory disease despite apparent clinical cure. At some stage, therefore, an antichlamydial agent, usually tetracycline or erythromycin, should be used.

4. Antigonococcal cover. Although the gonococcus is becoming less important in the development of pelvic inflammatory disease provision must still be made for its treatment. Penicillin or ampicillin

should be used, or spectinomycin if the organism produces beta lactamase (Curran 1979).

Even if these guidelines are followed closely there will be a wide range of possible regimes, and each physician will decide on his personal preference. For the present author this is:

Penicillin (intravenous) 3–5 million units 6-hourly

Gentamicin (intravenous) 60–80 mg 8-hourly

Metronidazole 1 g 12-hourly per rectum or intravenously

After three days and a satisfactory response the penicillin is stopped and replaced by oxytetracycline 500 mg 6-hourly by mouth, to be continued for 14 days. Assuming the response is good, the gentamicin is stopped after 7 days and the metronidazole after 14 days. This regime is the author's personal preference, and theoretically equally useful combinations can involve ampicillin, erythromycin, clindamycin, carbenicillin and cotrimoxazole. The newer cephalosporins would also seem appropriate.

Outpatient management

In the United Kingdom especially it is customary to treat mild and some moderate cases of pelvic inflammatory disease on an outpatient basis. The decision to do this must depend on the individual circumstances surrounding each woman, and proper case selection is vital. If this is done at least double therapy must be used; even if a single agent such as *Chlamydia trachomatis* is strongly suspected, single therapy is unwise.

In theory a combination of an oral tetracycline, oral co-trimoxazole and metronidazole taken by mouth or per rectum should provide 96% cover of possible infecting organisms. Slightly less good cover is obtained by omitting the co-trimoxazole or the metronidazole.

Even if managed as outpatients all women with pelvic inflammatory disease need very close supervision. They should be reviewed at least on a twice-weekly basis, and if there is any doubt that the condition is not improving then admission to hospital is mandatory.

The role of corticosteroids in the treatment of pelvic inflammatory disease

In the 1950s and 1960s some reports appeared suggesting that the immediate response to treatment and the eventual case outcome in pelvic inflammatory disease could be improved by the addition of corticosteroids to the antibiotic therapy (Hurtig 1957). This matter was fully investigated by Falk (1965) in a large prospective double-blind trial involving 283 patients. He concluded that, although the initial response to treatment appeared to be somewhat better if corticosteroids were used with antibiotics this was not a lasting effect, and certainly this regime conferred no lasting benefit on the patient. The practice has nothing to recommend it.

REFERENCES

Acosta A A, Mabray R, Kaufman R H 1971 Intrauterine pregnancy and coexistent pelvic inflammatory disease. Obstetrics and Gynecology 37: 282–285

Adducci J E 1981 Laparoscopy in the diagnosis and treatment of pelvic inflammatory disease with abscess formation. International Surgery 66: 359–360

Barlow D 1977 The condom and gonorrhoea. Lancet i: 811–832

Barski G, Cornefert F, Wallace R E 1959 Response of ciliated epithelia of different histological origin to virus infections in vitro. Proceedings of the Society for Experimental Biology and Medicine 100: 407–411

Bell T A, James J F 1980 Computer-assisted analysis of the therapy of acute salpingitis. American Journal of Obstetrics and Gynecology 138: 1048–1054

Carney F E, Taylor-Robinson D 1973 Growth and effect of Neisseria gonorrhoeae in organ cultures. British Journal of Venereal Diseases 49: 435–440

Cevenini R, Possati G, La Placa M 1982 C. trachomatis infection in infertile women. In: Mardh P A, Holmes K K, Oriel J D, Piot P, Schachter J (eds) Chlamydial infections Elsevier Biomedical, Amsterdam, pp 193–196

Chamberlain G, Carron-Brown J 1978 Gynaecological laparoscopy. Royal College of Obstetricians and Gynaecologists, London

Chow A W, Malkasion K L, Marshall J R, Guze L B 1975 The bacteriology of acute pelvic inflammatory disease. American Journal of Obstetrics and Gynecology 122: 876–879

Chow A W, Carlson C, Sorrell T C 1980 Host defenses in acute pelvic inflammatory disease. American Journal of Obstetrics and Gynecology 138: 1003–1005

Cohen M S, Black J R, Proctor R A, Sparling P F 1984 Host defences in the vaginal mucosa. In: Mardh P A, Taylor-Robinson D (eds) Bacterial vaginosis. Almqvist and Wiksell International, Stockholm, pp 13–22

Cunningham F G, Hauth J C, Gilstrap L C, Herbert W N P, Kappus S S 1978 The bacterial pathogenesis of acute pelvic inflammatory disease. Obstetrics and Gynecology 52: 161–164

Curran J W 1979 Management of gonococcal pelvic inflammatory disease. Sexually Transmitted Diseases 6: 174–180

Curtis A H 1921 Bacteriology and pathology of fallopian tubes removed at operation. Surgery, Gynecology and Obstetrics 33: 621–631

Curtis A H 1930 A cause of adhesions in the upper right quadrant. Journal of the American Medical Association 94: 1211

Edelman D A, Berger D A 1980 Contraceptive practice and tubo-ovarian abscess. American Journal of Obstetrics and Gynecology 138: 541–544

Eilard T, Brorsson J-E, Hamark B, Forssman L 1976 Isolation of chlamydia in acute salpingitis. Scandanavian Journal of Infectious Diseases 9 (suppl): 82–84

Elgi G E, Newton M 1961 Transport of carbon particles in the human female reproductive tract. Fertility and Sterility 12: 151–155

Eschenbach D A, Buchanan T M, Pollock H M et al 1975 Polymicrobial etiology of pelvic inflammatory disease. New England Journal of Medicine 293: 166–171

Eschenbach D A, Harnisch J P, Holmes K K 1977 Pathogenesis of acute pelvic inflammatory disease: role of contraception and other risk factors. American Journal of Obstetrics and Gynecology 128: 838–850

Falk H C 1946 Interpretation of the pathogenesis of pelvic infection as determined by cornual resection. Obstetrics and Gynecology 52: 66–73

Falk V 1965 Treatment of acute non-tuberculous salpingitis with antibiotics alone and in combination with glucocorticoids. Acta Obstetrica et Gynecologica Scandinavica 44 (suppl 6)

Falk V, Ludviksson K, Agren G 1980 Genital tuberculosis in women. American Journal of Obstetrics and Gynecology 138: 974–977

Fitz-Hugh T 1934 Acute gonococcic peritonitis of the right upper quadrant in women. Journal of the American Medical Association 12: 2094–2096

Fox C A, Wolff H S, Baker J A 1970 Measurement of intravaginal and intrauterine pressures during human coitus by radio-telemetry. Journal of Reproduction and Fertility 22: 243–251

Francioli P, Shio H, Roberts R B, Muller M 1983 Phagocytosis and killing of Neisseria gonorrhoeae by trichomonas vaginalis. Journal of Infectious Diseases 147: 87–94

Gilstrap L C, Herbert W N P, Cunningham F G, Hauth J C, Van Patten H G 1977 Gonorrhoea screening in male consorts of women with pelvic infection. Journal of the American Medical Association 238: 965–966

Ginsberg D S, Stern J L, Hamad K A, Genadry R, Speme M R 1980 Tubo-ovarian abscess; a retrospective view. American Journal of Obstetrics and Gynecology 138: 1055–1058

Gjonnaes H, Dalaker K, Anestad G, Mardh P-A, Kvile G, Bergan T 1982 Pelvic inflammatory disease. Etiologic studies with emphasis on chlamydial infection. Obstetrics and Gynecology 59: 550–555

Gnarpe H, Friberg H 1973 T-mycoplasmas on spermatozoa and infertility. Nature 245: 97–98

Gomez C I, Stenback W A, James A N, Criswell B S, Williams R P 1979 Attachment of N. gonorrhoeae to human sperm. British Journal of Venereal Diseases 55: 245–255

Grimes D A, Schulz K F, Cates W 1984 Prophylactic antibiotics for curettage abortion. American Journal of Obstetrics and Gynecology 150: 689–694

Gump D W, Gibson M, Ashikaga T 1982 Infertile women and C. trachomatis infection. In: Mardh P-A, Homes K K, Oriel J D, Piot P, Schachter J (eds) Chlamydial infections. Elsevier Biomedical, Amsterdam, pp 193–196

Hager W D 1983 Followup of patients with tubo-ovarian abscess in association with salpingitis. Obstetrics and Gynecology 61: 680–684

Hager W D, Eschenbach D A, Speme M R, Sweet R L 1983 Criteria for diagnosis and grading of salpingitis. Obstetrics and Gynecology 61: 113–114

Hare M J, Barnes C F J 1979 Fallopian tube organ culture in the investigation of bacteroids as a cause of pelvic inflammatory disease. In: Phillips I, Collier J (eds) Metronidazole. Royal Society of Medicine, London, pp 191–197

Heinonen P K, Teisala K, Punnonen R, Miettinen A, Lehtinen M, Paavonen J 1985 Anatomic sites of upper genital tract infection. Obstetrics and Gynecology 66: 384–390

Henry-Suchet J, Catalan F, Loffredo V et al 1980 Microbiology of specimens obtained by laparoscopy from controls and from patients with pelvic inflammatory disease or infertility with tubal obstruction. American Journal of Obstetrics and Gynecology 138: 1022–1025

Hurtig A 1957 Cortisone and specific antibiotics for resistant pelvic infections. American Journal of Obstetrics and Gynecology 73: 1183–1185

Hutchinson G R, Taylor-Robinson D, Dourmashkin R R 1979 Growth and effect of chlamydiae in human and bovine oviduct organ cultures. British Journal of Venereal Diseases 55: 194–202

Jacobson L, Westrom L 1969 Objectivised diagnosis of acute pelvic inflammatory disease. American Journal of Obstetrics and Gynecology 105: 1088–1098

Keith L G, Berger G S, Edelman D A et al 1984 On the causation of pelvic inflammatory disease. American Journal of Obstetrics and Gynecology 149: 215–223

Kelaghan J, Rubin G L, Ory H W, Layde P M 1982 Barrier-method contraceptives and pelvic inflammatory disease. Journal of the American Medical Association 248: 184–187

Landers D V & Sweet R L 1985 Current trends in the diagnosis and treatment of tubo-ovarian abscess. American Journal of Obstetrics and Gynecology 151: 1098–1110

Lip J, Burgoyne X 1966 Cervical and peritoneal flora associated with salpingitis. Obstetrics and Gynecology 28:561–563

Lundberg W I, Wall J E, Mathers J E 1973 Laparoscopy in evaluation of pelvic pain. Obstetrics and Gynecology 42: 872–876

McCormack W M, Alpert S, McComb D E, Nichols R, Semine D, Zinner S 1979 Fifteen month follow-up study of women infected with C. trachomatis. New England Journal of Medicine 300: 123–125

Mardh P-A 1980 An overview of infectious agents of salpingitis, their biology and recent advances in methods of detection. American Journal of Obstetrics and Gynecology 138: 933–951

Mardh P-A, Westrom L 1970 Tubal and cervical cultures in acute salpingitis with special reference to Mycoplasma hominis and T-strain mycoplasmas. British Journal of Venereal Diseases 46: 179–186

Mardh P-A, Ripa T, Svensson L, Westrom L 1977 Chlamydia trachomatis infection in patients with acute salpingitis. New England Journal of Medicine 296: 1377–1379

Moller B R, Ahrons S, Lavrin J, Mardh P-A 1982 Pelvic infection after elective abortion associated with Chlamydia trachomatis. Obstetrics and Gynecology 59: 210–213

Monif G R G, Welkos S L, Baer H, Thompson R J 1976 Cul-de-sac isolates from patients with endometritis-salpingitis-peritonitis and gonococcal endocervicitis. American Journal of Obstetrics and Gynecology 126: 158–161

Niebyl J R, Palmley T H, Speme M R, Woodruff J D 1978 Unilateral ovarian abscesses associated with the intrauterine device. Obstetrics and Gynecology 52: 165–168

Nogales-Ortiz F, Tarancon I, Nogales F 1979 The pathology of female genital tuberculosis. Obstetrics and Gynecology 53: 422–428

Noonan A S, Adams J B 1974 Gonorrhoea screening in an urban hospital family planning programme. American Journal of Public Health 64: 700–704

Osser S, Persson K 1982 Epidemiologic and serodiagnostic aspects of chlamydial salpingitis. Obstetrics and Gynecology 59: 206–209

Paavonen J, Saikku P, Vesterinen E, Ahok 1979 C. Trachomatis in acute salpingitis. British Journal of Venereal Diseases 55: 203–206

Paavonen J, Valtonen V V, Kasper D L, Malkamaki M, Makela P H 1981 Serological evidence for the role of Bacteroides fragilis and enterobacteriaceae in the pathogenesis of acute pelvic inflammatory disease. Lancet i: 293–295

Paavonen J, Aine R, Teisala K, Heinonen P K, Punnonen R 1985a Comparison of endometrial biopsy and peritoneal fluid cytologic testing with laparoscopy in the diagnosis of acute pelvic inflammatory disease. American Journal of Obstetrics and Gynecology 151: 645–650

Paavonen J, Kiviat N, Brunham R C et al 1985b Prevalence and manifestations of endometritis among women with cervicitis. American Journal of Obstetrics and Gynecology 152: 280–286

Paavonen J, Teisala K, Heinonen P K et al 1985c Endometritis and acute salpingitis associated with C. trachomatis and herpes simplex virus type 2. Obstetrics and Gynecology 65: 288–291

Paavonen J, Lehtinen M, Teisala K et al 1985d Haemophilus influenzae causes purulent salpingitis. American Journal of Obstetrics and Gynecology 151: 338–339

Patton D L, Brunham R C, Halbert S A, Wong S-P, Kuo C C, Holmes K K 1983 C. Trachomatis salpingitis in the pig-tailed macaque. In: Mardh P-A, Holmes K K, Oriel J D, Piot P. Schachter J (eds) Chlamydial Infection. Elsevier Biomedical, Amsterdam

Punnonen R, Terho P, Nikkanen V, Meurman O 1979 Chlamydial serology in infertile women by immunofluorescence. Fertility and Sterility 31: 656–659

Rank R G, Barron A L 1982 Prolonged genital infection with GPIC agent associated with immunosuppression treatment with estradiol. In: Mardh P-A, Holmes K K, Oriel J D, Piot P, Schachter J (eds) Chlamydial infections. Elsevier Biomedical, Amsterdam, pp 391–394

Rebello R, Green F H Y, Fox H 1975 A study of the secretory immune system of the female genital tract. British Journal of Obstetrics and Gynaecology 82: 812–816

Ripa K T, Moller B R, Mardh P-A, Freundt F A, Melson F 1979 Experimental acute salpingitis in grivet monkeys provoked by C. trachomatis. Acta Pathologica et Microbiologica Scandinavica Section B 87: 65–70

Robinson J, Burch B H 1984 An assessment of the value of the menstrual history in differentiating acute appendicitis from pelvic inflammatory disease. Surgery, Gynecology and Obstetrics 159: 149–152

Rubin G L, Ory H W, Layde P M 1982 Oral contraceptives and pelvic inflammatory disease. American Journal of Obstetrics and Gynecology 144: 630–635

Schachter J, Banks J, Sung M, Sweet R 1982 Hydrosalpinx as a

consequence of chlamydial salpingitis in the guinea pig. In: Mardh P-A, Holmes K K, Oriel J D, Piot P, Schachter J (eds) Chlamydial infections. Elsevier Biomedical, Amsterdam, pp 371–374

Senanayake P, Kramer D G 1980 Contraception and the etiology of pelvic inflammatory disease. American Journal of Obstetrics and Gynecology 138: 852–860

Simpson D M, Davis O P 1979 Properties of a gonococcal inhibitor produced by E. coli. Journal of General Microbiology 115: 471–477

Singh B, Cutler J, Vridjian H 1972 Effect of vaginal contraceptive and non-contraceptive preparations on T. pallidum and N. gonorrhoeae. British Journal of Venereal Diseases 48: 57–64

Smith M R, Soderstrom R 1976 Salpingitis: a frequent response to intrauterine contraception. Journal of Reproductive Medicine 16: 159–162

Sparkes R A, Purrier B G A, Wat P J, Elstein M 1981 Bacteriological colonisation of the uterine cavity: role of tailed intrauterine contraceptive device. British Medical Journal 282: 1189–1191

Spirtos N J, Bernstine R L, Crawford W L, Fayle J 1982 Sonography in acute pelvic inflammatory disease. Journal of Reproductive Medicine 27: 312–320

Stark J (1986) Personal communication

Street D A, Wells C, Taylor-Robinson D, Ackers J P 1984 Interaction between Trichonomas vaginalis and other pathogenic micro-organisms of the human genital tract. British Journal of Venereal Diseases 60: 31–38

Sutherland A 1982 Post menopausal tuberculosis of the female genital tract. Obstetrics and Gynecology 59: 545–575

Svensson L, Weström L, Ripa K T, Mardh P-A 1980 Differences in some clinical and laboratory parameters in acute salpingitis related to culture and serologic findings. American Journal of Obstetrics and Gynecology 138: 1017–1021

Svensson L, Weström L, Mardh P-A 1984 Contraceptives and acute salpingitis. Journal of the American Medical Association 251: 2553–2555

Sweet R L, Mills J, Hadley K W et al 1979 Use of laparoscopy to determine the microbiologic etiology of acute salpingitis. American Journal of Obstetrics and Gynecology 134: 68–74

Sweet R L, Draper D L, Schachter J, James J, Hadley W K, Brooks G F 1980a Microbiology and pathogenesis of acute salpingitis as determined by laparoscopy. American Journal of Obstetrics and Gynecology 138: 985–989

Sweet R L, Banks, Sung M, Donegan E, Schachter J 1980b Experimental chlamydial salpingitis in the guinea pig. American Journal of Obstetrics and Gynecology 138: 952–956

Sweet R L, Schachter J, Robbie M O 1983 Failure of beta-lactam antibiotics to eradicate C trachomatis in the endometrium despite apparent clinical cure of salpingitis. Journal of the American Medical Association 250: 2641–2645

Targum S D, Wright N H 1974 Association of the intrauterine device and pelvic inflammatory disease. American Journal of Epidermiology 100: 262–271

Taylor-Robinson D, Tuffrey M, Falder P 1982 Some aspects of animal models for Chlamydia trachomatis genital infections. In: Mardh P-A, Holmes K K, Oriel J D, Piot P, Schachter J (eds) Chlamydial infections. Elsevier Biomedical, Amsterdam, pp 375–378

Thadepalli H, Gorbach S L, Keith L 1973 Anaerobic infections of the female genital tract. American Journal of Obstetrics and Gynecology 117: 1034–1040

Thompson S E, Hager W D, Wong K H et al 1980 The microbiology and therapy of acute pelvic inflammatory disease in hospitalised patients. American Journal of Obstetrics and Gynecology 136: 179–186

Toth A, O'Leary W M, Ledger W 1982 Evidence for microbial transfer by spermatozoa. Obstetrics and Gynecology 59: 556–559

Treharne J D, Ripa K T, Mardh P-A, Svensson L, Weström L, Darougar S 1979 Antibodies to C. trachomatis in acute salpingitis. British Journal of Venereal Diseases 55: 26–29

Vessey M P, Yeates D, Flavel R, McPherson K 1981 Pelvic inflammatory disease and the intrauterine device: findings in a large cohort study. British Medical Journal 282: 855–857

Wang S P, Eschenbach D A, Holmes K K, Wager G, Grayston T 1980 Chlamydia trachomatis in Fitz-Hugh Curtis syndrome. American Journal of Obstetrics and Gynecology 138: 1034–1038

Washington A E, Gove S, Schachter J, Sweet R L 1985 Oral contraceptives, Chlamydia trachomatis infection and pelvic inflammatory disease. A word of caution about protection. Journal of the American Medical Association 253: 2246–2250

Weström L 1980 Incidence, prevalence and trends of acute pelvic inflammatory disease and its consequences in industrialised countries. American Journal of Obstetrics and Gynecology 138: 880–892

Wölner-Hanssen P, Mardh P-A 1984 In vitro tests of the adherence of Chlamydia trachomatis to human spermatozoa. Fertility and Sterility 42: 102–107

Wölner-Hanssen P, Mardh P-A, Moller B, Westrom L 1982 Endometrial infection in women with chlamydial salpingitis. Journal of Sexually Transmitted Diseases 9: 84–88

PART III

Diseases due to specific organisms

Syphilis
J K Oates and M R FitzGerald

Syphilis must be the most frequently described infectious disease of all time. In spite of the attention paid to it by doctors for hundreds of years it is still very much with us, presenting problems both of diagnosis and management. It is clear that this old and enduring enemy of mankind still has many lessons to teach us.

No epitome or definition of the disease has ever bettered that of the great American syphilologist Stokes, who defined syphilis as an infectious disease due to *Treponema pallidum*, of great chronicity, systemic from the outset, capable of involving practically every structure of the body in its course; distinguished by florid manifestations on the one hand and years of completely asymptomatic latency on the other; able to simulate many diseases in medicine and surgery; transmissible to offspring in man; transmissible to certain laboratory animals; and treatable to the point of presumptive cure.

HISTORY

The disease first became widespread in Europe towards the end of the 15th century and it received its unique, elegant and somehow rather sinister name from that of a swineherd, the subject of a poem written about the disease in 1530 by the man often described as the first epidemiologist, Hieronymus Frascatorius.

Much controversy surrounds the disease's origins and there are several theories to be considered. A favourite is that it was imported to Europe by Christopher Columbus and his sailors on their return from the Americas. Another theory suggests that the treponemes of syphilis and yaws are identical and that the different clinical pictures pro-

duced are in fact due to environmental influences. A less widely held view is that the organisms causing the endemic treponematoses are distinct but once again environment plays a major part in the type of illness produced. Of the two main theories the second is perhaps more likely to be correct as African slaves were introduced into Portugal at least half a century before Columbus's journeys and there is no doubt that these slaves moved widely about Europe.

Before leaving this brief historical note perhaps one should reflect on another fact about this illness—surely no other has so many names: the French disease, the English disease, the great pox, the sailor's revenge and many others. Clinicians, especially today, should remember another descriptive name for syphilis: 'the disease of exceptions'!

EPIDEMIOLOGY

There is much evidence showing a slow decline in both incidence and morbidity from about the middle of the 19th century onwards, though this was interrupted by sharp increases attributable to wars, revolutions and large population movements. The cause for this decline is not clear, though some authorities attribute it directly to the improvement in general socioeconomic conditions resulting from the Industrial Revolution.

Throughout the western world in recent years there has been a steady fall in cases of both early infectious and late syphilis. Public health measures and the advent of penicillin have contributed to this, and there is no doubt that an important factor in the decline of syphilis in the West must be the frequent use of antibiotic remedies for a host of symptomatic disorders, which probably leads to the suppression of many cases of early infectious syphilis and interrupts the chain of infection.

The exception to the generally low rate of incidence of the disease has been in the western male homosexual communities where syphilis is today a common illness. For example, in England in 1982 the male: female ratio of cases of primary and secondary syphilis was 5.3:1, whereas for new clinic cases of all sexually transmitted diseases, it was 1.3:1.

Syphilis is still a major disease and perhaps the size of the change in its prevalence has masked its continuing importance. In a Yale University autopsy series between 1917 and 1941, nearly 10% of subjects had clinical, laboratory or autopsy evidence of syphilis (Rosahn 1947) and a serological survey in Alabama in 1932 found one man in four to have positive serology. Fifty years later, in the fiscal year 1982, 33 164 cases of primary and secondary syphilis alone were reported in the USA. If such figures continue in a country with readily available medical care, it is no surprise that the disease remains common in many parts of Africa, South America, the Indian subcontinent, and the Pacific.

BIOLOGY

Causative agent

Syphilis is caused by *Treponema pallidum*, which was discovered by Schaudin and Hoffman in 1905. It is a member of the order Spirochaetales, the family Treponemataceae containing genera which are virulent for human beings; members of the genus *Treponema* are *T. pertenue* (yaws), *T. carateum* (pinta), *T. pallidum* var. *Bosnia* (endemic syphilis), and *T. pallidum* (Turner & Hollander 1957). Yaws and pinta are disfiguring cutaneous and osseous diseases of tropical countries. These treponemes appear to be identical morphologically, chemically and as far as can be tested immunologically. Some slight differences are apparent in rabbit inoculation experiments. Culture has long been unsuccessful and this has hampered study of these organisms (Fitzgerald 1981a).

T. pallidum is a thin, regular, close-coiled spiral organism varying in length between 5 and 15 μm (approximately the diameter of a red blood cell) with 6 to 18 spirals. Its ends are noticeably tapered. Electron microscopy shows it to be formed of an axial bundle surrounded by a number of spirally wound fibrils. It is composed of proteins, a polymer and two different lipids (Hovind-Hougen 1983). It divides by transverse fission roughly every 33 hours. The organism is actively motile and its characteristic movements enable it to be identified by dark field microscopy. The movements consist of rotation, propulsion and changes of shape. Rotation or 'corkscrew' movement appears to depend somewhat on the viscosity of the surrounding medium whilst propulsive movements tend to be slow and regular. Changes in shape include coil compression, expansion, angulation, with buckling-angulation where the organism bends at an acute or obtuse angle being perhaps the most typical movement. All in all, when the appearance of motile *T. pallidum* is compared with that of other treponemes and spiral organisms often found at sites of syphilitic infection, its appearance to the experienced eye is characteristic.

Metabolism and culture

Treponema pallidum was not grown in culture until the work of Fieldsteel et al in 1981 using rabbit epithelial cell monolayers. The organism requires microaerophilic conditions with increased carbon dioxide; it metabolises glucose and pyruvate aerobically, has a cytochrome system, and has superoxide dismutase and catalase activity (Austin et al 1981). Replication time is about 30 hours. Neither long-term culture nor subculture have been achieved and experimental work has had to be performed mainly on infected rabbits, using non-pathogenic laboratory strains such as the Reiter treponeme.

Viability

It is rapidly inactivated by heating, drying and contact with antiseptics whilst the wearing of rubber gloves will provide complete protection to the hands. Unfortunately many patients apply antiseptic creams to ulcerative genital lesions and this is likely to destroy surface organisms, making diagnosis by dark field much more difficult.

The agent is unlikely to survive for more than 48 hours in whole blood stored at usual refrigeration temperatures. By careful techniques *T. pallidum* can be kept viable for long periods at $-78°C$.

Transmission

Syphilis is usually transmitted by intimate sexual contact, the important exceptions being when the fetus is infected via the placenta, and accidentally in blood transfusion. Transmission requires exposure to moist mucosal or cutaneous lesions, so occurs only early in the infection. It is not particularly infectious and generally only about one-third of named contacts of a case will prove to have been infected.

COURSE OF DISEASE

Treponema pallidum may be able to penetrate intact mucous membrane but requires a break in the epidermal cells to effect an entry via the skin. Following penetration the organisms rapidly reach the regional lymphatics—this has been shown to be in well under 24 hours in experimental animals and is likely to be true of man. From the lymphatic glands they then gain access to the bloodstream and are carried round the body in a series of 'showers', being deposited eventually in most tissues. It is important to realise that the infection is systemic from the outset and that the blood of patients with incubating syphilis is infectious.

The host response involves both cellular and humoral immunity (Fitzgerald 1981b). At the site of inoculation an inflammatory response is mounted with a polymorph, lymphoctyte, and especially a plasma cell infiltrate, causing periarteritis. Within the blood vessels there is proliferation of the endothelial cells. An inflammatory indurated papule appears, which as a result of the endarteritis soon ulcerates to form a sore; it is common to find clinical enlargement of the local lymphatic glands at this stage. The chancre or primary lesion may appear from 9 to 90 days after infection, though 28 to 42 days is the average incubation period. In some patients the chancre produced is so small as to

escape notice though the subsequent course of the disease is exactly the same as those with prominent primary lesions; in women some chancres must escape notice for anatomical reasons.

Healing then occurs and usually takes several weeks, with a small scar if tissue loss as a result of ulceration has occurred. Apart from a little local discomfort from the chancre, the patient usually feels perfectly well at this stage.

The secondary stage of the disease usually follows up to 12 weeks later. The time interval can be as short as 1 month or longer than 6 months and is ushered in with both clinical symptoms and signs. The commonest signs are the development of a generalised, non-irritating, persistent rash along with lesions of the mucous membranes. Generalised enlargement of the lymph glands is frequently present along with an obvious or healing primary sore. Fever, malaise, headache and bone pains are common and the patient with secondary disease is often an ill patient. The humoral immune system is activated and both specific and non-specific antibodies are produced. Neither has a completely protective role but antigen–antibody complexes can be detected and occasionally cause renal damage when they lodge in the kidneys. All serological tests are strongly positive. If the patient is pregnant the risk of infection to the fetus is extremely high.

In the absence of therapy the rash and symptoms slowly subside over a period of weeks and the patient then enters a long period of latency which may persist for life, though the infection has not been eliminated. As many as 25% of patients have an infectious relapse of the secondary stage within the first year, and relapses may occur until the second year after infection. The fetus may be infected in successive pregnancies, although the danger is greatly reduced after 4 years.

In some individuals persistent chronic infection of the cardiovascular and/or central nervous system ensues until damage is of such a degree that signs and symptoms of disease of these systems develop. Several studies (Gjestland 1955; Schuman et al 1955) have shown that of patients with untreated syphilis roughly two-thirds will die of causes unconnected with the disease. About one-third develop clinical manifestations of late or tertiary syphilis. Of this group roughly two-thirds will suffer from cardiovascular or central nervous system syphilis and one-third benign or gummatous disease.

Thus although the principal morbidity and mortality of syphilis in adults is due to the late manifestations of the disease, the greatest risk of sexual transmission is in early syphilis which is arbitrarily defined as covering 2 years from infection. The same risks apply to the possibility of transmission of the disease to the fetus. As a result the diagnosis of early syphilis is a vital element in the control of this illness.

CLINICAL FEATURES OF PRIMARY SYPHILIS

Although syphilis is a very old disease and its clinical manifestations have not really changed at all, misdiagnosis is common largely because it is not suspected. It should be a clinical rule that is rarely broken that all ulcerative genital lesions are regarded as potentially syphilitic until proved otherwide.

The first sign of the disease is the chancre which appears at the site of inoculation. In most cases this will be the genital area but the possibilities of infection developing elsewhere as a result of oral/genital, genital/anal and oral/anal contact must be remembered. Lesions of the mouth, nipple and fingers are also well documented though distinctly uncommon in clinical practice. In fact, chancres have been noted on virtually every portion of the body's skin or mucous membranes. They are usually single, but may be multiple.

Genital sites

These may be on the labia majora, labia minora or in the periclitoral area. A favourite site is the labial fraenum where the labia minora join inferiorly. This is a common site of trauma sustained during sexual activity and the injury may be visible as a small split or tear, though often nothing can be seen. This concept of 'microtrauma' resulting from sexual intercourse is borne out by the frequency of genital warts and herpetic lesions appearing at this site. Chancres of the cervix are well known and are almost certainly underdiagnosed because of their site and the lack of symptoms.

Syphilitic lesions of the labia are frequently associated with considerable local oedema and although primary chancres are in general painless, some, perhaps as a result of other superadded infections, are distinctly painful.

Perianal and anal sites

Chancres in these areas may result from anal intercourse or perianal contact. They tend to occur at the junction of skin and mucosa and thus are often not visible unless the buttocks are separated and the anal margin is gently everted. Inevitably any lesion in this area is likely to receive a diagnostic label of 'piles' by the patient and regrettably, her doctor.

Clinical appearances (Plates 29, 44, 48)

The chancre develops as a red infiltrated papule of variable size of which the surface first erodes and then becomes ulcerated. Its edge is usually well defined and on palpation is often markedly indurated. Some lesions however ulcerate rapidly and are not very indurated. When ulceration has developed the floor of the lesion is often covered with yellowish grey viscid secretion. Later as healing progresses a scab may form covering the lesion. Some degree of enlargement of the regional lymph glands is present in the great majority and this swelling is usually painless and unilateral, firm, rubbery, and mobile.

It must be appreciated that the chancre is an evolving lesion and at the beginning and end of its existence it will be 'atypical'. When one adds to this the fact that other sexually transmitted infections causing ulceration such as herpes or chancroid may be present (see Plate 46), that secondary infection due to other organisms is far from rare, and that many patients will have applied a variety of preparations to them before presentation, it is not surprising to learn that perhaps a majority of chancres seen in clinical practice are atypical in appearance (Chapel 1978).

Diagnosis

The only positive way to be sure of a diagnosis of primary syphilis is by the demonstration of living

Treponema pallidum in a dark field preparation. This is best done by roughly abrading the lesion with a gauze swab until gentle bleeding is produced. If this is swabbed dry, clear serum soon exudes and a sample of this obtained on a clean glass cover slip is examined immediately by means of dark field microscopy. If the lesion has scabbed over, positive results can sometimes be obtained by removing the scab with a sterile needle and proceeding as above. Where the lesion has healed, treponemes may be obtained by injecting 0.5 ml or so of sterile saline into an enlarged regional lymphatic gland. The gland is massaged gently with the needle in situ, a little fluid withdrawn and then examined under the dark field (the microscopic appearances of *T. pallidum* are described earlier). The examination should be repeated on 3 successive days if a suspicious lesion is negative at first.

Successful dark field microscopy requires skill, patience and experience as well as a good quality microscope. Centres which do not use the technique regularly are likely to be less successful at performing it, and for them the development of a fluorescein conjugated monoclonal antibody to *T. pallidum* seems promising. Smears can be examined immediately or sent to a centre where fluorescence microscopy is available, and preliminary results suggest that this is at least as sensitive and specific as dark field microscopy.

The first serological test for syphilis to become positive is the fluorescent treponemal antibody test and this is of value especially where the patient is unlikely to have suffered from the illness before. Other specific tests can also be expected to be positive in about half of all established primary lesions. At least one-third of all chancres will be first seen when all serological tests are negative, so dark field microscopy is of paramount importance in diagnosis. Serological follow-up should be continued for 3 months even if dark ground preparations from a suspicious lesion are negative.

The existence of syphilis in a sexual partner is vital epidemiological evidence and should intensify the search for signs of the disease. If syphilis is a possibility, treponemeicidal antibiotics should not be used for treating intercurrent infections as they will delay diagnosis: spectinomycin or sulphonamides are satisfactory.

Differential diagnosis

This involves a consideration of any illness producing ulcerative lesions of the genitals and the performance of serological tests for syphilis, dark field preparations, and any tests indicated for the possible causes such as virus isolation for herpes.

The following are the commonest problems met with in practice:

Primary herpes simplex

In herpes the ulceration is usually multiple, preceded by vesiculation and is painful. There is tender lymphadenopathy. Confusion may be caused by a few lesions 'running together' to form a single large ulcer and by the occasional occurrence of double infections (see Plate 48).

Herpes virus can easily be isolated in tissue culture. Dark field preparations should always be performed to exclude *T. pallidum*. Fluorescent staining methods using monoclonal antibodies also give rapid and accurate diagnosis of herpetic infections.

Furuncles

Any area of skin with moisture and hair follicles will be subject to the development of furuncles and the genital area, especially the labia majora, is no exception. For a day or two after they break down and discharge purulent material, large furuncles (which may also be associated with a little adenopathy) can prove a difficult diagnostic problem. However, careful examination, local tenderness of the lesion plus a negative dark field preparation along with a fairly rapid resolution generally allow a confident diagnosis to be made.

Chancroid

This condition, which is common in Africa, the Far East and other tropical and subtropical zones, produces multiple painful ulcers which are often associated with inguinal buboes; sometimes single large ulcers develop which are also associated with prominent regional adenopathy. The condition is uncommon in the West, though recent work suggests it is not as rare as was once thought. Negative serological tests, dark fields and a rapid response following therapy with sulphonamides soon makes the diagnosis clear. The causative organism can be isolated with some difficulty on a specialised nutrient medium.

Lymphogranuloma venereum

The initial lesion is a small transient ulcer which is eventually accompanied by marked tender inguinal lymphadenopathy and often systemic illness. There is a high and rising titre to the causative organism, *Chlamydia trachomatis* type 'L'.

Granuloma inguinale

This uncommon tropical condition causes soft raised beefy lesions which are painless and heal by granulation, but persist for long periods and may be locally destructive. Diagnosis is by smear or biopsy showing the Donovan bodies of *Calymmatobacterium granulomatis*.

Behçet's disease

This multisystem disorder may present with genital ulceration and at this stage differential diagnosis depends upon excluding syphilis, herpes and chancroid with appropriate tests. The ulceration typically tends to be persistent and painful and to be associated with ulceration of the oral mucous membrane. A history of recurrent attacks extending over many months or even years may be given. The diagnosis is made on the clinical picture as there is no specific test (see Plates 50, 51).

Carcinoma

Chronic painless ulcers of the genitalia require positive exclusion of neoplasia. Vulval carcinoma is rare, but cervical lesions should be investigated with cytology, colposcopy, and biopsy.

Traumatic ulceration

Traumatic ulceration of the female genitals is rare but can result from the use of dildos and vibrators. Ulceration of the vaginal mucous membrane may result from the use of chemicals of which the best

known culprit is potassium permanganate tablets. These can cause deep ulceration with haemorrhage. Though such causes of ulceration are rare, patients are often loath to give an accurate history and these reasons should be considered when no obvious cause is present.

CLINICAL FEATURES OF SECONDARY SYPHILIS

The secondary stage commences some 6 to 12 weeks after the appearance of the primary lesion which is still present in over 30% of cases. Any organ of the body can be involved, and any mucous or cutaneous surface. Most patients develop constitutional symptoms and a skin rash, and these symptoms may precede or accompany the rash (Stokes et al 1944).

Constitutional features

A frequent pattern of symptoms is headache, mild general malaise, sore throat and a low-grade fever. Sometimes only malaise and fever may be present. A few patients will develop severe headache and bone pains which are especially noticeable at night. Nervous system involvement may occur causing true meningitis, cranial nerve palsies, or nerve deafness (Willcox & Goodwin 1971). Mild hepatitis is present in up to 10% of patients (Feher et al 1975), sometimes with hepatomegaly. There may be an immune complex nephropathy causing transient proteinuria, nephrotic syndrome, or nephritis (Bhorade et al 1971). Generalised lymphadenopathy is an important feature and occurs in over 50% of cases.

Rash (Plate 62)

In over 75% of patients there is a skin rash and in about 30% lesions of the mucous membrane of the oropharynx are present. The eruption of secondary syphilis is very variable and can mimic many rare and common skin diseases. In general terms the rash tends to be present for many weeks, does not itch or vesiculate, is symmetrically distributed and often affects the palms and soles. The lesions themselves may be thinly or profusely distributed and often appear in crops over a period of several weeks. The lesions when new tend to have a fresh pink colour which assumes a coppery hue as they age. They are greyish on dark skins. Some may be macular whilst others are noticeably infiltrated and papular or even pustular: the commonest appearance is slightly scaly discs which are 0.5 cm in diameter. In some patients the rash may be entirely macular and faint, indeed only being noted by the patient after a hot bath or as a manifestation of the Jarisch-Herxheimer reaction. Patchy hair loss ('moth-eaten alopecia') occurs but is uncommon.

Lesions may be present on the mucous membranes of the oropharynx. Here they have a very different appearance due to necrosis of the overlying mucous membrane, the end result being an irregular greyish patch with a dull red areolar margin. These lesions are known as mucous patches and are highly infectious. On the fauces the lesions adopt a serpiginous conformation whilst the swallowing of food and mastication tends to rub off the necrotic mucous membrane revealing an erosion: the 'snail track' ulcer. Other lesions may appear on the tonsil where deep ulceration may develop. Small erosive patches are common on the tongue and at the angles of the lips.

In areas of warmth and moisture such as the vulva and perianal region the papular lesions of the secondary eruption persist even though skin lesions elsewhere in the body fade. The lesions at these moist sites enlarge, taking on a bluish grey appearance with a superficial resemblance to warts. These are condylomata lata (Plate 45). Not infrequently, especially around the anus, these lesions may form large vegetative plaques of which the surface is superficially eroded, and covered with serous exudate rich in treponemes.

The rash usually heals spontaneously in 2–10 weeks, but it may relapse.

Diagnosis

It is possible to demonstrate treponemes in many of the secondary lesions of syphilis by dark field microscopy and this is particularly easy with condylomata lata and mucous patches, though in the latter site confusion with non-pathogenic treponemes present in the mouth can be a problem.

A lymphocytosis, a mild degree of anaemia, and a moderately raised sedimentation rate are frequently found at this time. However, the most important diagnostic tests are the serological tests for syphilis—both standard and specific—which are always positive at this stage of the disease. In the presence of negative serological tests, a diagnosis of secondary syphilis cannot be entertained.

Differential diagnosis

This usually involves considering the possibility of a number of infectious illnesses and a wide range of dermatological conditions. Amongst skin diseases, pityriasis rosea, measles and drug eruptions perhaps pose the most frequently encountered difficulties. Viral illnesses such as infectious mononucleosis and acute HIV infection should be excluded. When lesions are few, lichen planus, tinea, sarcoid and a host of dermatoses may have to be considered. Fortunately the clinical history, presence of mucosal lesions, epidemiological information and the serological tests always allow a positive diagnosis to be made. Occasionally, when syphilis has not been considered and serological tests not performed, a biopsy may indicate the diagnosis. This shows characteristic dermal changes of endarteritis and an inflammatory infiltrate in which plasma cells predominate. *Treponema pallidum* can be seen with special stains.

Difficulty in diagnosis (Chapel 1981) may be found when such constitutional symptoms as fever, meningitis or jaundice dominate the clinical picture and a widespread rash is not evident. If early syphilis is remembered as a possible cause of such symptoms, careful clinical examination will nearly always show some of the signs of the disease, such as a healing primary sore, a scanty skin eruption, lesions of the mucous membranes or generalised lymphadenopathy. The serological tests will always confirm any clinical suspicions.

SYPHILIS AND PREGNANCY

From the earliest description of syphilis, it was recognised that the disease frequently spread to newborn infants, though for centuries most medical men believed it to be spread by direct contact through breast feeding or 'wet nursing'. Some authorities, even in the 16th century however, considered hereditary syphilis to be a possibility but such a hypothesis was not clearly proven until the early years of this century when serological tests allowed the demonstration of the transmission of infection to an infant via an infected, though asymptomatic, mother. It is now known that if a pregnant woman with early syphilis is not treated, half the infants born will be premature, neonatal deaths or still births; the other half will be infected with congenital syphilis, and only very few will be born normal full term infants (Fiumara et al 1952). Unfortunately, syphilis can be acquired by the woman who is pregnant as easily as at any other time and the infection behaves in a similar fashion.

Treponemes are known to cross from the maternal to the fetal circulation as early as 9 weeks of gestation (Harter & Benirschke 1976). At this early stage the fetus's immunity is too immature to mount a histologically visible reaction, and it was previously and erroneously thought that infection did not occur in the first trimester. In fact the mother is at her most infectious to the fetus in early disease, and almost every pregnancy in the first year of infection will be involved. Later pregnancies will be affected less frequently and less severely and after 4 years there is little danger, even if the woman has not been treated.

Congenital syphilis, when not fatal, can result in lasting neurological and skeletal damage. Descriptions of its clinical features are beyond the scope of this book (they can be found in Nabarro 1954) but two features should be mentioned. Infants with early congenital syphilis or stillborn fetuses often have exudative rashes which are highly infectious and thus require careful nursing. The obstetrician also needs to note that the majority of congenitally infected infants show no signs at birth as the characteristic clinical features do not develop until 2–12 weeks later. Consequently antenatal diagnosis is even more important in places where postnatal care is limited.

SEROLOGICAL TESTS FOR SYPHILIS

An understanding of these is vital for the correct diagnosis, treatment and follow-up of all cases of syphilis. A confusingly large variety of tests exists, but many are obsolescent, unproven innovations, or adaptations for rapid analysis. The tests in routine use fall into two main groups depending on whether they detect non-specific or specific antibodies.

Non-specific tests

All these tests measure an antibody, formerly called reagin, to cardiolipin in the treponemes. Reactivity reflects activity of the disease and all the tests can be performed on serial dilutions to quantify progression of infection or response to treatment. They usually become positive 10–30 days after the appearance of the chancre. They are refinements of the original Wassermann reaction, first used in 1906, which was a complement fixation test and laborious to perform. These modifications are flocculation tests, can be read easily, and lend themselves to automation. Tests in common use today include the following:

Cardiolipin Wassermann reaction (CWR);

The venereal disease research laboratory slide test (VDRL test);

Rapid plasma reagin card test (RPR);

Automated reagin test (ART).

The VDRL slide or tube test uses a standard cardiolipin–lecithin–cholesterol antigen. Reactive sera produce flocculation which is readily visible with a low-power microscope. The VDRL is an excellent test, though antigen has to be freshly prepared and the test sera heated. It is easy to quantitate and is perhaps the test of choice for follow-up of treated patients.

The RPR and ART employ a stabilised suspension of antigen and charcoal on a card. When a reactive serum is employed the resulting antigen/antibody combination traps the charcoal enabling the result to be read by the naked eye. The ART, as its name suggests, is an automated test using the same principles, but is processed on an autoanalyser. It is particularly convenient for single tests and is also an excellent test in large-scale screening programmes.

Cardiolipin is widespread in the human body as it is a component of the inner wall of the mammalian mitochondrion (the usual source for test material is an extract of beef heart). False positive tests may therefore be obtained in a number of acute and chronic inflammatory conditions (Moore & Mohr 1952). These include acute febrile illnesses, immunisations and pregnancy, lepromatous leprosy, narcotic abuse, and connective tissue disease. These reactions usually have a low positivity and practical management consists of observing the patient and repeating the test with a treponemal test after 2 weeks and then again a few weeks later. A persistently positive VDRL test in isolation is an indication to assess the patient for other diseases (Catterall 1972).

Specific tests

These depend upon the detection of specific antibodies to pathogenic treponemes. The first of these tests, the *Treponema pallidum* immobilisation or TPI test, is no longer routinely performed as it is expensive, time-consuming and dangerous (it employs live *T. pallidum*). It has been replaced by the fluorescent treponemal antibody absorption test (FTA ABS). Test sera are first absorbed to remove group antibodies to non-pathogenic treponemes found in most normal people. The sera are then placed on slides which have on them the antigen in the form of a dried suspension of *T. pallidum*. Fluorescein labelled antihuman globulin is added and in positive sera the dried treponemes fluoresce brightly. This is a very sensitive test and the first to become positive in newly acquired disease.

The most commonly employed specific test is the *Treponema pallidum* haemagglutination test (TPHA) or micro haemagglutination test (TP MHA). This test uses tanned formalinised sheep red cells to carry the treponemal antigen. Positive results are shown by agglutination of the sensitised red cells compared with a control. This test is easy to perform but is not as sensitive as the FTA ABS in early disease (Sequeira & Eldridge 1973). It can easily be quantitated, although this is of little use clinically. An IgM TPHA test was developed with the objective of assessing the activity of early disease but this too has proved unhelpful.

False positive results can be caused by connective tissue disease, and transiently by genital herpes and infectious mononucleosis. The TPI very rarely gives false positives.

It should be noted that these specific treponemal tests may take many years to revert to normal—indeed they frequently remain positive for life, especially the TPHA. Thus a positive test may indicate an attack of the illness sustained many years ago.

Use and interpretation of serological tests

When primary infection has been suspected from the clinical findings or history of exposure, serological tests can be expected to confirm a diagnosis within 10–30 days in the majority of cases (Dyckman et al 1980) although seroconversion may take as long as 90 days. The FTA is positive in up to 90% of primary infections (Duncan et al 1974), typically becoming so within 10 days. The TPHA follows a few days later and in practice the TPHA is more useful as it is more readily available from most laboratories. Tests taken over the next 2 weeks should show the VDRL becoming positive at steadily increasing titre. It is positive in up to 70% of primary syphilis.

In secondary syphilis all serological tests are positive, the VDRL commonly in dilutions as high as 1:128 or higher. After treatment the VDRL declines in successive tests with a speed which relates to the duration of the untreated infection. After one year it is negative in 75% of treated primary cases and 40% of secondary cases and after 2 years negative in almost all treated primary cases. It remains persistently positive at low titre in about 25% of patients treated for secondary or early latent disease and this does not indicate that treatment has failed. Evidence of reinfection is suggested by a rising titre in the VDRL: retreatment is necessary and a search for infected contacts. Treatment failure is exceptionally rare with penicillin therapy and is suggested by a continuing high VDRL or persistent clinical signs. In these cases retreatment should be for neurosyphilis and ideally the cerebrospinal fluid (CSF) should be examined.

The vast majority of tests are done for screening asymptomatic patients. For screening populations at high risk, such as women attending sexually transmitted disease clinics, a combination of a specific and a non-specific test is necessary. Positive specific tests will be common and usually indicate previous treated disease, thus new infections will be signalled by a sustained rise in titre of the non-specific tests. Fluctuations in titre of one or two dilutions are generally of no significance as they are due to intercurrent infections or laboratory technique and will have settled when rechecked. The frequency of screening depends on circumstances but it is commonly done 3-monthly. Screening populations at low risk such as blood donors and antenatal patients in the developed world can be done satisfactorily with a specific test alone. Positive results are then confirmed with another specific test. As very few tests are positive and most patients will be tested on only one occasion, attention to the screening schedule and to laboratory technique is very important. Screening patients with other conditions is necessary because of the large number of medical, surgical, and dermatological entities in which syphilis can play a part. A combination of specific and non-specific tests is needed, but even when both are positive syphilis may be a coincidental event and the final diagnosis depends on the clinical and historical findings.

The possibility of human error should always be remembered. There should be good quality control in the laboratory (Wasley 1985) and the diagnosis of syphilis should never be made on one blood specimen alone.

Problems of serological diagnosis

The interpretation of syphilis serology is basically straightforward but there are certain areas where tests currently available give equivocal results (see Table 7.1). In early syphilis all tests may be negative even though treponemaemia exists: repeat tests are necessary. False positive non-specific tests may occur as described above and cause confusion if they occur when there is already a positive specific test from previous disease. No test will in itself show that adequate therapy has been given and this can be a particular problem when assessing old disease, where the same serological pattern can be given by latent, treated, or partially treated infections. A final problem, particularly in tropical countries, is that the same serological picture is given by both syphilis and other more benign treponemal conditions, and that these infections may often coexist.

Continuing research on serological tests may resolve some of these problems in years to come but at present they can only be decided clinically and

Table 7.1 Patterns of serological reaction

	Non-specific	Specific
Primary infection early	−	+/−
Primary infection later	+	+
Secondary infection	++/+	+
Treated infection	+/−	+
Untreated old infection	+/−	+
Reinfection	+	+
Biological false positive	+	−
Other treponemal disease	+/−	+

sometimes not even then. If there is real doubt as to whether an episode of syphilis has been adequately treated, it is generally the case that the risks of treating it are less than the potential dangers of untreated infection.

Lumbar puncture

The purpose of CSF examination is to exclude active neurosyphilis, which if present would indicate more prolonged and intensive treatment. It is worth doing if the infection is of more than 1 year's duration, or in follow-up if there are doubts about the effectiveness of therapy, such as when the reagin titre fails to fall or when a non-penicillin antibiotic has been used. Involvement of the central nervous system is indicated by an elevated CSF lymphocyte count and positive serological test for syphilis; the total protein may also be elevated.

TREATMENT OF EARLY SYPHILIS

Treponema pallidum is extremely sensitive to penicillin, which is the drug of choice for the treatment of the disease on the grounds of efficacy, low cost and few toxic effects.

The drug acts on the treponeme cell wall preventing repair, and all that is necessary is to maintain a continuous level of penicillin in the blood sufficient to delay these repair mechanisms, for a period of 8 to 10 days. Levels as low as 0.03iu/ml are quite sufficient, though interruption of treatment for 24 hours or more may allow treponemes to resume multiplication. These levels are generally easily exceeded by all standard treatment regimes.

The effectiveness of penicillin in treating early syphilis and preventing long-term complications has been established through more than 30 years' use and follow-up. Other antibiotics may heal early disease equally well but there are much fewer data on long-term effectiveness and little justification to depart from conventional regimes (Idsoe et al 1972).

Choice of penicillin

Aqueous procaine penicillin G 0.6–1.2 megaunits given intramuscularly daily for a period of 10 days will produce virtually a 100% cure rate (Kampmeier 1981). Although in use for 40 years, there is no evidence yet to suggest that *T. pallidum* has become any less sensitive to penincillin. The only caveat to be entered here is that inability to culture the organism has prevented accurate testing of its antibiotic sensitivities. Long-acting penincillin such as benzathine penicillin G may be employed as an alternative as 2.4 million units.

Penicillin allergy

Patients who give a history of sensitivity to this drug should be treated with tetracycline 500 mg by mouth 6-hourly for 15 days. Doxycycline 200 mg once daily is more convenient and may be as effective. Nursing mothers or those who cannot tolerate tetracyclines should be given erythromycin 500 mg by mouth every 6 hours for 15 days.

Both these drugs are effective but not as active initially as penicillin. For example, treponemes can often be recovered after 48 hours of treatment with tetracycline, whilst following penicillin they cannot be found at the end of the first day.

Jarisch-Herxheimer reaction

This is a reaction which commonly occurs after the onset of therapy for early syphilis (Aronson & Soltani 1976). It is thought to be due to a toxin liberated from degenerating treponemes (Bryceson 1976)—such a toxin has been identified from patients treated for *Borrelia recurrentis*, a spirochaetal infection where the Jarisch-Herxheimer reaction is much more severe. It occurs irrespective of the antibiotic used, starting a few hours after treatment with malaise, headache, and nausea. This is followed by fever and chills, and may be accompanied by an intensification of the rash of secondary syphi-

lis or pain and swelling in a primary lesion. The symptoms usually subside within 24 hours or less and treatment is simply reassurance of the patient (who should be warned in advance), bed rest, and aspirin. The danger is that it may be misdiagnosed as a penicillin reaction and treatment stopped.

Contact action

Any physician undertaking the treatment of early infectious syphilis must remember that it is his duty to trace, examine and treat sexual contacts. If he is unable to do this, he should make arrangements for others to undertake this task. Sexually transmitted disease clinics may well have contact tracers available and their special skills should be used. Normal practice is to try to identify all contacts within the previous 3 months for primary syphilis and 12 months for secondary syphilis. Wherever possible a definite diagnosis should be made in all contacts, but in some cases epidemiological treatment (that is, treatment on contact history rather than on evidence of disease) is best. The usual circumstances under which this is done are when exposure to the index case or others is likely to occur during the incubation period of the infection, or when the contact is likely to be lost to follow-up.

Follow-up of treated syphilis

Following treatment, both primary and secondary lesions heal within a few weeks, but as the natural history of both is to resolve spontaneously, serological follow-up is necessary to be certain that treatment has been successful.

In primary cases where the serological tests are negative initially, follow-up blood tests may be carried out at 3-monthly intervals for a year. If all are negative, the patient should be discharged. In cases with positive serological tests, these should be repeated at 3-monthly intervals. One of the standard non-treponemal tests such as the VDRL should be quantitated. Nearly all cases of primary disease will have negative tests 1 year after therapy and most secondary cases should show a considerable decrease in titre. Most secondary cases should be negative at 2 years and may be safely discharged, as can those who show a maintained and significant decrease in titre (say fourfold). Should the titre increase significantly, reinfection or possibly relapse should be suspected and the patient carefully examined. Where there are no signs of fresh disease and the increase in titre is considerable and maintained, examination of the CSF should be performed before retreating. It should be noted that reinfection is much commoner than treatment failure.

Treatment of syphilis in pregnancy

Much the best treatment is penicillin, following the regimes recommended for other patients. The object is to prevent congenital syphilis by giving the treatment as early as possible in pregnancy, and if this is done it is virtually always successful. The mother then needs monthly quantitative reagin tests for the rest of the pregnancy. If there is a fourfold rise in titre, she should be retreated promptly. Very rarely labour is precipitated during a Jarisch-Herxheimer reaction.

Therapy for penicillin-allergic mothers is unsatisfactory. Tetracycline is unsuitable because it is incorporated into growing bones and teeth, causing discoloration and hypoplasia of the primary dentition. Erythromycin has therefore been used but low blood levels are obtained in the fetus and there are several documented cases of infants developing neonatal syphilis after apparently successful treatment of the mother (Fenton & Light 1976). Cephalosporins would be effective in theory but have been little used in practice and there may be cross-allergy to penicillin with them. Patients who give a history of penicillin allergy not infrequently do so on uncertain grounds and every effort should be made to establish whether they are in fact allergic. If so, one course of action is to treat the mother with erythromycin and then treat the infant with penicillin at birth.

Prevention of syphilis in pregnancy

As syphilis in pregnancy is readily treatable, the occurrence of congenital syphilis is now an index of unsatisfactory antenatal care. In the developed world, cases are few and tend to be born to mothers who are young, poor, and educationally disadvantaged. In England, where sexually transmitted disease reporting is comprehensive, 12 cases of syphilis were reported in children under 2 years of age in 1982; in the USA in 1982 there were 176 reported cases under 1 year. In such countries syphilis is detected by screening of all women in pregnancy (Hare 1973). The practice in the United Kingdom is to perform the VDRL test at 16 and 32 weeks of gestation, although as Wright & Gerken (1981) pointed out, it would be more sensible to use the TPHA instead. Reducing neonatal syphilis here requires making sure that socially inadequate mothers still receive adequate antenatal attention.

In the poor countries of the world syphilis represents a very much greater problem. In 1982–1983 in Mozambique, a large survey (Liljestrand et al 1985) found 6.3% of pregnant mothers to be seropositive and syphilis to have caused 8.5% of stillbirths in the capital. These figures, although not as bad as those from the prepenicillin era (Browne 1922), indicate a major public health problem which would need action at all levels of health provision.

PREVENTION OF SYPHILIS

It would be desirable to have available an effective vaccine against syphilis, but none seems in prospect. Experiments with inactivated treponemes in rabbits have conveyed only limited immunity. It is now possible to produce treponemal antigens from *Escherichia coli* clones and this may provide material for more fruitful work (Norgard & Miller 1983). However, as the natural antibody response to syphilis does not succeed in eliminating the disease, it may be that approaches via humoral immunity will be unsuccessful. Prevention is therefore by use of barrier contraceptives and antiseptics, which can have only limited usefulness, and by tracing and treating infected cases.

For the individual, syphilis can most surely be prevented by avoiding sexual contact with persons who may be infected, and particularly casual contact. The only realistic way that this can be encouraged is by public education about the infection and its transmission. When an individual has run a risk or suspects she has an infection, she needs to have readily available rapid, accurate, and inexpensive diagnostic services where she can be tested and where confidentiality will be respected. Many of the symptoms of early syphilis are mild and short-lived and may readily be ignored by the patient, so anything that deters her from seeking care will favour the progression of the disease.

To prevent the continuing spread of syphilis, it is essential that every effort is made to trace and treat the contacts of every case detected. In addition, persons at high risk, such as prostitutes, should be screened regularly. Generally this is best done by making facilities readily available, as coercion is counterproductive.

By means such as these, the incidence of primary and secondary syphilis has been reduced to 4.6% per 100 000 in England in 1982, and 14.6 per 100 000 in the USA in the same year. A host of social, economic, and political factors interact in the control of syphilis, but accurate diagnosis and effective treatment of early disease will continue to be fundamental.

REFERENCES

Aronson I K, Soltani K 1976 The enigma of the pathogenesis of the Jarisch-Herxheimer reaction. British Journal of Venereal Diseases 52: 313–315

Austin F E, Barbieri J T, Corin R E, Grigas K E, Cox C D 1981 Distribution of superoxide dismutase, catalase, and peroxidase activities among Treponema pallidum and other spirochetes. Infection and Immunity 33: 372–379

Bhorade M S, Carag H B, Lee H J, Potter M D, Dunea G 1971 Nephropathy of secondary syphilis: a clinical and pathogical spectrum. Journal of the American Medical Association 216: 1159–1166

Browne F J 1922 Neonatal death. British Medical Journal 2: 590–593

Bryceson A D M 1976 Clinical pathology of the Jarisch-Herxheimer reaction. Journal of Infectious Diseases 133: 696–704

Catterall R D 1972 Presidential address to the MSSVD: systemic disease and the biologic false positive reaction. British Journal of Venereal Diseases 48: 1–12

Chapel T A 1976 The variability of syphilitic chancres. Sexually Transmitted Diseases 5: 68–70

Chapel T A 1981 Physicians' recognition of the signs and symptoms of secondary syphilis. Journal of the American Medical Association 246(3): 250–251

Duncan W C, Knox J M, Wende R D 1974 The FTA-ABS test in darkfield positive primary syphilis. Journal of the American Medical Association 228: 859–860

Dyckman J D, Storms S, Huber T W 1980 Reactivity of microhaemagglutination, fluorescent treponemal antibody absorption, and venereal disease research laboratory tests in primary syphilis. Journal of Clinical Microbiology 12(4): 629–630

Feher J, Somogyi T, Timmer M, Jozsa L 1975 Early syphilitic hepatitis. Lancet ii: 896–899

Fenton L J, Light I J 1976 Congenital syphilis after maternal treatment with erythromycin. Obstetrics and Gynecology 47: 492–494

Fieldsteel A H, Cox D L, Moeckli R A 1981 Cultivation of virulent Treponema pallidum in tissue culture. Infection and Immunity 32: 908–915

Fitzgerald T J 1981a Invitro cultivation of Treponema pallidum: a review. Bulletin of World Health Organization 59(5): 787–812

Fitzgerald T J 1981b Pathogenesis and immunology of Treponema pallidum. Annual Review of Microbiology 35: 29–54

Fiumara N J, Fleming W L, Downing J G, Good F L 1952 The incidence of prenatal syphilis at the Boston City Hospital. New England Journal of Medicine 247: 48–52

Gjestland T 1955 The Oslo study of untreated syphilis: an epidemiologic investigation of the natural course of syphilitic infection based on a restudy of the Boeck-Bruusgaard material. Acta Dermatovenereologica 35 (Suppl 34): 1–368

Hare M J 1973 Serological tests for treponemal disease in pregnancy. Journal of Obstetrics and Gynaecology of the British Commonwealth 80: 515–519

Harter C A, Benirschke K 1976 Fetal syphilis in the first trimester. American Journal of Obstetrics and Gynecology 124: 705–711

Hovind-Hougen K 1983 Morphology. In: Schell R F, Musher D M (eds) Pathogenesis and immunology of treponemal infection. Dekker, New York, pp 3–28

Idsoe O, Guthe T, Willcox R R 1972 Penicillin in the treatment of syphilis: the experience of three decades. Bulletin of World Health Organization 47 (suppl)

Kampmeier R H 1981 A survey of 251 patients with acute syphilis treated in the collaborative penicillin study of 1943–1950. Sexually Transmitted Diseases 8(4): 266–279

Liljestrand J, Bergstrom S, Nieuwenhuis F, Hederstedt B 1985 Syphilis in pregnant women in Mozambique. Genitourinary Medicine 61: 355–358

Moore J E, Mohr C F 1952 Biologically false positive serologic tests for syphilis: type, incidence and cause. Journal of the American Medical Association 150: 467–473

Nabarro D 1954 Congenital syphilis. Edward Arnold, London

Norgard M V, Miller J N 1983 Cloning and expression of Treponema pallidum (Nichols) antigen genes in Escherichia coli. Infection and Immunity 42(2): 435–445

Rosahn P D 1947 Autopsy studies in syphilis. Journal of Venereal Disease Information (Suppl 21): 1–67

Schaudinn F, Hoffman E 1905 Vorläufiger Bericht über das Vorkommen von Spirochaeten in syphilitischen Krankheitsprodukten und bei Papillomen. Arbeiten aus dem Kaiserlichen Gesundheitsamte 22: 527–530

Schuman S H, Olansky S, Rivers E, Smith C A, Rambo D S 1955 Untreated syphilis in the male Negro: background and current status of patients in the Tuskegee study. Journal of Chronic Diseases 2: 543–548

Sequeira P J L, Eldridge A E 1973 The treponemal haemagglutination test. British Journal of Venereal Diseases 49: 242–248

Stokes J H, Beerman H, Ingraham N R 1944 Modern clinical syphilology, 3rd edn. Saunders, Philadelphia

Turner T B, Hollander D H 1957 Biology of the treponematoses. World Health Organization Monograph Series 35: 1

Wasley G D 1985 Internal quality control in serological tests for syphilis. Genitourinary Medicine 61: 88–94

Willcox R R, Goodwin P G 1971 Nerve deafness in secondary syphilis. British Journal of Venereal Diseases 47: 401–406

Wright D J M, Gerken A 1981 Antenatal screening for syphilis. British Journal of Venereal Diseases 57(2): 147–148

Gonorrhoea
R N T Thin

SPREAD AND CONTROL OF GONORRHOEA

Factors influencing spread of gonorrhoea

Gonorrhoea is infectious whether or not symptoms are present. The fundamental factor in its spread is sexual partner change, and this depends on availability of partners. World population movement from rural to urban areas is a potent factor in increasing the number of available sexual partners. Increased travel within and between countries is also important. Other social factors include increasing affluence in many parts of the world, increased alcohol consumption, leisure time, and personal freedom. Prostitution is probably more important in Africa and the East than in the West. Compared to men, many women with uncomplicated anogenital gonorrhoea have no symptoms so may unknowingly spread the infection. The intrauterine contraceptive device and the contraceptive pill offer no barrier to infection, unlike the sheath and diaphragm. Modern single-dose antimicrobial treatment of gonorrhoea is so simple it may encourage the risk of infection, for patients may believe that cure is easy. There is no natural or acquired immunity.

High risk groups

Many patients throughout the world who acquire gonorrhoea are aged 18 to 24 years and in most countries there has been a marked increase in cases in girls aged 16 and 17 years. Other groups include travellers, prostitutes, members of armed forces, merchant seamen, air crew and everyone in entertainment.

Homosexuals have a high prevalence and any girl who is in contact with a bisexual man may be at risk. Sexually transmitted disease affects all socioeconomic groups; though no one is immune, it does appear to be more prevalent in lower socioeconomic groups than in higher groups, at least in some places.

Control

In Britain this is based on the nationwide clinic service which provides accurate diagnosis, effective treatment and careful follow-up to ensure cure. In addition, most clinics have health advisers who ensure that as many potentially infected contacts as possible are traced, examined and when necessary treated. Health workers also check that treated patients return for follow-up to make sure they are cured. Education is an important element in control, but in Britain this is more difficult to implement than clinical care.

In areas where the specialist clinic service is less satisfactory, screening women by taking cervical cultures may be a useful control measure. Cultures can be taken at family planning clinics, well women clinics, obstetric and gynaecological clinics, casualty departments and in general practices with appropriate laboratory support.

THE CAUSATIVE ORGANISM: NEISSERIA GONORRHOEAE

Neisseria gonorrhoeae is a gram-negative coccus usually seen in pairs, hence the term diplococcus. Each coccus has a characteristic kidney shape and each member of the pair lies with its concave surface facing its partner. Gram stain of heavily infected pus such as that obtained from a man with acute gonococcal urethritis may show many typical intracellular gram-negative diplococci. Secretions from other sites such as the female genital tract, the rectum and the pharynx contain other organisms which may cause confusion. These include *N. meningitidis* and saprophytic neisseria species in the pharynx, organisms such as *Mimae* and *Moraxella* which may appear in pairs intracellularly and extracellularly, and partly digested staphylococci and streptococci which may lose their usual gram-positive reaction. In the female, Gram stains may lead to false positive and false negative results, and culture is important.

Transport media

The gonococcus is a fastidious organism and must reach the laboratory in the optimum condition. Where the specimens can be collected close to the laboratory the ideal is to inoculate a plate of growth medium at once, put this straight into a suitable incubator, and transfer it quickly to the laboratory for definitive incubation. When clinic and laboratory are further apart, some form of transport medium must be found. Transport media include Stuart's medium which must be inoculated with a charcoal impregnated swab and Amies medium which is similar to Stuart's medium but the charcoal is in the medium. Transgrow medium (Martin & Lester 1971) is a modified growth medium which can be used for transport and growth of gonococci. It is a modification of Thayer-Martin medium (see below). There are various similar media including Jembec Neigon (Martin & Jackson 1975) and Microcult (Willcox & John 1976).

Growth media

As mentioned above, gonococci are fastidious organisms and in the female usually occur in small numbers in secretions containing many other micro-organisms which easily overgrow gonococci. Early growth media included McLeod's heated blood, or so-called chocolate agar which favoured overgrowth of other organisms. Selective or antibiotic-containing media were introduced by Thayer & Martin (1966) who described a medium containing vancomycin, colistin and nystatin. Phillips et al (1972) added trimethoprim, so-called VCNT medium, which inhibited *Proteus* species. The use of these media has greatly improved the yield of gonococci from secretions containing many other micro-organisms. Occasionally, very sensitive strains are inhibited by such media, but this disadvantage is greatly outweighed by the overall increase in yield. It is important for the clinician to know which medium is being used in a laboratory. Furthermore, different laboratories have found different concentrations of antibiotics give better results.

The colonies are initially recognised by their appearance, and inspection using an operating microscope has shown four main types of colonies (Kellog et al 1965) and an occasional fifth type (Jephcott & Reyn 1971). Types 1 and 2 are pathogenic and their organisms have pili. During subculture in the laboratory, Types 1 and 2 readily change to the non-pathogenic Types 3 and 4.

Identification

In addition to the colonial appearance gonococci are recognised by their reaction to oxidase reagent (1% tetramethyl-p-phenylene diamine hydrochloride in water). Typical colonies rapidly turn a pink colour which deepens to dark purple. Few other organisms show such a rapid reaction but the test is not specific (King et al 1980). Gram staining of these organisms shows typical gram-negative diplococci. Further identification can be undertaken by means of sugar fermentation reactions. A pure subculture must be prepared from the suspect colonies. This is inoculated into media containing the test sugars, usually glucose, maltose, sucrose and lactose. It is important to use serum-free medium as the base for this reaction (Flynn & Waitkins 1972) for serum may contain maltase which inactivates the maltose and can confuse the results by indicating the presence of gonococci instead of meningococci. The medium usually also contains an indicator to show the presence of fermentation (acid formation). Gonococci ferment glucose but not maltose, sucrose or lactose. Sugar fermentation tests take time and are difficult to perform, so some departments rely on a colonial appearance, Gram stain findings and oxidase reaction.

Rapid fermentation reactions

In the rapid fermentation tests, preformed enzyme is identified by adding a suspension of an overnight growth of the suspect organism to a buffered non-nutrient solution containing the sugar and a pH indicator. Some results have been disappointing, but Young et al (1976) described a satisfactory technique.

Identification by immunofluorescence

Immunofluorescent (IF) staining of gonococci can be done using specific antigonococcal antibody raised in rabbits and conjugated with fluorescein isothiocyanate. The conjugate can be used to stain smears of secretions taken from patients. Background fluorescence of leucocytes may be marked, but can be overcome by the use of a counterstain such as naphthalene black. Such staining can give useful results (Thin 1970) but has been more widely used to identify organisms in suspect colonies after overnight or 24-hour incubation (Thin et al 1971), thus speeding up the accurate identification of organisms in cultures. Unfortunately, cross reactions may occur with meningococci and saprophytic neisseria so this method cannot be used for samples taken from the pharynx.

Coagglutination

This is a rapid slide agglutination test which uses protein A producing staphylococci with rabbit antigonococcal antibodies bound to the protein. On mixing this reagent—which is available commercially as the Phadebact gonococcus test—with a suspension of gonococci, a readily visible agglutination is produced. This reaction is compared with a control in which the staphylococci have not been coated with specific antibodies. Experience is necessary to interpret some of the results (Barnham & Glynn 1978).

Enzyme immunoassay

A solid phase enzyme immunoassay has been the subject of a number of reports (Danielsson et al 1983; Hofman & Petzold 1983; Lind et al 1985). This technique, Gonozyme, developed by Abbot, is only suitable for the detection of antigen in sam-

ples of genital secretion. Though giving satisfactory results in high risk groups of men, its predictive values in women are unsatisfactory and at present it appears to be no substitute for culture in women.

Sensitivity tests

Antimicrobial sensitivity tests, especially for penicillin, are important in planning treatment in each locality, for epidemiological purposes, and in individual patients in whom the infection recurs and in whom treatment failure appears to be the cause. For the gonococcus the agar dilution technique is to be preferred to the disc diffusion method, although the latter is simpler.

Most isolates are still sensitive to penicillin though the proportion of relatively insensitive strains, usually now regarded as those requiring 0.125 μg penicillin or more per ml for inhibition, varies in different parts of the world. The proportion and the actual minimum inhibitory concentration (MIC) is higher in the Far East than in most other parts of the world. This problem will be considered further in the section on treatment.

Detection of penicillinase-producing gonococci

In 1976, the first isolate which produced penicillinase was reported in London (Phillips 1976). Since then the number of these isolates has increased dramatically in many places. All isolates with an MIC to penicillin of 0.125 μg/ml penicillin or higher should be tested for penicillinase production. Various techniques are available (WHO 1978); one of them depends upon the hydrolysis by penicillinase of the lactam bond of a chromogenic cephalosporin substrate producing a coloured product which can be readily recognized (O'Callaghan et al 1972). The test can be applied to colonies on a plate or to a suspension of organisms.

Serological tests

At present there is no serological test with sufficient sensitivity or specificity for the diagnosis of individual patients with gonorrhoea.

Infectivity

Gonorrhoea is generally regarded as being a highly infectious disease spread by genital contact. However, hard data are lacking. In a study of female contacts of men with urethral gonorrhoea Thin et al (1971) diagnosed gonorrhoea in 90% of the women after multiple examinations and sets of investigations. Subsequent studies failed to support this. Six years later at the same centre in London, Barlow et al (1976) diagnosed gonorrhoea in only 66% of 250 female contacts. This figure is supported by a case control study at another centre in London (Thin et al 1979) in which gonorrhoea was found in both partners in 64% of couples. No such data are available yet for other forms of contact such as orogenital or penoanal.

UNCOMPLICATED GONORRHOEA IN WOMEN

The gonococcus invades columnar epithelium, and the common sites of infection in the adult female are the lower cervical canal, the urethra and the rectum. Many women with uncomplicated gonorrhoea are symptom-free, but the actual proportion varies with the population under study. Thus few women attending a casualty or emergency department are asymptomatic, while many women attending a sexually transmitted disease clinic with a good contact tracing service will be symptom-free. Perhaps the overall figure is around 50% (King et al 1980). An added complication is the presence of concurrent trichomoniasis which may be the cause of the symptoms.

Incubation period

The incubation period of uncomplicated gonorrhoea in women is not clear. In contrast, in men with urethritis it is usually said to be 1 to 5 days but it may extend up to 31 days with a mean of 13.6 days (Barlow 1986).

Clinical features

Endocervicitis

Endocervicitis often produces no symptoms or signs. A profuse cervical discharge may be sufficient to lead to the complaint of vaginal discharge. There may be no change in the cervical secretion, but examination may show increased clear mucus,

cloudy mucus or a mucopurulent discharge. Occasionally there is lower abdominal discomfort or low backache. The cervical os may look normal or there may be reddening around the lips of the os or cervical ectopy, though this may have no relation to the gonorrhoea.

Urethritis

Urethritis may produce dysuria, namely a complaint of burning or scalding on micturition without a sensation of obstruction. Women only very occasionally notice a discharge from the urethra.

On examination, after cleaning the vulva, there is usually no abnormality of the urethral meatus. A purulent discharge and redness of the vulva are rare. Occasionally, when the appearances are normal, it may be possible to massage a mucopurulent discharge down the urethra with a gloved finger inserted into the vagina.

Rectal infections

Infections of the rectum may arise as a result of penoanal intercourse. More often they probably arise during defaecation; infected secretion on the vulva may flow back over the everted anal canal, or may be carried back by toilet paper immediately afterwards. Rectal infections may be more likely in those with a profuse discharge. There are usually no symptoms, but a few patients complain of pain or discomfort on defaecation or a rectal discharge. On examination with a proctoscope there is usually no abnormality to be seen; occasionally there is marked redness of the rectal mucosa and mucopus or a purulent discharge. If ulceration is present then other causes should be sought, such as primary syphilis or herpes simplex infection.

Diagnosis of uncomplicated gonorrhoea in women

The clinical features of gonorrhoea in the female, as in the male, are unreliable and this disease requires microbiological investigations for diagnosis. Careful collection of samples for the investigations is vital.

As indicated above, a bivalve Cusco speculum should be inserted into the vagina. It is usual to collect samples of vaginal secretion first, as outlined in Chapter 5. The cervix is then wiped clear of vaginal secretion and a sterile loop or swab is passed directly into the os without touching the vaginal walls. A smear for Gram staining is then made and a culture inoculated (see above). Other cervical investigations are then undertaken, such as a swab for chlamydia culture and a smear for Papanicolaou staining.

The speculum is then withdrawn, running the tip along the anterior vaginal wall to message any urethral exudate towards the meatus. This is then collected with a loop or swab, a smear made and culture inoculated as above.

Opinion seems divided about the need, desirability, or acceptability to the patient of passing a proctoscope. The writer considers it an important part of the examination of a site potentially infected by the gonococcus and other sexually transmissable agents. It is essential if anal lesions such as warts are present. Most patients agree to the procedure if it is explained and undertaken sympathetically. Lubricate the proctoscope with a small amount of jelly and pass in the direction of the anal canal and then the rectum. Note the appearance of the mucosa, any exudate or other lesions, collect any infected secretion for Gram stain and culture. If no secretion is visible sweep the swab or loop around the mucosa to collect as much material as possible.

Gram staining of genital and rectal secretions remains the only widely accepted routine technique for rapid presumptive diagnosis in the clinic. Even when samples are collected from urethra, cervix and rectum, the Gram stains will only give positive results in 55 to 65% of women with gonorrhoea (Young 1981). Thus, cultural diagnosis is most important.

Cervical culture should give positive results in at least 80% of cases. In a large series, positive results from the cervix were reported in 85% of cases (Barlow & Phillips 1978). The urethral culture gives positive results less often; Barlow & Phillips (1978) reported positive urethral culture results in 76% of cases but Thin & Shaw (1979) found only 56% of urethral cultures positive. Rectal cultures are probably positive in about 40% of cases, but the rectum is the only positive site in 5 to 10% of cases—hence it is important to examine this site.

No significant differences were reported between direct plating and Stuart's transport medium in which swabs were left for a maximum of 19 hours (Thin & Shaw 1979). This finding applied to urethral, cervical, and rectal specimens collected through a proctoscope. When material was collected by passing a swab directly up the anal canal, results using Stuart's medium were inferior to those obtained by direct plating (Thin & Shaw 1979). Another study (Bhattacharyya & Jephcott 1974) in women also found direct anal swabs gave fewer positive results than proctoscopically obtained rectal samples when both were inoculated into Stuart's medium. In contrast, in a study of rectal gonorrhoea in men, similar results were obtained from anal swabs and rectal swabs when both were directly plated (Deheragoda 1977). Other studies have shown greater losses as reviewed by Adler (1985).

Investigation of female contacts of men with gonorrhoea

One examination and investigation by means of Gram stain and culture from urethra, cervix and rectum should provide positive results in up to 97% of cases (Adler 1985). It is common practice to re-examine and investigate contacts with negative results to their first investigations, and up to 99% of women may be diagnosed by two such examinations (Barlow et al 1976). Most specialists, especially any supported by laboratories giving less satisfactory results, examine and investigate contacts a third time, as recommended by Chipperfield & Catterall (1976).

LOCAL COMPLICATIONS OF GENITAL GONORRHOEA

Infection may spread to any structure lined by columnar epithelium and communicating with the uncomplicated infection. Sites for local complications include:

Skene's glands;
Bartholin's glands;
Pelvic organs;
Bladder and vulva.

Skenitis

The two little paraurethral glands of Skene lie on each side of the terminal urethra and their ducts open into or beside the urethral meatus. They are rarely infected but when this does happen pus may be seen exuding from the duct. Occasionally the duct becomes blocked and a small paraurethral abscess may develop, presenting as a swelling in the lower anterior vaginal wall.

In all cases the routine investigations for gonococci must be undertaken, plus a Gram stain and culture of any secretion exuding from the paraurethral duct.

Occasionally the infection may become chronic when it presents as a persistent, less tender paraurethral swelling.

Bartholinitis

Bartholin's glands lie in the lower half of each labium major and their ducts open on the inner surface of each labium minor, often around the junction of the lower and middle third. The glands become infected via the duct which often becomes blocked and an abscess forms. The patient complains of pain and swelling. On examination there is swelling of the lower half of the affected labium major and in the acute stage there is overlying redness. There is often surrounding oedema but the actual abscess may be confirmed by gentle palpation when a little pus may exude from the duct. If severe, acute, and neglected, the abscess may discharge through the inner aspect of the labium minor or occasionally anteriorly through the labium major.

If neglected, chronic or recurrent, bartholinitis may progress to form a cyst.

In all cases secretion for Gram stain and culture must be collected from the cervix, urethra and rectum, and any pus exuding from the ducts must also be collected.

Pelvic infection: pelvic inflammatory disease

The most important local complication of gonorrhoea in the female is upward spread to the fallopian tubes (salpingitis) and onward to involve other pelvic structures—pelvic infection or pelvic inflammatory disease (PID). The spread probably occurs up the cervical canal through the uterus into the fallopian tubes. The condition is usually bilateral. The diagnosis is difficult to establish clinically and where facilities are available laparoscopy should be considered in all suspected cases. When

this procedure is undertaken cultures should be taken from the pelvis (in addition to the usual genital and rectal cultures). However, in many centres laparoscopy is not possible. PID probably occurs in about 10% of cases of genital gonorrhoea in west European societies (Rees & Annels 1969) but may be more prevalent in some areas of the world, such as parts of Africa (Osoba 1981). The condition may recur in 40% of women who have a subsequent episode of genital gonorrhoea. Endometritis may form part of the syndrome.

PID may be caused by various micro-organisms. *Chlamydia trachomatis* now causes more cases than *N. gonorrhoeae* and the two may coexist. Anaerobic organisms are also important, especially in the USA (Mardh 1984). There is evidence that the incidence of the condition is rising (CDSC 1983). Some cases follow parturition, abortion—both spontaneous and induced—and other gynaecological procedures. PID is more common in women fitted with an intrauterine contraceptive device and may be less common in women taking oral contraceptives than in women not using these methods (Weström et al 1976).

Onset is often during or shortly after a menstrual period. This is said to be the first or second period after infection (WHO 1978), or soon after infection, because the seasonal incidence is similar to the seasonal pattern of gonorrhoea in men (Thompson 1981). However, it has also been noted that 20 to 60% of partners of women with gonococcal PID have asymptomatic urethral gonorrhoea (Polterat & King 1981), suggesting that the latent period between uncomplicated infection and gonorrhoea may be longer.

Clinical features

The patient usually presents with lower abdominal pain, often described as intermittent, cramping, colicky, or spasmodic. The pain may be central, unilateral or bilateral. She may also have deep dyspareunia. There is often malaise, fever and if the pain is severe, nausea and vomiting. Many women, including those taking oral contraceptives, have menstrual changes; these changes include pain and increased, irregular and prolonged bleeding.

On examination there may be localised tenderness in one or both iliac fossae. In severe cases there may be rigidity of the lower abdominal wall. Signs of generalised peritonitis are rare but there may be tenderness over the lower hepatic border due to associated perihepatitis which may be more common than hitherto recognised. On bimanual pelvic examination there is tenderness in one or both lateral fornices; when bilateral it is usually more marked on one side than the other. When the patient has salpingitis no mass may be palpable but if a pyosalpinx, infection of the parametrium—often postpartum—or a pelvic abscess have formed, then a lateral pelvic mass may be felt. Sometimes an ovary may be involved in a larger abscess when a so-called tubo-ovarian abscess forms. A pelvic abscess may also develop in the pouch of Douglas, producing a tender boggy mass in the posterior fornix. The development of an abscess may suggest a mixed infection (Thompson 1981).

Careful studies of women with PID proven by culdoscopic or laparoscopic examination have shown many atypical features (Thompson 1981). There may be no symptoms or signs, vague lower abdominal discomfort, mild menstrual disturbance, or merely mild pelvic tenderness.

Gram stains and cultures must be taken from the urethra, cervix and rectum in the usual manner. If there is any doubt about the diagnosis, laparoscopy should be considered and pelvic cultures taken. Genital and rectal cultures, even cervical cultures, are not reliable indicators of gonococcal PID; pelvic cultures are preferable whenever possible. A culture should also be taken from the cervix for *Chlamydia trachomatis* and it is worthwhile taking blood for antichlamydial microimmunofluorescent antibodies if this test is available (Treharne et al 1979). An ultrasonic scan may help to delineate and differentiate a pelvic abscess from other causes of pelvic mass. The temperature, white cell count and erythrocyte sedimentation rate may be raised but results are unreliable.

Differential diagnosis

A gonococcal pelvic abscess must be differentiated as far as possible by microbiological investigation from a pelvic abscess due to other organisms and mixed infections are probably common. An abscess most also be differentiated from ectopic pregnancy, septic abortion, and torsion or rupture of an ovarian cyst.

Pelvic infection without a mass must be differentiated from urinary infection and bowel disorders. Some women fitted with an intrauterine contraceptive device complain of pain similar to that of PID.

Chronic pelvic inflammatory disease

As already noted, acute PID can recur and become chronic. This can become a major problem for some women with pain, dysmenorrhoea, menorrhagia and menstrual irregularity. There can be malaise, anaemia and depression. Subfertility and infertility may follow and gonococcal PID is a major factor in reproductive failure in some areas, especially in Africa (Osoba, 1981). After PID a patient is more likely to have a tubal pregnancy than a woman who has never had PID (Thompson 1981).

While not a complication of gonorrhoea itself, it is important to remember the common association between gonorrhoea and chlamydial infection; this may explain the poor response to antigonococcal therapy.

Bladder involvement

Infection may occasionally spread up the urethra and invade the trigone of the bladder, producing frequency and increased burning on micturition. Severe cystitis and upper urinary infection are extremely rare.

Vulvitis

Vulvitis due to gonorrhoea in adult women is rare.

GENERALISED COMPLICATIONS OF GONORRHOEA

These take various forms, of which today a relatively benign bacteraemia may be the most common. In the preantibiotic era a more severe septicaemia occurred with endocarditis from which myocarditis, pericarditis and meningitis followed. Acute septic monoarthritis also used to be commonly due to the gonococcus. Gonococcal perihepatitis, also called the Fitz-Hugh-Curtis syndrome, may be another manifestation of generalised spread.

Disseminated gonococcal infection

This form of spread, the bacteraemic form, is characterised by fever, joint pains and a rash. There is evidence that the strains which cause this spread have particular biological characteristics, including marked sensitivity to penicillin, particular nutritional requirements and resistance to the complement mediated antibacterial activity of normal human serum (WHO 1978). It must not be assumed that all causative strains will be sensitive to penicillin. In addition to bacterial dissemination, immune complexes may have a part in the pathogenesis of this condition (Lancet 1984).

It has been suggested that gonococci may disseminate in 1% of cases. Clinical bacteraemia is more common in women than in men, especially in women whose male partners have asymptomatic urethral gonorrhoea (Holmes et al 1976). Pregnancy, particularly during the second half, is a common pre-existing factor, and in non-pregnant women the condition commonly starts during or just after menstruation (Keiser et al 1968).

Clinical features

The fever is variable and often mild. Joint pains tend to be additive but are sometimes migratory as in rheumatic fever; the commonly affected joints include wrists, knees, ankles, elbows and small joints of the hands. There may be associated tenosynovitis. A small effusion and slight overlying erythema may develop but the joints do not have the appearance of acute septic arthritis. Skin lesions may be macular, papular, vesicular, pustular, haemorrhagic or have central necrosis. More than one type may be present and haemorrhagic pustules with an unusually wide surrounding erythematous 'flare' are common. The lesions may appear in crops in association with fever, are sparse, 1 to 12 in number, are usually on the limbs overlying joints but not necessarily the affected joints; they may be near tenosynovitis (Thompson 1981).

The findings in one prospective study of 49 patients suggest that there may be two forms of disseminated infection—one with suppurative arthritis and negative blood cultures, the other with tenosynovitis and skin lesions (see Lancet 1984).

Because of the variety of the features and lack of genital symptoms, patients may present to general practitioners, casualty officers, general physicians, rheumatologists or dermatologists as well as venereologists or genitourinary physicians. It is important for all concerned to realise that the diagnosis may be suspected from the clinical picture but can only be established by microbiological investigation. The usual Gram stains and cultures must be taken from the urethra, cervix and rectum, and a pharyngeal culture must be collected from all suspected cases, for in some patients this is the only site to yield a positive result (Holmes et al 1976). The gonococcus may be readily identified in specimens taken from these sites. Blood cultures, material from skin lesions and aspirated synovial fluid should all be examined for gonococci but rarely give positive results. The causative strains may be very sensitive to penicillin and other antimicrobials, so non-selective as well as selective media should be used in all cases of suspected gonococcal bacteraemia.

Endocarditis and meningitis are now rarely reported.

Differential diagnosis

Differentiate this condition from meningococcal bacteraemia, *Moraxella* septicaemia and mild staphylococcal septicaemia.

Mild gonococcal bacteraemia may progress to septicaemia, so manage all cases energetically.

Gonococcal septic monoarthritis

The gonococcus may still be a common cause of septic arthritis in young adults in a few parts of the world (Thompson 1981) and may follow untreated bacteraemia. The knee is the most commonly affected joint, but any large joint can become infected. The clinical picture is that of acute septic arthritis and the only clinical clue to the cause is the occasional presence of tenosynovitis. Synovial fluid should always be aspirated and examined by Gram stain and culture. Blood cultures should also be taken and whenever gonorrhoea is suspected genital, rectal and pharyngeal investigations must be undertaken.

Gonococcal periphepatitis (Fitz-Hugh Curtis syndrome)

Gonococci may spread directly from the pelvis to the perihepatic area along the paracolic gutters, via the lymphatics, or in the bloodstream.

The clinical features may be mild with little or no upper abdominal pain and slight hepatic tenderness, or severe with sudden onset of upper right abdominal pain, or pain in the right shoulder increased by deep inspiration, coughing or flexion of the trunk. There may be fever, nausea and vomiting, and on examination rigidity of the upper right abdominal wall and marked tenderness. There may be features of PID, but in a female with no genital symptoms the true diagnosis may not be recognised.

Routine microbiological investigations must be done. Peritoneoscopy will show perihepatitis and so-called violin string adhesions may be seen between the surface of the liver and the anterior abdominal wall and diaphragm. Other investigations are usually unhelpful.

Gonococcal perihepatitis must be distinguished from chlamydial perihepatitis by culture and circulating antichlamydial antibodies, hepatitis due to other causes such as hepatitis B virus, cholecystitis, peptic ulceration, subphrenic abscess, pyelonephritis, and renal calculus.

Gonococcal ophthalmia

Gonococci are occasionally carried to the eye via the fingers when they will produce a conjunctivitis, which if neglected may spread back into the eye. The diagnosis can only be established by Gram stain and culture of the exudate.

GONORRHOEA IN CHILDREN

Genital gonorrhoea is rare in children and occurs more often in girls than in boys.

Genital gonorrhoea

In prepubertal girls the immature vulval and vaginal epithelium is susceptible to the gonococcus. Vulvovaginal infection may occur in families where a parent is infected, there is poor hygiene and over-crowding, and especially where a girl shares a bed with an infected adult. There may be symptoms of vulvovaginitis such as irritation, dysuria, or a discharge. On examination the vulval and vaginal epithelium may be reddened and there may be a purulent discharge. Alternatively, there may be no symptoms or signs.

Secretion for Gram stain and culture should be taken from the urethral meatus and directly from the vagina without the use of a speculum.

Gonococcal vulvovaginitis must be differentiated from other causes, including poor hygiene and threadworms.

Urethral gonorrhoea may also be present in boys, and in all children sexual abuse must be considered when gonorrhoea is diagnosed.

Gonococcal ophthalmia neonatorum

Theoretically this is a preventable disease, for diagnosis and treatment of gonorrhoea in the mother during pregnancy should minimise the possibility of infection of the baby during parturition. However, it is impracticable to screen all pregnant women. In some areas screening has produced worthwhile results but on the whole in Britain the positive findings have been minimal (Lancet 1984). Pregnant women who are likely to have gonorrhoea include unmarried women, women with vaginal discharge, unco-operative women, and women receiving social security benefits (Schofield 1969). In Nigeria 17% of pregnant women were reported to have gonorrhoea by Osoba (1981). Gonococcal ophthalmia neonatorum was found in 1% of East African infants (see Lancet 1984). Guidelines for selective screening can be established by consultation between venereologist, obstetrician, paediatrician and microbiologist.

The incubation period for gonococcal ophthalmia is commonly regarded as being a few days but it may be as long as 30 days (Schofield & Shanks 1971). The condition is commonly bilateral. The conjunctivae redden, the lids may swell and become red, pus oozes from the eye and there is photophobia.

The diagnosis is established by taking material for Gram stain and culture for gonococci. Cultures should also be taken for chlamydia and bacterial pathogens.

It is important to investigate the mother and undertake contact tracing. The principal complication is spread of infection into the eye which may cause its destruction. Other sites, such as the pharynx, may also be infected and it is important to give systemic therapy to ensure cure.

Perinatal gonococcal infection

Gonorrhoea may also be associated with premature rupture of the membranes, prolonged labour, premature delivery, postpartum fever, and orogastric contamination of the newborn which may be associated with signs of sepsis, including pneumonia and meningitis. In some places this may be more common than gonococcal eye infection. Cervical culture at the 36th week of pregnancy may prevent this problem (Holmes et al 1976).

TREATMENT OF GONORRHOEA

The golden rule in clinical management of any disease is diagnosis before treatment. Gonorrhoea is a bacteriological diagnosis depending on results of Gram stains and cultures. The few exceptions to this rule include patients who are known to be contacts of gonorrhoea, whose Gram stain results are negative but in whom there is no time to wait for the results of cultures. Such cases include pregnant women about to deliver, travellers about to depart, and patients known to be promiscuous unreliable attenders. With these few exceptions, this section concerns patients in whom the diagnosis has been bacteriologically established. No further consideration will be given to abortive or epidemiological antigonococcal treatment. Antitreponemal antimicrobials should be avoided when treponemal disease is suspected but not proven, and the place of antigonococcal therapy in aborting incubating treponemal disease will not be considered.

In addition to antimicrobial therapy, the management of a patient with gonorrhoea involves contact action and follow-up after treatment. While the recommendation in the USA is to see the patients once 3–7 days after treatment (USPHS 1985), the practice in Britain is to examine patients more frequently. A good routine is to see each patient 1–3 days, 7 days and 14 days after treatment.

At each visit a Gram stain and culture should be taken from each previously infected site. A common practice is to take specimens from the urethral meatus and cervical os at each visit, but only to repeat rectal investigations if they were positive before treatment. It is good practice to take one rectal culture after treatment if this was omitted beforehand or was negative (USPHS 1985).

General measures

Patients should be advised to refrain from intercourse until bacteriological cure has been established. A time honoured practice is to advise abstention from alcohol. There are no controlled studies to establish the value of this advice but alcohol does stimulate mucus secretion via the autonomic system and this is contrary to the principle of rest which aids healing. Furthermore, alcohol leads to release of cortical inhibitors and clouds the memory, so advice to avoid intercourse may not be followed.

Treatment of uncomplicated rectogenital gonorrhoea in adults

It has been known for many years that uncomplicated rectogenital gonorrhoea responds rapidly to antimicrobial threapy. In men with urethral gonorrhoea symptomatic response to therapy starts within 24 hours and is usually complete within 3 days (Holmes et al 1967). Negative results are obtained to cultures taken from the urethra 5 to 9 hours after a single dose of procaine penicillin (plus probenecid in some cases: Holmes et al 1967; Rajan et al 1978). In one of the first reports of partial penicillin resistance (Cradock Watson et al 1958), it was noted that patients harbouring gonococci with an MIC to penicillin of 0.125 u/ml or more had a failure rate five times higher than that among patients infected with more sensitive strains. This form of penicillin resistance is now frequently described as partial resistance or diminished sensitivity.

Partial penicillin resistance is due to mutation of chromosomal genes and tends to be associated with partial resistance to other antimicrobials such as tetracycline, chloramphenicol, erythromycin, streptomycin and rifampicin. Resistance to spectinomycin, certain cephalosporins (including

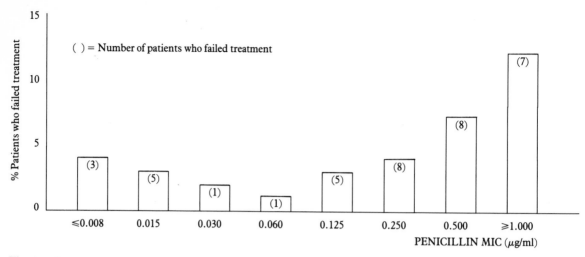

Fig. 8.1 Treatment failure rates rise with rising MIC's (Adapted from Jaffe et al 1976).

Table 8.1 Variation in partial penicillin resistance

Authors	Year	Location	No. of strains	% Partial resistance	MIC (mg/l)
Phillips et al	1976	London	264	30	0.125
Farthing et al	1985	London	558	62	0.12
Chitwarakorn et al	1985	Thailand	357	96	0.125
Sng et al	1984	Singapore	300	95	0.125

MIC = minimum inhibitory concentration.
For further details see Osoba (1981) and Sng et al (1984).

cefuroxime and cefoxitin and cefotaxime) and co-trimoxazole does not usually accompany partial resistance to penicillin.

The proportion of strains of gonococci showing partial resistance varies with time and place (Table 8.1). In 1969 in London, 35% of strains were reported to be partially resistent to penicillin (Phillips et al 1976), but has recently risen to 62% (Farthing et al 1985); much higher proportions have been reported from Africa and the Far East (Table 8.1). Areas with high percentages of partial resistance tend to have higher degrees of partial resistance. Treatment failure rate tends to rise with rising MICs, as shown in Figure 8.1.

In 1976 penicillinase (β-lactamase) producing gonococci were reported for the first time (Ashford et al 1976; Phillips 1976) and have since been found in many parts of the world (Siegel et al 1978), but far fewer strains with this form of resistance have been reported than with partial penicillin resistance. β-lactamase production is due to the presence of extrachromosomal plasmid-borne genes. Two such plasmids have been described (Perine et al 1977), one arising in the Far East and the other in Africa; it appears they may be transferred from other organisms such as coliforms or may arise by mutation. Like chromosomal mutation, these mutations tend to arise in the presence of low antimicrobial concentrations. Some isolates have a conjugating plasmid which facilitates the transfer of the β-lactamase plasmid. β-lactamase producing strains of gonococci tend to be sensitive to other antimicrobials, including spectinomycin and certain cephalosporins.

Reported β-lactamase producing isolates are still rare in Britain, at 2.2% of total cases (CDSC 1985) but are more common in areas such as the Far East with 40% in Bangkok (Chitwarakorn et al 1985) and 35% in Singapore (Sng et al 1984) while similar figures have been reported from Africa (Piot et al 1985).

In 1981 the first spectinomycin resistant isolate

was reported from the USA (Ashford et al 1981) and a few such isolates have been reported from London (Easman et al 1984). They appear to be more common in Africa (Piot et al 1985).

In 1983 a new form of total penicillin resistance was reported from the USA, namely chromosomally mediated resistance (Rice et al 1984). This is associated with resistance to other antimicrobials, such as tetracycline, so may prove more of a problem than β-lactamase mediated resistance. So far few isolates have been reported in Britain but more have been found in other countries (Piot et al 1985).

It remains vital to follow patients after treatment to ensure cure and to monitor antimicrobial sensitivity of the gonococcus.

Certain principles of treatment for uncomplicated rectogenital gonorrhoea have now emerged.

1. A single dose of antimicrobial should be given which rapidly achieves an effective concentration in blood and tissues, maintains it for about 9 hours, and then the level should fall rapidly to zero. This will minimise the low levels of antimicrobial which favour mutation and antimicrobial resistance.

2. The drug and dose chosen should be capable of achieving blood levels greater than the MICs of the partially resistant strains in the local gonococcal population for locally acquired infection. When the infection is acquired elsewhere, different treatment may be indicated, based on an estimate of the partial resistance.

3. In the event of treatment failure, there is no point in repeating the same dose of the same drug, or multiple (smaller) doses; these will only tend to promote antibiotic resistance. A larger dose of the same antimicrobial, or a different antimicrobial, should be given. This clinical situation usually arises before the results of invitro sensitivity tests are available. The drug chosen should be effective for partially resistant and β-lactamase producing strains. Spectinomycin, cefuroxime, cefoxitin and cefotaxime are likely to be the most effective.

Choice of first-line treatment

Penicillin is highly effective against sensitive gonococci; it is cheap and relatively non-toxic. Where *β-lactamase* producing strains remain rare, penicillin will be the drug of first choice for the treatment of uncomplicated gonorrhoea, unless the patient appears to be hypersensitive to it.

For many years, an injection of procaine penicillin was regarded as the treatment of choice, but it now appears that probenecid (which blocks the renal excretion of penicillin) should be given with penicillin (Holmes et al 1967; Thin 1974). A survey in the UK (Adler 1978) showed procaine penicillin 1.2 to 2.4 mu with or without probenecid was the most commonly used parenteral preparation. This survey also showed that oral therapy was more widely used, ampicillin in doses up to 3.5 g with or without probenecid being the most common treatment. Ampicillin 2 g plus probenecid 1 g in a single oral dose given under supervision has consistently given a cure rate of 95% or higher (using the 14-day rule described shortly) in the writer's experience over the last 8 years in London. It is generally accepted that treatment of first choice should give a cure rate of at least 95%.

Among the regimes currently recommended in the USA for first-line treatment (USPHS 1985) the following fulfil the criteria outlined:

Aqueous procaine penicillin G 4.8 mu intramuscularly with probenecid 1 g by mouth;
Either ampicillin 3.5 g or amoxycillin 3.0 g with probenecid 1 g.
In addition, WHO (1985) recommend aqueous crystalline pencillin G 5 mu intramuscularly with probenecid 1 g by mouth.

Patients who are hypersensitive to penicillin

Co-trimoxazole (Septrin, Wellcome; Bactrim, Roche) is a useful antimicrobial for the treatment of uncomplicated gonorrhoea in patients who are hypersensitive to penicillin. Cure rates of more than 95% have been reported from Britain with 5 tablets given 12-hourly for three doses and eight dispersible tablets in a single oral dose. Side-effects with this single oral dose are trivial and at present this appears to be the treatment of choice for patients who are hypersensitive to penicillin. An alternative recommended in the USA (USPHS 1985) is spectinomycin 2 g intramuscularly, but this is very much more expensive and is probably better kept for patients failing on treatment of first choice.

An alternative which was widely used at one time was kanamycin sulphate 2 g in a single dose by intramuscular injection. This gave good results; it is potentially ototoxic and nephrotoxic but such effects were extremely rare among the relatively healthy young adults treated for gonorrhoea.

Management of treatment failure

Treatment failure should be distinguished from reinfection whenever possible; there is little virtue in treating reinfection with expensive alternative antimicrobials. One arbitrary rule widely used to distinguish treatment failure from reinfection defined failure as reappearance of gonococci within 14 days of treatment in a patient who denied further sexual intercourse; recurrence in all other circumstances is regarded as reinfection (Evans 1966).

Treatment failure is often diagnosed before in vitro sensitivity results are available; they must be requested whenever there is recurrence. Thus treatment has to be decided from a knowledge of the probable MICs and this depends on knowing the sensitivity pattern in the area where the infection originated. The choice of treatment is likely to be increasing the dose of penicillin, or giving spectinomycin, or a cephalosporin such as cefuroxime, cefoxitin or cefotaxime. One useful routine is to give spectinomycin 2 g intramuscularly; if this fails the dose may increased to spectinomycin 4 g intramuscularly, but it would probably be wiser to change to cefuroxime 1.5 g intramuscularly with probenecid 1 g by mouth, cefoxitin 2 g intramuscularly or cefotaxime 0.5 g intramuscularly (Barlow & Phillips 1984). These regimens are all much more expensive than the first-line treatments advocated. Observation after therapy is especially important in these cases to minimise the spread of resistant strains.

Treatment of uncomplicated gonorrhoea in pregnancy

Treatments of choice in the pregnant woman with gonorrhoea are aqueous crystalline penicllin G, aqueous procaine penicillin G or ampicillin, each with probenecid, or spectinomycin in patients who are hypersensitive to penicillin.

While uncomplicated infections resolve satisfactorily with single dose of treatment, complications require a course of therapy.

Acute local complications of gonorrhoea in the female

Acute skenitis

Usually this resolves with ampicillin 2 g plus probenecid 1 g followed by ampicillin 500 mg plus probenecid 500 mg four times daily for 7 days.

Acute bartholinitis

Antimicrobial therapy is as for acute skenitis and the abscess is aspirated using a wide bore needle inserted into the medial aspect under local anaesthesia. Aspiration may have to be repeated.

If a second episode of acute bartholinitis occurs, antimicrobial therapy and aspiration should be repeated and the patient referred to a gynaecologist for marsupialisation of the gland.

Acute pelvic infection

Antimicrobial therapy should be based on known and possible microbial aetiology. A loading dose of penicillin, such as ampicillin 3.5 g plus probenecid 1 g or cefotaxime 1 g followed by oxytetracycline 500 mg four times daily or doxycycline 100 mg twice daily for 10 days plus metronidazole 400 mg twice a day for 5 to 10 days will cover gonococci, chlamydia and anaerobes (WHO 1985). The patient who is hypersensitive to penicillin may be given co-trimoxazole 8 dispersible tablets (3.8 g) at once followed by 4 tablets (1.9 g) 12-hourly for 2 to 4 days and 2 tablets (960 mg) 12-hourly to complete 10 days.

The management of an intrauterine contraceptive device in acute pelvic infection is not clear. In the writer's experience resolution is satisfactory if the device is left in position, at least in the first attack. The United States Public Health Service (1985) and World Health Organization (1985) recommend its removal after antimicrobial therapy has begun. Once removed, contraceptive counselling is required but very often these are the women who find other methods difficult and are therefore at risk to a tubal pregnancy and further infection.

β-lactamase producing gonococci may cause pelvic infection (and bartholinitis (Siegel et al 1978)). In such cases cefuroxime 1.5 g followed by cefuroxime 0.75 g 8-hourly intramuscularly or cefotaxime 1.0 g 12-hourly intramuscularly may be given until response is satisfactory, when an oral preparation may be given in the light of sensitivity results to complete 10 days of therapy.

Chronic local complications in the female

Chronic local complications in the female are also more likely to be non-gonococcal than gonococcal in origin.

Chronic skenitis

The glands should be destroyed by electrocautery.

Chronic bartholinitis

A cyst or recurrent abscess should be treated by excision or marsupialisation.

Chronic or recurrent pelvic infection

Care should be taken to obtain positive cultures whenever possible and to undertake quantitative sensitivity tests. The appropriate antimicrobial should then be given with a large loading dose as described for acute pelvic infection, and treatment continued for 2 to 4 weeks. Cultures should be taken at intervals and antimicrobial therapy adjusted according to the results of sensitivity tests. King et al (1980) recommend tetracyclines and metronidazole, as the aetiology is likely to be non-gonococcal.

Treatment of disseminated gonococcal infection

Strains of gonococci which cause disseminated gonococcal infection (DGI) apparently remain sensitive to pencillin, but a β-lactamase producing isolate has been implicated as the cause of DGI (Lancet 1984). As sensitivity results are not usually available when treatment starts, it is wise to start antimicrobial therapy as indicated for acute pelvic infection, but it should be continued for 12 to 14 days.

Another regimen which has been reported in the USA is to give crystalline penicillin G 2.5 mu intravenously over a 30-minute period every 6 hours for 3 days. This regimen of intravenous penicillin until improvement occurs with the addition of ampicillin 500 mg 4 times daily to complete 7 days' therapy is also recommended (USPHS 1985). For cases caused by β-lactamase producing organisms, one can give cefotaxime 500 mg 4 times daily intravenously for 7 days (USPHS 1985) although in the writer's experience intramuscular therapy is usually satisfactory.

Treatment of gonorrhoea in children

Ophthalmia neonatorum

This condition is an emergency and treatment should be vigorous. Though in the past penicillin drops were considered to be the main part of therapy it is now realised that systemic penicillin is more important. Give aqueous crystalline penicillin G 200 000 u every 3 or 4 hours for 24 hours. Pencillin eye drops may be given at the same time and continued 4 times daily for 5 days.

β-lactamase producing gonococci may cause gonococcal ophthalmia neonatorum; a case in Singapore responded to kanamycin 1 g intramuscularly and kanamycin eye drops (Pang et al 1979), while twins in London were given cefuroxime 100 mg/kg/day intramuscularly in three divided doses for 7 days (Dunlop et al 1980). Cefotaxime is an acceptable alternative (USPHS 1985).

Gonococcal genital infection in children

Treatment follows the principles already described for adults with the dose reduced according to the weight and age of the child.

Gonococcal vaccines

Though research into gonococcal vaccines has been under way for some time, many problems remain to be overcome before an effective vaccine will be available (WHO 1983).

REFERENCES

Adler M W 1978 Diagnostic treatment and reporting criteria for gonorrhoea in sexually transmitted diseases in England and Wales. 2 Treatment and reporting criteria. British Journal of Venereal Diseases 54: 15–23

Adler M W 1985 Criteria for the diagnosis of sexually transmitted diseases. In: Taylor Robinson D (ed) Clinical problems in sexually transmitted diseases. Martinus Nijhoff, Kluwer, Dordrecht, pp 1–14

Ashford W A, Golash R G, Hemming V G 1976 Penicillinase producing Neisseria gonorrhoeae. Lancet ii: 657–658

Ashford W A, Potts D W, Adams H J U et al 1981 Spectinomycin resistant penicillinase producing Neisseria gonorrhoeae Lancet ii: 1035–1037

Barlow D 1986 The carrier state: Neisseria gonorrhea. Journal of Antimicrobial Chemotherapy 18 (Suppl A): 73–79

Barlow D, Phillips I 1978 Gonorrhoea in women. Diagnostic, clinical and laboratory aspects. Lancet i: 761–764

Barlow D, Phillips I 1984 Cefotaxime in the treatment of gonorrhoea caused by β-lactamase producing Neisseria gonorrhoeae. Journal of Antimicrobial Chemotherapy 14 (suppl B): 291–293

Barlow D, Nayyar K, Phillips I, Barrow J 1976 Diagnosis of gonorrhoea in women. British Journal of Venereal Diseases 52: 326–328

Barnham M, Glynn A A 1978 Identification of clinical isolates of Neisseria gonorrhoeae by a coagglutination test. Journal of Clinical Pathology 31: 189–193

Bhattacharyya M N, Jephcott A E 1974 Diagnosis of gonorrhoea in women. Role of the rectal sample. British Journal of Venereal Diseases 50: 109–112

Chipperfield E J, Catterall R D 1976 Re-appraisal of Gram staining and cultural techniques in the diagnosis of gonorrhoea in women. British Journal of Venereal Diseases 52: 36–39

Chitwarakorn A, Ariyarit C, Panikabutra et al 1985 Treating gonococcal infections resistant to penicillin in Bangkok. Genitourinary Medicine 61: 306–310

Cradock Watson J E, Shooter R A, Nicol C S 1958 Sensitivity of strains of gonococci to penicillin, sulphamethiazole and streptomycin. British Medical Journal 1: 1091–1092

Communicable Diseases Surveillance Centre 1983 Sexually transmitted diseases surveillance in Britain 1981. British Medical Journal 286: 1500–1502

Communicable Diseases Surveillance Centre 1985 Sexually transmitted diseases surveillance in Britain 1985. British Medical Journal 291: 528–530

Danielsson D, Moi H, Forslin L 1983 Diagnosis of urogenital gonorrhoea with a solid phase enzyme immunoassay (Gonozyme). Journal of Clinical Pathology 36: 674–677

Deheragoda P 1977 Diagnosis of rectal gonorrhoea by blind anorectal swabs compared with direct vision swabs taken via a proctoscope. British Journal of Venereal Diseases 53: 311–313

Dunlop E M C, Rodin R, Seth A D, Kolator B 1980 Ophthalmia neonatorum due to β-lactamase producing Neisseria gonorrhoeae. British Medical Journal ii: 483

Easman C S F, Forster G E, Walker G D, Ison C A, Harris J R W Munday P E 1984 Spectinomycin as initial treatment for gonorrhoea. British Medical Journal 289: 1032–1034

Evans A J 1966 Relapse of gonorrhoea after treatment with penicillin or streptomycin. British Journal of Venereal Diseases 42: 251–262

Farthing C, Thin R N T, Smith S, Phillips I 1985 Two regimens of sulfamicillin in treating uncomplicated gonorrhea. Genito-

urinary medicine 61: 44–47

Flynn J, Waitkins S A 1972 A serum free medium for testing fermentation reactions in Neisseria gonorrhoeae. Journal of Clinical Pathology 25: 525–530

Hofman H, Petzold D 1983 Clinical evaluation of solid phase enzyme immunoassay for detection of N. gonorrhoeae antigen. European Journal of Sexually Transmitted Diseases I: 83–87

Holmes K K, Johnson D W, Floyd T M 1967 Studies of venereal disease. Probenecid—procaine penicillin G combination and tetracycline hydrochloride in the treatment of penicillin resistant gonorrhoea in men. Journal of American Medical Association 202: 461–473

Holmes K K, Counts G W Beatty H N 1971 Disseminated gonococcal infection. Archives of Internal Medicine 74: 979–985

Holmes K K, Eschenbach D A, Knapp J S 1976 Clinical epidemiology and change in clinical manifestations of gonococcal infections. In: Catterall R D, Nicol C S (eds) Sexually transmitted diseases. Academic Press, London, pp. 74–76

Jaffe H W, Biddle J W, Thornsberry C, Johnson R E, Kaufman R E, Reynolds G, Weisner P J 1976 National gonorrhea therapy monitoring study. New England Journal of Medicine 294: 5–9

Jephcott A E, Reyn A 1971 Neisseria gonorrhoeae colony variation. Acta Pathologica et Microbiologica Scandinavica 79: 609–613

Keiser H, Ruben F, Wolinsky E, Kushner I 1968 Clinical forms of gonococcal arthritis. New England Journal of Medicine 279: 234–241

Kellog D S, Peacock W E, Brown L, Pirkle C L 1963 Neisseria gonorrhoeae l. Virulence linked to colonial morphology. Journal of Bacteriology 85: 1274–1279

King A, Nicol C, Rodin P 1980 Venereal diseases. Bailliere Tindall, London

Lancet 1984 Disseminated gonococcal infection. Lancet i: 832–833

Lind L, Berthelsen L, Birkov O, Karlsmark T, Verdich J U, Weisman K 1985 The diagnosis of gonorrhoea by means of the Gonozyme test. European Journal of Sexually Transmitted Diseases 3: 37–42

Mardh P -A 1984 Microbial etiology of pelvic inflammatory disease. Sexually Transmitted Diseases 11: 428–429

Martin J E, Jackson R L 1975 Biological environmental chamber for the culture of Neisseria gonorrhoeae Journal of the American Venereal Diseases Association 2: 28–30

Martin J E, Lester A 1971 Transgrow; a medium for transport and growth of Neisseria gonorrhoeae and Neisseria meningitidis. Health Services and Mental Health Administration Report 86: 30–33

O'Callaghan C H, Morris A, Kirby S, Shingler A H 1972 Novel method for detection of β-lactamases by using a chromogenic cephalosporin substrate. Antimicrobial Agents and Chemotherapy 1: 283–288

Osoba A O 1981 Sexually transmitted diseases in tropical Africa; a review of the present situation. British Journal of Venereal Diseases 57: 89–94

Pang R, Teh L B, Rajan V S, Sng E H 1979 Gonococcal ophthalmia neonatorum caused by β-lactamase producing Neisseria gonorrhoeae. British Medical Journal 1: 380

Panikabutra K, Suvanmalik S 1973 Sensitivity to penicillin of Neisseria gonorrhoeae in Bangkok. British Journal of Venereal Diseases 49: 209–212

Perine P L, Thornsberry C, Schalla W et al Evidence for two

distinct types of penicillinase producing Neisseria gonorrhoeae. Lancet ii: 993–995

Phillips I 1976 β-lactamase producing penicillin resistant gonococcus. Lancet ii: 656–657

Phillips I, Humphrey D, Middleton A, Nicol C S 1972 Diagnosis of gonorrhoea by culture on a selective medium containing vancomycin, colistin, nystatin and trimethoprim (VCNT). British Journal of Venereal Diseases 48: 287–292

Phillips I, King A, Warren C, Watts B 1976 The activity of penicillin and eight cephalosporins on Neisseria gonorrhoeae. Journal of Antimicrobial Chemotherapy 2: 31–37

Piot P, Van Dyck E, Bogaerts J et al 1985 Susceptibility of N. gonorrhoeae to spectinomycin. Abstract WS-24-3, 14th International Congress of Chemotherapy, Kyoto

Polterat J J, King R D 1981 A new approach to gonorrhoea control. The asymptomatic man and incidence reduction. Journal of the American Medical Association 245: 578–580

Rajan V S, Pang R, Sng E H 1978 Inactivation of gonococci by procaine penicillin in vivo. British Journal of Venereal Diseases 54: 398–399

Rees E, Annels E H 1969 Gonococcal salpingitis. British Journal of Venereal Diseases 45: 205–215

Rice R R, Blount J H, Biddle J W, Jean Louis Y, Morse S A 1984 Changing trends in gonococcal antibiotic resistance in the United States 1983–1984. Morbidity and Mortality Weekly Report 33: 11SS–15SS

Schofield C B S 1969 Medicosocial background to gonococcal ophthalmia neonatorum. Lancet ii: 1102–1104

Schofield C B S, Shanks R A 1971 Gonococcal ophthalmia neonatorum despite treatment with antibacterial eye drops. British Medical Journal i: 257–259

Siegel M S, Perine P L, Westbrook W G, deJesus I 1978 Epidemiology of penicillinase producing Neisseria gonorrhoeae. In: Brooks G F, Gotslich E C, Holmes K K, Sawyer W D, Young F E (eds) Immunobiology of Neisseria gonorrhoeae. American Society for Microbiology, Washington D C, pp. 75–79

Siegel M S, Thornsberry C, Biddle J W, O'Mara P R, Perine P L, Weisner P J 1978 Penicillinase producing Neisseria gonorrhoeae; results of surveillance in the United States. Journal of Infectious Diseases 137: 170–175

Sng E H, Lim A L, Yeo K L 1984 Susceptibility to antimicrobials of N. gonorrhoeae isolated in Singapore; implications on the need for more effective treatment regimens and control strategies. British Journal of Venereal Diseases 60: 374–379

Thayer J D, Martin J E 1966 Improved selective medium for cultivation of N. gonorrhoeae and N. meningitidis. Public Health Report (Washington) 81: 559–562

Thin R N T 1970 Immunofluorescent method for diagnosis of gonorrhoea in women. British Journal of Venereal Diseases 46: 27–30

Thin R N 1974 Penicillin treatment of gonorrhoea in Edinburgh British Journal of Venereal Diseases 50: 57–60

Thin R N, Shaw E J 1979 Diagnosis of gonorrhoea in women. British Journal of Venereal Diseases 55: 10–13

Thin R N T, Williams I A, Nicol C S 1971 Direct and delayed methods of immunofluorescent diagnosis of gonorrhoea in women. British Journal of Venereal Diseases 47: 27–30

Thin R N, Rendell P, Wadsworth J 1979 How often are gonorrhoea and genital yeast infection sexually transmitted? British Journal of Venereal Diseases 55: 278–280

Thompson S E 1981 The clinical manifestations of gonococcal infections. In: Harris J R W (ed) Recent advances in sexually transmitted diseases 2. Churchill Livingstone, Edinburgh, pp 52

Treharne J D, Ripa K T, Mardh P -A, Svensson L, Weström L, Darougar S 1979 Antibodies to Chlamydia trachomatis in acute salpingitis. British Journal of Venereal Diseases 55: 26–29

United States Public Health Service 1985 Sexually transmitted disease treatment guidelines. Morbidity and Mortality Weekly Report 34: 755–1005

Weström L, Bengtsson L P, Mardh P -A 1976 The risk of pelvic inflammatory disease in women using intrauterine contraceptive devices as compared to non-users. Lancet ii: 221–224

Willcox R R, John J 1976 Simplified method for the cultural diagnosis of gonorrhoea British Journal of Venereal Diseases 52: 256–258

World Health Organization 1978 Neisseria gonorrhoeae and gonococcal infections. Technical Report Series 616 Geneva

World Health Organization 1983 Development of a gonococcal vaccine WHO/VDT/RES/GON/83.140 Geneva

World Health Organization 1985 Simplified approaches for sexually transmitted diseases control WHO/VDT/85.437 Geneva

Young H 1981 Advances in routine laboratory procedures for the diagnosis of gonorrhoea. In: Harris J R W (ed) Recent Advances in Sexually Transmitted Diseases 2. Churchill Livingstone, Edinburgh, p. 69

Young H, Paterson I C, McDonald D R 1976 Rapid carbohydrate utilisation test for the identification of Neisseria gonorrhoeae. British Journal of Venereal Diseases 52: 172–175

Trichomoniasis
M J Hare

INTRODUCTION

The trichomonads are flagellated protozoa, which are found in a wide range of animals, birds, reptiles, fish and some invertebrates. Although many members of the family are harmless commensals, some are pathogenic, and amongst these are found *Tritrichomonas foetus*, which cases a serious infection of cattle giving rise to infertility and abortion, and *Trichomonas gallinae* which causes a fungating infection in the digestive system of birds which is often fatal. The members of the group which occur in man are *Trichomonas vaginalis*, *T. tenax* and *Pentatrichomonas hominis*. The incidence of the last two has not been investigated in the United Kingdom; however reports from elsewhere suggest that the incidence is low and that they are non-pathogenic.

T. vaginalis was first described by Alfred Donné in 1836, the event being recorded in a preliminary publication addressed to the Academy of Sciences in Paris entitled 'Animalcules observés dans les matiéres purulentes et le produit des sécrétions des organes génitaux de l'homme et de la femme'. He gave the organism the name *Trichomonas* because of its similarities to two other protozoa, *Trichodes* and *Monas* (Thorburn 1974). In 1838 Ehrenberg added the specific *vaginalis*, recognising the vagina as the organism's normal habitat.

MORPHOLOGY (Low 1978)

T. vaginalis is a pyriform organism, ranging in length from 7 μm to 25 μm with an average of 13 μm. Giant and dwarf forms may occur. The nucleus is anterior, and lies under the fibrillar apparatus or blepharoplast. From this organelle emerge:

1. The axostyle, a prominent tubular structure which curves round the nucleus, passes through the cell and protrudes slightly at the posterior end;
2. Four anterior flagella;
3. A posterior flagellum which is attached to the end of the undulating membrane. The posterior flagellum of *T. vaginalis* does *not* extend as a free structure beyond the edge of the undulating membrane, which is a feature found in some other species. Movement of the posterior flagellum controls movement of the undulating membrane, and is the mode of propulsion of the organism.

Investigators disagree on the existence of a cystostome or cell mouth beside the blepharoplast. This seems to play no part in nutrition; trichomonads feed by osmosis and possibly by phagocytosis. They reproduce by longitudinal binary fission and do not form cysts.

For more detailed morphological descriptions and electron microscopic studies the reader is referred to the work of Neilson et al (1966) and of Ovcinnikov et al (1975). For laboratory study *T. vaginalis* may be kept in any standard culture medium; long term storage should be in liquid nitrogen (Walsey & Rayner 1970).

METHODS OF DETECTION AND DIAGNOSIS

Wet film examination

A drop of fresh genital exudate which is to be examined for *T. vaginalis* is diluted with normal saline and examined under a coverslip using direct light, dark field illumination or phase contrast microscopy. Active organisms are easily detected by this method, with the organism moving in an irregular fashion and its larger features being readily identified. Coutts & Silva-Inzunza (1965) suggested adding a small quantity of 5% aqueous fluorescein to discharge which need not be diluted; the organisms stain blue-green with their motility unaffected. Such preparations can be fixed by the addition of 10% formalin for later examination.

Stained films

For those who do not have immediate access to a microscope, fixed stained preparations are the easiest diagnostic method. Discharge is collected on a cotton wool swab or a cytology spatula, and spread over a slide. It is then either air-dried or fixed in alcohol depending on the staining method planned. Fixed slides may be transported distances or sent through the post to the laboratory where examination will be performed. Methods that may be used include:

1. Papanicolaou's method, when the primary examination is for premalignant disease of the cervix;
2. Gram's method with safranine counter stain;
3. Fontana's method;
4. Giemsa's method;
5. Leishman's method;
6. Acridine orange, using a fluorescent microscope (Fripp et al 1975);
7. Silver impregnation (Honigberg & Davenport 1954).

Culture methods

Material for culture may be placed directly into the culture medium from the patient, or stored in conventional transport media. Nielsen (1969) stresses that storage in such media as Stuart's transport medium should not be for longer than 24 hours. Culture media that can be used to grow the organism include:

1. Feinberg & Whittington (1957);
2. Squires & McFadzean (1962) (Modified Busby's Medium);

3. Cysteine-Peptone-Liver-Maltose (CPLM) medium (Johnson & Trussell 1943)
4. Lowe's semi-solid agar medium (Lowe 1972);
5. Diamond's medium (Diamond 1957);
6. Stenton's medium (Stenton 1957).

Lowe (1978) provides full technical data for most laboratory procedures.

COMPARISON OF THE ACCURACY OF DIAGNOSTIC METHODS

In the past there has been much discussion and disagreement concerning the usefulness of the various diagnostic methods. When organisms are plentiful, as in the infected discharge of women with vaginitis, the immediate wet film gives excellent results and provides an immediate diagnosis enabling immediate treatment. This test should certainly be available to all clinicians who might need to investigate such cases. However when the organism is not plentiful, and especially in male problem cases, other diagnostic tests should be used as well.

Rayner (1968) compared the value of wet preparations and culture in various media. Out of 72 infected women the diagnosis would have been missed in 14 if wet smears had been used alone; only 3 cases were missed on CPLM culture. Feinberg-Whittington medium was less than half as sensitive (38 of 72 infected cases missed). In a preceding part of the study Squires and MacFadzean's medium was shown to be much less sensitive than the Feinberg-Whittington (49 cases detected compared with 66). Rayner also conducted experiments to determine the minimal inoculation needed to initiate growth in each medium: this was 1–40 organisms for the CPLM medium, with 10 000–100 000 needed for the other two.

Lowe (1972) stated that he and Rayner had compared his semisolid medium against the CPLM medium and observed no significant differences. This put Lowe's medium at a considerable advantage as it is easier to prepare and store, and will act as a transport medium. He compared this medium with the commercially available Oxoid no. 2 medium (modified Squires & McFadzean) and found that the semisolid medium was more efficient, with an estimated 97% diagnostic accuracy compared with 85% for the Oxoid no. 2 medium. These results were in contrast with those of Hess (1969).

Greater problems are evident in attempting to assess the comparative efficiency of stained smears. Whereas in culture and wet preparations the diagnosis is based on the recognition of characteristic *motile* organisms, this motility is obviously lost on fixation, and the organism may become somewhat distorted in shape. Hence it can be argued that false positive diagnoses can be made, as well as false negatives.

Kean & Day (1954) compared the results obtained using 'hanging drop' preparations, culture in simplified trypticase serum and Papanicolaou cytology. Overall the culture method proved best, diagnosing 39 cases. The 'hanging drop' was positive in 30 cases and the Pap smear in 28, none of which were negative by culture. Oller (1965) similarly found culture most efficient (86%) compared with 78% for the Pap and 48% for the wet preparation. In his series 8 cases (7%) were diagnosed on Pap smear alone. Thin et al (1969) found almost complete agreement between Papanicolaou, Papperheim and wet smears. However Perl (1972) considered that in a very large number of cases the cytological diagnosis of trichomoniasis was in error, with a false positive rate as high as 48%. Hulka & Hulka (1967) conclude that culture methods are much superior to wet smear or Papanicolaou staining, with a false negative rate of 74% for the Pap smear in culture positive cases. There is clearly a great deal of disagreement concerning the value of the cytological method.

IMMUNOLOGICAL TESTS

Immunological tests are available for one other species of trichomoniasis, *Tritrichomonas foetus*, both on serum (Kerr & Robertson 1941) and on vaginal secretion (Pierce 1947). This organism causes a serious infection of cattle giving rise to infertility and abortion.

Wendlberger (1936) demonstrated complement fixing antibodies in 22 of 32 clinically infected women, but in no uninfected women or carriers.

Trussel & Wilson (1942) reported positive complement fixation in 47% of infected women, but in only 17% of controls. Trussell (1947) employed the technique of Kerr and Robertson and obtained satisfactory reactions with *T. vaginalis*. Lanceley (1958) claimed that immunologically *T. vaginalis* organisms could be divided into two groups, with different specimens being agglutinated by one but not both types of antisera. Kott & Adler (1961) tested 19 strains of *T. vaginalis* and claimed to distinguish 8 distinct serotypes. McEntegart et al (1958) conjugated antitrichomonal antibody prepared in rabbits with fluorescein isocyanate; the preparation worked well for staining with the pure culture of *T. vaginalis* but was less satisfactory in smears of infected vaginal discharge. Different degrees of fluorescent brilliance were observed with different strains of *T. vaginalis*. Kramer and Kucera (1966) used this fluorescent antibody method to demonstrate antibodies in the sera of patients with urogenital trichomoniasis. Since that time interest in the subject has waned, probably because of the introduction of very efficient methods of treatment.

TRANSMISSION OF TRICHOMONAS VAGINALIS

T. vaginalis was first reported in the male urethra in 1894 by three separate workers, Marchand, Mivra and Dock. It is usually accepted as being found most commonly in young, sexually active women, and because of this transmission during sexual intercourse is thought most likely. *T. vaginalis* was identified in all the female sexual partners of 56 men suffering from trichomonal urethritis (Catterall & Nicol 1960). The organism is much more difficult to identify in the male, but the reported rate of identified infestation amongst the male sexual partners of women with trichomoniasis varies between 18.6% and 90% (King 1964; Teokharov 1969). Because of the extremely common occurrence of the organism, and the implications of infidelity and promiscuity implied by sexual transmission, many workers have attempted to prove other methods of transfer to be possible.

Teokharov (1969) states that non-sexual infection of the adult female is possible but very rare, and reports that drying, high temperature or change in osmotic pressure will quickly kill the organism. He states that trichomonads die in water in between 10 and 30 minutes, unlike gonococci which may survive for 24 hours or more. Kessel and Thompson (1950) placed droplets of 0.5 ml of vaginal discharge containing *T. vaginalis* on wooden blocks: by direct smear and culture viable organisms lasted until the droplet dried out, that is for up to 6 hours. McCullugh in a letter to the Lancet in 1953 was emphatic that about 15% of cases of trichomoniasis were sexually acquired; in 80% of cases he claimed that lavatory seats were the vehicle, and suggested that the 'gap' seat would completely prevent infection. No figures were produced to support this view. Whittington (1957) took cultures from lavatory seats used by women attending a venereal disease clinic and known to be infected with *T. vaginalis*: in 4 of 30 cases infective material was left on the seat. Whether or not the patient sat on the seat (a fact recorded electrically) did not influence the chance of her depositing infected material. Whittington recorded that the parasite would survive for up to 45 minutes on seats of bakelite or polished wood, but less on absorbent wood. Burch et al (1959) demonstrated that trichomonads could be cultured after several hours from pieces of wet cloth used to wipe the external genitalia of women suffering from trichomoniasis and allowed to stand at room temperature in a moist environment. Burgess (1963) produced some evidence that splashing from the bowls of water closets could result in contamination of the genital area with trichomonad-infested urine from unflushed previous usage, although how often this might lead to actual infection is highly debatable. From all these reports one must conclude that the asexual transmission of the organism between adults remains hypothetical.

Accidental transfer from adults to children is also a matter of controversy. Worwag (1971) found *T. vaginalis* in the urine of 55% of the female infants of women with trichomoniasis, in contrast to none of the children with trichomonas-negative mothers. Similarly, 28.5% of the sons of such women were infected. Peter (1957) found the parasite in 1% of children up to one year of age. Crowther (1962) re-

ported two cases of trichomonal vaginitis occurring soon after birth in premature infants. Trussell & Wilson (1942) examined the female babies of 41 infected mothers: two were found to be infected in the vagina. Littlewood & Kohler (1966) described a severe urinary tract infection in a premature female infant which was proven to be due to *T. vaginalis*. Kurnatowska (1962) reported that 6 of 35 with vulvovaginitis harboured *T. vaginalis*; she attributed this to low standards of hygiene. Stein & Cope (1933) reported the disease in a mother and two daughters; they considered poor hygiene the reason for spread. It would seem that in neonates infection can occur at birth rarely: in young children with poor living conditions transfer can occur from parents. Recent awareness concerning the possible high incidence of sexual abuse of children may lead to a reappraisal of these past results.

CLINICAL PRESENTATION

Clinical presentation in women

T. vaginalis infection is a common cause for the clinical picture of classic vaginitis. In this condition the woman will present with symptoms of vaginal soreness and a discharge which will be green and offensive and possibly blood-stained. There may be dysuria, and intercourse may be painful or impossible. On superficial examination discharge may be soiling the vulval area, and causing erythema and a local skin reaction. The inguinal lymph nodes may be swollen and tender. Passage of a vaginal speculum will be most uncomfortable for the woman, and on opening the blades the lower one may become flooded with discharge. The whole of the vagina and the vaginal portion of the cervix will be obviously inflamed, with the typical 'strawberry' pattern shown in Plate 38. Gardner & Fernet (1964) described an even more florid form, vaginitis emphysematosa, which is characterised by gas-filled cystic cavities in the vaginal mucosa, but this is very rare. Urethritis will also be present in a high proportion of cases, and in a small minority trigonitis will lead to urinary symptoms. The odour will often be offensive. A rapid diagnosis can be made by identifying the organism in a 'wet' preparation of discharge, examined by microscope in the clinic.

The above pattern describes the acute and florid vaginitis caused by this organism, but probably the *majority* of cases are not typical. Any woman who presents with a vaginal discharge should be screened for the presence of *T. vaginalis*, at least by the examination of a 'wet' preparation of discharge. Whatever the nature of this discharge, if the organism is identified in it the woman should be treated.

More of a problem arises when the report of the presence of *T. vaginalis* is made solely from the examination of a Papanicolaou smear taken for cervical screening in an asymptomatic woman. Ideally one should back the diagnosis by 'wet' preparation or culture, but often such attempts give negative results. This raises the question as to whether it is wise or ethically correct to suggest to the woman that she undergoes treatment for a condition that causes her no symptoms, produces no clinical signs, has no significant complications or long term consequences and has been diagnosed by a method that may have a false positive rate. Also to be considered is the fact that the condition is almost certainly sexually transmitted, and therefore the decision to treat one patient should be accompanied by measures relating to her sexual partners. Each case must be judged on its own merits, but there would seem to be justification for doing nothing in many cases.

Clinical presentation in men

The reported incidence of trichomoniasis in men is less than one-tenth of that in women (Annual Reports of the Chief Medical Officer of the Department of Health and Social Security, HMSO London). The *actual* difference will be far greater, for the majority of women with trichomoniasis will not attend clinics for sexually transmitted disease but will be treated by gynaecologists and general practitioners, whilst the symptomatic male at least will almost certainly seek the advice of a genitourinary physician. The figure for England in 1982 was small—1620—and represents only 1.7% of the cases of non-gonococcal urethritis presenting, compared with the often quoted figure of 5%. If there is a clinical presentation it is as for non-gonococcal urethritis; but usually the consorts of women with vaginal trichomoniasis are asymptomatic, have no relevant signs, and the organisms cannot be recovered from them.

THE TREATMENT OF TRICHOMONIASIS

Metronidazole

Very few drugs have made as much impact on a disease as metronidazole on trichomoniasis, both from the welcome and lasting improvement it has made to patients' lives and the drastic fall in workload (and sometimes income) it has produced for those who look after them. This drug was introduced in 1960, and it rapidly became obvious that it was an extreme success. This is typified by the findings of Keighley (1971); writing 10 years after the introduction of the drug she reported a cure rate after one course of treatment of 488 out of 496 cases (98.3%). As all of her patients remained in prison for the seven day course of treatment one can surmise that compliance was excellent and the chances of reinfection minimal. The dose used, 400 mg twice daily, was slightly more than the usual one in the United Kingdom, 200 mg three times a day, but this latter also produced cure rates above 95%. In other countries the unitary dose (one tablet) was 250 mg and the recommended course of treatment in the United States was 250 mg three times daily for 10 days (Dykers 1975). In more recent years alternative regimes have been suggested in an attempt to counteract non-compliance with tablet taking over a prolonged period. Such regimes have included:

2 g as a single dose (Dykers 1975; Hager et al 1980)
4 g over 2 days (Davidson 1973)
1 g as a single dose (Austin et al 1982)

With the exception of the 1 g dose, for which the success rate was only 55%, all of these doses appear to be effective. Problems encountered, however, are an exaggeration of those side effects reported from prolonged treatment—nausea, vomiting, an unpleasant aftertaste from the tablets and unfavourable reaction with alcohol.

In the original treatment trials vaginal preparations and oral tablets were given together, until it was shown that the oral preparations were effective by themselves. Metronidazole is now marketed in suppository form, and Panja (1982) assessed the effectiveness of 2 g of the drug given rectally in a single treatment. The cure rate was reported as 94%, and in two (2%) of the women whose treatment failed, the suppositories caused diarrhoea before absorption could take place. Other side-effects were also common in this treatment group.

Various possible reasons for treatment failure have been put forward. The most significant of these is possible reinfection, and this will be discussed later in this chapter. Other postulated reasons include:

Inadequate dose for weight ratio. Austin et al (1982) reported that, with a single 1 g dose, heavier patients had a significantly higher failure rate than lighter ones. This was not observed in the group receiving a single dose of 2 g.

Malabsorption of the drug

Metronidazole-resistant trichomonads. Although in the early years resistant of *T. vaginalis* to metronidazole had not been reported, it is now recognised that this can occur (Waitkins & Thomas 1981). However this is a very uncommon occurrence.

Inactivation of metronidazole by other organisms. Edwards et al (1979) reported that a number of organisms present in the vagina both in health and disease could absorb and inactivate metronidazole and related drugs. Such organisms include *Streptococcus faecalis, Escherichia coli, Klebsiella faecalis* and *Proteus mirabilis*. (It is a shame that tests were not done on the *Bacteroides* group.) *Klebsiella aerogenes*, especially, absorbed and inactivated metronidazole in vitro; the less significant action of *E. coli* was however enhanced when it was in a mixed culture with *Str. faecalis*. Generally absorption and inactivation were three times as great in an anaerobic rather than an aerobic environment.

Zinc deficiency

Zinc appears to have an antitrichomonal effect, and low serum levels have been associated with persistent and recurrent infections (Willmott et al, 1983).

Other Nitroimidazole Compounds

As well as metronidazole a variety of other drugs in this group have been marketed in the United Kingdom and in other parts of the world. These include nimorazole, tinidazole, ormidazole, carmidazole and secridazole. None of them has been used in treatment on anything like the scale of metronidazole, and although they seem broadly to be equally effective, none of them have any real advantage over that drug. Nimorazole is marketed in the United Kingdom, and can be used in a variety of regimens in much the same way as metronidazole.

Local preparations

In the past a pentavalent arsenical preparation, acetarsol, was used for the treatment of trichomonal vaginitis. Results were fairly good, but the risk of toxicity led to its withdrawal. A mercurial preparation, hydrargaphen, also has the same effect. More recently, povidine iodine has been used, in the form of pessaries, vaginal jelly and vaginal cleanser. All of these preparations do not by themselves produce an acceptable cure rate, and the first two should probably be abandoned in any case. Povidine iodine may well have a place as an adjunct to nitroimidazole therapy in the treatment of problem cases.

Immunotherapy

Recently there has been described a completely new approach to the treatment of trichomoniasis based on the stimulation of the immune defence system. The vaccine concerned is prepared from so called 'aberrant lactobacilli'; the theory behind it being that the immunosystems of the vagina are sufficiently enhanced by this to provide greater resistance to all pathogenic organisms, with a resultant cure of present infection and prevention of future ones. Most authors who have undertaken research on this subject freely admit that the mode of action of this preparation is unknown; however, considerable claims are made for its success. Thus in a double blind study Harris (1984) treated 200 women with 2 g nimorazole, together with 'solco-trichovac' or a placebo. Although the initial response was no different between the two groups, those receiving active vaccination were significantly less likely to experience a recurrent attack within 8 months. Litschgi (1982) reported similar findings, with protection from vaccination extending to at least 1 year. Bonilla-Musoles (1984) studied a group of women with trichomoniasis treated only with vaccination and compared them with women treated with vaccination and metronidazole; although the combined treatment initially produced better responses, after 3 months the results were not significantly different. Similar claims have been made for the treatment of non-specific vaginitis.

This method is new and far from adequately understood. Nevertheless, it may hold considerable promise for future use.

The need to treat sexual partners

Since the early reports suggesting that *T. vaginalis* was transmitted commonly, if not exclusively, by the sexual route, it has been customary to treat sexual partners. This has been done on a far more universal scale than for most sexually transmitted diseases, but also at the same time far more casually. With the exception of those working in the field of genitourinary medicine (venereology) most doctors rarely enquire about the epidemiological aspect of the condition but instead write the woman a double prescription with the instruction that her 'husband' should take the second course. This custom has led to much comedy, some tragedy and a great deal of waste. No one would dream of treating syphilis, gonorrhoea or chlamydial infections in so cavalier a fashion—why trichomonal?

Most authors would agree that the need for prophylactic treatment of the male partner or partners is unproven. Westrom & Nicol (1963) demonstrated both the difficulty of isolating the organism from the male partners of infected women, and also the transient nature of infection in the male, possibly due to the high zinc concentration in the male genital tract (Krieger & Rein 1982). To demonstrate the organism in the male may well involve unpleasant techniques such as prostatic massage. No published work acceptably proves that treatment of the male sexual partner improves the initial cure prospects of the woman concerned, or her chances of avoiding a further attack.

In the environment of the clinic for sexually transmitted diseases, where proper contact tracing is expected and carried out properly, the location, examination and treatment of these men is probably appropriate. In general and gynaecological practice, however, the routine treatment of unseen male partners is to be deprecated. A better approach would be to treat the woman, suggesting that she returns in 3 weeks for test of cure and abstains from intercourse during that time. After that she resumes her sexual relation; should a recurrence then occur her partner or partners most be identified, interviewed and examined.

Treatment of the resistant case

The possible reasons for apparent treatment failure have been discussed in the section on metronidazole. When the likelihood of reinfection has been discounted, the organism should be examined for possible resistance to the nitroimidazole group of drugs, and blood taken from the patient after ingestion of a standard dose of one of these for blood levels. If the results of these do not provide the answer to the problem, the following empirical enhanced treatments may be tried:

Double dose nitroimidazole treatment;
Oral plus vaginal metronidazole;
Oral nitroimidazole plus local povidine iodine;
Oral nitroimidazole plus oral zinc;
Vaccination.

REFERENCES

Austin T W, Smith E A, Darwish R, Ralph E D, Pattison F L M 1982 Metronidazole in a single dose for the treatment of trichomoniasis. British Journal of Venereal Diseases 58: 121–123
Bonilla-Musoles F 1984 Immunotherapy in vaginal trichomoniasis: therapeutic and prophylactic effects of the vaccine Solco-Trichovac. Gynäkcologische Rundschau 24 (Suppl 3): 63–69
Burch T A, Rees C W and Rearden L V 1959 Survival of T. vaginalis. american Journal of Tropical Medicine and Hygiene 8: 312–320
Burgess J A 1963 Trichomonas vaginalis infection from

splashing in water closets. British Journal of Venereal Diseases 39: 248–249

Catterall R D, Nicol C S 1960 Is trichomonal infestation a venereal disease? British Medical Journal i: 1177–1179

Coutts W E, Silva-Inzunza E 1954 Vital staining of trichomonas vaginalis with fluorescein. British Journal of Venereal Diseases 30: 43

Crowther I A 1962 Trichomonal vaginitis in infancy. Lancet i: 1074

Davidson F 1973 Short-term, high dose metronidazole for vaginal trichomoniasis. Journal of Obstetrics and Gynaecology of the British Commonwealth 80: 368–370

Diamond L S 1957 The establishment of various trichomonads of animals and man in axenic cultures. Journal of Parasitology 43: 488

Donné A F 1836 Animalcules observés dans les matières purulentes et le produit des sécrétions des organes génitaux de l'homme et de la femme. Comptes Rendus Hebdomadaires des Séances de l'Academie des Sciences Paris 3: 385

Dykers J R 1975 Single dose metronidazole for trichomonal vaginitis. New England Journal of Medicine 23: 24

Edwards D I, Thompson E J, Tomusange J, Shanson D 1979 Inactivation of metronidazole by aerobic organisms. Journal of Antimicrobial Therapy 5: 315–316

Ehrenberg C G 1838 Die Infusionthierchen als vollkommene Organismen: ein Blick in das tiefere organische Leben des Natur. L Voss, Leipzig

Feinberg J G, Whittington M J 1957 A culture medium for T. vaginalis and Candida. Journal of Clinical Pathology 10: 327–329

Fripp P J, Mason P R, Super H 1975 A method for the diagnosis of trichomonas vaginalis using acridine orange. Journal of Parasitology 61: 966

Gardner H L, Fernet P 1964 Etiology of vaginitis emphysematosa. American Journal of Obstetrics and Gynecology 88: 680–694

Hager W D, Brown S T, Kraus, S J, Kleris G S, Perkins G J, Henderson M 1980 Metronidazole for vaginal trichomoniasis. Journal of the American Medical Association 244: 1219–1220

Harris J R W 1984 Double blind comparative study of T. vaginalis infection: Solco-Trichovac versus placebo. Gynäkologische Rundschau 24 (Suppl 3): 44–49

Hess J 1969 Review of current methods for the detection of T. vaginalis in clinical material. Journal of Clinical Pathology 22: 269–272

Honigberg B M, Davenport H A 1954 Staining flagellate protozoa by various silver protein compounds. Stain Technology 29: 241–245

Hulka B S, Hulka J F 1967 Dyskaryosis in cervical cytology and its relationship to trichomoniasis therapy. A double blind study. American Journal of Obstetrics and Gynecology 98: 180–187

Johnson G, Trussel R E 1943 Experimental basis for chemotherapy of T. vaginalis. Proceedings of the Society for Experimental Biology and Medicine (NY) 54: 245–248

Keen B H, Day E (1954) T. vaginalis infection. Evaluation of three diagnostic techniques with data on incidence. American Journal of Obstetrics and Gynecology 68: 1510–1518

Keighley E E 1971 Trichomoniasis in a closed community: efficiacy of metronidazole. British Medical Journal 1: 207–209

Kerr W R, Robertson M 1941 An investigation into the infection of cows with Trichomonas foetus by means of the agglutination reaction. Veterinary Journal 97: 351–356

Kessel J F, Thompson C F 1950 Survival of trichomonas vaginalis in vaginal discharge. Proceedings of the Society for Experimental Biology and Medicine 74: 755–758

King A J 1964 In: Recent Advances in Venereology. J and A Churchill Ltd, London, p. 477

Kott H, Adler S 1961 A serological study of Trichomonas sp parasitic in men. Transactions of the Royal Society of Tropical Medicine and Hygiene 55: 333–337

Kramer J, Kucera K 1966 Immunofluorescence demonstration of antibodies in urogenital trichomoniasis. Journal of Hygience, Epidemiology, Microbiology and Immunology 10: 85–87

Krieger J N, Rein M F 1982 Zinc sensitivity of T. vaginalis. In vitro studies and clinical implications. Journal of Infectious Diseases 146: 341–345

Kurnatowska A 1962 Detection and biological properties of T. vaginalis. Wiad Parcizyt 8: 165–177

Lanceley F 1958 Serological aspects of trichomonas vaginalis. British Journal of Venereal Diseases 34: 4–7

Litschgi M 1982 Incidence of recurrent infections after treatment of T. vaginalis with Solco Trichovac: a randomised double blind study. Geburtshilfe und Frauenheilkunde 42: 231–233

Littlewood J M, Kohler H G 1966 Urinary tract infection by T. vaginalis in a newborn baby. Archives of Disease in Childhood 41: 693–695

Lowe G H 1972 A comparison of culture media for the isolation of T. vaginalis. Medical Laboratory Technology 29: 389–396

Lowe G H 1978 The trichomonads. Public Health Monograph Series No 9 HMSO London

McCullagh W McK H 1953 The gap seat. Lancet i: 698

McEntegart M G, Chadwick C S, Nairn R C 1958 Fluorescent antisera in the detection of serological varieties of Trichomonas vaginalis. British Journal of Venereal Diseases 34: 1–6

Nielson M H, Ludvik J, Nielsen R 1966 On the ultrastructure of Trichomonas vaginalis Donné. Journal de Microscopie, Paris 5: 229–231

Nielson R 1969 Trichomonas vaginalis 1. Survival in solid Stuarts medium. British Journal of Venereal Diseases 45: 328–332

Oller L Z 1965 Routine exfoliature cytology for cancer and trichomonas detection at a clinic for venereal diseases. British Journal of Venereal Diseases 41: 304–308

Ovčinnikov N M, Delektorskij V V, Turanova E N, Yashkova G N 1975 Further studies of T. vaginalis with transmission and scanning electron microscopy. British Journal of Venereal Diseases 51: 357–375

Panja S K 1982 Treatment of trichomoniasis with metronidazole rectal suppositories. British Journal of Venereal Diseases 58: 257–258

Perl G 1972 Errors in diagnosis of T. vaginalis infections as observed among 1199 patients. Obstetrics and Gynecology 39: 7–9

Peter R 1957 In: Les Infestations a Trichomonas. Massan et Cie, Paris, p 155

Pierce A E 1947 The demonstration of an agglutinin in Trichomonas foetus in the vaginal discharge of infected heifers. Journal of Comparative Pathology 57: 84–88

Rayner C F A 1968 Comparison of culture media for the growth of T. vaginalis. British Journal of Venereal Diseases 44: 63–66

Squires S, McFadzean J A 1962 Strain sensitivity of trichomonas vaginalis to metronidazole. British Journal of Venereal Diseases 38: 218–219

Stenton P 1957 The isolation of trichomonas vaginalis. Journal of Medical Laboratory Technology 14: 228

Stein I F, Cope E S 1933 Trichomonas vaginalis. American Journal of Obstetrics and Gynecology 25: 819–825

Teokharov B A 1969 Non-gonococcal infections of the female

genitalia. British Journal of Venereal Diseases 45: 334–340

Thin R N T, Melcher D H, Tapp J W, Nicol C S, Hill J 1969 Detection of T. vaginalis in women: comparison of 'wet smear' results with those of two cervical cytological methods. British Journal of Venereal Diseases 45: 332–333

Thorburn A L 1974 Alfred François Donné 1801–1878 Discovery of trichomonas vaginalis and of leukaemia. British Journal of Venereal Disease 50: 377–380

Trussell R E, Wilson M 1942 Vaginal trichomoniasis: complement fixation, puerperal morbidity and early infection of newborn infants. American Journal of Obstetrics and Gynecology 42: 292–295

Trussell R E 1947 Trichomonas vaginalis and trichomoniasis. Thomas, Springfield

Waitkins S A, Thomas D J 1981 Isolation of T. vaginalis resistant to metronidazole. Lancet ii: 590

Wasley G D, Rayner C F A 1970 Preservation of T. vaginalis in liquid nitrogen. British Journal of Venereal Diseases 46: 323–325

Wendlberger J 1936 Zur pathogenität der T. vaginalis. Archiv für Dermatologie und Syphilis 174: 583–590

Weström T E T, Nicol C S 1963 Natural history of trichomal infection in moles. British Journal of Venereal Diseases 39: 251–257

Whittington M J 1957 Epidermology of infections with trichomonas vaginalis in the light of improved diagnostic methods. British Journal of Venereal Diseases 33: 80

Willmott F, Say J, Downey D, Hookham A 1983 Zinc and recalcitrant trichomoniasis. Lancet i: 1053

Worwag Z 1971 Wystepowanie rzesistka pochwowego w uklaclzie moczowym noworodkow plici meskiey. Wiadomosci Parazytologiczne 17: 351–358

Vaginal candidosis and related infections
D W Warnock, J D Milne and D C E Speller

VAGINAL CANDIDOSIS

Vaginal candidosis (candidiasis) is one of the most frequent infections seen in women. It is most common in pregnant women, but can occur in women of all ages, and it has been suggested that 75% of women will suffer one or more episodes during their lives (Sobel 1984). The conditions required for symptomatic infection are not well understood, and while most patients respond well to simple antifungal treatment, in some the infection is intractable and chronic, or recurrent, causing great distress to them and to their sexual partners (Hurley 1975). The number of cases of vaginal candidosis diagnosed among women attending sexually transmitted disease (STD) clinics in England and Wales increased throughout the 1970s (Cartwright 1980); on the other hand the prevalence of the condition in pregnant women throughout the world appears to have remained almost constant since the 1950s (Schnell 1982b).

Candida albicans is the most important cause of both superficial and deep forms of candidosis in man, although other members of the genus such as *C. tropicalis* and *C. parapsilosis* are sometimes involved. *C. albicans* has been reported as isolated from about 80–90% of women with vaginal candidosis (Oriel et al 1972; Gough et al 1985). The second most common fungus recovered from the genital tract of women with vaginitis is *Torulopsis glabrata*, now reclassified as *Candida glabrata*, which accounts for about 5% of vaginal infections (Oriel et al 1972). Infections with this fungus are apt to be mild and it is not often associated with florid clinical signs.

The status of Candida albicans as a vaginal pathogen

Candida albicans is found in the mouth and intestinal tract of a substantial proportion of the normal population, but it is still not clear to what extent it can be regarded as a normal inhabitant of the genital tract. Various reports suggest that asymptomatic vaginal colonisation occurs in about 5–10% of non-pregnant women and around 40% of pregnant women (Odds 1979; Schnell 1982b). Odds (1982) demonstrated regular diurnal variation in the amount of *C. albicans* recoverable from the lower genital tract of asymptomatic women. Other reports suggest that the isolation of *C. albicans* from the normal genital tract is an unusual finding.

In 1973, Carroll et al published details of a clinical and microbiological investigation of 303 pregnant women, 50 (16.5%) of whom were found to be harbouring *C. albicans*. Only one of these 50 women had a normal genital tract, which observation led Carroll et al to suggest that *C. albicans* is not part of the normal flora of the lower genital tract of pregnant women and that its isolation is an indication for prompt antifungal treatment. On the other hand, it must be said that careful clinical assessment led to the detection of clinical signs in a large proportion of the women (86%), most of whom (70%) were not harbouring *C. albicans*.

Hilton & Warnock (1975) studied 300 non-pregnant women attending the STD clinic in Bristol and found that 27 of the 80 patients (33%) with *C. albicans* had clinical signs of vulval or vaginal infection. In contrast, in a subsequent investigation of a similar group of women attending this clinic,

Gough et al (1985) found that 89 of 94 patients (95%) with *C. albicans* had clinical signs of vulval or vaginal infection. The isolation rate was similar in both investigations (28 and 31.3%). The most obvious difference between the investigations was that in the earlier work several clinicians assessed the patients and the relevant information was retrieved later, while in the later investigation one clinician examined all the patients and recorded the clinical findings in detail. There is an obvious parallel here with the work of Carroll et al (1973) and Hurley et al (1973) on pregnant women. In the former report, one clinician examined the patients and recorded the findings. In the latter work, which was performed in the same London hospital, clinical details were obtained later. As in the Bristol work, the isolation rates for *C. albicans* were similar in both reports (16.5 and 17%), but Carroll et al (1973) found that 49 of 50 women (98%) harbouring the fungus had clinical signs, while Hurley et al (1973) stated that 50% of women with *C. albicans* had neither symptoms nor clinical signs of vaginal infection.

It is clear that, in the select populations studied in these investigations (Carroll et al 1973; Gough et al 1985), the isolation of *C. albicans* from the lower genital tract is associated with symptoms and clinical signs. These findings tend to suggest that the fungus is not part of the normal microbial flora of this site, and that its isolation indicates a need for antifungal treatment. However, in both investigations, abnormalities were detected in a high proportion of women, most of whom were not harbouring *C. albicans* and some of whom had no infectious condition diagnosed. Therefore the causal association of *C. albicans* with the abnormalities has not been proven, and even the clinical importance of some of these 'abnormalities' is in doubt. If the status of the fungus as a vaginal inhabitant is to be established, then it will be important to perform detailed clinical and mycological assessment, with quantification, of an unselected population of normal women.

Mode of infection

Almost all human infections with *C. albicans* arise from the patient's own endogenous microbial flora or are acquired from another person. The fungus

has been found in inanimate habitats such as the soil, air or water, but its occurrence appears to be related to its more normal association with warm-blooded animals. In man *C. albicans* often forms part of the normal microbial flora of the mouth and intestinal tract. It can be recovered from the mouths of around 10–30% of normal persons, but much higher isolation rates have been recorded among selected groups of hospital patients.

C. albicans often appears in the intestinal contents of infants during the first month of life. It is often acquired at birth and it has been found that colonisation of the mouth precedes colonisation of the intestinal tract (Taschdjian & Kozinn 1957). The fungus may be found throughout the digestive tract and is prevalent in the mouth and rectum, where the flora can be sampled. Assessments of the prevalence of *C. albicans* in the rest of the gastro-intestinal tract have been carried out, albeit under unphysiological conditions. The findings of these investigations have been somewhat dissimilar, showing either a progressive increase through the mouth, small intestine and faeces (Stone et al 1973), or a higher prevalence in the mouth and faeces than in the jejunum (Cohen et al 1969).

The intestinal tract has long been considered an important source of vaginal infection or reinfection since most patients harbouring *C. albicans* in the genital tract are also harbouring this fungus in the mouth and anus (De Sousa & Van Uden 1960; Hilton & Warnock 1975; Miles et al 1977). The introduction of methods for differentiation of strains of *C. albicans* (Warnock et al 1979a; Odds & Abbott 1980) allowed investigations which established that most individuals harbour the same strain or strains of the fungus in different anatomical sites (Warnock et al 1979a, 1979b; Odds et al 1983a, 1983b). Moreover individuals who harbour *C. albicans* in a given site tend to retain the same strain for at least several weeks and often for months (Warnock et al 1979b; McCreight & Warnock 1982; McCreight et al 1985). Thus, most women with vaginal infection are also harbouring the same strain of *C. albicans* in the mouth and intestinal tract (Warnock et al 1979b; Odds et al 1983a). This finding has strengthened the suggestion that the intestinal tract is a source of vaginal reinfection.

Two reports (Rodin & Kolator 1976; Davidson 1977) have indicated that *C. albicans* can be recovered from the genital tract of a high proportion of contacts of men harbouring *C. albicans* on the penis. Typing the strains of *C. albicans* from male and female partners has revealed that both often harbour the same strain (Warnock et al 1979b; Odds et al 1983a). Thin et al (1977) calculated that sexual transmission of infection occurred in about 30–40% of their patients. However, unequivocal proof that the man is the source of vaginal infection, rather than the recipient, has still to be obtained. Although orogenital and anogenital contact are potential risk factors, further epidemiological investigation with typing of strains will be required to establish a causal relationship.

Pathogenesis of vaginal candidosis: the fungus

Candida albicans is the most frequent cause of superficial, mucosal and deep forms of candidosis in man. Similar strains of the fungus have been isolated from colonised persons and patients with different clinical forms of infection (Odds et al 1983a, 1983b). This is consistent with the notion of the fungus as an opportunistic pathogen that cannot establish an infection unless the host is impaired; thus, overt infection must be attributed more to alteration of the host than to the virulence of the pathogen. Although several factors, such as the formation of mycelium, have been suggested as contributing to the greater virulence of *C. albicans* as compared with other members of the genus, none of these features have so far been confirmed as virulence factors.

C. albicans is a dimorphic fungus which can grow in the form of budding yeast cells or hyphal filaments. Both forms are seen in infected tissues and it has been suggested that the formation of mycelium confers a pathogenic advantage on the fungus. It is clear that long hyphal forms are more resistant to phagocytosis than yeast cells. Hyphal forms are also more successful at penetrating host tissue and can therefore cause more mechanical damage to the host than yeast cells.

Sobel et al (1984) have described a strain of *C. albicans*, incapable of hyphal formation, that was less successful than other isolates in establishing vaginal colonisation in an animal model. Moreover, infection, when established, was milder, often transient and lower numbers of organisms were re-

covered from the animals. Mutants of this type may also lack other undetected virulence determinants, but, prima facie, hyphal formation appears to be a virulence factor, although it is not essential for infection to occur.

To cause mucosal infection, a microbial pathogen must first attach itself to the host epithelium. *C. albicans* yeast cells become attached to human vaginal and buccal epithelial cells in greater numbers than cells of other *Candida* species tested under identical conditions (King et al 1980). It has also been shown that *C. albicans* hyphal forms are attached in greater numbers than yeast cells to both vaginal and buccal epithelial cells (Kimura & Pearsall 1980; Sobel et al 1981). Segal et al (1984) have reported that *C. albicans* yeast cells from patients with vaginitis were more adherent than vaginal isolates from asymptomatic women. On the other hand, Kearns et al (1983) failed to detect consistent differences in the adhesion of *C. albicans* isolates from patients with oral candidosis and those from normal persons.

Transmission electron micrographs have shown that *C. albicans* can penetrate and proliferate within living intact vaginal epithelial cells (Garcia Tamayo et al 1982; Schnell 1982a). Hyphal forms have been seen up to 15 cell layers deep within the vaginal epithelium (Schnell 1982a). These findings have led Sobel (1984) to suggest that *C. albicans* can sojourn within the vaginal mucosa, protected from topical antifungal treatment, and can then emerge into the vaginal lumen some weeks or months later when the epithelial cells are shed. This hypothesis awaits verification, but it could help to account for the recurrence of vaginal infection after successful treatment in sexually inactive women who are not harbouring the fungus in other sites.

The mechanisms by which *C. albicans* produces symptoms of pruritus and vaginitis, often with minimal invasion of host cells, are not well understood. The fungus secretes an acid proteinase in vitro when proteins are the sole available source of nitrogen (Macdonald & Odds 1980, 1983; Kwon-Chung et al 1985) and this enzyme has been identified as an important virulence factor. Other hydrolytic enzymes, such as a phosphomonoesterase (Odds & Hierholzer 1973) and a phospholipase (Price & Cawson 1977) have been described, but these are located at the cell surface and not secreted. It is reasonable to suppose that secreted and cell-bound enzymes can damage the host, but whether they are important in the production of vaginitis has still to be established. Some men develop balanitis within a few hours of sexual contact with women with vaginal candidosis (Catterall 1966). This suggests that some form of allergic reaction could be involved and this could also have a role in women.

The recent identification of receptors for oestrogens and progesterone in *C. albicans* (Loose et al 1981, 1983; Powell & Drutz 1983; Powell et al 1984), together with reports that these hormones can stimulate fungal growth (Powell et al 1983) could be significant in an understanding of the pathogenesis of vaginal candidosis.

Pathogenesis of vaginal candidosis: the host

The fact that a certain proportion of women harbour *C. albicans* in the vagina with no apparent signs of infection has often led to suggestions that, in those women in whom signs are present, there is some underlying host defect. Such defects are well recognised in other forms of candidosis, but it has so far proved difficult to discover which host factors allow symptomatic vaginal infection with *C. albicans* to occur.

Persons colonised with *C. albicans* possess a number of defence mechanisms to prevent the fungus from establishing an infection. In the normal individual these mechanisms are sufficient to resist the fungus, but the balance between host and pathogen is a fine one. In the common, superficial forms of candidosis, trivial impairments of host defence are often sufficient to allow *C. albicans*, the most pathogenic member of the genus, to establish an infection. More serious impairment of the host can lead to lethal deep infection, often with less pathogenic members of the genus.

The intact epidermis of the host presents a substantial mechanical barrier to *C. albicans*. Cutaneous lesions are confined to sites that are moist because of maceration or occlusion and even then penetration is limited to the stratum corneum. If the fungus should succeed in penetrating the superficial epithelium of the host then a hyperkeratotic response will occur. In some patients with

congenital immunological defects, hyperkeratosis occurs on such a scale as to produce widespread, disfiguring, nodular lesions: this condition has been termed chronic mucocutaneous candidosis. Hyperkeratosis also appears to be responsible for the vaginal plaques that sometimes occur in women with florid vaginal candidosis.

If a microbial pathogen should succeed in establishing itself beneath the epithelium of the host, then inflammation will occur. Phagocytic cells form the earliest and most efficient mechanism for preventing the establishment of deep infection with *C. albicans*. Depletion of their numbers and defects in their function have been implicated as important predisposing factors in deep candidosis, but there is nothing to suggest that such factors are important in vaginal infection. Pus cells are often absent from vaginal secretions of women with symptomatic vaginal candidosis (Gough et al 1985).

Microbial cells that overcome the non-specific defence mechanisms of the host are faced, after an interval required for its activation, with the host's second defence mechanism, the immunological response. This consists of two distinct antigen recognition–elimination mechanisms: the T-cell mediated response and the B-cell mediated (humoral) response. It has been established that the former is more important in host protection against *C. albicans* infection. Thus, chronic mucocutaneous candidosis often occurs in individuals with underlying T-cell defects and often persists despite a strong humoral response (Valdimarsson et al 1973).

The precise role of the T-cell mediated response in host protection against vaginal infection with *C. albicans* is unclear. Hobbs et al (1977) found that 15 of 23 women with recurrent vaginal candidosis showed subnormal T-cell responses to *C. albicans* antigen. Witkin et al (1983) compared the T-cell responses of 6 patients with vaginal candidosis and 6 uninfected women. No differences were detected in tests with non-specific mitogens. In marked contrast, the patients' T-cells showed much reduced proliferation compared with the control subjects in tests with *C. albicans* antigen. Moreover, it was found that T-cells or serum from the infected patients suppressed the proliferative response of control T-cells to *C. albicans*, but not to mitogens. It appears, therefore, that some women with vaginal candidosis produce specific suppressor T-cells which inhibit the immunological response to *C. albicans*, but this needs further investigation. There is no justification at present for attempting immunostimulation (as with levamisole) in women with chronic vaginal candidosis (Hobbs et al 1977).

The role of the humoral immunological response in host protection against vaginal infection with *C. albicans* is also unclear. Anti-*C. albicans* IgA and IgG have been detected in the vaginal secretions of normal women as well as in women with symptomatic or asymptomatic infection with the fungus (Waldman et al 1972a; Milne & Warnock 1977; Gough et al 1984). These antibodies could be the product of a local immunological response in the genital tract: application of a *C. albicans* antigen to the cervical epithelium has been found to lead to the appearance of specific IgA and IgG in the vaginal secretions of normal women (Waldman et al 1972b). Gough et al (1984) found similar levels of specific IgA and IgG in the secretions of 64 non-pregnant women with vaginal candidosis and 158 similar uninfected women. Transudation from the circulation appeared to account for the anti-*C. albicans* IgA and IgG found in the secretions of uninfected women who had never had vaginal candidosis.

The role of anti-*C. albicans* IgA in the genital tract has still to be elucidated. In the gastrointestinal tract IgA is thought to prevent mucosal colonisation by reducing adhesion of the pathogen to host epithelium (Vudhichamnong et al 1982). *C. albicans* cells recovered from the genital tract of women with vaginal candidosis have been found to be coated with specific IgA (Gough et al 1984). The relevance of this observation to the pathogenesis of vaginal candidosis remains obscure.

Factors predisposing the host to vaginal candidosis

Although it has so far proved difficult to discover what host defects allow symptomatic vaginal infection with *C. albicans* to occur, this condition has been associated with a number of predisposing factors.

Vaginal candidosis is more common in the pregnant woman than in her non-pregnant counterpart. The condition occurs in about 20–30% of pregnant women during the first trimester and 30–45% during the third trimester. Recurrent infection is not unusual during gestation: according to one report, 45% of pregnant women require more than one course of treatment for the condition (Hurley & De Louvois 1979). Moreover, infection at this time seems to be the initiating event in a significant proportion of women with chronic or recurrent candidosis (Hurley 1981). No investigation has been performed to confirm the popular belief that vaginal candidosis clears without treatment after confinement. This assumption appears unjustified, for published findings are limited to the vaginal isolation rate of *C. albicans* which does show an abrupt decline in the puerperium (Jennison 1966). This could well be due to the cleansing action of lochial discharges (Hurley 1981). There is no work to show that symptomatic vaginal infection does not recur once the puerperium is over.

It has been established that the pregnant woman is more susceptible to vaginal infection with *C. albicans*, although the reasons for this remain unclear. In an early investigation, Bland et al (1937) induced vaginal infection in 10 of 12 pregnant women inoculated with the fungus as compared with 4 of 12 similar, but non-pregnant, women.

It has long been considered that the greater prevalence of both symptomatic and asymptomatic vaginal infection with *C. albicans* in pregnant women might be related to the increased proportion of large glycogen-rich vaginal epithelial cells which are produced under hormonal influence during gestation. Schnell (1982a) has suggested that if the glycogen released after cytolysis of these epithelial cells is converted to glucose or maltose, then this will produce an ideal environment for multiplication of *C. albicans*. Moreover, several investigations have demonstrated that sugars promote the attachment of *C. albicans* to epithelial cells (Douglas et al 1981; Samaranayake & MacFarlane 1981, 1982). The larger vaginal epithelial cells found during gestation might provide increased numbers of binding sites for *C. albicans*. Segal et al (1984) noted that *C. albicans* cells bind in greater numbers to vaginal epithelial cells obtained from pregnant women than to epithelial cells from non-pregnant women.

Vaginal candidosis is believed to be more prevalent among women with diabetes mellitus, a condition which has been implicated as a predisposing factor in other superficial and deep forms of candidosis. The factors which lead to increased fungal colonisation in diabetic patients are unclear, but the increased numbers of large vaginal epithelial cells and elevated vaginal glucose levels which occur in such women might be important. Segal et al (1984) found that attachment of *C. albicans* to vaginal epithelial cells from diabetic women was greater than attachment to epithelial cells from non-diabetic women.

Sobel (1984) has suggested that broad-spectrum antibiotic treatment is one of the most common precipitating factors in vaginal candidosis. The resident bacterial flora of the vagina is believed to form an important natural defence mechanism against colonisation with *C. albicans*. Thus, antibiotic treatment which leads to a reduction or alteration of this flora could permit the proliferation of *C. albicans* in the vagina. This could in turn account for the rapid onset of symptomatic vaginal infection with *C. albicans* following administration of antibiotics.

Oral contraception is still one of the most controversial predisposing factors associated with vaginal candidosis. Morton & Rashid (1977) claimed that the introduction of this form of contraception coincided with a profound change in the incidence of this infection. Thus, in one investigation involving more than 8000 women, it was found that vaginal candidosis was more common in women who had been using oral contraception for more than 12 months (Diddle et al 1969). However, most reports of a higher incidence of asymptomatic vaginal colonisation or symptomatic vaginal infection with *C. albicans* among women using oral contraception appeared at a time when the combined pills in common use contained at least 50 μg oestrogen. Most combined pills prescribed at present contain lesser amounts of oestrogen (30 μg) and several recent reports have indicated that vaginal colonisation or infection with *C. albicans* is no longer more prevalent among women using this form of contraception (Hilton & Warnock 1975; Goldacre et al 1979; Gough et al 1985).

The influence of serum iron on host defence against *C. albicans* infection has been the subject of much speculation. Abnormal iron metabolism has been proposed as an important factor in certain

patients with chronic mucocutaneous candidosis (Higgs & Wells 1972). However, Davidson et al (1977) found no significant difference in serum ferritin or serum iron levels in women with recurrent vaginal candidosis compared with an uninfected control group. These authors concluded that aberrations of iron metabolism were not predisposing factors in vaginal candidosis.

Many women have identified tight, insulating clothing as a precipitating factor in symptomatic vaginal candidosis. This has been confirmed by Elegbe & Elegbe (1983) who demonstrated an increased prevalence of vaginitis in Nigerian women wearing tight-fitting clothing as compared with women wearing loose-fitting or cotton clothing.

Clinical manifestations

Most women with vaginal candidosis complain of intense vulval and vaginal pruritus with or without vaginal discharge. The condition is often abrupt in onset and, in the non-pregnant woman, tends to begin during the week prior to menstruation. Some non-pregnant women complain of recurrent or increasing symptoms preceding each menstrual period. Pruritus is often more intense when the patient is warm in bed at night. Dysuria and dyspareunia are common.

Vulval erythema with fissuring is the most common clinical finding. This is often localised to the mucocutaneous margins of the vaginal introitus and the fourchette, but can spread to affect the labia majora and perineum. Vaginitis with discharge is another common clinical finding. The classical sign of florid vaginal candidosis in the pregnant woman is the presence of thick white adherent plaques on the vulval, vaginal or cervical epithelium. This is a useful sign in the non-pregnant woman as well. Often the discharge is thick and white and contains curds, but it can be thin or even purulent.

Vulvitis can be present without a concomitant vaginal infection. Chronic infection can lead to vulval lichenification.

C. albicans infection is but one of a number of causes of vulvovaginitis and vaginal discharge and must be distinguished from other conditions such as trichomoniasis and bacterial vaginosis. The clinical diagnosis of genital infection is difficult and clinical suspicion of candidosis must be confirmed with microbiological tests. It is important to remember that some patients with vaginal candidosis will also have other genital infections.

Methods of diagnosis

The diagnosis of vaginal candidosis depends on a combination of typical symptoms and signs and the demonstration of the fungus in smears or its isolation in culture. The latter is much more sensitive and reliable than the former (McLennan et al 1972; Thin et al 1975) and is required for definitive diagnosis of this condition. The successful diagnosis of vaginal candidosis depends on the combined efforts of both clinicians and microbiologists.

Specimens for mycological investigation are obtained after gentle insertion of a vaginal speculum lubricated with water. Swabs should be taken from discharge in the vagina and from the surface of the mid-vaginal mucosa. Swabs can be placed in transport medium or inoculated directly on to plates of glucose peptone or malt agar. It appears that culture will detect the presence of *C. albicans* in numbers above 10^3 cells per ml in the vaginal secretions (Odds 1982), and it has been shown that the fungus can survive on swabs stored for periods of up to 24 hours before plating out (Odds 1982). It is usual for swabs from patients with suspected candidosis to be inoculated on to plates containing chloramphenicol and incubated at 30°C or 37°C for 48 to 72 hours. Identification of isolates is based on morphological and biochemical tests, including germ tube production in serum and assimilation and fermentation reactions (English 1974).

Slide preparations should also be made from a sample of vaginal discharge. One wet-mount preparation should be made with either saline or 20% potassium hydroxide solution and a second slide should be Gram stained. The slides should be examined under the microscope for oval, budding cells and hyphal forms (the latter indicating *C. albicans*). It should be emphasised that for definitive diagnosis, isolation of the fungus in culture is required.

One promising recent development has been a slide latex agglutination test which detects *C. albicans* mannan antigen in vaginal secretions (Hopwood et al 1985). This test takes 3 minutes to perform and appears to compare well with traditional microbiological methods of diagnosis.

Treatment of vaginal candidosis

It is clear that the greatest problem in the management of vaginal candidosis lies in its treatment. Opinion is divided as to whether asymptomatic vaginal colonisation with *C. albicans* should be treated, or whether symptoms and clinical signs should condition treatment. It appears reasonable to treat even asymptomatic colonisation in the pregnant woman, but the situation in the non-pregnant woman is less clear. The optimum duration of treatment has not been established, nor has the optimum method. Patients often appear to prefer oral to topical treatment, but this cannot be justified if the drugs to be used have significant side-effects.

Topical treatment

Most women with vaginal candidosis respond to topical treatment, but there is a small group of patients who are subject to recurrent infection and require special management. These women will be considered later.

Since the 1950s it has been common practice to prescribe topical antifungal treatment for vaginal candidosis for a period of about 2 weeks. However, Masterton et al (1976) reported that 4% of their patients did not start treatment and half their patients did not complete a full fortnight's treatment, often abandoning it once symptomatic relief had been obtained. Masterton et al suggested that shorter, more intensive courses of antifungal treatment might be as effective a cure for vaginal candidosis as the traditional fortnight's course. It has since been demonstrated that the total dose of antifungal applied has more effect on the success of treatment than has the duration of treatment (Odds 1977; Gough 1979). Topical antifungal drugs have been found to persist in the vagina for a considerable period (Odds & Macdonald 1981).

There are at present two major groups of antifungal drugs that are used in the topical treatment of vaginal candidosis. The polyene antifungals include nystatin and natamycin. The imidazole derivatives are more recent introductions and include

Table 10.1 Treatment of vaginal candidosis with antifungal drugs

Drug name		Dosage		Duration of treatment
Nystatin	or	1 or 2 vaginal tablets (100 000 units each)		14 nights or longer
		4 or 8 g cream (100 000 or 200 000 units)		14 nights or longer
Natamycin		1 vaginal tablet	(25 mg)	20 nights or 10 mornings and evenings
Clotrimazole	or	1 vaginal tablet	(100 mg)	6 nights
	or	1 vaginal tablet	(200 mg)	3 nights
	or	1 vaginal tablet	(500 mg)	1 night
	or	5 g cream	(100 mg)	6 nights
	or	5 g cream	(100 mg)	3 mornings and evenings
		5 g cream	(500 mg)	1 night
Miconazole	or	1 vaginal tablet	(100 mg)	14 nights
	or	2 vaginal tablets	(100 mg each)	7 nights
	or	1 coated tampon	(100 mg)	5 mornings and evenings
	or	5 g cream	(100 mg)	14 nights
		10 g cream	(200 mg)	7 nights
Econazole		1 vaginal tablet	(150 mg)	3 nights
Isoconazole		2 vaginal tablets	(300 mg each)	1 night
Ketoconazole		1 oral tablet	(200 mg)	5 mornings and evenings
	or	10 ml oral suspension	(200 mg)	5 mornings and evenings

clotrimazole, miconazole, econazole and isoconazole. In addition, non-specific vaginal antiseptics are sometimes prescribed. Vaginal preparations of antifungal drugs are available in a number of formulations (Table 10.1).

Treatment of vaginitis should continue throughout menstruation. If vulvitis is present, a cream formulation for local application should also be prescribed. The male partner should be treated with an antifungal cream if signs of infection are present. There is no need to advise against intercourse once treatment has been started.

If further tests are performed to confirm cure, vaginal specimens should not be taken until at least 72 to 96 hours after the end of treatment. This is because antifungal drugs have been found to persist in vaginal secretions for at least 48 hours after insertion of a single vaginal tablet (Odds & Macdonald 1981).

Nystatin was the first polyene antifungal to be applied to the treatment of vaginal candidosis. It is still one of the cheapest and most popular agents for the treatment of oral or vaginal candidosis and is the compound most often used for comparison in trials of new drugs for the treatment of these conditions. If patients with vaginal candidosis are to be treated with nystatin, one or two vaginal tablets (100 000 units each) should be inserted high in the vagina at bedtime for 14 consecutive nights, regardless of an intervening menstrual period. If vulvitis is a problem, nystatin cream should also be applied for 2 weeks.

Four imidazole derivatives are available in a number of topical formulations for the treatment of vaginal candidosis: clotrimazole, miconazole, econazole and isoconazole (see Table 10.1). These drugs give similar high cure rates at the end of the course of treatment and with all the compounds there is a similar low relapse rate. These drugs are safe and side-effects after topical application are uncommon. Transient local irritation has been reported on occasion.

Clotrimazole is available as 100 mg, 200 mg and 500 mg vaginal tablets, as a 2% cream and as a 10% cream. If 100 mg vaginal tablets are prescribed, one should be inserted for 6 consecutive nights. If preferred, one 200 mg tablet can be inserted for 3 nights. The 500 mg vaginal tablets are a recent introduction: a single tablet should be inserted at night. Short-term treatment is effective if the patient is suffering from vaginal candidosis for the first time (Masterton et al 1977). It can also be recommended for patients who reject the discipline of regimens requiring more than 1 week of treatment. Women with recurrent candidosis may require a prolonged course of treatment before cure is achieved.

Miconazole is available in tablet form, tampon form or as 2% cream for the treatment of vaginal candidosis. Patients can be given two vaginal tablets (100 mg each) which should be inserted at night for 1 week. If coated tampons are prescribed (100 mg miconazole nitrate each), one should be inserted morning and evening for 1 week. If miconazole cream is to be used, one full applicator should be placed high in the vagina at bedtime for 10 to 14 nights, or two full applicators can be inserted for 7 nights. Local sensitisation has necessitated discontinuation of treatment in the occasional patient.

The recommended treatment regimen for econazole is one vaginal tablet (150 mg econazole nitrate) for 3 consecutive nights. Econazole cream should be applied in the morning and evening if vulvitis is present. Occasional irritation has been reported following treatment.

The most recent imidazole derivative to be used in the topical treatment of vaginal candidosis is isoconazole. Like econazole it is an analogue of miconazole and has an almost identical structure. The manufacturers' recommended treatment regimen for patients with vaginal candidosis is two vaginal tablets (300 mg isoconazole nitrate each) to be inserted together at night.

The large number of topical preparations available and the number of different regimens that have been recommended attest to the need for further improvements in the treatment of women with vaginal candidosis. Recommended treatment regimens (Table 10.1) are not clearly related to differences between the imidazole drugs themselves, and may owe more to commercial considerations than to careful comparisons. Shorter regimens achieve better patient compliance and may be useful in uncomplicated cases, but treatment courses of less than 6 nights should be reserved for first episodes.

Oral treatment

Increased patient compliance might be achieved if an oral drug could be used. This would dispense with the need for local vulval, vaginal and separate gastrointestinal treatment. Ketoconazole, the first imidazole derivative to be licensed for oral administration to women with vaginal candidosis, has proved an effective treatment for this condition (Bisschop et al 1979; Cauwenbergh 1984). However, it has almost ceased to be prescribed to British patients with superficial fungal infection since its occasional fatal effects on the liver were publicised (Lewis et al 1984).

Itraconazole and fluconazole are two recent triazole antifungals which are at present undergoing clinical trials and are being developed for the oral treatment of vaginal candidosis. Initial results appear encouraging.

No mention has been made so far of the use of flucytosine (5-fluorocytosine) in the treatment of vaginal candidosis. This is not an oversight. The use of this drug in this condition is to be deprecated. Even though it is well absorbed and distributed after oral administration, resistant strains of C. albicans often appear during treatment (Scholer & Polak 1984).

Management of recurrent vaginal candidosis

Vaginal infection with C. albicans is a common condition but most women with this infection respond well to a short course of local medication. In the occasional patient, a prolonged course of local treatment may be required. Patients with recurring vaginal infection, however, present a difficult problem (Hurley 1975). These women often suffer from depression and psychosexual difficulties are not uncommon. How should the clinician manage these problem patients? To recognise that there is indeed a problem is of prime importance: often patients have received repeated courses of antifungal treatment without their difficulties being investigated. The clinician must point out that our understanding of factors leading to chronic vaginal infection with C. albicans is limited and must remain resolute in prescribing well proven regimens of treatment. This entails a careful consideration of numerous different regimens because folklore abounds on the subject of vaginal candidosis! Potential precipitating factors should be investigated. It is, however, rare to find such abnormalities.

If psychosexual problems are present, these should be dealt with at once. The sequence of events leading to the establishment of these problems is often initiated by dyspareunia occurring during an episode of acute candidosis. This leads to the anticipation of being hurt again, and this in turn inhibits normal vaginal lubrication. The consequence is further dyspareunia and more local trauma. By the time the patient is seen in the clinic, sexual intercourse may have become impossible because of vaginismus in the woman or premature ejaculation or even impotence in the man who is afraid of hurting his partner. The only useful approach to this problem is psychotherapeutic treatment with 'sensate focus' exercises (Kaplan 1974).

Treatment of an acute episode of vaginal candidosis in a woman with recurrent infection should be as short as possible compatible with cure. If treatment is successful, can further infection be prevented? Since it has been demonstrated that one potential source of vaginal infection is the gastrointestinal tract of the woman herself, should an attempt be made to eliminate C. albicans from this site by prescribing oral nystatin? This is a course of action that is often recommended, but there is no real evidence that simultaneous oral treatment with this drug is a useful adjunct to local vaginal treatment. Vellupillai & Thin (1977) detected no significant difference between the effect of combined local and oral nystatin treatment compared with local nystatin treatment alone. The patients were assessed 2 weeks after the end of treatment. Milne & Warnock (1979) found that oral treatment with nystatin did not affect the rate of cure or relapse among patients receiving local treatment for vaginal infection with C. albicans. Of 41 women with intestinal tract colonisation prior to oral treatment, 20 were still colonised at the end of treatment 2 weeks later and 27 were colonised after a further 6 weeks.

The mouth is another potential source of C. albicans, but it remains to be established whether this reservoir should be eliminated. Since C. albicans can be transmitted to or from the male partner, treatment of the genitalia of the consort will also be required if all potential sources of reinfection are to be eradicated. The consort's mouth might also require to be treated if orogenital contact is part of the patient's sexual behaviour. It seems clear that if the objective is eradication of all potential sources of reinfection, the breadth of treatment required might be considerable and could well add to the patient's psychological problems.

Even if C. albicans can be eradicated with local antifungal treatment, reinfection will often occur. Oral treatment with an imidazole or triazole antifungal might be more successful but there is at present insufficient published information regarding the effect of prolonged courses of these drugs on oral and intestinal colonisation with C. albicans, and there is concern about the toxic effects of ketoconazole.

Sobel (1985) has investigated the usefulness of intermittent prophylactic treatment with oral ketoconazole in the management of recurrent vaginal candidosis. Patients were given a short course of treatment, commencing with the onset of menstruation, for 3 months and then observed for a further 9 months. Although 24% of patients relapsed during the first 3 months, and a further 32% relapsed during the following 3 months, 37.5% remained asymptomatic for 12 months. Moreover, most of the women who relapsed suffered fewer infections with C. albicans than during the 12-month period prior to prophylactic treatment. Davidson & Mould (1978) obtained similar beneficial results in a trial of intermittent prophylactic treatment with topical clotrimazole. These reports are encouraging, but further work is needed for confirmation and to ascertain the optimum method and duration of prophylactic treatment.

The long-term management of patients with recurrent candidosis must take into account factors that could precipitate an acute episode. Although a number of factors have been implicated, the incriminating evidence is in no instance conclusive. Uncontrolled diabetes mellitus with glycosuria and increased glucose concentrations in vaginal secretions can lead to symptomatic candidosis, but this is not common. The role of antibiotics as a precipitating factor in vaginal candidosis is not proven, but most clinicians are agreed that these drugs should be prescribed with circumspection to patients with recurrent candidosis. The role of oral contraception in vaginal candidosis is contentious. Most of the earlier reports claiming that oral contraception was implicated in this condition were based on investigations of patients taking combined pills which contained at least 50 μg oestrogen. Most combined pills prescribed at present contain lesser amounts of oestrogen (30 μg). This could well account for recent reports that vaginal colonisation is no more common among women on oral contraception than among other women. Thus, there appears to be no valid reason for depriving patients of this method of birth control because of vaginal candidosis.

CANDIDOSIS OF THE MALE GENITALIA

The role of sexual transmission as a means of vaginal inoculation with *C. albicans* was mentioned earlier. Asymptomatic fungal colonisation of the penis has been found to occur in about 15–18% of men attending STD clinics (Rodin & Kolator 1976; Davidson 1977), but colonisation is four times more prevalent among contacts of women with vaginal candidosis (Davidson 1977). Typing the strains of *C. albicans* recovered from male and female partners has shown that both often harbour the same strain (Warnock et al 1979b; Odds et al 1983a). These findings suggest that sexual transmission of the fungus does occur, but it is not clear how common this is, or to what extent the man is the source or the recipient of infection.

In 1961 Harvard described two men with acute balanitis from whom *C. albicans* was isolated. These cases were characterised by itching, inflamed, weeping mucosal surfaces of the glans penis and the prepuce, on which bright red macules, sometimes covered with white membranes were noted. Catterall (1966) described eight men with balanoposthitis due to *C. albicans*, six of whom had partners with vaginal candidosis. Catterall also described a further group of four men who complained of soreness and irritation of the glans penis commencing 6 to 24 hours after sexual intercourse. On examination these men were found to have multiple small circular erosions of the glans. No fungus was found in smears or isolated in culture. The condition resolved without treatment, but the female partners of all four men were found to have vaginal candidosis. It was suggested that the signs of infection in these men were the result of an allergic reaction.

Clinical manifestations and diagnosis

In men, genital candidosis most often presents as a balanitis or balanoposthitis. Patients often complain of soreness or irritation of the glans penis; less often there is a subpreputial discharge. On examination maculopapular lesions with diffuse erythema of the glans are often present; white peeling patches are sometimes seen on the surface of the glans. On occasion, there is oedema and fissuring of the prepuce. Itching, scaling cutaneous lesions are sometimes found on the penis and scrotum or in the groins.

An acute fulminating oedematous form of balanoposthitis with ulceration of the penis and fissuring of the prepuce is one of the common presenting signs of diabetes mellitus (Waugh et al 1978). This is most often seen in middle-aged or older men.

On occasion a male contact of a woman with vaginal candidosis will complain of soreness and irritation of the glans penis soon after intercourse and lasting for 24 to 48 hours. These cases are believed to be the result of an allergic reaction (Catterall 1966).

The diagnosis of candidal balanitis should not be made on clinical grounds alone as there are other causes of balanitis and balanoposthitis (Waugh 1982). Specimens for mycological investigation should be taken from the coronal sulcus.

Treatment

Genital candidosis in men should be treated with local applications of an antifungal cream. Nystatin cream should be applied morning and evening for at least 2 weeks. Waugh et al (1978) prescribed clotrimazole cream for 1 week, applied morning and evening, and obtained a cure in 55 of 58 men (95%) after 3 weeks. Miconazole and econazole creams can also be used. The female contacts should also be investigated.

INTRAUTERINE CANDIDOSIS

Although symptomatic candidosis of the lower genital tract is one of the most common infections encountered in pregnant women, opinions differ as to whether asymptomatic women should be given antifungal treatment. The chief justification for such treatment is to prevent the occurrence of chronic vaginal candidosis and to prevent infection of the fetus or of the infant during birth.

Candidosis acquired in utero and manifest at birth is a rare condition. It was first reported in 1958 when Benirschke & Raphael described chorioamnionitis and funiculitis due to *C. albicans* infection associated with an anencephalic fetus. Since then more than 50 other cases have been reported (Whyte et al 1982). In 1968 Schweid & Hopkins reported the first case of spontaneous abortion associated with fetal candidosis. Their patient had had an intrauterine contraceptive device in place for 13 months. She aborted at 13 weeks' gestation. Subsequent reports have emphasised the association between fetal candidosis and the presence of an intrauterine contraceptive device (Whyte et al 1982).

Clinical manifestations and diagnosis

The lesions resulting from candidosis acquired in utero have been well described (Aterman 1968). The infection appears as multiple small yellow-white pinpoint lesions scattered over the surface of the umbilical cord. In some instances the fungus affects the fetus and in live births such infections manifest as the characteristic lesions of congenital cutaneous candidosis (see below). Umbilical cord lesions are often associated with other lesions which are less characteristic and take the form of diffuse, generalised chorioamnionitis.

Histological investigation of fetal organs in cases of spontaneous abortion associated with fetal candidosis has revealed the presence of both morphological forms of *C. albicans* in the fetal membranes, lungs and gastrointestinal tract (Schweid & Hopkins 1968; Ho & Aterman 1970).

Mode of infection

Intrauterine candidosis is considered to be the result of ascending infection of the maternal genital tract. It is not clear whether *C. albicans* can penetrate the intact amniotic membranes or whether infection of the amniotic fluid is consequent upon overt or subclinical membrane rupture. Premature rupture of the membranes has not been noted in most reported cases (Whyte et al 1982). Indeed, in most cases the membranes ruptured during parturition while the clinical manifestions in the infant were such as to suggest that infection was well established before the onset of labour.

It is apparent that once the amniotic fluid is infected with *C. albicans*, involvement of the fetal skin, surface of the umbilical cord, fetal lungs and gastrointestinal tract is bound to occur. The observed distribution of lesions indicates that infection of the fetus follows infection of the amniotic fluid and that aspiration rather than haematogenous dissemination is involved.

NEONATAL CANDIDOSIS

Neonatal infection with *C. albicans* is a common paediatric problem. Oral thrush is the most prevalent form of neonatal candidosis, occurring in about 5% of infants. Although *C. albicans* can occur as an innocuous commensal in the mouth later in life, its presence in the mouth of neonates is associated with florid clinical signs of candidosis. Indeed Taschdjian & Kozinn (1957) demonstrated that in 99% of infants the detection of *C. albicans* in the mouth presaged the onset of clinical signs of oral thrush. The presence of this fungus in the intestinal contents of the newborn infant has been found to be associated with perianal lesions and rashes (Kozinn et al 1957; Taschdjian & Kozinn 1957). In most cases, however, *C. albicans* is not the principal cause of such rashes (Dixon et al 1969, 1972).

In 1960, Sonnenschein et al reported a case of candidosis in which widespread, diffuse, macular, papular, vesicular and pustular skin lesions that contained *C. albicans* arose on an infant soon after its birth. The condition was termed 'congenital cutaneous candidosis' and it was considered that the infection had arisen in utero. There have since been a number of reports of similar cases. The condition has a benign course and the lesions often clear after several weeks, or sooner with topical antifungal treatment.

Unifocal and multifocal forms of deep candidosis can occur in low-birth-weight infants requiring prolonged neonatal intensive care (Baley et al 1984; Johnson et al 1984). Meningitis occurs more often than in older patients (Faix 1984) and is sometimes associated with arthritis and osteomyelitis (Klein et al 1972; Rao & Myers 1979). Although uncommon, isolated renal infection can also occur and result in ureteric obstruction and renal failure (Pappu et al 1984). Prolonged total parenteral nutrition, central arterial and venous catheters and broad-spectrum antibacterial treatment have been cited as important predisposing factors.

Clinical manifestation and diagnosis

In infants with oral thrush, the characteristic white, raised lesions erupt on the buccal mucosa, the tongue, the gums and the mucosa of the throat. The lesions become confluent and form elevated white patches. On removal, an eroded, bleeding surface is left. The lesions are often painless although erosion and ulceration of the mucosa can occur.

The clinical manifestations of oral thrush are characteristic, but the diagnosis should be confirmed by the isolation of the fungus in culture from smears or scrapings of lesions and the detection of blastospores and mycelial forms on microscopic examination of smears or scrapings.

In infants with congenital cutaneous candidosis, the lesions which are present at birth or soon thereafter are a diffuse, maculopapular, vesicular rash distributed over the face, neck, trunk and limbs (Gellis et al 1976). Pustules are common and bullae appear on occasion. Pronounced desquamation follows the acute phase. There is no fever or other constitutional sign and the infant thrives despite the widespread skin involvement. Concomitant oral thrush is uncommon. Demonstration of blastospore and mycelial forms of C. albicans in direct smears and isolation of the fungus in cultures from the lesions establishes the diagnosis.

Elevated temperatures are common in disseminated neonatal candidosis, but there may be no focal signs. Even in meningitis, focal signs and meningism may be seen in less than 50% of cases (Chesney et al 1978; Rao & Myers 1979) and diagnosis depends on isolation of the fungus. C. albicans is often found in superficial sites, but diagnosis of disseminated infection requires isolation from deep sites or from blood. The discrimination between sepsis and transient candidaemia is important in older patients, as removal of indwelling intravascular catheters can lead to the resolution of transient infection in adults. This does not occur in infants and there are few published reports of candidaemia resolving in small infants without treatment (Baley et al 1984; Johnson et al 1984). Frequent culture of the urine as well as fundoscopic examination for signs of endophthalmitis (Baley et al 1981) is most useful because of the predilection of C. albicans for these sites. If cutaneous lesions occur, culture of these may confirm the diagnosis. C. albicans is often difficult to isolate from the cerebrospinal fluid and repeated cultures are often required. Large samples are recommended and should be obtained (if possible) from the ventricles in infants.

The clinical and radiological manifestations of candidal osteomyelitis and arthritis are similar to those of other infections at these sites (Yousefzadeh & Jackson 1980). Culture of joint effusions and necrotic tissue should permit the diagnosis.

The detection of C. albicans mannan antigen in the serum and cerebrospinal fluid of infants with disseminated candidosis has been reported as useful in the diagnosis of this condition (Schreiber et al 1984). Serial measurement of antigen levels could be useful in assessing the response to treatment.

Mode of infection

Neonatal oral candidosis is more common in infants born of mothers with vaginal candidosis than in other infants (Woodruff & Hesseltine 1938; Kozinn et al 1958; Schnell 1982b). This suggests that infection occurs when the infant takes in some of the vaginal contents during parturition. The presence of C. albicans in the mouth as soon as 24 hours after birth bears out this suggestion. It has been recommended that neonatal colonisation from the mother should be prevented by maternal screening at 34 weeks with topical antifungal treatment of positives (Schnell 1982b). On the other hand, prevalence of the fungus in the mouths of neonates in intensive care units tends to increase during subsequent days and weeks (Lay & Russell 1977) and it has been suggested that the hands of staff and mothers are a further potential source of oral candidosis in infants (Jennison 1966; Schnell 1982b). Occasional outbreaks have occurred from equipment, such as teats (Cremer & De Groot

1967). Disseminated forms of candidosis in infants appear to be haematogenous in origin.

Treatment

In most infants with oral thrush, the lesions clear within 2 weeks of commencing antifungal treatment. The condition can be treated with 1 ml nystatin suspension (100 000 units per ml) which should be dropped into the mouth after each feed or at 4 to 6 hour intervals. If swallowing is not possible, the mouth should be well swabbed with nystatin suspension. Other topical antifungals, such as miconazole gel, may also be useful.

The prognosis in congenital cutaneous candidosis is good and spontaneous cure often occurs after several weeks. The use of topical antifungal treatment (nystatin, amphotericin B, or an imidazole) will hasten the cure.

Disseminated neonatal candidosis should be treated with a combination of amphotericin B and flucytosine (Chesney et al 1978; Lilien et al 1978). Amphotericin B, in incremental doses up to 0.6 to 0.8 mg/kg/day, is given by slow intravenous infusion. It is essential in this serious condition to advance rapidly to therapeutic dose levels. Flucytosine, 150 mg/kg/day, may often be given by mouth; there is an intravenous preparation available. If meningitis does not rapidly respond to this regimen, small doses of amphotericin B may be given intraventricularly (McDougall et al 1982).

Intravenous miconazole has been used in the treatment of neonatal candidosis, but McDougall et al (1982) reported failure of this drug in two patients who later responded to the amphotericin B–flucytosine combination. De Mol et al (1982) reported failure of intravenous and intrathecal miconazole to sterilise the cerebrospinal fluid of an infant with *C. albicans* meningitis and osteomyelitis. The child responded to a short course of amphotericin B.

CONCLUSION

This chapter has emphasised the central role of vaginal infection with *C. albicans*, both as one of the most common forms of human candidosis and as responsible in most cases for infection in consorts and offspring. Recent investigations have increased our understanding of the pathogenesis of vaginal candidosis, and of the different modes of transmission of the causal fungus. More work, however, will be required before treatment regimens and methods of prevention can be planned on an altogether rational basis. Just as diagnosis and management of vaginal candidosis require close collaboration between the clinician and the microbiologist, so improved understanding of this condition will require the co-operation of microbiologists, immunologists and clinicians.

REFERENCES

Aterman K 1968 Pathology of Candida infection of the umbilical cord. American Journal of Clinical Pathology 49: 798–804

Baley J E, Annable W L, Kliegman R M 1981 Candida endophthalmitis in the premature infant. Journal of Pediatrics 98: 458–461

Baley J E, Kliegman R M, Fanaroff A A 1984 Disseminated fungal infections in very low-birth-weight infants: clinical manifestations and epidemiology. Pediatrics 73: 144–152

Benirschk K, Raphael S I 1958 Candida albicans infection of the amniotic sac. American Journal of Obstetrics and Gynecology 75: 200–202

Bisschop M P J M, Merkus J M W M, Scheijgrond H, Van Cutsem J, Van de Kuy J 1979 Treatment of vaginal candidiasis with ketoconazole, a new orally active antimycotic. European Journal of Obstetrics, Gynecology and Reproductive Biology 9: 253–259

Bland P B, Rakoff A E, Pincus I J 1937 Experimental vaginal and cutaneous moniliasis: clinical and laboratory studies of certain monilias associated with vaginal, oral and cutaneous thrush. Archives of Dermatology and Syphilology 36: 760–780

Cartwright R Y 1980 Opportunistic mycoses of various body sites. In: Speller D C E (ed) Antifungal chemotherapy. Wiley, Chichester, pp 365–404

Carroll C J, Hurley R, Stanley V C 1973 Criteria for diagnosis of candida vulvovaginitis in pregant women. Journal of Obstetrics and Gynaecology of the British Commonwealth 80: 258–263

Catterall R D 1966 Urethritis and balanitis due to Candida. In: Winner H I, Hurley R (eds) Symposium on Candida infections. Churchill Livingstone, London, pp 113–118

Cauwenbergh G 1984 Ketoconazole, international experience in vaginal candidosis. In: Eliot B W (ed) Oral therapy in vaginal candidosis (Medicine Publishing Foundation Symposium Series 13). Medical Education Services, Oxford, pp 33–36

Chesney P J, Justman R A, Bogdanowicz W M 1978 Candida meningitis in newborn infants: a review and report of combined amphotericin B-flucytosine therapy. Johns Hopkins

Medical Journal 142: 155–160

Cohen R, Roth F J, Degado E, Ahearn D G, Kalser M H 1969 Fungal flora of the normal human small and large intestine. New England Journal of Medicine 280: 638–641

Cremer G, De Groot W P 1967 An epidemic of thrush in a premature nursery. Dermatologia 135: 107–114

Davidson F 1977 Yeasts and circumcision in the male. British Journal of Venereal Diseases 53: 121–122

Davidson F, Mould R F 1978 Recurrent genital candidosis in women and the effect of intermittent prophylactic treatment. British Journal of Venereal Diseases 54: 176–183

Davidson F, Hayes J P, Hussein S 1977 Recurrent genital candidosis and iron metabolism. British Journal of Venereal Diseases 53: 123–125

De Mol P, Laureys W, Dorchy H 1982 Neonatal meningitis due to Candida albicans, associated with osteomyelitis; failure to respond to miconazole. Journal of Infection 5: 195–197

De Sousa H M, Van Uden N 1960 The mode of infection and reinfection in yeast vulvovaginitis. American Journal of Obstetrics and Gynecology 80: 1096–100

Diddle A W, Gardner W H, Williamson P J, O'Connor K A 1969 Oral contraceptive medications and vulvovaginal candidiasis. Obstetrics and Gynecology 34: 373–379

Dixon P N, Warin R P, English M P 1969 Role of Candida albicans infection in napkin rashes. British Medical Journal 2: 23–27

Dixon P N, Warin R P, English M P 1972 Alimentary Candida albicans and napkin rashes. British Journal of Dermatology 86: 458–462

Douglas L J, Houston J G, McCourtie J 1981 Adherence of Candida albicans to human buccal epithelial cells after growth on different carbon sources. FEMS Microbiology Letters 12: 241–243

Elegbe I A, Elegbe I 1983 Quantitative relationships of Candida albicans infections and dressing patterns in Nigerian women. American Journal of Public Health 73: 450–452

English M P 1974 Identifying yeasts. Medical Laboratory Technology 31: 327–333

Faix R G 1984 Systemic Candida infections in infants in intensive care nurseries: high incidence of central nervous system involvement. Journal of Pediatrics 105: 616–622

Garcia Tamayo J, Castillo G, Martinez A J 1982 Human genital candidosis. Histochemistry, scanning and transmission electron microscopy. Acta Cytologica (Baltimore) 26: 7–14

Gellis S S, Feingold M, Kozinn P J, Tariq A A, Reale M R, Rudolph N 1976 Picture of the month: congenital cutaneous candidiasis. American Journal of Diseases of Children 130: 291–292

Goldacre M J, Watt B, Loudon N, Milne L J R, Loudon J D O, Vessey M P 1979 Vaginal microbial flora in normal young women. British Medical Journal 1: 1450–1453

Gough D 1979 The influence of dosage and duration of administration of miconazole on the cure and relapse of candidal vaginitis. Royal Society of Medicine International Congress and Symposium Series 7: 15–20

Gough P M, Warnock D W, Richardson M D, Mansell N J, King J M 1984 IgA and IgG antibodies to Candida albicans in the genital tract secretions of women with or without vaginal candidosis. Sabouraudia: Journal of Medical and Veterinary Mycology 22: 265–271

Gough P M, Warnock D W, Turner A, Richardson M D, Johnson E M 1985 Candidosis of the genital tract in non-pregnant women. European Journal of Obstetrics, Gynecology and Reproductive Biology 19: 237–246

Harvard B M 1961 Acute monilial balanitis. Journal of Urology 85: 374–376

Higgs J M, Wells R S 1972 Chronic mucocutaneous candidiasis: associated abnormalities of iron metabolisms. British Journal of Dermatology 86 (suppl 8): 88–102

Hilton A L, Warnock D W 1975 Vaginal candidiasis and the role of the digestive tract as a source of infection. British Journal of Obstetrics and Gynaecology 82: 922–926

Ho C Y, Aterman K 1970 Infection of the fetus by Candida in a spontaneous abortion. American Journal of Obstetrics and Gynecology 106: 705–710

Hobbs J R, Brigden D, Davidson F, Kahan M, Oates J K 1977 Immunological aspects of candidal vaginitis. Proceedings of the Royal Society of Medicine 70 (suppl 4): 11–13

Hopwood V, Evans E G V, Carney J A 1985 Rapid diagnosis of vaginal candidosis by latex particle agglutination. Journal of Clinical Pathology 38: 455–458

Hurley R 1975 Inveterate vaginal thrush. Practitioner 215: 753–756

Hurley R 1981 Recurrent Candida infection. Clinics in Obstetrics and Gynaecology 8: 209–214

Hurley R, De Louvois J 1979 Candida vaginitis. Postgraduate Medical Journal 55: 645–647

Hurley R, Leask B G S, Faktor J A, De Fonseka C I 1973 Incidence and distribution of yeast species and Trichomonas vaginalis in the vagina of pregnant women. Journal of Obstetrics and Gynaecology of the British Commonwealth 80: 252–257

Jennison R F 1966 Candida infections in a maternity hospital. In: Winner H I, Hurley R (eds) Symposium on candida infections. Churchill Livingstone, London, pp 102–112

Johnson D E, Thompson T R, Green T P, Ferrieri P 1984 Systemic candidiasis in very low-birth-weight infants (<1500 grams). Pediatrics 73: 138–143

Kaplan H S 1974 The new sex therapy. Bailliere Tindall, London

Kearns M J, Davies P, Smith H 1983 Variability of the adherence of Candida albicans strains to human buccal epithelial cells: inconsistency of differences between strains related to virulence. Sabouraudia 21: 93–98

Kimura L H, Pearsall N N 1980 Relationship between germination of Candida albicans and increased adherence to human buccal epithelial cells. Infection and Immunity 28: 464–468

King R D, Lee J C, Morris A L 1980 Adherence of Candida albicans and other Candida species to mucosal epithelial cells. Infection and Immunity 27: 667–674

Klein J D, Yamaguchi T, Horlick S P 1972 Neonatal candidiasis, meningitis and arthritis: observations and a review of the literature. Journal of Pediatrics 81: 31–34

Kozinn P, Taschdjian C L, Dragutsky D, Minsky A 1957 Cutaneous candidiasis in early infancy and childhood. Pediatrics 20: 827–834

Kozinn P J, Taschdjian C L, Wiener H, Dragutsky D, Minsky A 1958 Neonatal candidiasis. Pediatric Clinics of North America 5: 803–815

Kwon-Chung K J, Lehman D, Good C, Magee P T 1985 Genetic evidence for role of extracellular proteinase in virulence of Candida albicans. Infection and Immunity 49: 571–575

Lay K M, Russell C 1977 Candida species and yeasts in mouths of infants from a special care unit of a maternity hospital. Archives of Disease in Childhood 54: 794–796

Lewis J H, Zimmerman H J, Benson G D 1984 Hepatic injury associated with ketoconazole treatment. Gastroenterology 86: 503–513

Lilien L D, Ramamurthy R S, Pildes R S 1978 Candida albicans meningitis in a premature neonate successfully treated with 5-fluorocytosine and amphotericin B: a case report and review of the literature. Pediatrics 61: 57–61

Loose D S, Schurman D J, Feldman D 1981 A corticosteroid binding protein and endogenous ligand in C. albicans indicating a possible steroid-receptor system. Nature (London) 293: 477–479

Loose D S, Stevens D A, Schurman D J, Feldman D 1983 Distribution of a corticosterone-binding protein in Candida and other fungal genera. Journal of General Microbiology 129: 2379–2385

McCreight M C, Warnock D W 1982 Enhanced differentiation of isolates of Candida albicans using a modified resistogram method. Mykosen 25: 589–598

McCreight M C, Warnock D W, Martin M V 1985 Resistogram typing of Candida albicans isolates from oral and cutaneous sites in irradiated patients. Sabouraudia: Journal of Medical and Veterinary Mycology 23: 403–406

Macdonald F, Odds F C 1980 Inducible proteinase of Candida albicans in diagnostic serology and in the pathogenesis of systemic candidosis. Journal of Medical Microbiology 13: 423–435

Macdonald F, Odds F C 1983 Virulence for mice of a proteinase-secreting strain of Candida albicans and a proteinase-deficient mutant. Journal of General Microbiology 129: 431–438

McDougall P N, Fleming P J, Speller D C E, Daish P, Speidel B D 1982 Neonatal systemic candidiasis: a failure to respond to intravenous miconazole in two neonates. Archives of Disease in Childhood 57: 884–886

McLennan M T, Smith J M, McLennan C E 1972 Diagnosis of vaginal mycosis and trichomoniasis. Reliability of cytologic smear, wet smear and culture. Obstetrics and Gynecology 40: 231–234

Masterton G, Henderson J N, Napier I R, Moffett M 1976 Vaginal candidosis. British Medical Journal 1: 712–713

Masterton G, Napier I R, Henderson J N, Roberts J E 1977 Three-day clotrimazole treatment in candidal vulvovaginitis. British Journal of Venereal Diseases 53: 126–128

Miles M R, Olsen L, Rogers A 1977 Recurrent vaginal candidiasis. Importance of an intestinal reservoir. Journal of the American Medical Association 238: 1836–1837

Milne J D, Warnock D W 1977 Antibodies to Candida albicans in human cervicovaginal secretions. British Journal of Venereal Diseases 53: 375–378

Milne J D, Warnock D W 1979 Effect of simultaneous oral and vaginal treatment on the rate of cure and relapse in vaginal candidosis. British Journal of Venereal Diseases 55: 362–365

Morton R S, Rashid S 1977 Candidal vaginitis: natural history, predisposing factors and prevention. Proceedings of the Royal Society of Medicine 70 (suppl 4): 3–6

Odds F C 1977 Cure and relapse with antifungal therapy. Proceedings of the Royal Society of Medicine 70 (suppl 4): 24–28

Odds F C 1979 Candida and candidosis. Leicester University Press, Leicester

Odds F C 1982 Genital candidosis. Clinical and Experimental Dermatology 7: 345–354

Odds F C, Abbott A B 1980 A simple system for the presumptive identification of Candida albicans and differentiation of strains within the species. Sabouraudia 18: 301–317

Odds F C, Hierholzer J C 1973 Purification and properties of a glycoprotein acid phosphatase from Candida albicans. Journal of Bacteriology 114: 257–266

Odds F C, Macdonald F 1981 Persistence of miconazole in vaginal secretions after single applications. Implications for the treatment of vaginal candidosis. British Journal of Venereal Diseases 57: 400–401

Odds F C, Abbott A B, Reed T A G, Willmott F E 1983a Candida albicans strain types from the genitalia of patients with and without candida infection. European Journal of Obstetrics, Gynecology and Reproductive Biology 15: 37–43

Odds F C, Abbott A B, Stiller R L, Scholer H J, Polak A, Stevens D A 1983b Analysis of Candida albicans phenotypes from different geographical and anatomical sources. Journal of Clinical Microbiology 18: 849–857

Oriel J D, Partridge B M, Denny M J, Coleman J C 1972 Genital yeast infections. British Medical Journal 4: 761–764

Pappu L D, Purohit D M, Bradford B F, Turner W R, Levkoff A H 1984 Primary renal candidiasis in two preterm neonates. Report of cases and review of literature on renal candidiasis in infancy. American Journal of Diseases of Children 138: 923–926

Powell B L, Drutz D J 1983 Confirmation of corticosterone and progesterone binding activity in Candida albicans. Journal of Infectious Diseases 147: 359

Powell B L, Drutz D J, Huppert M, Sun S H 1983 Relationship of progesterone- and estradiol-binding proteins in Coccidioides immitis to coccidioidal dissemination in pregnancy. Infection and Immunity 40: 478–485

Powell B L, Frey C L, Drutz D J 1984 Identification of a 17B-estradiol binding protein in Candida albicans and Candida (Torulopsis) glabrata. Experimental Mycology 8: 304–313

Price M F, Cawson R A 1977 Phospholipase activity in Candida albicans. Sabouraudia 15: 179–185

Rao H K, Myers G J 1979 Candida meningitis in the newborn. Southern Medical Journal 72: 1468–1471

Rodin P, Kolator B 1976 Carriage of yeasts on the penis. British Medical Journal 1: 1123–1124

Samaranayake L P, MacFarlane T W 1981 The adhesion of the yeast Candida albicans to epithelial cells of human origin in vitro. Archives of Oral Biology 26: 815–820

Samaranayake L P, MacFarlane T W 1982 The effect of dietary carbohydrates on the in-vitro adhesion of Candida albicans to epithelial cells. Journal of Medical Microbiology 15: 511–517

Schnell J D 1982a Investigations into the pathoaetiology and diagnosis of vaginal mycoses. Chemotherapy 28 (suppl 1): 14–21

Schnell J D 1982b Epidemiology and the prevention of peripartal mycoses. Chemotherapy 28 (suppl 1): 66–72

Scholer H J, Polak A 1984 Resistance to antifungal agents. In: Bryan L E (ed) Antimicrobial drug resistance. Academic Press, New York, pp 393–459

Schreiber J R, Maynard E, Lew M A 1984 Candida antigen detection in two premature neonates with disseminated candidiasis. Pediatrics 74: 838–841

Schweid A I, Hopkins G B 1968 Monilial chorionitis associated with an intrauterine contraceptive device. Obstetrics and Gynecology 31: 719–721

Segal E, Soroka A, Schechter A 1984 Correlative relationship between adherence of Candida albicans to human vaginal epithelial cells in vitro and candidal vaginitis. Sabouraudia: Journal of Medical and Veterinary Mycology 22: 191–200

Sobel J D 1984 Pathogenesis of vaginal candidosis. In: Eliot B W (ed) Oral therapy in vaginal candidosis (Medicine Publishing Foundation Symposium Series 13). Medical Education Services, Oxford, pp 1–13

Sobel J D 1985 Management of recurrent vulvovaginal candidiasis with intermittent ketoconazole prophylaxis. Obstetrics and Gynecology 65: 435–440

Sobel J D, Myers P G, Kaye D, Levison M E 1981 Adherence of Candida albicans to human vaginal and buccal epithelial cells. Journal of Infectious Diseases 143: 76–82

Sobel J D, Muller G, Buckley H R 1984 Critical role of germ tube formation in the pathogenesis of candidal vaginitis. Infection and Immunity 44: 576–580

Sonnenschein H, Clarke H L, Taschdjian C L 1960 Congenital cutaneous candidiasis in a premature infant. American Journal of Diseases of Children 99: 81–85

Stone H H, Geheber C E, Kolb L D, Kitchens W R 1973 Alimentary tract colonization by Candida albicans. Journal of Surgical Research 14: 273–276

Taschdjian C L, Kozinn P J 1957 Laboratory and clinical studies on candidiasis in the newborn infant. Journal of Pediatrics 50: 425–433

Thin R N, Atia W L, Parker J D, Nicol C S, Canti G 1975 Value of Papanicolaou-stained smears in the diagnosis of trichomoniasis, candidiasis and cervical herpes simplex virus infections in women. British Journal of Venereal Diseases 51: 116–118

Thin R N, Leighton M, Dixon M J 1977 How often is genital yeast infection sexually transmitted? British Medical Journal 2: 93–94

Valdimarsson H, Higgs J M, Wells R S, Yamamura M, Hobbs J R, Holt P J L 1973 Immune abnormalities associated with chronic mucocutaneous candidiasis. Cellular Immunology 6: 348–361

Vellupillai S, Thin R N 1977 Treatment of vulvovaginal yeast infection with nystatin. Practitioner 219: 897–901

Vudhichamnong K, Walker D M, Ryley H C 1982 The effect of secretory immunoglobulin A on the in vitro adherence of the yeast Candida albicans to human oral epithelial cells. Archives of Oral Biology 27: 617–621

Waldman R H, Cruz J M, Rowe D S 1972a Immunoglobulin levels and antibody to Candida albicans in human cervicovaginal secretions. Clinical and Experimental Immunology 10: 427–434

Waldman R H, Cruz J M, Rowe D S 1972b Intravaginal immunization of humans with Candida albicans. Journal of Immunology 109: 662–664

Warnock D W, Speller D C E, Day J K, Farrell A J 1979a Resistogram method for differentiation of strains of Candida albicans. Journal of Applied Bacteriology 46: 571–578

Warnock D W, Speller D C E, Milne J D, Hilton A L, Kershaw P I 1979b Epidemiological investigation of patients with vulvovaginal candidosis. Application of a resistogram method for strain differentiation of Candida albicans. British Journal of Venereal Diseases 55: 357–361

Waugh M A 1982 Clinical presentation of candidal balanitis: its differential diagnosis and treatment. Chemotherapy 28 (suppl 1): 56–60

Waugh M A, Evans E G V, Nayyar K C, Fong R 1978 Clotrimazole in the treatment of candidal balanitis in men; with incidental observations on diabetic candidal balanoposthitis. British Journal of Venereal Diseases 54: 184–186

Whyte R K, Hussain Z, de Sa D 1982 Antenatal infections with Candida species. Archives of Disease in Childhood 57: 528–535

Witkin S S, Yu I R, Ledger W J 1983 Inhibition of Candida albicans-induced lymphocyte proliferation by lymphocytes and sera from women with recurrent vaginitis. American Journal of Obstetrics and Gynecology 147: 809–811

Woodruff P W, Hesseltine H C 1938 Relationship of oral thrush to vaginal mycosis and incidence of each. American Journal of Obstetrics and Gynecology 36: 467–471

Yousefzadeh D K, Jackson J H 1980 Neonatal and infantile candidal arthritis with or without osteomyelitis: a clinical and radiographical review of 21 cases. Skeletal Radiology 5: 77–90

Oculogenital chlamydia*
J Schachter

In western industrialized societies *Chlamydia trachomatis* is recognised as one of the most common of the sexually transmitted agents (Schachter et al 1975a). For many years this organism was considered a 'large virus'. It was mainly of interest to ophthalmologists because it caused trachoma (the world's leading cause of preventable blindness) in many developing countries and was also responsible for sporadic cases of conjunctivitis in industrialised communities (Jones 1975). Indeed ophthalmologists recognised the genital tract reservoir for *C. trachomatis* in the first decade of this century. During the following 50 to 60 years most research on oculogenital *C. trachomatis* as a cause of human disease was undertaken by opthalmologists. Thus chlamydial cervical infections and non-gonococcal urethritis were described by 1910 (Lindner 1911). These conditions were related epidemiologically to a non-gonococcal form of opthalmia neonatorum (inclusion conjunctivitis of the newborn (ICN); Thygeson & Mengert 1936).

Aetiological diagnosis was always cytological (i.e. inclusion demonstration). Later complications such as salpingitis were also noted in women whose infants had developed ICN. Only with the advent of modern tissue culture isolation procedures has it become possible to study large groups of patients. This has resulted in the expanding clinical syndromes associated with these infections.

While these studies have indicated a high prevalence of chlamydial infections and identified serious systemic complications, it has been disappointing that characteristic clinical entities have not been defined so that many of the chlamydial infections still fit into the background of 'non-specific genital tract disease'. Thus accurate diagnosis requires the availability of microbiological procedures for chlamydial diagnosis which are still not readily available. This is particularly unfortunate because these infections are relatively easy to treat and have a major public health impact. It is currently estimated in the United States that chlamydial infections are twice as prevalent as gonococcal infections and probably cost about the same in terms of public health dollars spent to deal with the infections and their complications (NIAID 1981).

MICROBIOLOGY

Chlamydiae have been placed in their own order (Chlamydiales) and their own family (Chlamydiaceae) on the basis of a unique growth cycle (Page 1974). The organism is an obligate intracellular parasite and it selectively induces phagocytosis by a susceptible host cell. The infectious particle—the elementary body—attaches to the surface of the susceptible cell and is ingested in a phagocytic process. It remains within a phagosome throughout the growth cycle. Approximately 8 hours after ingestion the elementary body has reorganised into a metabolically active and dividing particle called the reticulate body or initial body. This particle will predominate for approximately another 18 to 24 hours into the growth cycle, during which it synthesises its own macromolecules and divides by binary fission. At approximately 24 to 30 hours into the growth cycle the reticulate bodies again undergo a reorganisation, this time into the elementary bodies which are released when the cell bursts. Once released into the extracellular environment

---

* This term refers to non-lymphogranuloma venereum *Chlamydia trachomatis* strains.

they can initiate infection in other susceptible host cells.

There are two species in the genus *Chlamydia*. *Chlamydia psittaci* is the causative agent of psittacosis and is virtually ubiquitous amongst avian species; it is a common pathogen in domestic mammals where it causes a number of diseases of economic importance. This organism causes zoonotic infections, although there is some evidence suggesting that certain *C. psittaci* strains may circulate among humans. *C. trachomatis*, on the other hand, is (with the exception of a few strains of rodent origin) a strictly human pathogen which depends on person to person transmission for its persistence. There are two biotypes within the genus *C. trachomatis*. The biotypes may also be identified on serological grounds (Grayston & Wang 1975). The lymphogranuloma venereum biotype (serotypes L1, L2 and L3) causes the serious systemic sexually transmitted infection, lymphogranuloma venereum. The other *C. trachomatis* serotypes (often referred to as the oculogenital chlamydiae) cause trachoma, inclusion conjunctivitis and the common genital tract infections. Serotypes A, B, Ba and C are associated with hyperendemic blinding trachoma. Serotypes D to K are associated with sporadic cases of conjunctivitis but are the common genital tract pathogens. Thus, there are 15 serotypes currently recognised. The lymphogranuloma venereum strains are much more invasive in vivo and appear to be much less selective in terms of susceptible cells or in cell receptors.

The *Chlamydia* are recognised as bacteria, despite the fact that they are obligatory intracellular parasites, because they contain both nucleic acids (RNA and DNA) and have a complex cell wall structure similar in constituents to the gram-negative cell wall (although muramic acid is lacking; Moulder 1964, 1966; Schachter & Caldwell 1980). They are sensitive to a wide variety of broad-spectrum antibiotics and have limited metabolic capabilities. They, however, do not generate their own adenosine triphosphate. It is likely that this defect restricts them to an intracellular life cycle because they need the host cell's adenosine triphosphate to fuel their own metabolic processes. All chlamydiae are sensitive to tetracyclines and macrolides and appear to be resistant to the action of aminoglycosides.

LABORATORY DIAGNOSIS

There are several methods of diagnosing chlamydial infections of the female genital tract (Schachter 1985). *Chlamydia trachomatis* infection produces typical intracytoplasmic inclusions which can be demonstrated by cytological methods. Cytologic tests, such as Giemsa stain, are time consuming and relatively insensitive. Papanicolaou stain is not useful for chlamydial diagnosis. The introduction of monoclonal antibody technology provides considerable improvement in cytological diagnosis and may make chlamydial diagnostic tests much more widely available. Other non-culture methods of diagnosis have been introduced. These include antigen detection by enzyme immunoassay procedures.

Chlamydial infections are also accompanied by abundant antibody responses that can be measured by a number of serological tests. Because of a high background of antibody in sexually active populations, serological tests are not particularly useful (including those which measure antibody in local secretions) in routine diagnosis. It is difficult to demonstrate rising titres because of the natural history of the infections (patients are often seen as chronic carriers rather than in acute stages of infection) and the predictive value of positive tests tends to be relatively low (Schachter et al 1979).

The agent can be isolated in appropriate cell culture systems. It is clear that the tissue culture isolation procedures represent the diagnostic method of choice. Isolation is probably more expensive in most settings than the non-culture methods of diagnosis. In expert hands, it is more sensitive than the non-culture methods and has the obvious advantage of not having any false positive results. However, the necessity for maintaining a tissue culture laboratory has severly restricted access to this methodology.

Isolation

The most commonly used isolation techniques use McCoy cells (a murine cell line which carries an erroneous label of a human synovial cell line) which have been treated with an antimetabolite such as cycloheximide to restrict the cell's growth and provide an advantage to the chlamydiae (Ripa & Mardh 1977). Clinical specimens to be tested generally are swabs or scrapings collected from the anatomical sites being sampled. It is imperative that adequate samples of epithelial cells are collected because culture of discharges is inadequate. Biopsy specimens may also be collected. Specimens are usually collected into a transport medium which contains antibiotics (aminoglycosides and antifungals) which are inactive against *C. trachomatis* but can inhibit the growth of other bacteria or fungi commonly found in these sites. The specimen is then transported to the laboratory where it is inoculated into cell monolayers by centrifugation to enhance contact between cell monolayer and organism. After an appropriate incubation period (24 to 72 hours, depending on stains being used) the monolayers are stained by iodine, Giemsa or immunofluorescent procedures to detect the intracytoplasmic inclusions (Darougar et al 1972; Thomas et al 1977; Schachter 1985). This procedure requires a tissue culture laboratory but can be performed readily in any setting where virus diagnosis is available. While it is the most sensitive diagnostic test, the sensitivity is clearly less than 100%, probably of the order of 75 to 85%.

Cytology

Inclusions can be demonstrated by immunofluorescent or Giemsa stain. The Giemsa technique is the classical procedure which was originally used by ophthalmologists to define the epidemiology of human infection with *C. trachomatis*. These procedures are relatively insensitive (immunofluorescence is superior to Giemsa), being positive at best in only 40 to 60% of cervical samples that would yield chlamydiae (Schachter & Dawson 1977). Adequate samples of epithelial cells must be obtained since the organism cannot be identified after the cells have burst and the particles have been released into the discharge. These procedures are not recommended for routine diagnosis as they are time consuming, requiring up to 30 minutes for evaluation of a single slide. Some workers have reported that Papanicolaou stain can be used to detect *C. trachomatis* infections of the cervix. Several studies have failed to confirm the utility of Papanicolaou stain for chlamydial diagnosis, so currently this procedure cannot be recommended.

The monoclonal antibody techniques do not stain antichlamydial intracellular inclusions, but rather detect free elementary bodies. Thus, these procedures combine antigen detection with a morphological criterion for chlamydial identification. Because there is always the possibility that other small round particles may non-specifically bind the conjugated antibody, the manufacturers of these tests have suggested relatively conservative criteria, such as identification of 10 fluorescent particles before a specimen can be called positive. In expert hands these tests appear to be >90% sensitive compared to culture, with specificities ranging from 95 to 99%. The tests do produce some false positive results (reactions with a number of bacteria have been identified) and the importance of false positive reactions becomes more important as the prevalence of infection decreases. Thus, currently it seems prudent to recommend that these tests only be used in high prevalence settings, where the predictive value of a positive test will be high. Of greater concern is the question as to whether the extremely good results obtained in highly specialised microbiology laboratories can be transferred into a routine laboratory setting. If not, there can be considerable problems from misidentification of chlamydial infections.

Antigen detection by non-cytological means

Enzyme immunoassays for chlamydial antigens are commercially available using either monoclonal antibodies or polyclonal antibodies as indicators of chlamydial antigens. These tests have not yet had a broad experience and it is difficult to make recommendations. In highly qualified laboratories they appear to be of equal or somewhat less sensitivity as compared to the fluorescein-conjugated monoclonal antibody test and are less sensitive than culture. If the tests have a reasonable performance profile they will be better suited for processing large numbers of specimens, such as would be collected in venereal disease clinics or large screening studies.

Serology

Although complement fixation tests and enzyme immunoassay tests, among others, have been developed to measure antibodies to *C. trachomatis*, most of the available serological information on these infections has been gleaned through the use of the microimmunofluorescence test, which is still the test of choice (Wang & Grayston 1970). This procedure can measure the class-specific (IgG, IgM, IgA or secretory) antibody response to chlamydial antigens. Simplified forms of the test have been described using, as antigen, elementary bodies of a single broadly reacting serotype or inclusions in cell culture (Thomas et al 1976; Richmond & Caul 1977). However the procedure which yields the most information (but is technically more difficult) uses all 15 serotypes either individually or pooled according to serotype relatedness (Wang et al 1975). Although the technique cannot be recommended for routine diagnosis because of high background prevalence rates of antibodies, it is clear that much higher antibody levels of both IgG and IgM antibody are seen in women with systemic infection as compared to those with superficial infection. Thus women with salpingitis will have higher antibody titres than will women with uncomplicated cervical infection, while women with Fitz-Hugh Curtis syndrome will have the highest antibody titres of all. In general, titres of the IgG class ≥1:1000 with IgM titres ≥1:32 may support the diagnosis of a chlamydial salpingitis. In several studies ≥20% of acute salpingitis cases were found to seroconvert (four-fold rises in titre) to *C. trachomatis* antigens (Eschenbach et al 1975; Paavonen 1980; Ripa et al 1980; Sweet et al 1980; Mardh et al 1981a).

DISEASES OF THE MALE GENITAL TRACT

It is imperative that the clinician dealing with infection in the female genital tract should be aware of the diseases seen in the male. In many instances disease of the male genital tract will be the only objective indicator of a possible chlamydial infection in the female sex partner. For practical purposes these organisms are always sexually transmitted and thus a symptomatic male partner can identify a female candidate for presumptive therapy.

The most common manifestation of chlamydial infection in the male is non-gonococcal urethritis (NGU). Approximately one-third to one-half of men with NGU will be found to have chlamydial infection (Schachter 1978; Judson 1981; Oriel & Ridgway 1982). In addition, men with gonorrhoea have a high rate (20 to 40%) of concomitant infection with *C. trachomatis*. Most of these men with double infections will go on to develop postgonococcal urethritis if their gonorrhoea is treated with penicillins (Oriel et al 1976). Thus, for practical purposes, any woman who has a male partner with urethritis may be considered a candidate for antichlamydial therapy. Approximately one-third of female partners of men with either gonorrhoea or NGU will have chlamydial infection. If they are partners of men who have proven chlamydial infections, more than 60% of these women will yield chlamydiae from their cervical cultures.

Epididymitis in the young sexually active male is almost always caused by gonococcal or chlamydial infection (Berger et al 1978). This is usually associated with anterior urethral inflammation. Thus non-gonococcal epididymitis in the male is also a signal for presumptive treatment of female partners.

INFECTION OF THE NEONATE

The newborn infant passing through an infected birth canal is at risk for acquiring chlamydial infection. The first such disease associated with this infection was inclusion conjunctivitis of the newborn, first specifically attributed to chlamydiae in 1907 (Lindner 1911). The incubation period of conjunctivitis is typically between 5 and 19 days postpartum. The disease is characterised by mucopurulent discharge and pseudomembrane formation may occur. It is usually a self-limiting disease and will disappear in several months if untreated. It is not a blinding condition, although some scarring of the conjunctiva or corneal lesions may develop.

The potential for the exposed infant to develop pneumonia was not recognized until 1974 and a characteristic clinical syndrome termed chlamydia pneumonia of infants has been described (Schachter et al 1975c; Beem & Saxon 1977). Chlamydia pneumonia generally occurs in infants between 2 weeks and 4 months of age and is characterised by an afebrile protracted course associated with a staccato cough and positive radiological findings. Identification of chlamydial infection in the infant always indicates a need for treatment of the mother and her sex partner.

The risks to the infant have been studied in a number of prospective studies in the United States where it is currently estimated that 10 to 20% of exposed infants will develop pneumonia, and between one-third and one-half will develop conjunctivitis (Schachter & Grossman 1981). Serological evidence of chlamydial infection may be found in 60 to 70% of the exposed infants. Chlamydia pneumonia in infants has been described from a number of countries but appears to be far more common in the United States. The reason for this is not clear, but it may reflect the different health care delivery systems that are involved. It is also possible that there are socioeconomic factors and coexistent infections that may be involved in the pathogenesis of this disease. Possibly, radiological confirmation is more often sought for these infants in the medical centre settings where these studies have been performed. These infants should be treated systemically with 40 mg/kg erythromycin ethylsuccinate in 4 daily divided doses for at least 2 weeks. Systemic therapy is indicated for conjunctivitis or pneumonia, since topical treatment shows very high failure rates for conjunctivitis (Rowe et al 1979). Some workers have found a relatively high failure rate with systemic treatment (Rees et al 1981). It is not known whether this is actual drug failure or a compliance problem.

Because chlamydial conjunctivitis is far more common than gonococcal ophthalmia neonatorum, it has been recommended that erythromycin ocular prophylaxis be used instead of silver nitrate (Credé) prophylaxis because erythromycin is effective against *Chlamydia trachomatis* and gonococcal infections, while silver nitrate, although highly effective against gonococci, is not active against chlamydiae. This is a recommendation which must be studied in areas where antibiotic-resistant *Neisseria* present a problem. Ocular prophylaxis may be effective in preventing ICN but it will not prevent subsequent development of chlamydia pneumonia, which is a more threatening and more expensive condition. In high prevalence settings it has been shown that routine screening of pregnant women for cervical chlamydial infection and treatment of the infected women with erythromycin form a cost-

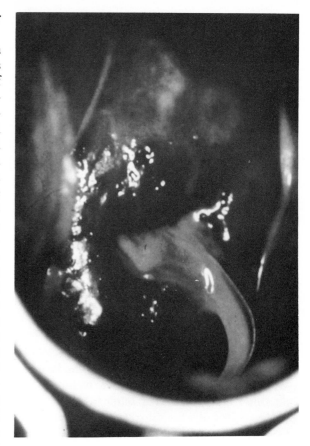

Fig. 11.1 Mucopurulent cervicitis associated with *Chlamydia trachomatis* infection (courtesy E. Rees).

effective approach to eradicating the maternal infection and preventing perinatal transmission.

DISEASES OF THE FEMALE GENITAL TRACT

Cervicitis

The cervix is the most commonly infected site within the female genital tract. *Chlamydia trachomatis* grows only in the cells within the squamocolumnar junction and thus it causes an endocervicitis rather than an ectocervicitis. Asymptomatic infections are quite common and there are no pathognomonic findings which indicate a chlamydial infection (Oriel et al 1978). Chlamydial infections are often described as causing hypertrophic cervical erosions with a mucopurulent endocervical discharge (Rees et al 1977; Fig. 11.1). Ectopy is often seen. The cervix will be erythematous and friable and will bleed easily upon being swabbed. Inflammatory cells will be seen in smears. Rees and colleagues found that only *C. trachomatis* and *Neisseria gonorrhoeae* were associated with mucopurulent endocervicitis. Because of lack of unanimity in the description of the clinical findings, efforts have been made to provide an objective diagnosis of mucopurulent endocervicitis. A swab test has been described: a white swab being rotated within the endocervical canal will have a greenish hue which correlates with the presence of inflammatory cells and a second swab rubbed against the cervix within the zone of ectopy will turn red as a result of bleeding due to friability (Brunham et al 1984). These two findings can provide a presumptive diagnosis of mucopurulent endocervicitis and call for antichlamydial therapy. The predictive value of this test for chlamydial infection is in the range of 30 to 50%. The treatment of choice for chlamydial infections in women is tetracycline, with 2 g/day for 7 days being curative in more than 95% of cases. Erythromycin at equivalent doses is recommended for those women who are tetracycline-intolerant. *C. trachomatis* does not cause vaginitis—it does not appear to grow in squamous cells.

Dunlop and colleagues have described a follicle-like appearance in the chlamydia-infected cervix which is similar to the follicular reaction seen in the conjunctiva (Dunlop et al 1964). Hare and colleagues have confirmed this observation with cervical biopsies showing true follicles with germinal centres generally under an area of metaplastic epithelium (Hare et al 1981; Plates 26 and 27).

Acute salpingitis

It is clear that the most serious complication of chlamydial infection in women is acute salpingitis. The best evidence for a chlamydial aetiology in salpingitis has come from studies in Scandinavia (Mardh et al 1981c). Most recent studies from that part of the world suggest that from one-fifth to one-half of acute salpingitis is caused by *C. trachomatis* (with some temporal variation). In Lund, Sweden, 30% of women with acute salpingitis had chlamy-

dial infection of the fallopian tube as determined by needle biopsy from that site; serological evidence of chlamydial infection was found in 80% of patients with acute salpingitis as compared to only 8% of pregnant women (Mardh et al 1977, 1981). The antibody titres appear to correlate with the severity of tubal inflammation as determined by laparoscopy. Treharne and colleagues found evidence of chlamydial infection in 67% of women with acute salpingitis and their study also found a correlation between antibody level and severity of tubal inflammation (Treharne et al 1979). Cervical cultures from salpingitis cases in Finland have also yielded high rates of chlamydial infection with data suggesting that younger women were at higher risk (Paavonen 1980).

In the United States, however, the chlamydial recovery rates from peritoneal cultures have ranged from 0 to 10% of cases with acute salpingitis (Eschenbach et al 1975; Sweet et al 1980; Thompson et al 1980). Serological data from two laboratories suggested that approximately 20% of acute salpingitis has a chlamydial aetiology (Eschenbach et al 1975; Sweet et al 1980). The discrepancy between the results in Scandinavia and those in the United States may be based on two major factors. Firstly, that gonococcal infection is a far more common cause of salpingitis in the United States than in Scandinavia where control programmes for gonorrhoea appear to have been more successful. Thus, the chlamydiae probably emerge as major pathogens in a population that has reduced levels of gonococcal salpingitis. In addition, there is a methodological difference in these studies; Swedish investigators culture needle aspirates of the fallopian tube or a biopsy of the fimbria taken at time of laparoscopy. In the United States the specimens have been collected by culdocentesis (which may not reflect tubal involvement) or by swabbing of the fimbria. Because in other chlamydial infections the culture of discharges is inadequate and it is imperative that an adequate sample be collected from the involved site, it is possible that needle biopsy of fallopian tubes of women with salpingitis in the United States would result in higher chlamydial recovery than has been detected to date.

It is also likely that there are differences in the populations being studied. In Sweden the practice appears to be to admit all patients with acute salpingitis, while in the United States it is likely that only more severe cases would be hospitalised and the use of intraperitoneal specimen collection has generally been restricted to more severe cases presenting at emergency rooms. Svensson and colleagues have noted that chlamydia infection of the fallopian tube appears to be associated with a milder clinical disease, these women are more often afebrile and have had milder symptoms for a longer period of time (Svensson et al 1980). Thus the symptoms associated with chlamydial infection may be milder than those associated with gonococcal or anaerobic salpingitis.

The likelihood that both speculations are correct is supported by results of studies performed in San Francisco where more invasive culturing techniques were used and less stringent diagnostic criteria were used to accept a diagnosis of acute salpingitis. When women with milder disease were admitted to the hospital and had chlamydial cultures peformed from the endometrium, the recovery rate for the organism increased to approximately 25% (Sweet et al 1983). Of particular interest is the observation that only 14% of these women yielded the organism from the cervix, indicating that the endometrium may be a better sampling site. Thus, it is likely now that in the United States, if these results can be generalised, approximately one in four cases of acute salpingitis is associated with a chlamydial infection. Many of these women had gonococcal infections or other bacteria were detected in fallopian tube or endometrial culture. Of particular interest was the observation that treatment with cephalosporins as single drug therapy resulted in a dramatic clinical response but left the women with relatively asymptomatic endometrial infections with Chlamydia. That finding is consistent with the clinical observations of the 'pure' chlamydial salpingitis described in Scandinavia. Most salpingitis cases are of polymicrobial aetiology, and it is likely that different organisms cause different parts of the clinical picture. It has become obvious that cases of salpingitis must be treated with more than one antimicrobial compound in order to provide coverage for all potential pathogens.

It has also been observed that oral contraceptive usage may be associated with milder salpingitis (Svensson et al 1984). Contraceptives have been shown to protect against the development of gonococcal salpingitis. It is not clear whether a similar role, however, occurs in the case of chlamydial salpingitis. Many studies have found that young women on oral contraceptives have higher rates of chlamydial infection than those using other or no methods of contraception. The need for further study in this subject has been pointed out because, if oral contraceptives have a neutral effect on ascending chlamydial infection, their widespread use would probably lead to more cases of chlamydial salpingitis simply because there would be more cases of cervical infection with a relatively constant rate of ascending infection (Washington et al 1985).

Fitz-Hugh Curtis syndrome

The Fitz-Hugh Curtis syndrome, or acute perihepatitis, with inflammation affecting the anterior surface of the liver and adhesions between the liver and diaphragm, is a consequence of acute salpingitis. It is generally distinguished from acute salpingitis on clinical grounds of acute and severe upper quadrant abdominal pain, as compared to lower abdominal pain commonly found in uncomplicated salpingitis. Neisseria gonorrhoeae was considered to be the cause of the Fitz-Hugh Curtis syndrome, although historically this was always based on the association of cervical infection in the affected women, occasionally on tubal infection, and until very recently, never on recovery of the gonococcus from the surface of the liver. Muller-Schoop et al reported that 9 of 11 patients with perihepatitis and peritonitis had very high titres of antibody to Chlamydia trachomatis (Muller-Schoop et al 1978). A number of other workers from Scandinavia and the United States and England have confirmed those results. Wang and associates noted that approximately half of the women with uncomplicated salpingitis in Seattle had antibodies to C. trachomatis (9 out of 19) as compared to 17 of 19 with Fitz-Hugh Curtis syndrome (Wang et al 1980). Of particular interest was that the geometric mean positive titre for these salpingitis cases was 1:138, while that of the Fitz-Hugh Curtis cases was 1:724. C. trachomatis has been isolated from the affected liver surface (Wolner-Hanssen et al 1982). It thus seems likely that most cases of the Fitz-Hugh Curtis syndrome are caused by C. trachomatis and antichlamydial therapy would be indicated. Cervical cultures often do not reflect the microbiology of the affected fallopian tube and undoubtedly the peritoneum. It would seem reasonable to apply antimicrobial coverage for both gonococcal and chlamydial infections in Fitz-Hugh Curtis cases.

Endometritis

The endometrium may be involved in women with generalised pelvic inflammation. It is uncertain as to whether endometrial chlamydial infection occurs as part of a pathway involving cervix to oviduct spread (as is likely to be the case for women with salpingitis) or whether there is a discrete self-limited chlamydial endometritis (Mardh et al 1981b). A number of other studies have reported recovery of the organism from non-pregnant women with endometritis and it would seem likely that chlamydial endometritis may well exist as a distinct entity, although it is obviously impossible to tell whether it is part of a progressive disease process.

The acute urethral syndrome

The acute urethral syndrome, which is defined as frequency and dysuria in any woman whose bacterial cultures of urine show $<10^5$ organisms, is a relatively common condition. Chlamydiae have been associated with this syndrome for a number of years and chlamydial infection of the female urethra has been documented (Dunlop et al 1972). More recently, Stamm and associates, in efforts to elucidate the aetiology of this condition, have usefully partitioned it into a number of subsets which can be defined on the basis of laboratory findings (Stamm et al 1980). The subset of women whose urine contained polymorphonuclear leucocytes and was bacteriologically sterile was found in most instances to have chlamydial infection. Thus, a sterile pyuria in a woman with frequency and dysuria would be an indication for treatment for chlamydial infection. It should be noted that these results have been obtained in young college-age women. While one may feel safe in generalising for that group, it would be unwise to assume that similar results apply to other age groups and socioeconomic set-tings unless the results are validated in the appropriate setting.

Proctitis

Chlamydia trachomatis is recognised as a contributive cause to proctitis in homosexual men (Quinn et al 1981). Rectal infections also occur in women. Systematic studies have not been performed, but from the disease distribution in men it is clear that both ulcerative and hypertrophic forms of proctitis may be due to chlamydia infection (Plate 42). Lymphogranuloma venereum strains will cause more severe disease (Schachter & Dawson 1978).

Dysplasia

Chlamydial infection of the cervix may be associated with abnormal cytology. The usual finding will be of an inflammatory pattern but metaplastic cells are common. A number of retrospective studies have suggested an excess of antichlamydial antibody in women with dysplasia as compared to women with normal Papanicolaou smears (Schachter et al 1975b, 1982; Paavonen et al 1979). This area requires further investigation.

Infertility

Punnonen and colleagues noted that women with abnormal hysterosalpingograms often (21/23 or 91%) had antibody titres against *C. trachomatis*, whereas only 50% of infertile patients with patent tubes had such antibodies and only 29% of pregnant women had antibodies to *C. trachomatis* (Punnonen et al 1979). This general finding has been confirmed in many studies performed in several parts of the world. Virtually every study that has examined the subject has found an excess of antichlamydial antibody in women with tubal factor infertility as compared to controls. Of particular interest in some of these studies has been the observation that approximately half of the women with occluded tubes and evidence of chlamydial infection have no previous history of acute salpingitis. This is consistent with the spectrum of chlamydial salpingitis which can involve very mild disease, but apparently the outcome in terms of fertility can still be bad. Some studies have also noted an excess of ectopic pregnancies in women with evidence of chlamydial infection and this is an area which requires further study.

Henry-Suchet and colleagues recovered *Chlamydia* from women undergoing tubal surgery for treatment of infertility due to tubal obstruction. They noted that while there were no marked signs of tubal inflammation, half of their patients had antibodies to *C. trachomatis* and approximately 20% yielded the organism from the involved sites (Henry-Suchet et al 1980). Thus it would appear that chlamydial infection may result in infertility either as a late sequela of acute salpingitis or as a result of chronic tubal infection.

Complications of pregnancy

In the past it was noted that women whose infants developed inclusion conjunctivitis of the newborn had a relatively high rate of postpartum salpingitis. More recently, preliminary data have suggested that women who were chlamydia-positive in the first trimester of their pregancies showed a higher rate of postpartum endometritis after a vaginal delivery (Wager et al 1980). Another study showed a significant excess of fetal wastage in women whose infection was identified during their first visit (Martin et al 1982). It is clear that these studies must be repeated using larger numbers and with appropriate control for other agents which may be responsible for these conditions. In a prospective study we have been performing in San Francisco we have not confirmed these findings.

Harrison and colleagues (1983) have found that many of the complications seen could be attributed to coexistent *Mycoplasma hominis* infection, but that a subset of women with chlamydial infection (those with IgM antibody) had an excess prematurity rate. That suggests that the simple presence of *C. trachomatis* in the endocervical canal may not be a risk factor for adverse pregnancy outcome.

Bartholinitis

Evidence suggesting a chlamydial aetiology for some cases of bartholinitis has been developed. It is uncertain as to what proportion of this disease may be attributed to chlamydiae. Most of the reported cases had concomitant chlamydial and gonococcal

infection (Davies et al 1978). It would certainly seem reasonable to consider *Chlamydia* in the aetiology of bartholinitis in cases where gonococci are not recovered or where symptoms may persist following penicillin treatment.

TREATMENT

Chlamydia trachomatis infections will respond to treatment with tetracyclines, erythromycin, or sulphonamides (Schachter 1978). Optimal regimens have yet to be defined. Many workers prefer to treat chlamydial infections with 2 g tetracycline daily for 7 days, since this regimen is also adequate for most gonococcal infections and will treat the organisms (presumably *Ureaplasma urealyticum*) that are apparently involved in the aetiology of nongonococcal urethritis. A dosage of 1 g/day for 7 or 14 days is also effective for chlamydiae. Similar dosages of erythromycin may be used. Sulphonamides, although active against *C. trachomatis*, are not used as often since they require specific diagnosis and may not be indicated for some of the conditions with which chlamydiae are associated. In other words, they may not be active against other causes of the same condition. Sulphonamide-trimethoprim combinations will also be effective, but have not been adequately evaluated. Sulphonamide therapy of 1 to 2 weeks would be effective. For example, Bowie has found that sulphisoxazole for 10 days at 2 g/day is effective (Bowie et al 1982).

PRESUMPTIVE TREATMENT

It has been pointed out that there are no pathognomonic signs for chlamydial infection and that accurate identification of infected women is dependent on microbiological diagnosis. Even the routine treatment of female partners of men with urethritis or of women with gonorrhoea with antichlamydial therapy would miss most of the infected women (Willcox et al 1979). Thus, chlamydial diagnostic tests should be routinely used in clinics catering for sexually active women. The author heartily endorses this viewpoint. However, it is clear that chlamydial diagnosis will not be routinely available in many clinic settings until improved diagnostic methodology is developed. It is also clear that there are a number of subsets of patients who are at particularly high risk for chlamydial infection (Stamm & Holmes 1981). If considered on demographic grounds, age is inversely related to chlamydial infection rate and the young sexually active women (usually of teen age) of lower socioeconomic class (which often implies being of a minority race) are at highest risk for chlamydial infection. A number of surveys have found that 20% or more of sexually active teenagers in inner city populations are carrying chlamydiae in their cervix. Also, women on birth control pills have higher carrier rates (although it is not clear whether this is because of different behavioural patterns or whether the ectopy associated with pill usage makes such

women more susceptible to chlamydial infection, or perhaps allows a better sample to be collected for the isolation attempts). It is clear that a high index of suspicion should be used by clinicians dealing with this type of population, and although obviously one cannot suggest routine treatment with tetracycline of all sexually active teenagers on birth control pills, it is likely that antichlamydial therapy should be used whenever it may be indicated for any reason in this setting. There are also clinical findings which associate with chlamydial infection. Thus, a woman who has sterile pyuria or a mucopurulent endocervicitis, or who has gonorrhoea or a male partner with urethritis will be at high risk for chlamydial infection and should be treated on presumptive grounds.

REFERENCES

Beem M O, Saxon E M 1977 Respiratory-tract colonization and a distinctive pneumonia syndrome in infants infected with Chlamydia trachomatis. New England Journal of Medicine 296: 306–310

Berger R E, Alexander E R, Monda G D, Ansell J, McCormick G, Holmes K K 1978 Chlamydia trachomatis as a cause of acute 'idiopathic' epididymitis. New England Journal of Medicine 298: 301–304

Bowie W R, Manzon L M, Borrie-Hume C J, Fawcett A, Jones H D 1982 Efficacy of treatment regimens for lower urogenital Chlamydia trachomatis infection in women. American Journal of Obstetrics and Gynecology 142: 125–129

Brunham R C, Paavonen J, Stevens C E, Kiviat N, Kuo C-C, Holmes K K 1984 Mucopurulent cervicitis—the ignored counterpart in women of urethritis in men. New England Journal of Medicine 311(1): 1–6

Darougar S, Jones B R, Kinnison J R, Vaughn-Jackson J D, Dunlop E M C 1972 Chlamydial infection: advances in the diagnostic isolation of Chlamydia, including TRIC agent from the eye, genital tract, and rectum. British Journal of Venereal Diseases 48: 416–420

Davies J A, Rees E, Hobson D, Karayiannis P 1978 Isolation of Chlamydia trachomatis from Bartholin's ducts. British Journal of Venereal Diseases 54: 409–413

Dunlop E M C, Jones B R, Al-Hussaini M K 1964 Genital infection in association with TRIC virus infection of the eye. British Journal of Venereal Diseases 40: 33–42

Dunlop E M C, Darougar S, Hare M J, Treharne J D, Dwyer R St C 1972 Isolation of Chlamydia from the urethra of a woman. British Medical Journal 2: 386

Eschenbach D A, Buchanan T M, Pollock H M et al 1975 Polymicrobial etiology of acute pelvic inflammatory disease. New England Journal of Medicine 293: 166–171

Grayston J T, Wang S-P 1975 New knowledge of chlamydiae and the diseases they cause. Journal of Infectious Diseases 132: 87–105

Hare M J, Toone E, Taylor-Robinson D et al 1981 Follicular cervicitis—colposcopic appearances and association with Chlamydia trachomatis. British Journal of Obstetrics and Gynaecology 88: 174–180

Harrison H R, Alexander E R, Weinstein L, Lewis M, Nash M, Sim D A 1983 Cervical Chlamydia trachomatis and mycoplasmal infections in pregnancy. Journal of the American Medical Association 250(13): 1721–1727

Henry-Suchet J, Catalan F, Loffredo V et al 1980 Microbiology of specimens obtained by laparoscopy from controls and from patients with pelvic inflammatory disease or infertility with tubal obstructions: Chlamydia trachomatis and Ureaplasma urealyticum. American Journal of Obstetrics and Gynecology 138: 1022–1025

Jones B R 1975 The prevention of blindness from trachoma. Transactions of the Ophthalmological Societies of the United Kingdom 95: 16–33

Judson F N 1981 Epidemiology and control of nongonococcal urethritis and genital chlamydial infections: a review. Sexually Transmitted Diseases 8(2): 117–126

Lindner K 1911 Gonoblennorrhoe, Einschlussblennorrhoe, und Trachoma. Albrecht von Graefe's Archives of Ophthalmology 78: 380

Mardh P-A, Ripa K T, Svensson L, Weström L 1977 Chlamydia trachomatis in patients with acute salpingitis. New England Journal of Medicine 296: 1377–1379

Mardh P-A, Lind I, Svensson L, Weström L, Moller B R 1981a Antibodies to Chlamydia trachomatis, Mycoplasma hominis and Neisseria gonorrhoeae in sera from patients with acute salpingitis. British Journal of Venereal Diseases 57: 125–129

Mardh P-A, Moller B R, Ingerslev H J, Nussler E, Weström L, Wölner-Hanssen P 1981b Endometritis caused by Chlamydia trachomatis. British Journal of Venereal Diseases 57(3): 191

Mardh P-A, Moller B R, Paavonen J 1981c Chlamydial infection of the female genital tract with emphasis on pelvic inflammatory disease: a review of Scandinavian studies. Sexually Transmitted Diseases 8(2): 140–155

Martin D H, Koutsky L, Eschenbach D A et al 1982 Prematurity and perinatal mortality in pregnancies complicated by maternal Chlamydia trachomatis infections. Journal of the American Medical Association 247: 1585–1588

Moulder J W 1964 The psittacosis group as bacteria. Wiley, New York

Moulder J W 1966 The relation of psittacosis group (chlamydiae) to bacteria and viruses. Annual Review of Microbiology 20: 107–130

Muller-Schoop J W, Wang S-P, Munzinger J, Schlapfer H U, Knoblauch M, Ammann R W 1978 Chlamydia trachomatis as a possible cause of peritonitis and perihepatitis in young women. British Medical Journal 1: 1022–1024

National Institute of Allergy and Infectious Diseases 1981 Sexually transmitted diseases: 1980 status report. US Government Patent Office, Washington, DC (publ. no. 81-2213)

Oriel J D, Ridgway G L 1982 Genital infection by Chlamydia trachomatis. Edward Arnold, London

Oriel J D, Ridgway G L, Reeve P, Beckingham D C, Owen J 1976 The lack of effect of ampicillin plus probenecid given for genital infections with Neisseria gonorrhoeae on associated infections with Chlamydia trachomatis. Journal of Infectious Diseases 133: 568–571

Oriel J D, Johnson A L, Barlow D, Thomas B J, Nayyar D, Reeve P 1978 Infection of the uterine cervix with Chlamydia trachomatis. Journal of Infectious Diseases 137: 443–451

Paavonen J 1980 Chlamydia trachomatis in acute salpingitis. American Journal of Obstetrics and Gynecology 138: 957–959

Paavonen J, Vesterinen E, Meyer B et al 1979 Genital Chlamydia trachomatis infections in patients with cervical atypia. Obstetrics and Gynecology 54: 289–291

Page L A 1974 Order II chlamydiales. In: Buchanan R E, Gibbons N E (eds) Bergey's manual of determinative bacteriology, 8th edn. Williams & Wilkins, Baltimore, pp 914–928

Punnonen R, Terho P, Nikkanen V, Meurman O 1979 Chlamydial serology in infertile women by immunofluorescence. Fertility and Sterility 31: 656–659

Quinn T C, Goddell S E, Mkrtichian E et al 1981 Chlamydia trachomatis proctitis. New England Journal of Medicine 305: 195–200

Rees E, Tait I A, Hobson D, Johnson F W A 1977 Chlamydia in relation to cervical infection and pelvic inflammatory disease. In: Holmes K K, Hobson D (eds) Nongonococcal urethritis and related infections. American Society for Microbiology, Washington, DC, pp 67–76

Rees E, Tait A, Hobson D, Karayiannis P, Lee N 1981 Persistence of chlamydial infection after treatment for neonatal conjunctivitis. Archives of Disease in Childhood 56: 193–198

Richmond S J, Caul E O 1977 Single-antigen indirect immunofluorescence test for screening venereal disease clinical populations for chlamydial antibodies. In: Holmes K K, Hobson D (eds) Nongonococcal urethritis and related infections. American Society for Microbiology, Washington, DC, pp 259–265

Ripa K T, Mardh P-A 1977 Cultivation of Chlamydia trachomatis in cycloheximide-treated McCoy cells. Journal of Clinical Microbiology 6: 328–331

Ripa K T, Svensson L, Treharne J D, Westrom L, Mardh P-A 1980 Chlamydia trachomatis infection in patients with laparoscopically verified salpingitis: results of isolation and antibody determinations. American Journal of Obstetrics and Gynecology 138: 960–964

Rowe S, Aicardi E, Dawson C R, Schachter J 1979 Purulent ocular discharge in neonates: significance of Chlamydia trachomatis. Pediatrics 63: 628–632

Schachter J 1978 Chlamydial infections. New England Journal of Medicine 298: 428–435, 490–495, 540–549

Schachter J 1985 Chlamydiae (psittacosis-lymphogranuloma venereum-trachoma group). In: Lennette E H (ed) Manual of clinical microbiology, 4th edn. American Society for Microbiology, Washington, DC, pp 856–862

Schachter J, Caldwell H D 1980 Chlamydiae. Annual Review of Microbiology 34: 285–309

Schachter J, Dawson C R 1977 Comparative efficiency of various diagnostic methods for chlamydial infection. In: Holmes K K, Hobson D (eds) Nongonococcal urethritis and related infections. American Society for Microbiology, Washington, DC, pp 337–341

Schachter J, Dawson C R 1978 Human chlamydial infections. PSG, Littleton

Schachter J, Grossman M 1981 Chlamydial infections. Annual Review of Medicine 32: 45–61

Schachter J, Hanna L, Hill E C et al 1975a Are chlamydial infections the most prevalent venereal disease? Journal of the American Medical Association 231: 1252–1255

Schachter J, Hill E C, E B, Coleman V R, Jones P, Meyer K F 1975b Chlamydial infection in women with cervical dysplasia. American Journal of Obstetrics and Gynecology 123: 753–757

Schachter J, Lum L, Gooding C A, Ostler B 1975c Pneumonitis following inclusion blennorhea. Journal of Pediatrics 87: 799–780

Schachter J, Cles L, Ray R, Hines P 1979 Failure of serology in diagnosing chlamydial infections of the female genital tract. Journal of Clinical Microbiology 10(5): 647–649

Schachter J, Hill E C, King E B et al 1982 Chlamydia trachomatis and cervical neoplasia. Journal of the American Medical Association 248: 2134–2138

Stamm W E, Holmes K K 1981 Chlamydial infections: what should we do while waiting for a diagnostic test? Western Journal of Medicine 135: 226–229

Stamm W E, Wagner K F, Amsel R et al 1980 Causes of the acute urethral syndrome in women. New England Journal of Medicine 303: 409–415

Svensson L, Weström L, Ripa K T, Mardh P-A 1980 Differences in some clinical and laboratory parameters in acute salpingitis related to culture and serologic findings. American Journal of Obstetrics and Gynecology 138: 1017–1021

Svensson L, Weström L, Mardh P-A 1984 Contraceptives and acute salpingitis. Journal of the American Medical Association 251(19): 2553–2555

Sweet R, Draper D, Schachter J, James J, Hadley W, Brooks G 1980 Microbiology and pathogenesis of acute salpingitis as determined by laparoscopy: what is the appropriate site to sample? American Journal of Obstetrics and Gynecology 138: 985–989

Sweet R L, Schachter J, Robbie M 1983 Failure of beta lactam antibiotics to eradicate Chlamydia trachomatis in the endometrium despite apparent clinical cure of acute salpingitis. Journal of the American Medical Association 250(19): 2641–2645

Thomas B J, Reeve P, Oriel J D 1976 Simplified serological test for antibodies to Chlamydia trachomatis. Journal of Clinical Microbiology 4: 6–10

Thomas B J, Evans R T, Hutchinson G R, Taylor-Robinson D 1977 Early detection of chlamydial inclusions combining the use of cycloheximide-treated McCoy cells and immunofluorescence staining. Journal of Clinical Microbiology 6: 285–292

Thompson S E, Hager W D, Wong K-H et al 1980 The microbiology and therapy of acute pelvic inflammatory disease in hospitalized patients. American Journal of Obstetrics and Gynecology 126: 179–186

Thygeson P, Mengert W F 1936 The virus of inclusion conjunctivitis: further observations. Archives of Ophthalmology 15: 377–410

Treharne J D, Ripa K T, Mardh P-A, Svensson L, Weström L, Darougar S 1979 Antibodies to Chlamydia trachomatis in acute salpingitis. British Journal of Venereal Diseases 55: 26–29

Wager G P, Martin D H, Koutsky L et al 1980 Puerperal infectious morbidity: relationship to route of delivery and to antepartum Chlamydia trachomatis infection. American Journal of Obstetrics and Gynecology 138: 1028–1033

Wang S-P, Grayston J T 1970 Immunologic relationship between genital TRIC, lymphogranuloma venereum, and related organisms in a new microtiter indirect immunofluorescence test. American Journal of Ophthalmology 70: 367–374

Wang S-P, Grayston J T, Alexander E R, Holmes K K 1975 Simplified microimmunofluorescence test with trachoma-lymphogranuloma venereum (Chlamydia trachomatis) antigens for use as a screening test for antibody. Journal of Clinical Microbiology 1: 250–255

Wang S-P, Eschenbach D A, Holmes K K, Wager G, Grayston J T 1980 Chlamydia trachomatis infection in Fitz-Hugh Curtis syndrome. American Journal of Obstetrics and Gynecology 138: 1034–1038

Washington A E, Gove S, Schachter J, Sweet R L 1985 Oral contraceptives, Chlamydia trachomatis infection and pelvic inflammatory disease. Journal of the American Medical Association 253(1): 2246–2250

Willcox J R, Fisk P G, Barrow J, Barlow D 1979 The need for a chlamydial culture service. British Journal of Venereal Diseases 55: 281–283

Wolner-Hanssen P, Svensson L, Weström L, Mardh P-A 1982 Isolation of Chlamydia trachomatis from the liver capsule in Fitz-Hugh Curtis syndrome. New England Journal of Medicine 306(2): 113

Mycoplasmal infection of the female genital tract and its complications
D Taylor-Robinson and P E Munday

MYCOPLASMAS IN THE HUMAN GENITOURINARY TRACT

Originally mycoplasmas were called pleuro-pneumonia-like organisms (PPLO). They do not exceed 300 μm in diameter, being the smallest free-living micro-organisms, and characteristically produce fried-egg-like colonies on agar medium. The size of the colonies varies, as indicated below.

The first report of the isolation of a mycoplasma from a human subject was by Dienes & Edsall in 1937 who recovered organisms, apparently in pure culture, from an abscess of Bartholin's duct. Of course, there was no identification of mycoplasma species at that time but the organisms were probably *Mycoplasma hominis* because this is the large-colony forming species most frequently recovered from the genital tract. So far, mycoplasmas of 12 different species have been isolated from human subjects and at least four of these are found predominantly in the genitourinary tract (Table 12.1).

M. hominis is commonly found in the genitourinary tract but less frequently in the oropharynx or elsewhere. T-strain mycoplasmas, or T-mycoplasmas, were first described by Shepard in 1954. The prefix T (T for tiny) was coined by him to denote the small colonies produced by these organisms on agar medium. Later they were found to have the ability, unique among mycoplasmas, to hydrolyse urea and those of human origin were placed in a new genus and species, *Ureaplasma urealyticum* (Shepard et al 1974). These organisms are referred to trivially as ureaplasmas and are also found commonly in the genitourinary tract but infrequently in the oropharynx or elsewhere.

M. fermentans was isolated first from patients with balanitis (Ruiter & Wentholt 1952). However, it seems to be rare in the genitourinary tract, perhaps only 1% or less of all isolates being identified as belonging to this species (Mardh & Weström 1970a). *M. primatum* (DelGiudice et al 1971) is isolated also rarely (Thomsen 1974). Confirmation of the rarity of isolation of these species was obtained by using the epi-immunofluorescence technique to identify every colony produced by inoculating clinical specimens on agar medium (Taylor-Robinson & Furr unpublished observations). *M. pneumoniae*, a cause of primary atypical pneumonia, has been recovered from a tubo-ovarian abscess (Thomas et al 1975) and also from the lower genital tract (Csutortoki et al 1975), presumably as a result of orogenital contact. It is not surprising, therefore, that other mycoplasmas such as *M. salivarium*, normally resident as commensals in the oropharynx, are recovered very occasionally from the genital tract (Foy et al 1975; Gump et al 1975). Most mycoplasmas, because of their rarity, are not obvious contenders for causing disease. However, *M. hominis* and *U. urealyticum* are different in this respect and, therefore, their possible role in disease is considered in some detail. *M. genitalium* is the micro-organism discovered most recently. It was isolated from the urethra of men with non-gonococcal urethritis (Taylor-Robinson et al 1981; Tully et al 1981). Little is known about its incidence and distribution but serological and other data concerning its possible role in pelvic inflammatory disease will be mentioned.

COLONISATION OF FEMALES

Colonisation of infants and children

Infants become colonised with genital mycoplasmas usually during passage through the birth canal. This can be deduced from the fact that infants deli-

Table 12.1 The metabolism, occurrence and disease association of mycoplasmas isolated from human subjects

Mycoplasma	Metabolism of	Frequency of isolation from the		Cause of disease
		Respiratory tract	Genitourinary tract	
Mycoplasma buccale	Arginine	Rare	—*	No
Mycoplasma faucium	Arginine	Rare	—	No
Mycoplasma fermentans	Glucose, arginine	—	Rare	No
Mycoplasma genitalium	Glucose	?	?	?
Mycoplasma hominis	Arginine	Rare	Common	Yes
Acholeplasma laidlawii	Glucose	Rare	—	No
Mycoplasma lipophilum	Arginine	Rare	—	No
Mycoplasma orale	Arginine	Common	—	No
Mycoplasma pneumoniae	Glucose	Rare†	Very rare	Yes
Mycoplasma primatum	Arginine	—	Rare	No
Mycoplasma salivarium	Arginine	Common	Rare	No
Ureaplasma urealyticum	Urea	Rare	Common	Yes

*No reports of isolation; †except in disease outbreaks.

vered by Caesarean section are rarely colonised in comparison with those born vaginally (Klein et al 1969). Ureaplasmas have been isolated from the genitalia of up to one-third of infant girls, and *Mycoplasma hominis* from a smaller proportion (Klein et al 1969; Foy et al 1970a; Braun et al 1971). Neonatal colonisation by mycoplasmas tends not to persist but the few female infants that are still colonised (<5%) at 1 year of age may carry the organisms into adult life (Hammerschlag et al 1978). Children who have been sexually abused are much more likely to be colonised in the vagina (predominantly) and throat by genital mycoplasmas than are other children.

Colonisation of adults

A variety of factors may actually or apparently affect colonisation.

Sexual experience

The proportion of women who are colonised by *M. hominis* and by ureaplasmas increases after puberty, which is probably a reflection of sexual contact. Indeed, the frequency of colonisation increases with increasing numbers of sexual partners. In one study (McCormack et al 1972a) *M. hominis* was isolated from the vagina of less than 2% of sexually mature young women without a history of sexual contact and ureaplasmas from less than 6%, whereas *M. hominis* was isolated from about 17% and ureaplasmas from 75% of those who had had inter-

course with three or more partners. This observation is in keeping with the rare finding of genital mycoplasmas in the urine of nuns (Archer 1968; Kundsin et al 1971) but frequently in women attending venereal disease clinics (Hunter et al 1981; Munday et al 1981; Young et al 1981), who, almost invariably, have had sexual experience. The extent to which genital mycoplasmas persist in the absence of reinfection in women is difficult to assess. Because of repeated sexual contact, persistence may be more apparent than real.

Race

This appears to exert some influence on colonisation by genital mycoplasmas because mycoplasmas have been isolated more frequently from black women than from white women (Foy et al 1970b; Braun et al 1971; McCormack et al 1973b). The extent to which this may be due to a difference in sexual experience rather than to a real racial predisposition to colonisation is not clear but after taking the factor of sexual experience carefully into account, W M McCormack (personal communication) found that black women were more often colonised by *M. hominis* and ureaplasmas than were other women.

Socioeconomic status

This also seems to have an effect, presumably indirectly, on genital mycoplasmal colonisation. Thus, Ford (1967) reported large-colony forming mycoplasmas to be twice as common among women in jail as among patients of private gynaecologists. Furthermore, McCormack et al (1973b) isolated *M. hominis* and ureaplasmas much more frequently from patients attending prenatal and gynaecology clinics at a municipal hospital than from those visiting private obstetricians and gynaecologists in the same area. This apparent socioeconomic difference may be a reflection of a difference in sexual activity, but other factors, such as contraception or vaginal douching, could be involved.

Contraception

The evidence that different means of contraception influence mycoplasmal colonisation of the female lower genital tract is conflicting. Some workers (Gregory & Payne 1970; McCormack, 1974) found *M. hominis* more often in women who used intrauterine devices than in those who did not. Furthermore, some workers (Gregory & Payne 1970; Young et al 1981) have reported that oral contraceptives have no influence on colonisation by *M. hominis* and ureaplasmas, whereas others (Mardh & Weström 1970b; McCormack et al 1973b; P E Munday, unpublished data) have found these organisms more frequently in women using oral contraceptives. The lack of uniform opinion is illustrated further by the observations of Gump et al (1975) who reported that neither intrauterine nor oral contraceptives had a significant effect on genital colonisation by *M. hominis* or ureaplasmas.

Menstruation

This could affect colonisation by genital mycoplasmas and the ability to isolate them but, surprisingly, has received scant attention in this respect. Indeed, the only information of any relevance is by Singer & Ivler (1975) who recorded that they had isolated genital mycoplasmas from women attending a family planning clinic more frequently after the midcycle (75%) than at midcycle (56.5%) and by P E Munday (unpublished data) who recovered ureaplasmas a little more often (87%) in the first week of the cycle than in the last week (75%).

Pregnancy

There are no studies in which pregnant and nonpregnant women have been matched for sexual experience but most workers have recovered both *M. hominis* and ureaplasmas apparently more frequently from pregnant women (Csonka et al 1966; Jones 1967b; Archer 1968; Mardh & Westrom 1970b, 1970c). Other workers (Harwick et al 1970; de Louvois et al 1975) consider that colonisation by *M. hominis* increases between the first and third trimesters of pregnancy. If this is so, it could be due to the microbiological and pH changes which are known to occur in the vagina during pregnancy providing conditions more conducive to mycoplasmal growth. On the other hand, Ross et al (1981) found that there was no difference in the isolation rate for ureaplasmas during the course of pregnancy, although there was a reduction in the rate immediately after childbirth which was attributable, no doubt, to the natural lavage by amniotic fluid and the products of conception.

Menopausal changes

Menopausal changes seem to be associated with a decrease in the incidence of genital mycoplasmas (Csonka et al 1966; Archer 1968; Mardh & Weström 1970b, 1970c). It must be admitted, however, that the various factors, already mentioned, which could influence the results have not always been controlled.

Anatomical considerations

It seems that the bladder, uterus and fallopian tubes of healthy women are usually free of mycoplasmas. In the lower genital tract, the organisms may be recovered from the endocervix but possibly not as often as from the vagina, the posterior fornix, or even the periurethral area (Dunlop et al 1969; McCormack et al 1972b). In this regard, it appears that mycoplasmas, unlike chlamydiae, do not have a predilection for columnar epithelium. In adults, the urethra may be infected or it may be contaminated superficially by vaginal secretions. It is not surprising, therefore, that some investigators (Csonka et al 1966; Archer 1968; Hunter et al 1981) have isolated ureaplasmas from urine as frequently as from cervical swabs.

Observations based on serology

Newborn infants, some of whom are colonised by genital mycoplasmas, frequently possess serum antibodies, measured by the metabolism inhibition technique, to genital and other mycoplasmas (D Taylor-Robinson & T Feizi unpublished observations; Taylor-Robinson & McCormack 1979). These antibodies are probably maternal in origin and not due to a response to colonisation, since the antibody titres parallel the maternal antibody titres and antibody disappears about 6 months after birth. At or soon after puberty, antibodies to large-colony forming mycoplasmas (Taylor-Robinson et al 1965; Jones & Sequeria 1966; Purcell et al 1969; Mardh & Weström 1970c) and ureaplasmas (Purcell et al 1966) increase in frequency consistent with the acquisition or activation of genital mycoplasmas at this time. The infrequent occurrence of metabolism inhibiting antibody to ureaplasmas in the sera of nuns and its common occurrence in the sera of other groups of women correlates with the rate of isolation of ureaplasmas from women in the various groups (Kundsin et al 1973).

The frequency and titre of antibody to genital mycoplasmas are influenced not only by vaginal mycoplasmal colonisation but also by haematogenous spread of mycoplasmas which occurs during pregnancy and after childbirth and its complications. Rises in the titre of *M. hominis* antibody in the sera of women after childbirth have been correlated with the presence of mycoplasmas in the genital tract. Almost 90% of women colonised with *M. hominis* and 40% colonised with ureaplasmas have been found to have significant changes in the titres of antibodies to these mycoplasmas throughout an apparently normal pregnancy (Lin et al 1978). Furthermore, the antibody titres may be related to the number of pregnancies, the lowest titres being found in primigravidae.

ROLE OF MYCOPLASMAS IN LOWER GENITAL TRACT DISEASE

The results of isolation and serological studies have shown that *Mycoplasma hominis* and ureaplasmas occur with considerable frequency in the genital tract of apparently healthy women. Of course, this

is an argument against these micro-organisms being prominent causes of genital tract disease and is a factor that must be taken into account in designing studies to evaluate their significance.

Bartholin's gland abscess

Mycoplasmas of human origin were first isolated from an abscess of Bartholin's gland (Dienes & Edsall 1937) and *M. hominis* and ureaplasmas have been isolated subsequently from the same site. In these studies, however, abscess rupture or surgical intervention before specimens were obtained may have resulted in colonisation or contamination of the abscesses by mycoplasmas present in the vagina, thus leading to spurious ideas about the organisms causing them. This criticism was overcome by Lee et al (1977) who examined percutaneous aspirates from intact abscesses. Of 34 abscesses, 24 (71%) contained bacteria, only 1 contained *M. hominis* (together with other vaginal organisms) and none contained ureaplasmas, despite the fact that genital mycoplasmas were isolated from the vaginas of most patients. Clearly, the case for genital mycoplasmas causing abscesses of Bartholin's gland is poor.

Vaginitis, vaginosis and cervicitis

Unfortunately many workers have failed to define accurately the clinical condition under investigation and in some cases grouped together patients with a variety of conditions probably of differing aetiologies. Earlier workers used the term 'vaginitis' to indicate any abnormal vaginal findings or discharge: 'cervicitis' was rarely defined. The term 'vaginosis' has recently been introduced to describe an abnormal vaginal discharge in the absence of inflammatory changes in the vaginal wall. In the following discussion, the terminology chosen by the authors has been respected, in the main.

Isolation studies. The mycoplasmas isolated in many of the early studies were not identified specifically, although it is likely that most of them were *M. hominis*. The results of numerous studies, summarised previously (Taylor-Robinson et al 1969), indicated that isolations were made from persons with vaginitis or cervicitis more than twice as frequently as from those considered free of disease. Apart from the difficulty of clinical categorisation mentioned above, control groups were often selected inappropriately, thus making the interpretation of these studies difficult. Furthermore, it is possible that another micro-organism caused the disease and at the same time provided conditions favourable for the growth of mycoplasmas. Indeed, unidentified large-colony forming mycoplasmas or *M. hominis* are more frequently isolated when there is infection by other micro-organisms such as *Trichomonas vaginalis*, *Neisseria gonorrhoeae*, *Chlamydia trachomatis*, *Gardnerella vaginalis* or *Candida albicans* (Taylor-Robinson et al 1969; Mendel et al 1970; Dattani et al 1982; Hanna et al 1985). A mixed flora, by replacing lactobacilli, causes a rise in vaginal pH and this may be conducive to the growth of mycoplasmas. The diminution in the number of lactobacilli in pregnancy may have the same effect (de Louvois et al 1975).

In many early studies, non-specific vaginitis was defined as vaginitis in a patient from whom *N. gonorrhoeae*, *T. vaginalis* and *C. albicans* were not isolated. In these studies, *M. hominis* was isolated from one-third (Bercovici et al 1962; Mendel et al 1970) to about one-half or more (Csonka et al 1966; Mardh & Weström 1970a, 1970c) of such women. The isolation rate of more than 50% noted by the Swedish workers (Mardh & Weström 1970a, 1970c) for women who had clinical and cytological signs of lower genital tract infections was about 10 times that for women without such signs. The difference in these isolation rates may suggest an aetiological relationship, but the sexual experience of the women in the two groups and the possible role of other bacteria (see below) is unknown. De Louvois et al (1975) observed that the isolation rate for *M. hominis* was increased in pregnant women suspected of having vulvovaginitis, a finding they thought was worth further investigation.

More recently there has been a revival of interest in 'non-specific vaginitis', a condition first described by Gardner & Dukes (1955). The syndrome which Gardner described was defined by positive criteria, namely the presence of an offensive homogeneous, non-pruritic grey discharge and data were presented to support the claim that a newly discovered micro-organism, then named *Haemophilus vaginalis*, was the sole aetiological agent. Controversy surrounded both the clinical disease and the presumptive aetiological agent for many years. There is now, however, widespread agreement that the disease, defined by specific clinical criteria, should be called bacterial vaginosis (BV; Weström et al 1984). Since it is clear that *H. vaginalis* (now renamed *Gardnerella vaginalis*) is not the sole aetiological agent, a number of workers have investigated the possible role of mycoplasmas in this condition. Pheifer et al (1978) isolated *M. hominis* from 63% of a group of symptomatic women with an abnormal vaginal discharge (compatible with a diagnosis of BV) compared with 10% of a similar group of women without abnormal findings. Further analysis of the data suggested that, of the many micro-organisms studied, only *G. vaginalis* and *M. hominis* were associated with the disease. Dattani et al (1982) also found that *G. vaginalis* and *M. hominis* were isolated more frequently from women with 'non-specific vaginitis'. Similar data were obtained by Paavonen et al (1983a) and P E Munday and C A Ison (unpublished data).

Ureaplasmas, in contrast to *M. hominis*, have been less consistently associated with vaginitis and vaginosis. For example, in comparison with women in control groups, ureaplasmas were not isolated more frequently from patients with non-specific, trichomonal or monilial vaginitis in one study (Romano & Romano 1968) or from patients with gonococcal or chlamydial infections in another (Hunter et al 1981). In another study (Mardh & Weström 1970b), the frequency of ureaplasmas in the lower genital tract of women with signs of infection was not different from that in a carefully matched group without signs. Although Kundsin et al (1973) isolated ureaplasmas from 80% of women with genitourinary tract infections, including 'cervicitis' and 'vaginitis', compared to 51% of private practitioners' patients with reproductive problems who were otherwise asymptomatic, the difference may well reflect a difference in sexual attitudes, women in the latter group probably being more selective in their sexual contacts. However, despite any past negative findings, the role of ureaplasmas in BV needs to be explored further, because Gravett & Eschenbach (1986) mention that women with BV have a 1000-fold increase in the intravaginal concentration of anaerobic bacteria, a 100-fold increase in *G. vaginalis* and a 100-fold increase in ureaplasmas.

There are few data suggesting an association between cervicitis per se and genital mycoplasmas. Thus, Hare et al (1981, 1982) found that follicular cervicitis and cervical dysplasia were significantly associated with the isolation of *Chlamydia trachomatis* but not with the isolation of ureaplasmas or *M. hominis*. Furthermore, Paavonen et al (1982) could find no association between the isolation of *M. hominis* from the cervix and mucopurulent cervicitis, but more recently Paavonen et al (1986) not only significantly associated *C. trachomatis* with the condition but ureaplasmas also, at least on a qualitative basis. Obviously, the relationship needs to be investigated further with quantitative estimations of the numbers of organisms.

Antibiotic studies. Antibiotics which affect one micro-organism but not another have been used in efforts to resolve the possible contribution of mycoplasmas, especially *M. hominis* in lower genital tract infections. This approach is likely to be only partially successful because the large number of micro-organisms involved makes it difficult or impossible to find an antibiotic which selectively inhibits only one of them. It is not surprising, therefore, that the results of some of the studies have been conflicting. In patients infected with *Trichomonas vaginalis* and *M. hominis*, treatment that eliminated only *T. vaginalis* led to clinical improvement, whereas treatment that eliminated only *M. hominis* did not (Bercovici et al 1962), suggesting that the latter micro-organism was unimportant. However, in a study of 12 patients who had both micro-organisms, treatment with metronidazole eradicated *T. vaginalis* but not *M. hominis* and did not result in clinical cure (Weström & Mardh 1971). Pheifer et al (1978) also used metronidazole to treat patients suffering from 'non-specific vaginitis'. The drug eliminated *Gardnerella vaginalis* from most patients and this correlated with clinical improvement: surprisingly, *M. hominis* was also eliminated from many patients but without clinical improvement, again suggesting the unimportance of this mycoplasma. Blackwell et al (1983) also commented on the disappearance of *M. hominis* from patients who were given metronidazole. Tetracyclines, which inhibit *M. hominis* in vitro, have frequently been given to women who harbour this mycoplasma, often with disappearance of the abnormal cytological picture and eradication of the micro-organism. For example,

'dirty' vaginal smears attributed to *M. hominis* disappeared after such treatment (Mardh et al 1971). In contrast, Pheifer et al (1978) used doxycycline to treat BV but, despite eliminating *M. hominis*, they failed to effect clinical improvement.

Serological studies. Antibody to *M. hominis*, measured by the indirect haemagglutination technique, has been found almost three times more often in the sera of women with lower genital tract infections than in those of healthy controls. Paavonen et al (1983a) found that the mean level of serum IgG antibody against *M. hominis* was higher among women with BV than among controls. Moreover, metabolism inhibiting antibody to several ureaplasmas has been found more often in a group of women with lower genital tract infections than in other groups of women (Kundsin et al 1973). However, these differences are not, of course, proof that an aetiological relationship exists.

In conclusion, the results of the various studies do not suggest that *M. hominis* or ureaplasmas are of great importance in vaginitis or cervicitis. There is no doubt, however, that *M. hominis* is an important constituent of the abnormal vaginal flora found in BV and that ureaplasmas may be also. While the results of antibiotic studies suggest that *M. hominis* is not an aetiological agent in BV but merely flourishes in the particular environment generated by other micro-organisms, particularly *Gardnerella vaginalis* and anaerobes, its contribution to the pathological changes is not clear. It is possible that a small number of patients with true 'non-specific vaginitis' might have disease caused by *M. hominis*.

COMPLICATIONS OF LOWER GENITAL TRACT INFECTION

Endometritis and pelvic inflammatory disease

Micro-organisms present in the vagina and lower cervix may ascend directly or be carried haematogenously to the normally sterile regions of the upper genital tract, causing inflammation in the endometrium, fallopian tubes and adjacent pelvic structures. It is possible that *Mycoplasma hominis* may have a role in plasma cell endometritis, because Paavonen et al (1983b) found an association between this condition and the prevalence and titre of antibody to *M. hominis*. There was no association, however, between endometritis and the isolation of *M. hominis* from the cervix. Other aspects of endometritis in relation to recurrent abortion and infertility are discussed below.

Like non-gonococcal urethritis in men, non-gonococcal pelvic inflammatory disease (PID) does not have a single cause and the possibility that infection by genital mycoplasmas might be one cause has received attention from numerous investigators.

Isolation studies. There have been numerous reports (Taylor-Robinson & Csonka 1981) concerned with the isolation of large-colony forming mycoplasmas, including *M. hominis*, from inflamed fallopian tubes, tubo-ovarian abscesses, and pelvic abscesses or fluid. However, the most thorough and relevant studies have been carried out by Swedish investigators (Mardh & Weström, 1970a; Mardh et al 1975; Weström & Mardh 1975) who examined 50 women with salpingitis diagnosed laparoscopically, 50 carefully matched women without symptoms or signs of genital tract infection, and 50 women with lower genital tract infections. The absence of salpingitis was confirmed laparoscopically in 34 of these 100 patients. *M. hominis* was isolated from fallopian tube specimens taken from 4 (8%) women with salpingitis but not from similar specimens from women without signs of salpingitis. In addition, there were more isolations of *M. hominis* from cervical and urethral cultures of patients with salpingitis than from the control patients. Although *Neisseria gonorrhoeae* was isolated from the cervix or urethra of 17 of the 50 patients with salpingitis and from the tubes of 2 of them, the latter isolations were not concurrent with those of *M. hominis*. Sweet et al (1980) and Lind et al (1985) failed to isolate *M. hominis* from the tubes of 24 and 25 women with PID, respectively, but the former workers did isolate from the pouch of Douglas and subsequently have done so from the endometrium of 40% of cases of acute PID (Sweet 1986). Eschenbach et al (1975) also isolated this mycoplasma from the pouch of Douglas, 2 of 54 aspirates being culture-positive. Such studies would seem to be easier to interpret than those involving isolation attempts from the vagina or cervix (Moller et al 1981b). The fact that Eschenbach et al (1975) isolated *M. hominis* from endocervical swabs

from women with non-gonococcal acute PID only a little more often than from women without PID, that is 64% as against 54%, should not be taken to imply that *M. hominis* is not involved.

Ureaplasmas have been studied less extensively in acute PID but have been isolated from the endometrium of 15% of women (Sweet 1986), directly from the fallopian tubes of 4% (Mardh & Weström 1970a) and about 9% (Sweet 1986) of patients, respectively, from pelvic fluid (Solomon et al 1973; Eschenbach et al 1975) and from a tubo-ovarian abscess (Braun & Besdine 1973). *M. pneumoniae* has also been isolated from such an abscess (Thomas et al 1975). The significance of these findings is unclear but it seems likely that the recovery of *M. pneumoniae* must be a rare and chance event and that ureaplasmas will be found to be of less importance than *M. hominis*.

Serological studies. In some of the early studies (Melen & Gotthardson 1955; Lemcke & Csonka 1962), complement fixing antibody against large-colony forming mycoplasmas, presumably *M. hominis*, and *M. hominis* itself, was found in higher titre in the sera of some patients with salpingitis than in those from other groups of women serving as controls. Furthermore, the *M. hominis* isolation studies of the Swedish workers were given added significance by serological investigations on the same patients. Indirect haemagglutinating (IHA) antibody to *M. hominis* was found in the sera of 54% of patients with salpingitis, compared to 10.5% of healthy women (Mardh & Weström 1970c). In addition, a significant rise or fall in antibody titre was detected during the course of disease in the sera of 9 of 16 women who had *M. hominis* in the lower genital tract, 3 of them also having the organisms in their fallopian tubes (Mardh & Weström 1970c). An increased level of IgM antibody was found in 34% of the patients with acute salpingitis (Mardh 1970) and this was associated with the isolation of *M. hominis* and with the presence of IHA antibody to the mycoplasma. Other workers (Eschenbach et al 1975), who used a different serological procedure, also detected a larger number of antibody responses to *M. hominis* in groups of patients with acute PID than in selected control groups. More recently, two series of PID patients were tested for antibodies to *M. hominis*, *Chlamydia trachomatis* and *Neisseria gonorrhoeae* (Mardh et al

1981; Moller et al 1981b). Antibody to *M. hominis* was found in about 40% of the patients and a rise in antibody titre in 17–30%. These responses did not overlap completely with those to the chlamydiae and gonococci. In addition, Miettinen et al (1983) detected antibody responses to *M. hominis* in 23% of patients with PID and failed to isolate chlamydiae or gonococci from the cervix. The fact that some antibody responses to *M. hominis* occur in patients from whom this mycoplasma is not isolated from the cervix (Moller et al 1981b) suggests that cervical culture may be misleading in studying the aetiology of PID. A problem remains because Lind et al (1985) found antibody responses to *M. hominis* in only those patients who had evidence of chlamydial or gonococcal salpingitis and, on this basis, they did not regard the mycoplasma as a primary pathogen.

PID has been seen to develop after hysterosalpingography and in one case was associated serologically with *M. hominis* (Moller et al 1984a).

Antibody responses to ureaplasmas have been detected less often than responses to *M. hominis* in patients with PID (Mardh & Weström 1970b; Eschenbach et al 1975). This could indicate, of course, that ureaplasmas are less important than *M. hominis* or simply that antibody responses to ureaplasmas are more difficult to detect, a suggestion made with some justification.

Mycoplasma genitalium is difficult to isolate and this creates a problem in defining its role in inflammatory conditions. The serological approach, however, has shown some promise. Thirty-one women with acute PID, in whom serum antibodies to *Chlamydia trachomatis* and *M. hominis* could not be detected, were examined for antibodies to *M. genitalium* by a microimmunofluorescence technique. About 40% of them had a fourfold or greater change in the titre of antibody during the 1-month period after the onset of disease, suggesting that *M. genitalium* might be implicated (Moller et al 1984b).

Organ culture and animal model studies. Pieces of tissue and whole organs can be maintained in a culture system more or less in the same physiological condition as they occur in vivo. In fallopian tube organ cultures, ciliary activity may be assessed and used as an index of cell viability. *Neisseria gonorrhoeae* produces profound damage to the epithelium of such cultures (Taylor-Robinson et al 1975)

whereas *Mycoplasma hominis*, despite multiplying and persisting in the cultures, has been found to cause little more damage than swelling of some of the cilia (Mardh et al 1976). This may be due to the effect of ammonia produced by mycoplasmal metabolism. Ureaplasmas of human origin have been inoculated into fallopian tube organ cultures without obvious damage being observed (Taylor-Robinson & Carney 1974).

The failure of *M. hominis* and ureaplasmas to damage organ cultures appreciably does not necessarily mean that they are avirulent. The tissues in this system are separated from the immune mechanisms of the host which may play an important part in pathogenesis. This would seem to be the case, because the introduction of *M. hominis* into the oviducts of grivet monkeys produced a self-limited acute salpingitis and parametritis accompanied by an antibody response (Moller et al 1978). Other experiments (Moller & Mardh 1980) suggest that the organisms spread from the lower genital tract to the oviducts via the lymphatics and blood vessels rather than canalicularly via the uterus. In contrast, ureaplasmas have not produced disease in grivet monkeys (Moller et al 1981a). This cannot be said, however, for *M. genitalium*, which has produced salpingitis accompanied by an antibody response in grivet monkeys and marmosets following oviduct inoculation (Moller et al 1985a). The changes were similar to those produced by *Chlamydia trachomatis* and support the serological evidence for *M. genitalium* being involved in PID.

In conclusion, the isolation of *M. hominis* from a site which is normally sterile, accompanied by an antibody response, in addition to the findings in grivet monkeys inoculated experimentally, suggest that this mycoplasma has a primary pathogenic role in some cases of acute PID. Moller (1983) attributes 25% of all cases to *M. hominis*. Despite this, the significance of *M. hominis* and *M. genitalium* is not as clear as that of some other micro-organisms capable of causing the condition, nor is the role, if any, of the ureaplasmas. Serological studies are relatively easy to undertake and are rewarding if sera are tested for antibodies to *M. hominis*, *M. genitalium*, ureaplasmas, *N. gonorrhoeae* and *C. trachomatis* rather than against a single micro-organism. However, the relative contribution of *M. hominis* and ureaplasmas is likely to be determined best by a combined serological and cultural approach in geographically different areas, in which specimens obtained during laparoscopy from inflamed fallopian tubes are examined not only for genital mycoplasmas but also for *N. gonorrhoeae*, *C. trachomatis* and aerobic and anaerobic bacteria.

Infertility

It is not appropriate to discuss male infertility, but since fertility depends on the sum of the fertility of each partner it is sometimes necessary to refer to 'couples'.

As discussed previously, there are several indications that *M. hominis* has a primary pathogenic role in some cases of acute PID. Thus, this mycoplasma has the potential for causing infertility as a consequence of tubal disease and, indeed, antibody to *M. hominis* has been found three times more often in infertile women following PID than in a control group of women (Moller et al 1985b). Nevertheless, the extent to which infertility may be attributed to *M. hominis* after *M. hominis*-associated PID is unknown. The role of genital mycoplasmas in unexplained infertility has been debated for more than a decade and will be discussed under the following two headings.

Isolation studies. Although Gnarpe & Friberg (1972, 1973) isolated ureaplasmas more often from genital specimens taken from infertile than from fertile couples, these findings have not been confirmed consistently by other investigators. Thus, de Louvois et al (1974) isolated ureaplasmas from 53% of one partner or both partners of fertile couples but from no more than 57% of infertile couples. Similar data have been recorded by others (Matthews et al 1975; Andre et al 1978; Rehewy et al 1978; Nagata et al 1979). It must be admitted, however, that the criteria for selection of the infertile couples were not the same in all studies, which makes comparisons difficult.

A determination of mycoplasmas in the uterus may have greater relevance than an assessment of those in the cervix or vagina, provided the method of sample collection does not contaminate the endometrium from the lower genital tract. The extent to which this may have occurred in various studies is difficult to know. Nevertheless, it is of interest that ureaplasmas have been recovered more often

from endometrial specimens from infertile women than from fertile women (Koren & Spigland 1978; Stray-Pedersen et al 1978, 1982). However, in one of these studies (Stray-Pedersen et al 1982), the endometrial isolation rate for women with unexplained infertility was about the same as that for women in whom the cause of infertility was known. It is important to emphasise that an assessment of all the possible causes of infertility is essential in attempting to determine the possible role of microorganisms in the condition. This was an important ingredient in the detailed study by Cassell et al (1983b). They identified one clinicopathological entity, that is infertility associated with 'male factor', in which the prevalence of ureaplasmal infection of the female lower genital tract, but not of the endometrium, was over twice that observed in other groups of infertile women. No other clinical subpopulation with single or multiple diagnoses which did not include male factor had an increased prevalence of infection. Since male factor infertility involved 20% or less of infected infertile couples the possible role of ureaplasmas was small and it is, of course, still a moot point as to whether they are aetiologically involved. Certainly Gump et al (1984) do not believe that ureaplasmas or *M. hominis* interfere with the function or numbers of spermatozoa once they reach the cervical mucus.

Antibiotic studies. Uncontrolled antibiotic trials in which treatment of infertile ureaplasma-colonised persons was associated with conception in some instances are reviewed in detail elsewhere (Taylor-Robinson & McCormack 1979, 1980) and will not be considered further. Only one (Harrison et al 1975) of another five small studies mentioned previously (Taylor-Robinson & McCormack 1979, 1980) and one more recently (Upadhyaya et al 1983) was properly controlled and none of them provides support for the hypothesis that ureaplasmas are an important cause of unexplained infertility. More recently, Toth et al (1983) recorded that among 129 couples in which the men had negative ureaplasmal cultures after doxycycline treatment, the 3-year rate of successful pregnancy was 60%, in contrast to the 5% pregnancy rate among 32 couples in which cultures from the men remained positive after treatment. Busolo et al (1984) also gave doxycycline for 30 days to couples and reported that conception occurred in 5 of 19 who became ureaplasma-negative but not in any of 22 who, curiously, remained ureaplasma-positive. While these observations are seemingly provocative, a lack of adequate controls again means that their significance is in doubt. The antibiotic approach will only carry weight when a subpopulation with which ureaplasmas might be involved as a cause of infertility is defined, as emphasised by Cassell et al (1983b), and a large, properly controlled, double-blind study in which couples are randomly assigned to receive antimicrobial agent or placebo is conducted. Otherwise, there is no doubt that a causal relationship could be overlooked.

In conclusion, the role of genital mycoplasmas in human infertility is unresolved. Whether the risk of sterility after PID can be attributed at all to *M. hominis* is unknown. There are some recent interesting observations on the possible aetiological role of ureaplasmas in infertility but placebo-controlled treatment studies designed to evaluate this role need to be carefully thought out, otherwise a small effect of ureaplasmas might be overlooked. Finally, over-riding emphasis should not be placed on the eradication of infection, because this may not necessarily reverse damage that the organisms have caused.

Obstetric complications

Postpartum fever

Like other micro-organisms present in the vagina, genital mycoplasmas can be found almost immediately but transiently in the bloodstream after vaginal delivery and this is not associated with postpartum fever (McCormack et al 1975). However, there have been many reports (Taylor-Robinson & McCormack 1979) of individual patients with postpartum fever from whom *M. hominis* has been isolated from the blood a day or more after delivery and in whom an antibody response has nearly always been detected (McCormack et al 1973a; Wallace et al 1978). Genital mycoplasmas are seldom recovered from the blood of afebrile postpartum women (Wallace et al 1978) which further suggests that *M. hominis* causes postpartum fever, presumably by causing uterine infection. In one large study (Platt et al 1980), 23 of 535 women delivered vaginally had postpartum fever with

which *M. hominis* was the only micro-organism significantly associated. Furthermore, fever occurred most often in those who had a low or absent titre of antibody to *M. hominis* at delivery. These observations were corroborated by those of another study (Lamey et al 1982) in which genital mycoplasmas were isolated from the blood of 16 (12.8%) of 125 febrile puerperal women but from none of 60 afebrile women. The isolates were almost equally divided between *M. hominis* and the ureaplasmas. The recovery of the latter from the blood of febrile women has been commented on again by Eschenbach (1986) and it seems that they may be implicated too. Most patients have a low-grade fever for a day or two after delivery, are not severely ill, and recover uneventfully even without antibiotic therapy (Wallace et al 1978).

In conclusion, *M. hominis* is one of the causes of postpartum fever, but further studies are needed to define more fully its contribution to contemporary postpartum fever in relation to that of other micro-organisms. Ureaplasmas may be important in this regard also.

Postabortion fever

The most striking evidence for a role of *M. hominis* in fever after abortion comes from a prospective study (Harwick et al 1970) in which this mycoplasma was isolated from the blood of 4 of 51 women who had febrile abortions but not from 53 women who had afebrile abortions or from 102 normal pregnant women. A fourfold or greater rise in the titre of antibody to *M. hominis* was detected in the sera of half the women who became febrile after abortion but in only 2 of 14 women who had abortions and remained afebrile. In addition, others (Jones 1967a; Taylor-Robinson & McCormack 1979) have detected antibody responses to this mycoplasma after abortions. Thus, *M. hominis* appears to cause some cases of fever after abortion, although the observations are fewer than in the case of postpartum fever. As in the latter, the patients recover whether or not appropriate antibiotic treatment is given.

Arthritis after delivery

Since mycoplasmaemia occurs particularly after childbirth and abortion it is perhaps not surprising that there have been reports of the isolation of *M. hominis* from synovial fluids of mothers who developed arthritis soon after childbirth (Verinder 1978). In these cases, the temporal association and response to tetracycline therapy suggests a causal relationship. The possibility of *M. hominis* infection should be considered in patients with postpartum arthritis whose condition does not respond to penicillin.

Spontaneous preterm labour

The aetiology of preterm labour is multifactorial (Turnbull & Anderson 1978). Infection is thought to be one of the factors and has been a centre of interest recently (Minkoff 1983). Lamont et al (1986) studied the association between infection and preterm labour by examining prospectively 72 women in labour between 26 and 34 weeks' gestation and 26 controls of the same gestational age. Abnormal bacterial colonisation, the presence of ureaplasmas, a heavy growth of *M. hominis* and chorioamnionitis were all found significantly more often in the preterm labour group. However, infection appeared to be the result rather than the cause of ruptured membranes. Others (Hillier et al 1986) have noted an association between bacterial vaginosis and preterm labour, and among the various micro-organisms involved, ureaplasmas were associated independently with preterm delivery. Of course, to what extent, if any, the association of the organisms is a causal one is unknown. It has been postulated that the production of phospholipase A_2 by some micro-organisms with the subsequent release of arachidonic acid from cell membranes and the production of prostaglandins might be responsible for the initiation of labour.

The association of genital mycoplasmas with low birth weight occurring at full term is discussed below.

Intra-amniotic infection

In the USA, clinically evident intrauterine infection is said to occur in about 1% of pregnancies (Sweet & Gibbs 1985). This figure seems high, but whatever the prevalence, the condition leads to increased maternal morbidity and perinatal mortality and morbidity. The terms chorioamnionitis, amnionitis, intrapartum infection and amniotic fluid infection have also been applied. Subclinical infection of amniotic fluid is discussed in the following section.

Occasionally intra-amniotic infection (IAI) occurs without rupture of the membranes or labour and sometimes following a surgical procedure or as a complication of diagnostic amniocentesis or intrauterine transfusion. However, the ascent of micro-organisms from the lower genital tract with the onset of labour or with rupture of membranes is the most common cause of infection.

The micro-organisms involved are usually urinary tract pathogens associated with the intestinal flora (Gibbs et al 1982; Gravett et al 1982). However, there are individual case reports (see Taylor-Robinson 1978) of the recovery of genital mycoplasmas from the amniotic fluid of infected patients, and Shurin et al (1975) reported an association between the isolation of *M. hominis* and/or ureaplasmas and placental inflammation, but did not correlate isolation with maternal or neonatal infection. In a controlled study, however, Blanco et al (1983) found that 18 (35%) of 52 amniotic fluids collected via a transcervical catheter from patients with IAI contained *M. hominis* compared with 8% of 52 matched control fluids. Of course, the transcervical approach is not without the problem of contamination. Fifteen of the 18 fluids also contained pathogenic bacteria and ureaplasmas were isolated from an equal proportion (50%) of clinically infected and uninfected patients. Patients with IAI and *M. hominis* in the fluid responded clinically to antibiotic therapy which was not directed against this mycoplasma and *M. hominis* was isolated from some of the patients in the control group without apparent sequelae. In a further study, Cassell et al (1986) isolated ureaplasmas from 50% of amniotic fluids taken at the time of delivery from women with clinical IAI and from a similar proportion of matched controls; the organisms were isolated from the blood of 11 (13.6%) of 81 women with IAI and from 8 (18.2%) of 44 controls. The pathogenic potential of the genital mycoplasmas in this setting is, therefore, still unclear.

Habitual spontaneous abortion and stillbirth

Isolation studies. Several of the earlier workers who studied this subject pointed to the more frequent recovery of genital mycoplasmas from the lower genital tract of women who had spontaneous pregnancy losses than from women who did not. The report of Quinn et al (1983c) is no exception. They isolated ureaplasmas and/or *M. hominis* from 84.5% of couples with histories of pregnancy wastage but from only 25% of those with successful deliveries. However, in a prospective study, Munday et al (1984) isolated *M. hominis* most often from the cervices of women who had threatened abortions but this mycoplasma and ureaplasmas were found no more often in women who went on to abort than in those who had uncomplicated pregnancies. Further, in prospective studies of two large unselected groups of pregnant women (Harrison 1986), endocervical ureaplasmas were not found to be associated with spontaneous abortion although association with a small subgroup was not ruled out. Of course, endometrial rather than cervical ureaplasmas may be the more relevant indicator of the importance of genital mycoplasmas. In this regard, it is worth noting that Stray-Pedersen et al (1978) isolated ureaplasmas more often from the endometrium of women who had repeated spontaneous abortion (28%) than from the same site of women comprising a control group (7%), using an aspiration technique which would seem to be less likely to result in contamination from the cervix than curettage.

The other approach has been to examine the aborted products of conception. Contamination of the products by vaginal mycoplasmas at the time of birth is a problem which was not accounted for in the early studies and led to uninterpretable information. Some later workers, for example Quinn et al (1985), have taken steps to avoid contamination. The latter workers found genital mycoplasmas in 79% of perinatal deaths compared to 32% of controls, although the groups were very small. Furthermore, some of the mycoplasmas isolated from aborted fetuses and stillborn infants have come from the lungs, brain, heart and viscera, so that not all the isolations can be attributed to superficial contamination. The presence of genital mycoplasmas in the heart and viscera of an aborted fetus may be indicative of haematogenous spread, possibly due to invasion through the umbilical vessels. Their presence in the respiratory tract (see below) is probably due to aspiration of infected amniotic fluid. Mycoplasmal infection of the fluid may occur before rupture of the membranes (Taylor-Robinson

1978; Cassell 1982; Cassell et al 1983a). Repeated amniocentesis could lead to infection of the fluid, but whatever the cause, subclinical infection as opposed to clinical IAI would not seem to be a common event. Thus, Thomsen et al (1984) found that only 1 of 297 fluids contained ureaplasmas; these fluids were taken by transabdominal amniocentesis before membrane rupture in women in three geographical locations. Although it cannot be denied that subclinical infection of the fluid could be of serious consequence for the fetus, this is still problematical. Whatever the mode of entry to the fetus there is, as yet, no answer to the question of whether abortion occurs because mycoplasmas invade the fetus and cause its death, or because it dies from another cause, the mycoplasmas being subsequent unimportant invaders.

Serological studies. Antibody to *M. hominis* has been detected more frequently in women after abortion than in pregnant women before delivery (Jones 1967a) and, as mentioned previously, an antibody response to *M. hominis* may occur after an abortion (Jones 1967a; Harwick et al 1970; Taylor-Robinson & McCormack 1979). However, since genital mycoplasmas often enter the circulation after a normal pregnancy and stimulate an antibody response (Lin et al 1978), an increased frequency of antibody or a rise in the titre of antibody does not necessarily provide supportive evidence for *M. hominis* causing abortions. In the case of the ureaplasmas, Quinn et al (1983c) reported that 43% of aborted fetuses had serum metabolism inhibiting antibody titres which were fourfold greater than those detected in their mothers, whereas this difference was seen only in the case of 15% of normal infants. This observation, reaffirmed later (Quinn 1986), was taken to mean that a sizeable proportion of the fetuses were sufficiently infected to have produced antibody. Its significance, however, must await further study.

Antibiotic studies. Since mycoplasmas are sensitive to tetracyclines and other antibiotics, fetal loss, if caused by these organisms, might be prevented by appropriate antimicrobial therapy. Successful pregnancies have been recorded (Kundsin 1970; Stray-Pedersen et al 1978) in treated women who had been colonised by ureaplasmas and who had had frequent spontaneous abortions. However, because such treatment was uncontrolled and other micro-organisms, especially *Chlamydia trachomatis*, were not studied, it is inadvisable to draw the conclusion that the ureaplasmas were responsible for the reproductive failures. Quinn et al (1983b) gave doxycycline before conception to 62 ureaplasma-positive women who had previously had spontaneous abortions and reported a reduction in the pregnancy loss rate from 96 to 48% and a further reduction to 16% in women who were given erythromycin from the second or third month until the end of pregnancy. Nevertheless, this trial was small and not well controlled and considerable caution still needs to be exercised in interpreting the results of this or any other study, because it has been well documented (Hawkins 1974) that patients who have habitual spontaneous abortions frequently have a normal delivery when brought under hospital care.

Involvement of the fetus

Low birth weight

In studies (Elder et al 1971) conducted before it was recognised that there was an association between prenatal exposure to tetracycline and staining of the primary teeth, women who were treated with a placebo for 6 weeks during pregnancy gave birth to infants weighing 2500 g or less significantly more often than did women who were treated with tetracycline. It was postulated that tetracycline-sensitive micro-organisms might be responsible and mycoplasmas were among those considered.

Isolation studies. The first direct evidence for an association between mycoplasmas and birth weight was obtained in a study at the Boston City Hospital, USA (Klein et al 1969). It was found that the rates of nasal or pharyngeal colonisation of unselected newborn infants with genital mycoplasmas, mainly ureaplasmas, were roughly inversely proportional to birth weight. In a subsequent prospective study (Braun et al 1971), urine and cervical specimens obtained from 484 pregnant women at their first clinic visit were examined. Women who were colonised with ureaplasmas gave birth to infants with a significantly lower mean birth weight (3099 g) than those who were not colonised (3297 g). Embree et al (1980) have also found this association. However, others (Foy et al 1970b; Harrison et al 1979; Ross et al 1981; Upadhyaya et

al 1983; Munday et al 1985) have been unable to associate ureaplasmal colonisation with low birth weight. Indeed, Ross et al (1981) found that Caucasian women colonised by ureaplasmas had larger babies than those born to non-colonised women. This difference was not seen for babies born to Asian women and the authors speculated that race and social class were more important than the ureaplasmas in affecting the size of the infant. Gilbert et al (1986) noted that women with ureaplasmal bacteriuria were more likely to develop pre-eclampsia than those without, but the birth weights of their infants were not, on average, reduced.

Harrison (1986) reported on the endocervical carriage of ureaplasmas and their association with abnormal pregnancy outcome in two large unselected groups of women studied prospectively. Ureaplasmas were not found to be associated with spontaneous abortion or preterm low birth weight in univariate analysis, nor with low birth weight or postpartum endometritis/fever either in univariate analysis or by conditional logistic regression. He pointed out, however, that an association might exist in subgroups of infected women and outlined the need and the difficulties of defining such subgroups.

The association between *M. hominis* and low birth weight is less striking than for ureaplasmas and low birth weight in the Boston area (Foy et al 1970b; Braun et al 1971; Embree et al 1980; Ross et al 1981), although an association has been recorded by some investigators (di Musto et al 1973; Romano et al 1976).

Serological studies. Recent observations in the Boston area (Kass et al 1981) have provided additional support for the association of ureaplasmas with low birth weight. Serological tests were undertaken on 246 ureaplasma-positive women. Of those delivering infants weighing <2500 g, 30% had a more than fourfold rise in the titre of antibody whereas only 7.3% with infants of >2500 g had such a rise.

Antibiotic studies. In a double-blind trial of erythromycin in pregnant women (Kass et al 1981), 250 mg of the antibiotic or a placebo were given four times daily for 6 weeks. Treatment during the second trimester had no effect on birth weight. However, women treated with erythromycin during the third trimester delivered infants with a greater mean birth weight (3331 g) than did women in the placebo group (3187 g) and only 2 of 64 treated women delivered infants weighing ≤2500 g compared with 10 of 84 in the placebo group.

In conclusion, the association between genital mycoplasmas and low birth weight has not been seen in all populations. However, there seems no doubt that in a few of the populations studied, the association between low birth weight and mycoplasmal infection, particularly with ureaplasmas, is a real phenomenon. It is feasible that the organisms cause chorioamnionitis in the later stages of pregnancy and that this results in impaired fetal nutrition or early labour or both. On the other hand, it cannot be concluded that genital mycoplasmas are directly responsible for low birth weight, because it is possible that women who have a predisposition to smaller babies are selectively colonised. Clearly, however, in view of the importance of low birth weight in perinatal morbidity and mortality, the phenomenon warrants further investigation.

Involvement of the newborn

Occasionally, colonisation or infection of the newborn by genital mycoplasmas will have occurred in utero. More often, passage through a birth canal colonised by genital mycoplasmas, mostly ureaplasmas, results in colonisation of the infant (Klein et al 1969; Foy et al 1970a; Braun et al 1971), as discussed previously. Thus, an opportunity is provided for the subsequent development of disease of the skin (Hoogendijk et al 1965; Sacher et al 1970) and of other sites, as indicated below.

Neonatal conjunctivitis

M. hominis has been isolated from the eyes of babies with neonatal conjunctivitis and proposed as a cause of the disease (Jones & Tobin 1968). However, as pointed out previously (Tyrrell & Taylor-Robinson 1968), an aetiological relationship is not proven and cannot be deduced without knowing, in the same study, the extent to which other micro-organisms, particularly *C. trachomatis*, are responsible for the disease.

The proportion of pregnant women who are infected in the lower genital tract by ureaplasmas will vary from one population to another. However, in one hospital where the ureaplasmal isolation rate for women attending an antenatal clinic was about 40% (Ross et al 1981), conjunctival colonisation with ureaplasmas was detected in only about 2% of newborn infants (Prentice et al 1977). This may be due to the closure of the eyes before birth and/or an inherent insusceptibility of the conjunctival mucosa to ureaplasmal infection, as suggested by the failure to infect the eyes of chimpanzees with ureaplasmas of human origin (Taylor-Robinson, unpublished observations). In any event, ureaplasmal colonisation would seem to occur rarely and, so far, has not been associated with conjunctivitis.

Neonatal pneumonia

M. hominis was suggested as a possible cause of the respiratory distress syndrome (RDS; Steytler 1970), and, in one case, infection of amniotic fluid by this mycoplasma after rupture of the membranes appeared to be responsible (Brunell et al 1969). In another case, this mycoplasma seemed to be the cause of respiratory distress, fever and pneumonia occurring within a few hours of birth; isolation from blood was accompanied by an antibody response and the patient responded slowly to tetracycline (Unsworth et al 1985). There are also other studies in which the genital mycoplasmas have been associated with neonatal respiratory disease, that of Dische et al (1979) being an example. They recovered *M. hominis* and ureaplasmas from the fetal lung. Since ureaplasmas are present in the female genital tract more frequently than *M. hominis*, the possibility that they may be a more significant cause of RDS deserves attention. However, studies by Taylor-Robinson et al (1984) and Rudd & Carrington (1985), based on the isolation of ureaplasmas, failed to demonstrate a pathogenic role for them. In the former study, these organisms were isolated from the throats and gastric aspirates of babies without RDS almost as frequently as from those who suffered from it. This finding does not suggest an aetiological involvement, and was supported by the almost total failure to isolate ureaplasmas from babies born by Caesarean section, 40% of whom developed RDS. It could be argued, however, that the data do not enable a distinction to be made between colonisation and infection and that the latter could be occurring in infants with

RDS. In this regard, it is of interest that Quinn et al (1983a) and Quinn (1986) have reported that, at birth, higher metabolism-inhibiting antibody titres to some ureaplasmas exist in the sera of neonates with RDS than in the sera of normal infants. In addition, some of the neonates with RDS were reported to have a higher antibody titre than that of the mother, suggesting infection in utero. However, Rudd et al (1986) are critical of these serological findings and summarise their own (Rudd et al, 1984) and those of Gallo et al (1983) which are less supportive of an association between ureaplasmas and RDS. If the serological findings of Quinn and colleagues are, indeed, indicative of ureaplasmal infection, its exact site and whether it is responsible for RDS remain open questions.

Neonatal meningitis

The few reported cases of meningitis in which *M. hominis* has been isolated from cerebrospinal fluid (Wealthall 1975; Gewitz et al 1979; Hjelm et al 1980) or brain (Siber et al 1977) have resulted presumably from infection in utero, or from colonisation at birth with subsequent infection. Such infection seems to be more likely if there is an anatomical abnormality, such as spina bifida, and the possibility should be considered in cases of neonatal central nervous system disease in which the results of bacteriological staining and culture techniques are negative.

SUMMARY

Twelve different mycoplasma species have been isolated from human subjects, at least four of which have been found predominantly in the genitourinary tract. The frequency of occurrence of the newly discovered *Mycoplasma genitalium* is, as yet, unknown, but it may be involved in some cases of acute salpingitis. Of the others, *M. hominis* and *Ureaplasma urealyticum* (ureaplasmas) are found most frequently, but rarely before puberty. After this time, the frequency of colonisation of the lower genital tract depends on a variety of factors, perhaps the most important of which is sexual experience. The association of these mycoplasmas with disease is sometimes difficult to assess, in particular proving a negative association. It is, therefore, unwise to be too dogmatic. Nevertheless, *M. hominis* does not seem to be an important cause of bartholinitis, vaginitis, or cervicitis, although its role in association with other micro-organisms needs to be elucidated, particularly in the context of bacterial vaginosis. The significance of ureaplasmas in the latter condition and in cervicitis needs further exploration. Mycoplasmas may spread from the lower genital tract and there is evidence to show that *M. hominis* causes some cases of acute salpingitis, postpartum and postabortion fever, and occasionally arthritis after delivery. There is little evidence to implicate ureaplasmas in these conditions apart, possibly, from postpartum fever. Neither the ureaplasmas nor *M. hominis* have been shown conclusively to cause infertility. *M. hominis* and ureaplasmas, together with various bacteria, have been associated with preterm labour but whether the association is a causal one is unknown. Furthermore, ureaplasmas are not a major cause of spontaneous abortion but their role in some cases of recurrent abortion has not been discounted. In some studies, ureaplasmas have been associated with low birth weight, but it seems unlikely that they are a direct cause of the diminished weight. Although mycoplasmas in the genital tract might affect the infant after birth, they have not been associated with neonatal conjunctivitis and there is scanty evidence for the role of ureaplasmas in neonatal pneumonia or the respiratory distress syndrome. However, *M. hominis* has caused neonatal pneumonia and meningitis occasionally.

REFERENCES

André D, Sepetjian M, Mikaelian S, Fouillet C 1978 Rôle des mycoplasmes dans la stérilité: étude de 150 femmes stériles. Journal de Gynécologie Obstétrique et Biologie de la Réproduction (Paris) 7: 51–56

Archer J F 1968 'T' strain mycoplasma in the female uro-genital tract. British Journal of Venereal Diseases 44: 232–234

Bercovici B, Persky S, Rozansky R, Razin S 1962 Mycoplasma (pleuropneumonia-like organisms) in vaginitis. American Journal of Obstetrics and Gynecology 84: 687–691

Blackwell A L, Fox A R, Phillips I, Barlow D 1983 Anaerobic vaginosis (non-specific vaginitis): clinical, microbiological, and therapeutic findings. Lancet ii: 1379–1382

Blanco J D, Gibb R S, Malherbe H, Strickland-Cholmley M, St Clair P J, Castaneda Y S 1983 A controlled study of genital mycoplasmas in amniotic fluid from patients with intra-amniotic infection. Journal of Infectious Diseases 147: 650–653

Braun P, Besdine R 1973 Tuboovarian abscess with recovery of T-mycoplasma. American Journal of Obstetrics and Gynecology 117: 861–862

Braun P, Lee Y -H, Klein J O et al 1971 Birth weight and genital mycoplasmas in pregnancy. New England Journal of Medicine 284: 167–171

Brunell P A, Dische R M, Walker M B 1969 Mycoplasma, amnionitis, and respiratory distress syndrome. Journal of American Medical Association 207: 2097–2099

Busolo F, Zanchetta R, Lanzone E, Cusinato R 1984 Microbial flora in semen of asymptomatic infertile men. Andrologia 16: 269–275

Cassell G H 1982 The pathogenic potential of mycoplasmas: Mycoplasma pulmonis as a model. Review of Infectious Diseases 4 (Suppl): 18–34

Cassell G H, Davis R O, Waites K B et al 1983a Isolation of Mycoplasma hominis and Ureaplasma urealyticum from amniotic fluid at 16–20 weeks of gestation: potential effect on outcome of pregnancy. Sexually Transmitted Diseases 10 (Suppl): 294–302

Cassell G H, Younger J B, Brown M B et al 1983b Microbiologic study of infertile women at the time of diagnostic laparoscopy: association of Ureaplasma urealyticum with a defined sub-population. New England Journal of Medicine 308: 502–505

Cassell G H, Waites K B, Gibbs R S, Davis J K 1986 Role of Ureaplasma urealyticum in amnionitis. Pediatric Infectious Diseases 5 (Suppl): 247–252

Csonka G W, Williams R E O, Corse J 1966 T-strain mycoplasma in non-gonococcal urethritis. Lancet i: 1292–1296

Csutortoki V, Stipkovits L, Varga L 1975 Mycoplasma pneumoniae in gynaecologic diseases. Acta Microbiologica Academiae Scientarium Hungaricae 22: 353

Dattanl I M, Gerken A, Evans B A 1982 Aetiology and management of non-specific vaginitis. British Journal of Venereal Diseases 58: 32–35

DelGiudice R A, Carski T R, Barile M F, Lemcke R M, Tully J G 1971 Proposal for classifying human strain Navel and related simian mycoplasmas as Mycoplasma primatum sp. n. Journal of Bacteriology 108: 439–455

de Louvois J, Blades M, Harrison R F, Hurley R, Stanley V C 1974 Frequency of mycoplasma in fertile and infertile couples. Lancet i: 1073–1075

de Louvois J, Hurley R, Stanley V C 1975 Microbial flora of the lower genital tract during pregnancy: relationship to morbidity. Journal of Clinical Pathology 28: 731–735

Dienes L, Edsall G 1937 Observations on the L-organism of Klieneberger. Proceedings of the Society for Experimental Biology and Medicine 36: 740–744

di Musto J C, Bohjalian O, Millar M 1973 Mycoplasma hominis type 1 infection and pregnancy. Obstetrics and Gynecology 41: 33–37

Dische M R, Quinn P A, Czegledy-Nagy E, Sturgess J M 1979 Genital mycoplasma infection: intrauterine infection: pathologic study of the fetus and placenta. American Journal of Clinical Pathology 72: 167–174

Dunlop E M C, Hare M J, Jones B R, Taylor-Robinson D 1969 Mycoplasmas and 'nonspecific' genital infection. II. Clinical aspects. British Journal of Venereal Diseases 45: 274–281

Elder H A, Santamarina B A G, Smith S, Kass E H 1971 The natural history of asymptomatic bacteriuria during pregnancy: the effect of tetracycline on the clinical course and the outcome of pregnancy. American Journal of Obstetrics and Gynecology 111: 441–462

Embree J E, Krause V W, Embil J A, MacDonald S 1980 Placental infection with Mycoplasma hominis and Ureaplasma urealyticum. Clinical correlation. Obstetrics and Gynecology 56: 475–481

Eschenbach D A 1986 Ureaplasma urealyticum as a cause of postpartum fever. Pediatric Infectious Diseases 5 Suppl: 258–261

Eschenbach D A, Buchanan T M, Pollock H M et al 1975 Polymicrobial etiology of acute pelvic inflammatory disease. New England Journal of Medicine 293: 166–171

Ford D K 1967 Relationships between mycoplasma and the etiology of nongonococcal urethritis and Reiter's syndrome. Annals of the New York Academy of Sciences 143: 501–504

Foy H M, Kenny G E, Levinsohn E M, Grayston J T 1970a Acquisition of mycoplasmata and T-strains during infancy. Journal of Infectious Diseases 121: 579–587

Foy H M, Kenny G E, Wentworth B B, Johnson W L, Grayston J T 1970b Isolation of Mycoplasma hominis, T-strains and cytomegalovirus from the cervix of pregnant women. American Journal of Obstetrics and Gynecology 106: 635–643

Foy H M, Kenny G E, Bor E, Hammar S, Hickman R 1975 Prevalence of Mycoplasma hominis and Ureaplasma urealyticum (T-strains) in urine of adolescents. Journal of Clinical Microbiology 2: 226–230

Gallo D, Dupuis K W, Schmidt N J 1983 Broadly reactive immunofluorescence test for measurement of immunoglobulin M and G antibodies to Ureaplasma urealyticum in infant and adult sera. Journal of Clinical Microbiology 17: 614–618

Gardner H L, Dukes C D 1955 Haemophilus vaginalis vaginitis. A newly defined specific infection previously classified 'nonspecific vaginitis'. American Journal of Obstetrics and Gynecology 69: 962–976

Gewitz M, Dinwiddie R, Rees L et al 1979 Mycoplasma hominis. A cause of neonatal meningitis. Archives of Disease in Childhood 54: 231–233

Gibbs R S, Blanco J D, St Clair P J, Castaneda Y S 1982 Quantitative bacteriology of amniotic fluid from women with clinical intraamniotic infection at term. Journal of Infectious Diseases 145: 1–8

Gilbert G L, Garland S M, Fairley K F, McDowall D M R 1986 Bacteriuria due to ureaplasmas and other fastidious organisms during pregnancy: prevalence and significance. Pediatric Infectious Diseases 5 Suppl: 239–243

Gnarpe H, Friberg J 1972 Mycoplasma and human reproductive failure. I. The occurrence of different mycoplasmas in couples with reproductive failure. American Journal of Obstetrics and Gynecology 114: 727–731

Gnarpe H, Friberg J 1973 T-mycoplasmas as a possible cause for reproductive failure. Nature 242: 120–121

Gravett M G, Eschenbach D A 1986 Possible role of Ureaplasmas urealyticum in preterm premature rupture of the fetal membrane. Paediatric Infectious Diseases 5 (Suppl): 253–257

Gravett M G, Eschenbach D A, Speigel-Brown C A, Holmes K K 1982 Rapid diagnosis of amniotic-fluid infection by gas-liquid chromatography. New England Journal of Medicine 306: 725–728

Gregory J E, Payne F E 1970 Mycoplasma in the uterine cervix. American Journal of Obstetrics and Gynecology 107: 220–226

Gump D W, Horton E, Phillips C A, Mead P B, Forsyth B R 1975 Contraception and cervical colonization with mycoplasmas and infection with cytomegalovirus. Fertility and Sterility 26: 1135–1139

Gump D W, Gibson M, Ashikaga T 1984 Lack of association between genital mycoplasmas and infertility. New England Journal of Medicine 310: 937–941

Hammerschlag M R, Alpert S, Rosner I et al 1978 Microbiology of the vagina in children: normal and potentially pathogenic organisms. Pediatrics 62: 57–62

Hanna N F, Taylor-Robinson D, Kalodiki-Karamanoli M, Harris J R W, McFadyen I R 1985 The relation between vaginal pH and the microbiological status in vaginitis. British Journal of Obstetrics and Gynaecology 92: 1267–1271

Hare M J, Toone E, Taylor-Robinson D et al 1981 Follicular cervicitis-colposcopic appearances and association with Chlamydia trachomatis. British Journal of Obstetrics and Gynaecology 88: 174–189

Hare M J, Taylor-Robinson D, Cooper P 1982 Evidence for an association between Chlamydia trachomatis and cervical intraepithelial neoplasia. British Journal of Obstetrics and Gynaecology 89: 489–492

Harrison H R 1986 Cervical colonization with Ureaplasma urealyticum and pregnancy outcome: prospective studies. Pediatric Infectious Diseases 5 Suppl: 266–269

Harrison R F, de Louvois J, Blades M. Hurley R 1975 Doxycycline treatment and human infertility. Lancet i: 605–607

Harrison R F, Hurley R, de Louvois J 1979 Genital mycoplasmas and birth weight in offspring of primigravid women. American Journal of Obstetrics and Gynecology 133: 201–203

Harwick H J, Purcell R H, Iuppa J B, Fekety F R 1970 Mycoplasma hominis and abortion. Journal of Infectious Diseases 121: 260–268

Hawkins D F 1974 Sex hormones in pregnancy. In: Hawkins D F (ed) Obstetric therapeutics. Bailliere Tindall, London. pp 106–151

Hillier S L, Krohn M J, Kiviat N, Martius J, Eschenbach D A 1986 The association of Ureaplasma urealyticum with preterm birth, chorioamnionitis, post-partum fever, intrapartum fever and bacterial vaginosis. Pediatric Infectious Diseases 5 Suppl: 349

Hjelm E, Jonsell G, Linglov T, Mardh P -A, Moller B R, Sedin G 1980 Meningitis in a newborn infant caused by Mycoplasma hominis. Acta Paediatrica Scandinavica 69: 415–418

Hoogendijk J L, De Bruijne J I, Herderschee D 1965 Infectie door Mycoplasma hominis bij een pasgeborene. Nederlands Tijdschrift voor Geneeskunde 109: 1433–1434

Hunter J M, Young H, Harris A B 1981 Genitourinary infection with Ureaplasma urealyticum in women attending a sexually transmitted diseases clinic. British Journal of Venereal Diseases 57: 338–342

Jones D M 1967a Mycoplasma hominis in abortion. British Medical Journal 1: 338

Jones D M, 1967b Mycoplasma hominis in pregnancy. Journal of Clinical Pathology 20: 633–635

Jones D M, Sequeira P J L 1966 The distribution of complement-fixing antibody and growth-inhibiting antibody to Mycoplasma hominis. Journal of Hygiene (London) 64: 441–449

Jones D M, Tobin B 1968 Neonatal eye infections due to Mycoplasma hominis. British Medical Journal 3: 467–468

Kass E H, McCormack W, Lin J-S, Rosner B 1981 Genital mycoplasmas as a hitherto unsuspected cause of excess premature delivery in the underprivileged. Clinical Research 29: 575A

Klein J O, Buckland D, Finland M 1969 Colonization of newborn infants by mycoplasmas. New England Journal of Medicine 280: 1025–1030

Koren Z, Spigland I 1978 Irrigation technique for detection of Mycoplasma intrauterine infection in infertile patients. Obstetrics and Gynecology 52: 588–590

Kundsin R B 1970 Mycoplasma in genitourinary tract infection and reproductive failure. Progress in Gynecology 5: 275–282

Kundsin R B, Kirsch A, Parreno A 1971 Mycoplasma isolation from the urine and metabolic inhibition of T strains in nuns. Bacteriological Proceedings 77

Kundsin R B, Parreno A, Kirsch A 1973 T-strain mycoplasma isolation and serology in women. British Journal of Venereal Diseases 49: 381–384

Lamey J R, Eschenbach D A, Mitchell S H, Blumhagen J M, Foy H M, Kenny G E 1982 Isolation of mycoplasmas and bacteria from the blood of postpartum women. American Journal of Obstetrics and Gynecology 143: 104–111

Lamont R F, Taylor-Robinson D, Newman M, Wigglesworth J, Elder M G 1986 Spontaneous early preterm labour associated with abnormal genital bacterial colonisation. British Journal of Obstetrics and Gynaecology 93: 804–810

Lee Y -H, Rankin J S, Alpert S, Daly A K, McCormack W M 1977 Microbiological investigation of Bartholin's gland abscesses and cysts. American Journal of Obstetrics and Gynecology 129: 150–153

Lemcke R, Csonka G W 1962 Antibodies against pleuropneumonia-like organisms in patients with salpingitis. British Journal of Venereal Diseases 38: 212–217

Lin J -S L, Radnay K, Kendrick M I, Rosner B, Kass E H 1978 Serologic studies of human genital mycoplasmas: distribution of titers of mycoplasmacidal antibody to Ureaplasma urealyticum and Mycoplasma hominis in pregnant women. Journal of Infectious Diseases 137: 266–273

Lind K, Kristensen G B, Bollerup A C et al 1985 Importance of Mycoplasma hominis in acute salpingitis assessed by culture and serological tests. Genitourinary Medicine 61: 185–189

McCormack W M 1978 Personal Communication

McCormack W M 1974 Factors associated with vaginal colonization with genital mycoplasmas (abstract) In: Proceedings of 14th Interscience Conference on Antimicrobial Agents and Chemotherapy, San Francisco. American Society of Microbiology, Washington, p 385

McCormack W M, Almeida P C, Bailey P E, Grady E M, Lee Y -H 1972a Sexual activity and vaginal colonization with genital mycoplasmas. Journal of the American Medical Association 221: 1375–1377

McCormack W M, Rankin J S, Lee Y -H 1972b Localization of genital mycoplasmas in women. American Journal of Obstetrics and Gynecology 112: 920–923

McCormack W M, Lee Y -H, Lin J -S, Rankin J S 1973a Genital mycoplasmas in postpartum fever. Journal of Infectious Diseases 127: 193–196

McCormack W M, Rosner B, Lee Y -H 1973b Colonization with genital mycoplasmas in women. American Journal of Epidemiology 97: 240–245

McCormack W M, Rosner B, Lee Y -H, Rankin J S, Lin J -S 1975 Isolation of genital mycoplasmas from blood obtained shortly after vaginal delivery. Lancet i: 596–599

Mardh P -A 1970 Increased serum levels of IgM in acute salpingitis related to the occurrence of Mycoplasma hominis. Acta Pathologica Microbiologica Scandinavica 78B: 726–732

Mardh P -A, Weström L 1970a Tubal and cervical cultures in acute salpingitis with special reference to Mycoplasma hominis and T-strain mycoplasmas. British Journal of Venereal Diseases 46: 179–186

Mardh P -A, Weström L 1970b T-mycoplasmas in the genitourinary tract of the female. Acta Pathologica Microbiologica Scandinavica 78B: 367–374

Mardh P -A, Weström L 1970c Antibodies to Mycoplasma hominis in patients with genital infections and in healthy controls. British Journal of Venereal Diseases 46: 390–397

Mardh P -A, Stormby N, Weström L 1971 Mycoplasma and vaginal cytology. Acta Cytologica 15: 310–315

Mardh P -A, Weström L, Colleen S 1975 Infections of the genital and urinary tracts with mycoplasmas and ureaplasmas. In: Danielsson D, Juhlin L, Mardh P -A (eds) Genital infections and their complications. Almqvist and Wiksell, Stockholm 53–62

Mardh P -A, Weström L, von Mecklenburg C, Hammar E 1976 Studies on ciliated epithelia of the human genital tract. I Swelling of the cilia of Fallopian tube epithelium in organ cultures infected with Mycoplasma hominis. British Journal of Venereal Diseases 52: 52–57

Mardh P -A, Lind I, Svensson L, Weström L, Moller B R 1981 Antibodies to Chlamydia trachomatis, Mycoplasma hominis and Neisseria gonorrhoeae in sera from patients with acute salpingitis. British Journal of Venereal Diseases 57: 125–129

Matthews C D, Elmslie R G, Clapp K H, Svigos J M 1975 The frequency of genital mycoplasma infection in human fertility. Fertility and Sterility 26: 988–990

Melen B, Gotthardson A 1955 Complement fixation with human pleuro-pneumonia-like organisms. Acta Pathologica et Microbiologica Scandinavica 37: 196–200

Mendel E B, Rowan D F, Graham J H M, Dellinger D 1970 Mycoplasma species in the vagina and their relation to vaginitis. Obstetrics and Gynecology 35: 104–108

Miettinen A, Paavonen J, Jansson E, Leinikki P 1983 Enzyme immunoassay for serum antibody to Mycoplasma hominis in women with acute pelvic inflammatory disease. Sexually Transmitted Diseases 10 (Suppl): 289–293

Minkoff H 1983 Prematurity: Infection as an etiologic factor. Obstetrics and Gynecology 62: 137–144

Moller B R 1983 The role of mycoplasmas in the upper genital tract of women. Sexually Transmitted Diseases 10 (Suppl): 281–284

Moller B R, Mardh P -A 1980 Experimental salpingitis in grivet monkeys. Modes of spread of infection to the Fallopian tubes. Acta Pathologica Microbiologica Scandinavica 88B: 107–114

Moller B R, Freundt E A, Black F T, Fredericksen P 1978 Experimental infection of the genital tract of female grivet monkeys by Mycoplasma hominis. Infection and Immunity 20: 248–257

Moller B R, Black F T, Freundt E A 1981a Attempts to produce gynaecological disease in grivet monkeys with Ureaplasma urealyticum. Journal of Medical Microbiology 14: 475–478

Moller B R, Mardh P -A, Ahrons S, Nussler E 1981b Infection with Chlamydia trachomatis, Mycoplasma hominis and Neisseria gonorrhoeae in patients with acute pelvic inflammatory disease. Sexually Transmitted Diseases 8: 198–202

Moller B R, Allen J, Toft B, Brogaard Hansen K, Taylor-Robinson D 1984a Pelvic inflammatory disease after hysterosalpingography associated with Chlamydia trachomatis and Mycoplasma hominis. British Journal of Obstetrics and Gynaecology 91: 1181–1187

Moller B R, Taylor-Robinson D, Furr P M 1984b Serological evidence implicating Mycoplasma genitalium in pelvic inflammatory disease. Lancet i: 1102–1103

Moller B R, Taylor-Robinson D, Furr P M, Freundt E A 1985a. Acute upper genital-tract disease in female monkeys provoked experimentally by Mycoplasma genitalium. British Journal of Experimental Pathology 66: 417–426

Moller B R, Taylor-Robinson D, Furr P M, Toft B, Allen J 1985b Serological evidence that chlamydiae and mycoplasmas are involved in infertility of women. Journal of Reproduction and Fertility 73: 237–240

Munday P E 1979 Unpublished data

Munday P E, Furr P M, Taylor-Robinson D 1981 The prevalence of Ureaplasma urealyticum and Mycoplasma hominis in the cervix and anal canal of women. Journal of Infection 3: 253–257

Munday P E, Ison C A 1982 Unpublished data

Munday P E, Porter R, Falder P F et al 1984 Spontaneous abortion—an infectious aetiology? British Journal of Obstetrics and Gynaecology 91: 1177–1180

Munday P E, Carder J M, Falder P F, Taylor-Robinson D, Porter R, Lewis B V 1985 The role of sexually transmitted micro-organisms in pregnancy wastage and perinatal morbidity. In: Morisset R, Kurstal R E (eds) Advances in sexually transmitted diseases. VNU Science Press, Utrecht, p 11–15

Nagata Y, Iwasaka T, Wada T 1979 Mycoplasma infection and infertility. Fertility and Sterility 31: 392–395

Paavonen J, Brunham R, Kiviat N et al 1982 Cervicitis-etiologic, clinical, and histopathologic findings. In: Mardh P-A, Holmes K K, Oriel J D, Piot P, Schachter J (eds) Chlamydial infections. Elsevier, Amsterdam, pp 141–145

Paavonen J, Miettinen A, Stevens C E, Chen K C S, Holmes K K 1983a Mycoplasma hominis in nonspecific vaginitis. Sexually Transmitted Diseases 10 (suppl) 271–275

Paavonen J, Miettinen A, Stevens C E et al; 1983b Mycoplasma hominis in cervicitis and endometritis. Sexually Transmitted Diseases 10 (suppl): 276–280

Paavonen J, Critchlow C W, DeRouen T et al 1986 Ureaplasma urealyticum associated with mucopurulent cervicitis. Pediatric Infectious Diseases 5 Suppl: 354

Pheifer T A, Forsyth P S, Durfee M A, Pollock H M, Holmes K K 1978 Nonspecific vaginitis: role of Haemophilus vaginalis and treatment with metronidazole. New England Journal of Medicine 298: 1429–1434

Platt R, Lin J S -L, Warren J W, Rosner B, Edelin K C, McCormack W M 1980 Infection with Mycoplasma hominis in postpartum fever. Lancet ii: 1217–1221

Prentice M J, Hutchinson G R, Taylor-Robinson D 1977 A microbiological study of neonatal conjunctivae and conjunctivitis. British Journal of Ophthalmology 61: 601–607

Purcell R H, Taylor-Robsinson D, Wong D, Chanock R M 1966 Color test for the measurement of antibody to T-strain mycoplasmas. Journal of Bacteriology 92: 6–12

Purcell R H, Chanock R M, Taylor-Robinson D 1969 Serology of the mycoplasmas of man. In: Hayflick L (ed) The mycoplasmatales and the L-phase of bacteria. Appleton-Century-Crofts, New York, pp 221–264

Quinn P A 1986 Evidence of an immune response to Ureaplasma urealyticum in perinatal morbidity and mortality. Journal of Pediatric Infectious Diseases 5 Suppl: 282–287

Quinn P A, Rubin S, Li H C S, Nocilla D M, Read S E, Chipman M 1983a Serological evidence of Ureaplasma urealyticum infection in neonatal respiratory disease. Yale Journal of Biology and Medicine 56: 565–572

Quinn P A, Shewchuk A B, Shuber J et al 1983b Efficacy of antibiotic therapy in preventing spontaneous pregnancy loss among couples with genital mycoplasmas. American Journal of Obstetrics and Gynecology 145: 239–244

Quinn P A, Shewchuk A B, Shuber J et al 1983c Serologic evidence of Ureaplasma urealyticum infection in women with spontaneous pregnancy loss. American Journal of Obstetrics and Gynecology 145: 245–250

Quinn P A, Butany J, Chipman M, Taylor J, Hannah W 1985 A prospective study of microbial infection in stillbirths and early neonatal death. American Journal of Obstetrics and Gynecology 151: 238–249

Rehewy M S E, Jaszczak S, Hafez E S E, Thomas A, Brown W J 1978 Ureaplasma urealyticum (T-mycoplasma) in vaginal fluid and cervical mucus from fertile and infertile women. Fertility and Sterility 30: 297–300

Romano N, Romano F 1968 Reperto e significato di Micoplasmi nelle infezioni infiammatorie del tratto vaginale. Giornale di Malattie Infettive Parassitarie 20: 585–591

Romano N, Scariata G, Cadili G, Carolle F 1976 Mycoplasmas in pregnant women and in newborn infants. Bollettino dell' Istituto Sieroterapico Milanese 55: 568–572

Ross J M, Furr P M, Taylor-Robinson D, Altman D G, Cold C R 1981 The effect of genital mycoplasmas on human fetal growth. British Journal of Obstetrics and Gynaecology 88: 749–755

Rudd P T, Carrington D 1985 A prospective study of chlamydial, mycoplasmal and viral infections in a neonatal intensive care unit. Archives of Disease in Childhood 59: 120–125

Rudd P T, Brown M B, Cassell G H 1984 A prospective study of mycoplasma infection in the preterm infant. Israel Journal of Medical Science 20: 898–901

Rudd P T, Waites K B, Duffy L B, Stagno S, Cassell G H 1986 Ureaplasma urealyticum and its possible role in pneumonia during the neonatal period and infancy. Pediatric Infectious Diseases 5 Suppl: 288–291

Ruiter M, Wentholt H M M 1952 The occurrence of a pleuropneumonia-like organism in fuso-spirillary infections of the human genital mucosa. Journal of Investigative Dermatology 18: 313–325

Sacher I, Walker M, Brunell P A 1970 Abscess in newborn infants caused by mycoplasma. Pediatrics 46: 303–304

Shepard M C 1954 The recovery of pleuropneumonia-like organisms from Negro men with and without nongonococcal urethritis. American Journal of Syphilis 38: 113–124

Shepard M C, Lunceford C D, Ford D K et al 1974 Ureaplasma urealyticum gen. nov., sp. nov.: proposed nomenclature for the human T (T-strain) mycoplasmas. International Journal of Systematic Bacteriology 24: 160–171

Shurin P A, Alpert S, Rosner B et al 1975 Chorioamnionitis and colonization of the newborn infant with genital mycoplasmas. New England Journal of Medicine 293: 5–8

Siber G R, Alpert S, Smith A L, Lin J-S L, McCormack W M 1977 Neonatal central nervous system infection due to Mycoplasma hominis. Journal of Pediatrics 90: 625–627

Singer G R, Ivler D 1975 Nongonococcal urethritis and the menstrual cycle. New England Journal of Medicine 293: 780

Solomon F, Caspi E, Bukovsky I, Sompolinsky D 1973 Infections associated with genital mycoplasma. American Journal of Obstetrics and Gynecology 116: 785–792

Steytler J G 1970 Studies on endogenous infection by vaginal mycoplasma based on positive cord-blood cultures. South African Journal of Obstetrics and Gynaecology 8: 14–22

Stray-Pedersen B, Eng J, Reikvam T M 1978 Uterine T-mycoplasma colonization in reproductive failure. American Journal of Obstetrics and Gynecology 130: 307–311

Stray-Pedersen B, Bruu A-L, Molne K 1982 Infertility and uterine colonization with Ureaplasma urealyticum. Acta Obstetricia et Gynecologica Scandinavica 61: 21–24

Sweet R L 1986 Colonization of the endometrium and fallopian tubes with Ureaplasma urealyticum. Pediatric Infectious Diseases 5 Suppl: 244–246

Sweet R L, Gibbs R S 1985 Intraamniotic infections (intrauterine infection in late pregnancy). In: Sweet R L, Gibbs R S (eds) Infectious diseases of the female genital tract. Williams & Wilkins, Baltimore, pp 263–276

Sweet R L, Mills J, Hadley K W et al 1980 Use of laparoscopy to determine the microbial etiology of acute salpingitis. American Journal of Obstetrics and Gynecology 134: 68–72

Taylor-Robinson D 1978 Mycoplasmas in relation to amniocentesis. In: McGarrity G J, Murphy D G, Nichols W W (eds) Mycoplasma infection of cell cultures. Plenum, New York, pp 159–165

Taylor-Robinson D 1980 Unpublished observations

Taylor-Robinson D, Carney F E 1974 Growth and effect of mycoplasmas in Fallopian tube organ cultures. British Journal of Venereal Diseases 50: 212–216

Taylor-Robinson D, Csonka G W 1981 Laboratory and clinical aspects of mycoplasmal infections of the human genitourinary tract. In: Harris J R W (ed) Recent advances in sexually transmitted diseases. Churchill Livingstone, London, pp 151–186

Taylor-Robinson D, Feizi T 1967 Unpublished observations

Taylor-Robinson D, Furr P M 1976 Unpublished observations

Taylor-Robinson D, McCormack W M 1979 Mycoplasmas in human genitourinary infections. In: Barile M F, Razin S, Tully J G, Whitcomb R G (eds) The mycoplasmas, vol 2. Academic Press, New York, pp 307–366

Taylor-Robinson D, McCormack W M 1980 Medical progress: the genital mycoplasmas. New England Journal of Medicine 302: 1003–1010, 1063–1067

Taylor-Robinson D, Ludwig W M, Purcell R H, Mufson M A. Chanock R M 1965 Significance of antibody to Mycoplasma hominis type 1 as measured by indirect haemagglutination. Proceedings of the Society for Experimental Biology and Medicine 118: 1073–1083

Taylor-Robinson D, Addey J P, Hare M J, Dunlop E M C 1969 Mycoplasmas and 'non-specific' genital infection. I. Previous studies and laboratory aspects. British Journal of Venereal Diseases 45: 265–273

Taylor-Robinson D, Johnson A P, McGee Z A 1975 Use of organ cultures and small laboratory animals for the study of gonococcal infections. In: Danielsson D, Juhlin L, Mardh P-A (eds) Genital infections and their complications. Almqvist and Wiksell, Stockholm, pp 243–252

Taylor-Robinson D, Tully J G, Furr P M, Cole R M, Rose D L, Hanna N F 1981 Urogenital mycoplasma infections of man: a review with observations on a recently discovered mycoplasma. Israel Journal of Medical Sciences 17: 524–530

Taylor-Robinson D, Furr P M, Liberman M M 1984 The occurrence of genital mycoplasmas in babies with and without respiratory distress. Acta Paediatrica Scandinavica 73: 383–386

Thomas M, Jones M, Ray S, Andrews B 1975 Mycoplasma pneumoniae in a tubo-ovarian abscess. Lancet ii: 774–775

Thomsen A C 1974 The isolation of Mycoplasma primatum during an autopsy study of the mycoplasma flora of the human urinary tract. Acta Pathologica et Microbiologica Scandinavica 82B: 653–656

Thomsen A C, Taylor-Robinson D, Brogaard Hansen K 1984 The infrequent occurrence of mycoplasmas in amniotic fluid from women with intact fetal membranes. Acta Obstetricia Gynecologica Scandinavica 63: 425–429

Toth A, Lesser M L, Brooks C, Labriola D 1983 Subsequent pregnancies among 161 couples treated for T-mycoplasma genital-tract infection. New England Journal of Medicine 308: 505–507

Tully J G, Taylor-Robinson D, Cole R M, Rose D L 1981 A newly discovered mycoplasma in the human urogenital tract. Lancet i: 1288–1291

Turnbull A C, Anderson A B M 1978 Reviews in perinatal medicine, vol 2. Raven Press, New York, pp 103–142

Tyrrell D A J, Taylor-Robinson D 1968 Sticky eye and Mycoplasma hominis. British Medical Journal 3: 801–802

Unsworth P F, Taylor-Robinson D, Shoo E E, Furr P M 1985 Neonatal mycoplasmaemia: Mycoplasma hominis as a significant cause of disease? Journal of Infection 10: 163–168

Upadhyaya M, Hibbard B M, Walker S M 1983 The role of mycoplasmas in reproduction. Fertility and Sterility 39: 814–818

Verinder D G R 1978 Septic arthritis due to Mycoplasma hominis. A case report and review of the literature. Journal of Bone and Joint Surgery (London) 60: 224

Wallace R J Jr, Alpert S, Brown K, Lin J-S L, McCormack W M 1978 Isolation of Mycoplasma hominis from blood cultures in patients with postpartum fever. Obstetrics and Gynecology 51: 181–185

Wealthall S R 1975 Mycoplasma meningitis in infants with spina bifida. Developmental Medicine and Child Neurology (Suppl 35) 17: 117

Weström L, Mardh P-A 1971 The effect of antibiotic therapy on mycoplasmas in the female genital tract: in vitro and in vivo studies on the sensitivity of Mycoplasma hominis and T-mycoplasmas to tetracyclines and other antibiotics. Acta Obstetricia Gynecologica Scandinavica 50: 25–31

Weström L, Mardh P-A 1975 Acute salpingitis. Aspects on aetiology, diagnosis, and prognosis. In: Danielsson D, Juhlin L, Mardh P-A (eds) Genital infections and their complications. Almqvist and Wiksell, Stockholm, pp 157–167

Weström L, Evaldson G, Holmes K K, Van der Meijden W, Rylander E, Fredriksson B 1984 Taxonomy of vaginosis: bacterial vaginosis—a definition. In: Mardh P-A, Taylor-Robinson D (eds) Bacterial vaginosis. Almqvist and Wiksell, Stockholm, pp 259–260

Young H, Tuach S, Bain S S R 1981 Incidence of Ureaplasma urealyticum infection in women attending a clinic for sexually transmitted disease. Journal of Infection 3: 258–265

Infection with herpes virus and cytomegalovirus
C B J Woodman

INTRODUCTION

The incidence of herpes genitalis continues to increase with 13 653 new cases being reported by sexually transmitted disease clinics in England and Wales in 1983; this was a major increase over the preceding 5 years. Although much of this can be accounted for by patients with recurrent lesions in search of a cure, there is also a real rise in the number of new cases (Hindley & Adler 1985). As this is a chronic infection with a tendency to recur and as with each recurrence virus is shed, we can only expect the genital reservoir of herpes simplex virus (HSV) in the community to increase inexorably. In addition to the considerable personal morbidity, social and sexual disruption associated with episodes of recurrent herpes genitalis, HSV has been implicated as a likely cofactor in the aetiology of cervical cancer. While herpes neonatorum is frequently a fatal infection, congenital cytomegalovirus infection remains the most common intrauterine infection with an incidence ranging between 0.4 and 2.2% of all live births (Stagno et al 1982b).

HERPES SIMPLEX VIRUS

Organism

HSV is a relatively large virus consisting of a nucleoprotein core containing DNA and surrounded by a capsid; the virus particle is enclosed within a glycoprotein-containing lipoprotein envelope. The two types of HSV have 50% of their genome in common and consequently share a number of structural and non-structural antigens (Hoeness &

Watson 1977). While possessing considerable immunological crossreactivity, they can be differentiated on the basis of serological and biochemical tests (Plummer et al 1974), or the use of polyacrilamide gel electrophoresis to identify type-specific polypeptides (Heine et al 1971).

Following entry and replication of the virus at a mucocutaneous surface it is thought to move centripetally along axonal or perineuronal vascular or lymphatic channels to the local sensory ganglia where a productive infection is produced (Cook & Stevens 1973; Klein 1982). Following on the acute phase a state of latent infection is established. In response to as yet undefined stimuli, acting either on the skin surface or directly on the ganglia, reactivation of viral synthesis occurs resulting in the development of a clinical recurrence (Klein 1982).

Clinical course (Plates 28, 47–49)

The first attack of herpes genitalis is usually an acutely painful and distressing episode. It is characterised by the presence of vesicles which subsequently break down to form shallow ulcers. Lesions may involve the labia, perineum and perianal areas, occasionally extending out on to the buttocks. Inguinal lymphadenopathy is usual. Occasionally the combination of herpetic urethritis and swollen ulcerated labia may warrant admission to hospital for catheterisation. A low grade pyrexia and general malaise are characteristic features of the acute attack. Meningism may occasionally be a prominent feature.

The frequency with which recurrent herpes genitalis follows on the initial clinical episodes has been the subject of few studies. We have reported 17 out of 20 patients as having experienced at least one recurrence within 12 months of their first attack (Woodman et al 1983). Silvestri et al (1982) found a similar rate of recurrence in 38 patients followed for 6 months after their first attack. In the largest prospective study to date. Corey et al (1982) reported that 59% of 137 patients with initial clinical disease had experienced a recurrence within a mean period of follow-up of 7 months.

The latter authors reported that type 1 initial disease was significantly less likely to be followed by the development of recurrent disease. Indirect evidence supporting this is provided by the infrequency with which type 1 has been isolated from people with recurrent herpes genitalis (Kwana et al 1976; Peutherer et al 1982). However, Mindel (1982) has recently reported 7 of 15 patients with initial type 1 infection developing further attacks within 6 months and Barton et al (1982) have reported isolating HSV 1 from 5 of 14 patients with recurrent disease.

There have been no prospective studies defining the frequency, duration or longevity of recurrent herpes genitalis. While further attacks frequently occur at the site of the original lesions, the involvement of secondary areas along the same dermatome is common. Recurrences usually last between 3–7 days, are usually milder and without the systemic symptoms that characterise the first attack. Occasionally successive attacks without any apparent healing interval may occur over a period of 6–10 weeks, a condition approximating to 'status herpeticus'.

While the avoidance of stress, local trauma, alcohol or fatigue is claimed by some patients to reduce the frequency of their attacks, the vast majority of patients continue to have recurrences irrespective of these variables.

Transmission of infection

While herpes genitalis is usually acquired following close sexual contact with a partner who has active herpetic lesions, asymptomatic shedding of the virus may be an important vector in the transmission of this infection.

Duenas et al (1971) isolated virus in the genital secretions of 24 prostitutes, only 2 of whom had clinically apparent lesions. Adam et al (1979) recovered virus from 5 of 50 women with recurrent herpes genitalis at a time when they were symptomatically and clinically free from disease. Rawls et al (1971) recovered virus from the cervix of 30% of sexual contacts of men with herpes genitalis. At the time of examination 7 of these 10 women were asymptomatic. HSV has occasionally been isolated from urethral swabs taken from men with established disease in the absence of visible external lesions (Jeansson & Holin 1970). The virus has been grown from prostatic tissue and seminal vesicles, suggesting a possible role for these organs as genital reservoir for the virus (De Ture et al 1976). However, the same investigators were unable to demonstrate the virus in seminal fluid of 30 men with recurrent herpes genitalis (De Ture et al 1978). These observations reflect our own clinical experience and offer an explanation for the significant minority of patients who claim to have acquired the infection without being exposed to active lesions.

Not surprisingly, fewer studies defining the rate of asymptomatic excretion in more general populations exist. Tejani et al (1979) found only one clinically unsuspected case following attempted virus isolation from genital tract secretions in 1092 consecutive patients admitted to their unit in labour. The frequency of asymptomatic viral shedding in subjects yet to experience the first clinical manifestation of this infection awaits definition.

Acquisition of type 1 genital infection following orogenital contact with a partner experiencing oral cold sores has been documented (Whitney et al 1978). We have reported 5 of 22 patients presenting with primary genital herpes in whom this seemed the likely route of infection; all 5 isolates were subsequently found to be type 1 HSV (Woodman et al 1983). A number of studies have shown that initial type 1 genital infection is almost invariably a true primary infection (Kwana et al 1976; Reeves et al 1981; Peutherer et al 1982). In addition it has been reported that the level of immunity against type 1 HSV has declined among British schoolchildren (Duckworth 1979). It is therefore tempting to speculate that the first contact with HSV type 1 may occur with increasing frequency, with the onset of sexual activity. This may explain the increasing incidence with which genital infection is being caused by HSV 1.

Genital infection has been documented in children in circumstances suggesting that it might have been acquired other than by sexual contact (Scott et al 1952; Brain 1956). In addition it has been shown that HSV can survive on cloth samples under hot humid conditions for up to 4 hours (Montefiore et al 1980). Further work will be necessary to determine whether this relatively delicate virus is able to exist outside the body in sufficient titre to allow fomites transmission to be a significant vector in the transmission of this infection.

Diagnosis

The most useful adjunct to clinical diagnosis is virus isolation. A premoistened cotton tipped swab taken from the lesion should be transported with due expedition to the laboratory. If a delay is anticipated the swab should be stored at 4°C.

HSV can be identified in a wide range of cell lines. In the author's laboratory, baby hamster kidney cells are used and a characteristic cytopathological effect is frequently observed within 24 hours. In approximately 5% of isolates this may not appear until the third day after inoculation. Recently Darougar et al (1986) have suggested that examination of all inoculated cell cultures by immunofluorescence after 48 hours will provide a rapid result, with a greater degree of accuracy than the longer, conventional test.

Electron microscopic examination of vesicular fluid will rapidly identify a herpes virus. This may be sufficient when taken in conjunction with the clinical picture. However, this is a relatively insensitive method and virus must be present in high titres before it can be detected. In addition, varicella zoster and cytomegalovirus have identical particle morphology. While the cytological characteristics of HSV are now well defined, a number of studies have shown examination of stained preparations to be a relatively insensitive method of diagnosis when compared with virus isolation (Vontver et al 1971; Naib et al 1973).

Immunology

The two types of HSV share many common antigens and consequently infection with either will produce both type-specific and type-common antibodies (Hoeness et al 1979). Attempts have been made to predict the type specificity of human sera from the ratio of type 1/type 2 antibody activity. However, infection with both virus types, as may occur when a person with oral herpes contracts a genital infection, may result in indeterminate values (Skinner et al 1976; Grossman et al 1981). This problem may be overcome by reacting the serum to be tested with type-specific antigen preparations (Skinner et al 1976), or by making each serum type-specific by absorption with heterologous antigen (Patterson 1979). However, these methods are too cumbersome, tedious or expensive for routine diagnostic use.

Humoral immunity

Few studies have defined the immune response to the first symptomatic episode of herpes genitalis. This may represent the first contact with either type of HSV and thus constitute a true primary infection. Conversely an initial clinical episode may follow on previous episodes of oral cold sores or possibly asymptomatic genital infection when pre-existing antibodies may be found in acute phase sera. The immunological response differs in the two groups. Reeves et al (1981) have shown that whereas seroconversion could be demonstrated in all true primary infections, 44% of patients experiencing an initial clinical episode of herpes genitalis failed to show a significant rise in complement fixing or neutralising antibody titre. It seems clear therefore, that the humoral response following the first symptomatic episode of herpes gentalis is influenced by previous exposure to type 1 or type 2 HSV; in these situations it may not always be possible to confirm serologically an initial clinical episode.

It has been reported that IgG antibodies appear about the first week following the onset of the initial infection, and persist indefinitely, remaining relatively unchanged despite episodes of recurrent disease (Lopez & O'Reilly 1977; Kurtz 1974). However, in the author's laboratory we have found 21 of 70 patients with recurrent herpes genitalis of some years standing to have no detectable neutralising antibodies against type 1 or type 2 HSV using a complement-independent assay (Woodman 1968). While the majority of these patients were subsequently found to have antibodies detectable by radioimmunoassay (Woodman unpublished data) their failure to seroconvert in terms of neutralising antibodies suggests caution in attributing a diagnostic significance to an immunological profile.

Cell mediated immunity

The occurrence of severe and disseminated herpetic infections in conditions associated with a primary or acquired deficiency of the cell mediated immune response emphasises the role for this arm of the immune system in preventing or curtailing infection with HSV. Regrettably our knowledge of the cell mediated immune response has to date not thrown any light on the quintessential problems as to why some patients who are seropositive and thus presumably harbour the virus in their ganglia have none or few recurrences, while others have frequent episodes of recurrent disease.

What information we have is related to the role of the cell mediated response in active disease. Corey et al (1978) studied the lymphocyte transformation response in 36 patients with initial clinical disease. The duration of virus excretion was inversely related to the magnitude of the mean stimulation index, a shorter duration of infection being associated with a correspondingly greater stimulation index. O'Reilly et al (1977) found a deficiency in lymphokine production using the macrophage inhibition factor test in lymphocytes taken from patients during episodes of recurrent disease.

Local immune response

This aspect of the immune system has received little attention in patients with herpes genitalis. This is surprising, as neutralising and immunoprecipitating antibodies against HSV have been found in cervical mucus (Coughlan & Skinner 1977) and our awareness that the secretion of IgA as mucosal surfaces occurs independently of the humoral antibody system (Ogra & Ogra 1973).

HERPES GENITALIS IN PREGNANCY

The increasing number of women entering pregnancy with a history of herpes genitalis constitutes a potential threat to the neonatal population and has necessitated a reappraisal of the obstetric management of these patients.

Herpes neonatorum is a potentially devastating infection which is commoner in premature infants and may be caused by type 1 or type 2 HSV. Of infected infants, 50% will die and 50% of the remainder will have a residual neurological deficit (Nahmias et al 1971). While there have been only 66 reported cases in England and Wales between 1973 and 1980 (PHLS: Communicable Disease Reports), studies in the United States have quoted incidence figures between 1 in 3500 and 1 in 30 000 pregnancies (Nahmias et al 1975).

Infection is usually acquired following passage of the neonate through an infected birth canal, although ascending infection in the presence of ruptured membranes has also been documented (Light & Linemann 1974). There have been a few case reports suggesting a haematogenous route of transmission. These have been based on the pattern of congenital malformations of infants delivered to women who had experienced an initial episode of herpes genitalis during their first trimester (Charles 1980).

However, as a similar array of anomalies may be produced by cytomegalovirus infection and as HSV has only rarely been isolated from amniotic fluid (Zervoudakis et al 1980), intrauterine transmission with resultant fetal pathology must, at most, be a rare event. Failure to recover virus from amniotic fluid is scarcely surprising as 60% of women having a diagnostic amniocentesis performed for other reasons were found to possess neutralising antibodies against HSV in their liquor (Cox et al 1982).

The prevention of neonatal infection requires identification of the woman shedding virus from her genital tract at the time of onset of labour and her subsequent delivery by Caesarean section. The American National Institute of Allergic and Infectious Disease (NIAID) has reported on 56 cases of herpes neonatorum. At the time of delivery 70% of the mothers have no symptoms or signs of active infection. One-third of these however, had experienced previous episodes of herpes genitalis during that pregnancy, or had a sexual partner suffering from the disease (Whitley et al 1980). This has prompted an evaluation of the efficacy of screening in these high risk groups. Vontver et al (1982) have reported on 80 patients with recurrent herpes genitalis swabbed from the 28th week of pregnancy. Of 199 culture proven episodes, 7% occurred in the absence of external genital lesions. Grossman et al (1981) found 7 of 58 patients to be asymptomatically excreting virus when swabs were taken weekly during the last 4 weeks of pregnancy.

However, a number of questions pertaining to the epidemiology of this infection remain unanswered. Despite the imprecision of our data relating to the general prevalence of herpes genitalis, the incidence of the neonatal infection seems unaccountably low and indeed a number of studies have documented the passage of neonates through infected birth canals apparently unscathed (Nahmias et al 1971). An answer to this enigma may lie in the immunological status of the infant at risk. In the absence of an active infection, neonatal antibody against HSV is IgG in type and is presumably acquired from the transplacental diffusion of maternal antibody. Bradley et al (1982) have shown a close correlation between maternal and neonatal titre of neutralising antibodies against type 1 and type 2 HSV. These authors have reported 16 of 25 infants (64%) with neonatal herpes as having low or absent neutralising antibody titres against either virus type. In contrast only 2% of 41 healthy infants born to mothers with recurrent herpes genitalis had comparable titres. However, the NIAID study found no correlation between the presence of neutralising antibody and the severity of the ensuing infection (Whitley et al 1980).

It seems clear, therefore, that women with active genital lesions at term should be delivered by Caesarean section. The use of virological monitoring in the last few weeks of pregnancy may identify those women who are asymptomatically shedding virus. Their current virological status provides a rational basis for selecting the route of delivery in these patients.

The possibility of drug treatment in pregnancy is discussed later in this chapter.

HERPES SIMPLEX VIRUS AND CERVICAL CANCER

It is 15 years since Naib et al first proposed on epidemiological grounds an association between type 2 HSV and carcinoma of the cervix uteri (Naib et al 1972). In the interim, more than 50 seroepidemiological studies have tended to confirm this association by demonstrating higher prevalence of antibodies against HSV-2 in women with cervical carcinoma. This association has been sustained when investigators have sought to overcome the difficulties posed by immunological crossreactivity by identifying type-specific antibodies in human sera (Skinner et al 1976). As retrospective studies are susceptible to difficulties in rigorous case control matching, a number of prospective studies warrant further attention.

In 1963 Nahmias initiated a large-scale prospective study where to date approximately 600 women with evidence of previous exposure to HSV-2 have been enrolled. These patients have been found to have at least a fourfold increased risk of developing cervical carcinoma. Coleman et al (1983) have followed 114 patients with mild cervical dysplasia over a 4-year period. Of women with antibodies to type 2, 23% progressed to severe dysplasia, as compared with 9% with only type 1 antibody. Catalano & Johnson (1971) examined sera which had been obtained 10 years previously from 1040 women and reported that type 2 antibodies were five times more common in women who developed the disease than in women who remained disease-free. Case control differences have also been observed when other immunological parameters have been measured. Murphy et al (1984) found increased titres of neutralising antibody to type 2 HSV in the cervical mucus of patients with pre-invasive cancer as compared to a control group matched for age, socioeconomic status and number of sexual partners.

HSV can transform certain cell lines. This transformation follows the acquisition of new genetic information and produces an alteration in the biochemical or morphological characteristics of the cell, and may convert a normal cell to one showing many of the features of neoplastic cells. These cells may be shown to be oncogenic when injected into animals (Skinner 1976; Duff & Rapp 1981; McNab 1974). The fate of the viral genome has been the object of some conceptual concern. While some investigators have found varying amounts of viral DNA, only for it to disappear in subsequent cell passages, others have failed to find any (Knipe

1982). Following the identification of the gene sequence within the viral genome responsible for the transformation process, it has been possible, using this DNA fragment as an in situ hybridisation probe, to detect the frequency with which viral DNA sequences occur in transformed cells (Reyes et al 1979). Using this technique it has been shown that each cell contains less than one copy of DNA fragment per cell (Galloway & McDougall 1981). Thus transformed cells do not consistently contain even one copy of the transforming DNA sequence. This provides support for the 'hit and run' theory which suggests that HSV merely initiates or catalyses a transformation process, the continuation of which is not dependent on further replication of the viral genome (Skinner 1976).

The finding of virus coded material in cervical neoplastic tissue has provided more direct evidence of an aetiological role for the virus in cancer of this organ. Dreesman et al (1981) have shown antisera prepared against two HSV-2-DNA binding proteins to react using an immunoperoxidase test with tissue sections cut from cervical carcinoma. Frenkel et al (1971) have demonstrated HSV-specific RNA in a case of squamous carcinoma. McDougall et al (1980) were able to demonstrate this in cervical intraepithelial neoplasia, but not in invasive disease. Eglin (1981) has recently used a modification of the in situ hybridisation technique to give quantitative data. He has reported 72% of biopsies from patients with cervical intraepithelical neoplasia and 60% of cases of invasive carcinoma to contain HSV-specific RNS, as compared to 2% of non-neoplastic controls.

It is of course arguable that the presence of parts of the viral genoma in a neoplastic cell does not imply a purposeful integration of viral DNA into the cell genome. Indeed, such an integration, when demonstrated, may be merely opportunistic. It is therefore worth considering those models which appear to demonstrate a direct cause and effect relationship between HSV and cancer of the cervix. Wentz et al (1981) have reported the development of cervical lesions in mice following prolonged exposure to ultraviolet or formalin inactivated type 1 or type 2 HSV. The yield of invasive carcinoma in mice vaginally challenged with ultraviolet inactivated HSV-2 was 60%. At no stage during the study did it appear that an active infection

had taken place. The cervical lesions produced included adenocarcinoma, squamous and adenosquamous tumours. Chien et al (1974), using a type 2 HSV isolate from a patient with carcinoma of the cervix, showed invasive carcinoma of the cervix to have developed in 3–5% of mice who survived infection with the live virus. It is interesting to note that prior immunisation of these mice with a subunit vaccine was subsequently shown to reduce the incidence of cervical lesions from 52% to 19% following exposure to this virus (Hilton et al 1978).

It would of course be absurd to suggest that HSV is implicated in all cases of cervical cancer. However, a considerable weight of evidence has accumulated implicating it as at least the most likely cofactor in the aetiology of this cancer.

TREATMENT

The patient with herpes genitalis requires counselling and reassurance. The risks of infecting a sexual partner following sexual congress at a time when lesions are present must be explained and encouragment given to redefine relationships in this light. There is frequently anxiety concerning the possible sequelae of herpes genitalis, providing an opportunity to emphasise the value of cervical cytology and explain the role of current obstetric practices in preventing herpes neonatorum.

A plethora of discarded chemotherapeutic agents attest our inability to control or eradicate this infection. The most promising recent addition to the antiviral armentarium is acyclovir. This nucleoside analogue is a substrate for the viral enzyme thymidine kinase. The phosphorylated end product of this enzyme reaction inhibits DNA polymerase, disrupting DNA synthesis. While antiviral agents such as adenine arabinoside, idoxyuridine and trisodium phosphonformate have been shown to inhibit viral replication in vitro, their efficacy in reducing the duration and severity of genital lesions has not been established (Hilton et al 1978; Silvestri et al 1982; Wallen 1982).

Mindel et al (1982) have reported that intravenous administration of acyclovir shortened the duration of viral and accelerated lesion healing in the initial disease; Nilsen et al (1982) reported a similar response using an oral preparation to treat patients with initial and recurrent disease. Kinghorn et al (1986) also demonstrated the beneficial effect of oral acyclovir in first episode genital herpes, and also showed that there was benefit in adding cotrimoxazole to this regime to control superadded bacterial infection. Topical application has been less successful; while the duration of viral shedding was reduced in those experiencing a first attack, acyclovir did not prevent the development of fresh lesions and was only of marginal benefit in patients with recurrent disease (Corey et al 1982). Mindel et al (1986) showed the oral preparation to be strikingly effective in the prevention of recurrence after first attacks.

Acyclovir is not recommended for use in pregnancy, and obviously with the present state of knowledge it should not be used unless the mother's life is threatened. Two cases have been published where it has been used with successful outcome for mother and baby (Lagrew et al 1984; Grover et al 1985). Kingsley presented data (unpublished) from the Wellcome Foundation in Paris in 1986, stating that up to 1 May 1986 this company was aware of over 100 cases where the drug had been used in pregnancy, over half of these being in the first trimester. The outcomes of 95 pregnancies were known. Eleven first trimester pregnancies had been terminated by elective abortion, and in two cases spontaneous abortion had occurred. Of 82 live born babies one had a cardiac abnormality requiring surgery; as exposure to the drug was only 3 days before birth this could not have been the cause. Fifteen babies had minor problems, none of which seemed to be due to the drug therapy. Despite the encouraging findings reported, the manufacturer has no plans to change the recommendations concerning pregnancy.

There have been a number of reports of acyclovir-resistant strains appearing in people previously treated with the agent (Burns et al 1982; Crumpacker et al 1982). It is more disappointing perhaps that a recent study has shown that genital isolates from people yet to be treated were relatively resistant to this drug (Parris & Harrington 1982).

Mendelson et al (1986) assessed the value of recombinant interferon on first attacks and recurrences of genital herpes: there was a trend towards beneficial effects but this hardly reached statistical value.

It is surprising that more effort has not been invested in attempting to prevent this infection by immunisation. Indeed, a successful vaccine might be expected not only to curtail the further transmission of this virus, but in view of the evidence incriminating it as a likely cofactor in the aetiology of cervical carcinoma, to go some way towards reducing the prevalence of this condition.

While a number of animal studies have shown the considerable protective efficacy of immunisation using live or killed virus, or subunit vaccine preparation, the use of 'vaccines' in herpes genitalis has been directed not at the potentially more attainable goal of preventing infection, but at modifying the anticipated clinical course in patients with established disease. More than 40 years ago, Franks vaccinated patients with recurrent HSV infection using a formaldehyde inactivated vaccine and reported a decrease in frequency and duration of attacks in 13 of 14 patients (Franks 1940). Hull & Peck (1966), using a rabbit kidney cell vaccine, reported a 50% improvement over a 6-month period in vaccinated patients. However, this improvement was not sustained over a longer period of follow-up. While the preparations used were relatively crude vaccines and the studies themselves poorly controlled, these results provide use of immunomodulators in patients with established disease.

The possible oncogenic potential of whole virus vaccines has resulted in the development of subunit, DNA-free vaccines. Cappel et al (1982) have recently reported on the immunogenicity of a subunit vaccine prepared from HSV. The vaccine elicited cell-mediated and humoral immunity in a group of healthy volunteers with no history of previous infection. Interestingly, vaccination of a group of patients with recurrent disease produced a rise in neutralising antibody in some and induced the formation of cytotoxic antibodies in others. The intriguing observation that the immune response in patients with recurrent disease is not satiated but is capable of further responding to vaccine induced antigenic stimulation confirms the previous observations of Skinner et al (1982).

Recently a subunit vaccine prepared from an HSV-1 infected human embryo long cell extract has been used to protect people at risk of contracting this infection. Skinner et al (1982) have reported on the outcome in 60 patients vaccinated because their regular sexual partners had recurrent herpes genitalis. Vaccination was followed by a significant rise in neutralising antibodies against type 1 and type 2 HSV in 70% of patients, and the appearance of immunoprecipitating antibodies in 40%. Only 1 of 60 patients had contracted this infection after a mean period of follow-up of 1 year. While this study was not placebo controlled, the author reports that 8 of 20 historical controls matched for age, frequency of recurrences in the index case and contraceptive practices had contracted the infection within this period of time—a transmission rate of 40%. Woodman et al (1983) reported on 22 patients vaccinated following the initial clinical episode of herpes genitalis. To date, after a mean period of follow-up of 10 months, only 7 patients have developed a further episode of recurrent disease, in contrast to 17 of 20 unvaccinated patients. While it is of course imperative to validate these results by the appropriate double-blind placebo controlled studies, there is every reason to believe that vaccination will offer considerable protection to those at risk of contracting this infection and may modify the anticipated clinical course in patients vaccinated following the initial clinical episode.

CONCLUSION

While antiviral agents that shorten the duration of genital lesions are a welcome innovation, they appear unlikely to influence the development of recurrent disease. There are therefore cogent and compelling reasons for attempting to prevent the further transmission of this infection. Experience with other antiviral vaccines suggests that this may be achieved by immunisation of those at risk. The early clinical experience with a subunit vaccine reported above suggests that this goal may be within reach.

In the future vaccination may be offered to certain high risk groups, for example, the regular sexual partners of patients with herpes genitalis. The concept of a high risk group may have to be redefined in the light of the increasing importance of orogenital transmission and the potential risks implicit in asymptomatic excretions.

Finally, in view of the putative association between HSV type 2 and cervical carcinoma, it may be appropriate to give serious consideration to the possibility of immunising the adolescent population.

CYTOMEGALOVIRUS

Organism

Cytomegalovirus (CMV) is a DNA virus which replicates primarily in vivo in human epithelial cells. Examination of clinical isolates of CMV by endonuclease restriction techniques has revealed considerable diversity in the virus genome (Kilpatrick et al 1977). This is reflected in differences in biological characteristics in vitro, variation in the pattern of viral structural polypeptides and some strain-specific serological responses (Weller 1981). However, the clinical significance of these variations is unclear as strains do not appear to exhibit any predilection for specific sites of infection nor do they appear to differ in their pathogenic potential.

Whilst few people escape infection with CMV the vast majority of infections are asymptomatic. CMV mononucleosis is the most commonly described syndrome in young adults. It is characterised by fever and hepatomegaly in the absence of cervical lymphadenopathy or pharyngitis. The peripheral blood film shows many atypical lymphocytes but the Paul-Bunnell test is negative and serological evidence of recent CMV infection can be demonstrated (Jordan et al 1973). In common with asymptomatic primary infections, viral shedding occurs in saliva, urine, semen and cervical secretion for months and even years (Sullivan & Hanshaw 1982). Cessation of this may be followed by episodic recurrences with further asymptomatic viral excretion from a number of sites.

The fate of the virus in the interim is a matter of some conjecture. There is evidence to suggest that the leucocyte may represent a possible site of latent infection. While the virus has frequently been isolated from blood during the acute phase of CMV mononucleosis, it has always been found in the leucocytes rather than the plasma fraction. However, while cell-free virus may be isolated from a number of body sites, leucocyte lysates have failed to yield infectious virus. This can only be demonstrated by the cultivation of intact leucocytes on a permissive cell line, suggesting that the virus exists within the leucocyte in a latent stage (Olding et al 1975; Rinaldo et al 1977). However, the particular cell type responsible for harbouring the virus remains to be identified. Further support for this proposed site of latency is provided by the observation that seroconversion may follow transfusion of fresh blood (Caul et al 1971). This ability to transmit CMV is lost when blood is stored or leucocyte-free units are used. In addition, CMV has occasionally been isolated from the leucocytes of healthy blood donors (Diosi et al 1969).

Serological evidence of previous exposures to CMV has been found in all populations sampled. Its prevalence increases with age and varies with the geographical setting and socioeconomic status of the population studied. In developing countries virtually everyone has acquired the infection by the time of puberty (Schopfer et al 1978; Stagno et al 1982a). While it has been shown that 70% of people from the lower income groups of industrialised societies will have seroconverted at this stage, this falls to 30–37% in the upper echelons of these societies (Stagno et al 1982b).

It seems likely that transmission of this virus requires intimate contact. This is facilitated by the persistent or episodic excretion of virus from a number of body sites. It may be acquired following contact with infected genital secretions at the time of delivery, as CMV has been isolated from the cervix of between 11 and 27% of pregnant women (Stagno et al 1982a). While the incidence of cervical shedding of CMV increases with the stage of gestation, the eventual levels attained do not significantly differ from a similar non-pregnant population. This progression has been shown to reflect a diminution in cervical excretion of virus during early pregnancy, an effect possibly mediated by maternal hormones (Knox et al 1975; Stagno et al 1975). CMV has been isolated from the milk of between 15 and 50% of breast feeding mothers and constitutes an important vector of transmission in the first year of life (Hayes et al 1972; Stagno et al 1980a). Close contact with other children who may be excreting virus in urine, faeces or saliva expedites the transmission of CMV in the ensuing years. As CMV has been shown to be excreted in semen in

addition to being recovered from cervical secretions, it seems likely that venereal transmission results in a further contraction of the ranks of the non-immune, with the onset of sexual activity.

Diagnosis

A primary CMV infection can be diagnosed if seroconversion can be shown to have occurred. While the most widely used method of antibody detection is the complement fixation test, certain reservations exist regarding the interpretation of its clinical significance. Titres of complement fixing antibody have been shown to fluctuate widely, with some patients previously found to be sero-positive subsequently having low or undetectable titres (Wayner et al 1975). In addition the sera of some patients have been shown to react selectively with complement fixing antigen prepared from different strains of CMV. This may explain the failure to detect complement fixing antibody in the sera of 15% of congenitally infected infants actively excreting virus (Stagno et al 1975a). It would, therefore, appear that failure to detect antibodies using this technique does not necessarily imply lack of previous exposure to the virus. In contrast, IgG fluorescent antibodies appear to be a reliable indicator of previous infection. The titres of these antibodies have been reported as remaining stable over long period of time (Stagno et al 1975b, Wayner et al 1975).

Alternatively, a primary CMV infection may be inferred if IgM-specific antibodies can be demonstrated in serum. This approach obviates the necessity of documenting previous sero-negativity. IgM-specific antibody can be detected by the fluorescent antibody technique of radioimmunoassay. The latter technique appears the more sensitive with serum-specific antibodies detectable in 90% of women with primary infection and in 87% of congenitally infected infants (Griffiths et al 1982a, b). IgM fluorescent antibodies frequently fail to discriminate between primary and previous infections.

Virus isolation is the most specific method of making a diagnosis of CMV infection. CMV can be isolated from tears, saliva, bronchoscopic aspirate, urine, semen, cervical secretion and stools. Clinical specimens should ideally be processed within a few hours. Failing this, storage at 4°C is optimum.

CMV grows preferably in monolayers of human fibroblasts with a characteristic cytopathic effect appearing between 24 hours and 4 weeks, depending on the size of the infecting inoculum. The usefulness of electron microscopy is restricted by the morphological homogeneity of the herpes viruses and the need for the virus to be present in sufficient titre to permit detection.

INTRAUTERINE INFECTION

The incidence of congenital CMV infection ranges between 0.4 and 2.2%. However, only between 5 and 10% of those shedding virus at birth will be symptomatically infected. This illness will be fatal in 20% and 90% of the survivors will develop major sequelae (Diosi et al 1969). The stigmata include sensorineural deafness, chorioretinitis, optic atrophy and intellectual impairment. In addition, it has been reported that between 5 and 15% of those asymptomatically infected at birth will subsequently manifest some loss of hearing or neurological impairment (Melish & Hanshaw 1973; Hanshaw et al 1976).

The congenital infection may be acquired following a primary maternal infection, or as a result of reactivation or viral synthesis in a woman with latent disease. A primary maternal infection does not inevitably lead to intrauterine infection; the risk of this has been estimated as between 25 and 50% (Diosi et al 1969; Stern & Tucker 1973; Griffiths & Baboonian 1984). Congenital CMV infection has been reported in the offspring of between 1.4 and 1.6% of women (Caul et al 1971; Stagno et al 1982a) adjudged to be serologically immune as a result of previous exposure to CMV. While maternal immunity does not appear to prevent congenital CMV infection, it does appear to protect against its harmful sequelae. To date there has only been one case report of a congenitally infected neonate developing these sequelae, being born to a mother who was sero-positive prior to that pregnancy (Ahlfors et al 1981). In addition, there have been a number of studies showing the risks to infants of mothers with recurrent disease to be negligible (Caul et al 1971; Stagno et al 1982a).

In view of the incomplete protection afforded by maternal humoral antibodies attention has been focused on the role for the cell mediated immune system. A number of studies have shown this to be deficient in congenitally infected infants. This has been manifest as a failure of lymphocytes to transform or produce interferon in response to challenge with CMV antigen (Reynolds et al 1979; Starr et al 1979). Similarly, a reduction in the leucocyte migration inhibition index has been described (Fiorilli et al 1982). While symptomatically infected infants have been shown to have a more severely depressed lymphocyte transformation response, absent responses have been demonstrated in congenitally infected but asymptomatic neonates. Many of the mothers of these infants themselves have an impaired cell mediated immunity response against CMV using this test (Reynolds et al 1979). However, a number of investigators have suggested that this may reflect a specific reduction in the cell mediated immunity response to CMV in pregnancy. Recently, a small group of sero-positive women were shown to have a dramatic decline in their lymphocyte transformation response to CMV during their second and third trimesters, these levels only beginning to return to normal 90–120 days postpartum. This decline occurred in the absence of maternal productive infection and none of the offspring were infected. Other parameters of the cell mediated immunity response remained unchanged during the study period (Gehtz et al 1981). It seems clear that the role of cell mediated immunity response in mitigating the effects of congenital infection, while conceptually attractive, awaits further definition.

With the exception previously mentioned, all cases of symptomatically infected infants occurred following primary maternal infections. Schopfer has reviewed a number of prospective studies documenting primary maternal infection during pregnancy and concluded that the risk of severe fetal disease in women seroconverting during pregnancy was between 2 and 4% (Schopfer at al 1978). Griffiths & Baboonian (1984) reported the results of a 7-year study involving nearly 11 000 pregnancies. In this group 56 women experienced primary seroconversion. Fetal loss occurred in 4 cases out of the 26 where seroconversion occurred early in pregnancy. After birth, 46 infants from these women were tested; 9 had congenital infection. Two of these have developed intellectual impairment attributable to CMV infection. Peckham et al (1983) reported similar results and in their series some of the affected babies were born to mothers who had had recurrent rather than primary infections.

TREATMENT

Antivirals

A number of antiviral agents have been used to treat the various manifestations of this infection. While administration of cytosine arabinoside, adenine arabinoside and, more recently, acyclovir, may produce a quantitative reduction or transient cessation of viral excretion, this has not been reflected in any improvement in the eventual clinical outcome and rates of excretion have rapidly returned to their previous levels once treatment was discontinued (Chien et al 1974; Plotkin et al 1982). A similar partial and transient inhibition of viral replication has been observed following administration of interferon to congenitally infected infants and renal transplant patients (Arvin et al 1976; Chessman et al 1979).

Vaccination

It is clear that while maternal immunity does not prevent congenital infection it does appear to protect against its harmful sequelae. Our current knowledge suggests that symptomatic infection only follows a primary infection in pregnancy. Immunisation of the female population prior to puberty might therefore be expected to reduce the incidence of this disease considerably.

Experience with two live attenuated vaccines prepared from different strains of CMV have been reported; Elek & Stern (1974) reported on the administration of such a vaccine prepared from the AD-169 strain as producing a rise in complement fixing antibodies and being free from adverse reactions; the humoral response to this vaccine was subsequently shown to persist for at least a year (Neff et al 1979). Using the Town strain of CMV Plotkin et al (1982) have shown a significant change in the cell mediated immunity response in addition to the appearance of humoral antibodies. In neither set of studies was vaccination followed by a productive infection, despite frequent attempts to isolate the virus.

It remains to be established by large-scale prospective studies whether the protective effect of these vaccines parallels their undoubted immunogeneity. Reservations have been expressed about the possible confounding effects of strain variation. In this respect it is perhaps disappointing that immunisation of renal transplant patients showed no protective effect against acquisition of exogenous CMV (Frazer et al 1979). However, this may be explained by a reduction in vaccine induced immunity in addition to natural immunity brought about by immunosuppressive regimens.

CONCLUSION

The available data suggest that symptomatic congenital infection only follows on a primary maternal infection. Unlike rubella, the vast majority of CMV infections are asymptomatic. Therefore, the identification of women seroconverting during pregnancy would require serial assessments of antibody status: a logistically difficult, time consuming exercise which may be frustrated by undocumented seroconversion in early pregnancy.

It is accepted that only a proportion of women experiencing a primary infection will give birth to infected infants, and that at least 50% of these will have no permanent sequelae. Therefore, while the use of invasive techniques such as amniocentesis or fetoscopy may provide virological or serological confirmation of fetal CMV infection, this will not identify the infant likely to be symptomatically infected at birth.

It would appear that a reduction in the morbidity attributable to congenital CMV infection is most likely to be achieved by the successful immunisation of the sero-negative adolescent population.

REFERENCES

Adam I, Kaufmann R, Hirkovic R, Melnick J 1979 Persistence of virus shedding in asymptomatic women after recovery from

herpes genitalis. Obstetrics and Gynecology 54: 171–173

Ahlfors K, Harris S, Svanberl L 1981 Secondary maternal

cytomegalovirus infection causing symptomatic congenital infection. New England Journal of Medicine 305: 284

Arvin A M, Yaegar A S, Meffigan T C 1976 Effect of leucocyte interferon on urinary excretion of CMV by infants. Journal of Infectious Diseases 133: A205–A210

Barton I G, Kinghorn G R, Najem S, Al-Omar L S, Potter C W 1982 Incidence of HSV 1 and HSV 2 isolated from a group of patients with herpes genitalis in Sheffield. British Journal of Venereal Diseases 58: 44

Bradley J S, Yeager A S, Dyson D C, Hensleigh P A, Medeeris A L 1982 Neutralisation of herpes simplex virus by antibody in anmiotic fluid. Obstetrics and Gynecology 60: 318–321

Brain R T 1956 The clinical vagaries of herpes virus. British Medical Journal 1061–1067

Burns W H, Saral R, Santos G V et al 1982 Isolation and characterisation of resistant herpes simplex virus after acyclovir therapy. Lancet i: 421–423

Cappel R, Sprecher S, Rickaer F, DeCupyer F 1982 Immune response to a DNA free herpes simplex vaccine in man. Archives of Virology 73: 61–67

Catalano W L, Johnson L D 1971 Herpes virus antibody and carcinoma in situ of the cervix. Journal of the American Medical Association 217: 447–451

Caul E O, Clarke S K R, Mott M G, Perham J G M, Wilson S E 1971 Cytomegalovirus infections after open heart surgery. Lancet i: 777

Charles D 1980 In: Infections in Obstetrics and Gynaecology. W B Saunders, Philadelphia

Chessman S H, Rubin R H, Stewart J A et al 1979 Controlled clinical trial of prophylactic human leucocyte interferon in renal transplantation. New England Journal of Medicine 300: 1345

Chien L R, Cannon N J, Whitler R J et al 1974 Effect of adenine arabinoside on cytomegalovirus infections. Journal of Infectious Diseases 130: 32–39

Coleman D V, Morse A, Beckwith P, Anderson M C 1983 Prognostic significance of HSV antibody status in women with dysplasia of uterine cervix. British Journal of Obstetrics and Gynaecology 90: 421–427

Cook M L, Stevens J G 1973 Pathogenesis of herpetic neuritis and ganglionitis in mice: evidence for intraxonal transport of infection. Journal of Infection and Immunology 7: 272

Corey L, Reeves W C, Holmes K K 1978 Cellular immune response in genital herpes simplex virus infection. New England Journal of Medicine 299: 986–991

Corey L, Nahmias A J, Guinan M E et al 1982 A trial of topical acyclovir in genital herpes simplex virus infection. New England Journal of Medicine 306: 1313

Coughlan B M, Skinner G R B 1977 Antibody activity to type 1 and type 2 HSV in human cervical mucus. British Journal of Obstetrics and Gynaecology 84: 622

Cox D, Hawkins S, Hartley C E, Mylotte M J, Skinner G R B 1982 Antibody activity against herpes simplex virus in amniotic fluid. British Journal of Obstetrics and Gynaecology 89: 226–230

Crumpacker C S, Schnipper L E, Marlowe S I et al 1982 Resistance to antiviral drugs of herpes simplex virus isolated from a patient treated with acyclovir. New England Journal of Medicine 306: 343–346

Darougar S, Walpita P, Thaker U, Goh B T, Dunlop E M C 1986 A rapid and sensitive culture test for the laboratory diagnosis of genital herpes in women. Genito-Urinary Medicine 62: 93–96

De Ture F A, Drylie D M, Kaufmann H E, Centifanto Y W 1976 Herpes virus type 2: isolation from seminal vesicles and testes. Urology 7: 541–544

De Ture F A, Drylie D, Kaufmann H E, Centifanto Y W 1978 Herpes virus type 2: study of semen in male subjects with recurrent infections. Journal of Urology 120: 449–451

Diosi P, Moldovan E, Tomesu N 1969 Latent cytomegalovirus infection in blood donors. British Medical Journal 4: 660

Dreesman G R, Burek J, Adam E et al 1981 Expression of herpes virus induced antigen in human cervical cancer. Nature (London) 283: 591–593

Duckworth R 1979 Symposium: oral herpes simplex infection. Journal of the Royal Society of Medicine 72: 126–129

Duenas A, Adam I, Melnick J 1971 Herpes virus type 2 in a prostitute population. American Journal of Epidemiology 95: 483

Duff R, Rapp F 1981 Properties of hamster embryo fibroblasts transformed in vitro after exposure to ultraviolet irradiated HSV type 2 Journal of Virology 8: 469–477

Eglin R 1981 Detection of RNA complementary to herpes simplex virus DNA in human cervical squamous cell neoplasms. Journal of Cancer Research 41: 3597

Elek S D, Stern H 1974 Development of a vaccine against mental retardation caused by cytomegalovirus infection in utero. Lancet i: 1–5

Fiorilli M, Sirianni M C, Ianetti P, Pana A, Divizia M, Alun E 1982 Cell mediated immunity in human cytomegalovirus infection. Journal of Infection and Immunity 36: 1162

Franks S B 1940 Formalised herpes virus therapy and neutralising substance in herpes simplex. Journal of Investigative Dermatology 1: 267–282

Frazer J P, Friedman H M, Grossman R A et al 1979 Live cytomegalovirus vaccination of renal transplant candidates: preliminary trial. Annals of Internal Medicine 91: 676

Frenkel N, Roizman B, Cassai L, Nahmias A 1971 A DNA fragment of herpes simplex and its transcription in human cervical cancer tissues. Proceedings of the National Academy of Sciences 69: 3784–3789

Galloway D A, McDougall J K 1981 Transformation of rodent cells by a cloned DNA fragment of herpes simplex virus type 2. Journal of Virology 38: 749–760

Gehtz R C, Christianson W R, Linner K M, Conroy M M, McCue S A, Balfour H H 1981 Cytomegalovirus specific humoral and cellular immune response in human pregnancy. Journal of Infectious Diseases 143: 391–395

Griffiths P, Baboonian C 1984 A prospective study of primary cytomegalovirus infection during pregnancy. British Journal of Obstetrics and Gynaecology 91: 307–315

Griffiths P, Stagno S, Pass R E, Smith R J, Alford C 1982a Infection with cytomegalovirus during pregnancy: specific IgM antibodies as a marker of recent infection. Journal of Infectious Diseases 145: 647–653

Griffiths P, Stagno S, Pass R E, Smith R J, Alford C 1982b Congenital cytomegalovirus infection: diagnostic and prognostic significance of the detection of specific immunoglobulin M antibodies in cord serum. Paediatrics 69: 544–549

Grossman J H, Wallen W C, Serer J L 1981 Management of genital herpes simplex virus infection during pregnancy. Obstetrics and Gynecology 58: 1–4

Grover L, Kane J, Kravitz J, Cruz A 1985 Systemic acyclovir in pregnancy. Obstetrics and Gynecology 65: 284–287

Hanshaw J B, Schneir A P, Moxley A W, Gaer L, Abel V, Schnier B 1976 School failure and deafness after 'silent' congenital cytomegalovirus infection. New England Journal of Medicine 295: 468

Hayes K, Danks D, Gibas H, Jack L 1972 Cytomegalovirus in human milk. New England Journal of Medicine 287: 177

Heine J W, Honess R W, Cassai E, Roizan B 1971 Proteins specified by herpes simplex virus. The virion polypeptides of type 1 strains. Journal of Virology 14: 640–651

Hilton A L, Bushel T E, Waller B, Blight J 1978 A trial of adenine arabinoside in genital herpes. British Journal of Venereal Diseases 54: 50–52

Hindley D J, Adler M W 1985 Genital herpes: an increasing problem? Genito-Urinary Medicine 61: 56–58

Hoeness R W, Watson D H 1977 Unity and diversity in the herpes viruses. Journal of General Virology 37: 15

Hoeness R W, Powell K L, Robinson D J, Sim C, Watson D A 1979 Type specific and type common antigens in cells infected with herpes simplex virus type 1 and on the surface of naked and enveloped particles of the virus. Journal of General Virology 22: 159

Hull R N, Peck F B 1966 Vaccination against herpesvirus infections. Proceedings of the first international conference on vaccines against viral and rickettsial diseases of man. Scientific Publications 147 Pan American Health Organisation pp 265–275

Jeansson S, Holin L 1970 Genital herpes virus hominis infection: venereal disease? Lancet i: 1064

Jordan C, Rousseall W, Stewart J, Noble G, Chin T 1973 Spontaneous cytomegalovirus mononucleosis. Annals of Internal Medicine 79: 153

Kilpatrick B A, Huang E S, Pagano J J 1977 Human cytomegalovirus genome: partial denaturation map and organisation of genome sequences. Journal of Virology 24: 261

Kinghorn G R, Abeywickrene I, Jeavons M et al 1986 Efficacy of oral treatment with acyclovir and cotrimoxazole in first episode genital herpes. Genito-Urinary Medicine 62: 33–37

Klein R J 1982 The pathogenesis of acute, latent and recurrent herpes simplex virus infections. Archives of Virology 72: 143

Knipe D M 1982 Cell growth transformation by herpes simplex virus. In: J Melnick (ed) Progress in Medical Virology vol 28 Karger, Basel, pp 114–137

Knox G E, Reynolds D W, Cohen S, Alford C A 1975 Alteration of the growth of cytomegalovirus herpes simplex type 1 by epidermal growth factor—a contaminant of crude human chorionic gonadotrophin preparations. Journal of Clinical Investigation 61: 1635

Kurtz J B 1974 Specific IgG antibody responses in herpes simplex virus infection. Journal of Medical Microbiology 7: 333

Kwana T, Kanaguch T, Sakumoto S 1976 Clinical and virological studies in genital herpes. Lancet ii: 964

Lagrew D C, Furlow T G, Hager W D, Yarrish R L 1984 Disseminated herpes simplex virus infection in pregnancy. Journal of the American Medical Association 252: 2058–2059

Light I J, Linemann C C 1974 Neonatal herpes simplex infection following delivery by Caesarean section. Obstetrics and Gynecology 44: 496

Lopez C, O'Reilly R J 1977 Cell mediated immune response in recurrent herpes virus infections. Journal of Immunology 118: (suppl 3) 895

McDougall J R, Galloway D A, Fenoglio C M 1980 Cervical carcinoma; detection of herpes simplex virus RNA in cells undergoing neoplastic change. International Journal of Cancer 25: 1–8

McNab J C M 1974 Transformation of rat embryo cells by temperature sensitive mutants of herpes simplex virus. Journal of General Virology 24: 143–153

Melish M E, Hanshaw J B 1973 Congenital cytomegalovirus infection: developmental progress of infants detected by routine screening. American Journal of Diseases in Children 126: 190

Mendelson J, Clecner B, Eiley S 1986 Effect of recombinant interferon alpha 2 on clinical course of first episode genital herpes and subsequent recurrences. Genito-Urinary Medicine 62: 97–101

Mindel A 1982 Free communication: 31st General Assembly of the International Union against the Venereal Diseases and the Treponematoses

Mindel A, Adler M V, Sutherland S, Fiddian A P 1982 Intravenous acyclovir treatment for primary genital herpes. Lancet i: 697–700

Mindel A, Weller I V D, Faherty A, Sutherland S, Fiddian A P, Adler M W 1986 Acyclovir in first attacks of genital herpes and the prevention of recurrences. Genito-Urinary Medicine 62: 28–32

Montefiore D, Sogbetun A O, Anong C A 1980 Herpes virus hominis type 2 infection in Ibadan. British Journal of Venereal Diseases 56: 49–53

Murphy J, Murphy D, Mylotte M, Coughlan B, Skinner G R B 1984 Neutralising antibody against type 1 and type 2 herpes simplex virus in cervical mucus of women with cervical intraepithelial neoplasia. Medical Microbiology and Immunology (Berlin) 174: 73–80

Nahmias A J, Josey W E, Naib Z, Luce C, Duffey A 1970 Antibodies to herpes virus hominis types 1 and 2 in humans. American Journal of Epidemiology 91: 539

Nahmias A J, Josey W E, Naib Z M et al 1971 Perinatal risk associated with maternal genital herpes simplex infection. American Journal of Obstetrics and Gynecology 110: 825–837

Nahmias A, Vinsintine A, Reimer C et al 1975 Herpes simplex virus infection of the fetus and newborn. In: Gershon A (ed) Infections of the fetus and newborn infant, 1st edn. Liss, New York pp 63–76

Naib Z M, Nahmias A J, Josey W E 1972 Cytology and histopathology of cervical herpes simplex infection. Journal of Cancer Research 29: 1026–1031

Naib Z M, Nahmias A J, Josey W E, Zaki A S 1973 Relationship of cytopathology of genital herpes virus infection of cervical anaplasia. Journal of Cancer Research 33: 1452

Neff B, Wiebel R, Buynak E, McClean A, Hilleman M 1979 Clinical and laboratory studies of live cytomegalovirus vaccine. Proceedings of the Society for Experimental Biology and Medicine 160: 32–37

Nilsen A E, Ansen T, Halds A M et al 1982 Efficacy of oral acyclovir in the treatment of initial and recurrent genital herpes. Lancet ii: 571–573

Ogra P L, Ogra S S 1973 Local antibody response to polio vaccine in human female genital tract. Journal of Immunology 110: 1307

Olding L B, Jensen F C, Oldstone M B 1975 Pathogenesis of cytomegalovirus infection. Journal of Experimental Biology 141: 561

O'Reilly R J, Chibbard A, Anger E et al 1977 Cell mediated immune responses in patients with recurrent herpes simplex virus infections. Journal of Immunology 108: 1095–1102

Parris D S, Harrington J E 1982 Herpes simplex variants resistant to high concentrations of acyclovir exist in clinical isolates. Antimicrobiological Agents and Chemotherapy 22: 71–77

Patterson W R 1979 Antibody to herpes simplex virus type 2 specified antigens in sera of women with and without squamous cell carcinoma of the cervix. Disease Abstracts International (B) 39: 4197

Peckham C S, Chin K S, Coleman J C, Henderson K, Hurley R, Preece P M 1983 Cytomegalovirus infection in pregnancy. Lancet i: 1352–1355

Peutherer J F, Smith I, Robertson D 1982 Genital infection with herpes simplex virus type 1. Journal of Infection 4: 33

Plotkin S A, Starr S E, Bryan C K 1982 In vitro and in vivo responses of cytomegalovirus to acyclovir. American Journal of Medicine 73a (Suppl 1A): 257

Plummer G, Goodheart G R, Miyagi M, Skinner G R B, Thouless M E, Wildy P 1974 Herpes simplex viruses: discrimination of types and correlation between different characteristics. Journal of Virology 60: 206–216

Rawls W E, Gardner H L, Flanders R W et al 1971 Genital herpes in two social groups. American Journal of Obstetrics and Gynecology 110: 682–689

Reeves W C, Corey L, Adams H G 1981 Risk of recurrence after first episodes of genital herpes. New England Journal of Medicine 305: 315

Reyes G R, La Fenina R, Hayward S D, Hayward G S 1979 Morphological transformation by DNA fragments of human herpes viruses: evidence for two distinct transforming regions in HSV types 1 and 2 and lack of correlation with biochemical transfer of the thymidine kinase gen. Cold Spring Harbor Symposium on Quantitative Biology, vol 44. Viral oncogens, pp 529–641

Reynolds D W, Dean P H, Pass R H, Alford C A 1979 Specific cell mediated immunity in children with congenital and neonatal cytomegalovirus infection and their mothers. Journal of Infectious Diseases 140: 493

Rinaldo C R, Black P H, Hirsh H S 1977 Interaction of cytomegalovirus with leucocytes from patients with mononucleosis due to cytomegalovirus. Journal of Infectious Diseases 136: 667

Schopfer K, Lauber E, Krech U 1978 Congenital cytomegalovirus infection in newborn infants of mothers infected before pregnancy. Archives of Disease in Children 53: 536

Scott T F M, Coriell L, Blank H et al 1952 Some comments on herpetic infection in children with special emphasis on unusual manifestations. Journal of Pediatrics 41: 835–843

Silvestri D, Corey L, Holmes K 1982 Ineffectiveness of topical IDU in dimethylsulfoxide for therapy for herpes genitalis. Journal of the American Medical Association 246: 953

Skinner G R B 1976 Transformation of primary hamster embryo fibroblasts by type 2 herpes simplex virus: evidence for a hit and run phenomenon. British Journal of Experimental Pathology 51: 361–376

Skinner G R B, Thouless M E, Edwards J et al 1976 Serorelatedness of type 1 and type 2 herpes simplex virus: type specificity of antibody response. Journal of Immunology 31: 481–494

Skinner G R B, Woodman C B J, Buchan S A, Harley C, Fuller A E 1982 Preparation of imunogenicity of vaccine AcNFU, S MRC5 towards prevention of herpes genitalis in human subjects. British Journal of Venereal Diseases 58: 381–386

Skinner G R B, Woodman C, Hartley C, Buchan A et al 1982 Early experience with antigenoid vaccine Ac NFU, S MRC towards prevention or modification of herpes genitalis. In: Development of biological standardisation 52. Karger, Basle pp 113–127

Stagno S, Reynolds D, Tsiantos A et al 1975a Cervical cytomegalovirus excretion in pregnant and non-pregnant women: suppression in early gestation. Journal of Infectious Diseases 131: 522

Stagno S, Reynolds D, Tsiantos A, Fucillo D, Long W, Alford C A 1975b Comparative serial virologic and serologic studies of symptomatic and subclinical and naturally acquired cytomegalovirus infection. Journal of Infectious Diseases 132: 568

Stagno S, Reynolds D, Pass R F, Alford C A 1980 Breast milk and the risk of cytomegalovirus infection. New England Journal of Medicine 302: 1073–1076

Stagno S, Pass R E, Dworsky M E et al 1982a Congenital cytomegalovirus infection. New England Journal of Medicine 306: 945

Stagno S, Pass R E, Dworsky M E, Alford C A 1982b Maternal cytomegalovirus infection and perinatal transmission. Journal of Clinical Obstetrics and Gynaecology 25: 563

Starr S E, Tolpin M D, Friedman H M, Paucker K, Plotkin S A 1979 Impaired cellular immunity to cytomegalovirus in congenitally infected infants and their mothers. Journal of Infectious Diseases 140: 500

Stern H, Tucker S M 1973 Prospective study of cytomegalovirus in pregnancy. British Medical Journal 2: 268

Sullivan J L, Hanshaw J B 1982 In: Glazer R, Gotlie-Stmasky T (ed) Human cytomegalus infections in human herpes virus infections: clinical aspects. Marcel Dekker, New York, pp 87–103

Tejani N, Klein S, Kaplan M 1979 Subclinical herpes simplex genitalis infections in the perinatal period. American Journal of Obstetrics and Gynecology 135: 547

Vontver L, Reeves W C, Rattray M et al 1979 Clinical course and diagnosis of genital herpes simplex virus infection and evaluation of topical surfactant therapy. American Journal of Obstetrics and Gynecology 133: 548

Vontver L A, Hickok D E, Brown Z et al 1982 Recurrent genital herpes simplex virus infection in pregnancy: infant outcome and frequency of asymptomatic recurrences. American Journal of Obstetrics and Gynecology 143: 75

Wallen J H 1982 Free communication: Thirty First General Assembly of the International Union against the Venereal Diseases and Trepenomatoses. June 1982

Waner J, Weller T H, Kevy S W 1975 Patterns of cytomegalovirus compliment—fixing antibody activity; a longitudinal study of blood donors. Journal of Infectious Diseases 127: 538–543

Weller T H 1981 Clinical spectrum of cytomegalovirus infection. In: Nahmias A J (ed) The human herpes viruses Elsevier, New York, pp 20–30

Wentz W B, Reagan J W, Heggi A, Fu Y, Anthony D 1981 Induction of uterine cancer with inactivated herpes simplex virus types 1 and 2. Journal of Cancer Research 48: 1783–1790

Whitley R J, Nahmias A J, Vinsintine A M et al 1980 The natural history of herpes simplex virus infection of mother and newborn. Journal of Pediatrics 66: 489

Whitney J E, Skinner G R B, Buchan A 1978 Acquisition of type 1 herpes simplex vulvitis within a monogamous relationship. British Journal of Venereal Diseases 54: 121

Woodman C B J, Buchan A, Fuller A et al 1983 Efficacy of vaccine Ac NFU, (5) MRC 5 given after an initial clinical episode in the prevention of herpes genitalis. British Journal of Venereal Diseases 59: 311–313

Woodman C B J 1987 unpublished data

Zervoudakis I, Silverman F et al 1980 Herpes simplex virus in the amniotic fluid of an unaffected fetus. American Journal of Obstetrics and Gynecology 55: 165

Condyloma acuminata and molluscum contagiosum
P J Lynch

CONDYLOMA ACUMINATA

Condyloma acuminata is the general term used for viral warts which occur on mucous membranes and surrounding skin of the genitalia and anus. The prevalence of these troublesome and contagious lesions is increasing rapidly and they are assuming new importance because of their recently recognised association with epithelial malignancy.

The aetiological agent

Anogenital warts arise as a result of a viral infection. Although the putative virus has not been cultured, viral particles can be identified microscopically and bacteria-free inoculations can successfully transfer the infection from person to person. Even without the advantage of cultured organisms, morphological and biochemical studies are quite detailed and sophisticated. Electron microscopy of human warts reveals, within the nuclei of mid-epidermal cells, spherical viral particles 55 nm in diameter formed in the shape of an icosahedron. Biochemical studies indicate this virus has a molecular weight of $5.0-5.3 \times 10^6$ daltons. The virion contains a dense central core and a surrounding protein shell known as a capsid. The core is formed of double-stranded DNA which primarily exists as a closed circle. In most instances the viral DNA remains as an episome, unintegrated with host cell DNA. Considerable new information has recently become available based on successful cloning and analysis of endonuclease derived fragments of viral DNA (Smith & Campo 1985).

This wart virus has been assigned to the papovavirus family with the other papillomaviruses (Table 14.1). As of late 1985 more than 35 distinct types of

Table 14.1 Classification of papovaviruses

I. Papoviridae (family)
  A. Papillomaviruses (genus)
    1. Human papillomavirus (HPV)
    2. Animal papillomavirus (rabbit, bovine, canine, etc.)
  B. Polyomaviruses (genus)
    1. Human BK polyomavirus
    2. Human JC polyomavirus
    3. Monkey SV40 virus
    4. Other animal polyomaviruses

Table 14.2 Selected HPV types and clinical correlates

HPV 1, 2, 4	Plantar and hand warts
HPV 3	Flat warts
HPV 3, 5, 8	Epidermodysplasia verruciformis
HPV 6, 11, 16, 18	Anogenital warts
HPV 11	Laryngeal papillomatosis

human papillomaviruses (HPV) have been recognised. The most important of these, together with their clinical correlates, are listed in Table 14.2. These different types are identified on the basis of their nucleotide sequence and annealing properties as determined by endonuclease fragmentation patterns and hybridisation studies. Four of these HPV types (HPV 6, 11, 16, 18) account for the majority of HPV recovered from anogenital lesions (Gissmann et al 1983, 1984; Ferenczy et al 1985).

Type and location of anogenital warts

Several morphological types of anogenital warts are recognised (Oriel 1971a). The prototypic venereal wart is a non-keratotic, elongated, sessile papule 2–3 mm in diameter and 10–15 mm in length. Such lesions can exist singularly or in clusters (Fig. 14.1). In women this type of wart is most often found on the labia minora, around the clitoris and at the vaginal introitus. Less often they occur on

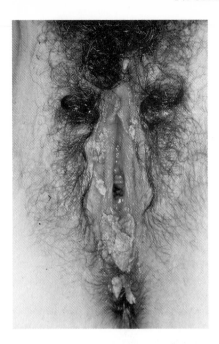

Fig. 14.1 Sessile condyloma acuminata on the labia and interior to the anus. Confluent growth has occurred at the anterior four-chette.

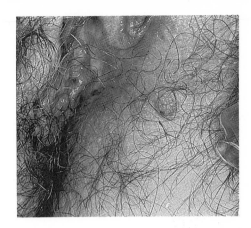

Fig. 14.2 A keratotic verruca vulgaris is present on the perivulvar skin.

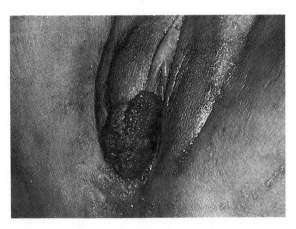

Fig. 14.3 A nodular giant condyloma acuminata is present on the labia. Microscopic examination revealed areas of carcinoma in situ.

the labia majora, the walls of the vagina and on the cervix. In men these sessile warts are most often located on the inner surface of the prepuce and within the coronal sulcus. In both sexes the urinary meatus, the perineum, the anus and the perianal tissue may be involved. The second clinically distinctive type of anogenital wart is that of a squared-off, keratotic papule 4–8 mm in diameter. This variety of wart is similar in appearance to the typical common hand wart (verruca vulgaris). Such lesions, when they occur in the groin, are located on dry, non-mucosal surfaces such as the pubis, inner thighs (Fig. 14.2) and, in men, the penile shaft and scrotum. The third clinical variety of venereal wart is a minute, flat topped, non-keratotic papule. These are similar in appearance to common flat warts (verruca plana). These lesions are most often found in men on the glans and shaft of the penis (Levine et al 1984) and, in women, on the labia and cervix (Nyeem et al 1982). In both sexes, urethral lesions may be present (Keating et al 1985; Libby et al 1985). Because they are often less than 2 mm in diameter, recognition often depends on acetic acid swabbing and magnified observation such as is carried out with ordinary colposcopy. The fourth

morphological type of anogenital wart is a larger nodular lesion 1 to several cm in diameter (Fig. 14.3). These, too, are non-keratotic and usually have a pebbly, strawberry-like surface. Such lesions are most often located on mucosal or modified mucosal epithelium. When these 'giant condyloma' possess features of histological atypia or unregulated epithelial growth they are called Buschke-Lowenstein tumours or verrucous carcinomas (Partridge et al 1980; Ananthakrishnan et al 1981). Finally, several patterns of vaginal wall involvement have been described (Roy et al 1981). Most of these vaginal warts are variations on the morphology described above but a distinctive, diffuse, cobblestone involvement is recognised.

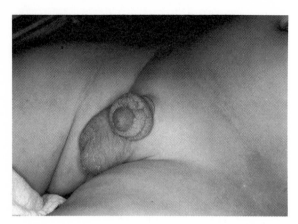

Fig. 14.4 Confluent growth of condyloma acuminata has occurred at the circumcision site of a 5-month-old boy.

The appearances of wart virus infection of the uterine cervix are described in chapter 5 and shown in plates 30–33.

Age and sex

Anogenital warts are found primarily in sexually active individuals and thus are most commonly seen between the ages of 16 and 25 (Oriel 1971a). Individuals with anal lesions are, on average, several years older than those with genital and perigenital warts (Oriel 1971b). The age distribution curve is almost identical to that determined for gonorrhoea and other sexually transmitted diseases. However, the occasional presence of anogenital warts in neonates and young children (Sait & Garg 1985; Stringel et al 1985) indicates that infection at other ages does occur (Fig. 14.4). Men were thought to be affected somewhat more often than women but recent evidence, to include the prevalence of cervical warts, suggests that the opposite may in fact be true (Chuang et al 1984).

Incidence and prevalence

Fifty years ago condyloma acuminata were thought to be uncommon lesions. However, within the last decade, probably due both to better identification and to changes in sexual behaviour, a veritable epidemic has occurred. In England there has been a consistent 10% annual increase throughout the last decade (Chief Medical Officer 1981, 1985) and in the United States the Centers for Disease Control

(1983) report a 500% increase in the last 15 years. Furthermore recent information, based on cervical culposcopy and cytology, suggests that the prevalence of HPV infection of the cervix is about 2% in women of reproductive age (Meisels et al 1981; Schneider et al 1985). It is likely that, with the exception of non-gonococcal urethritis, HPV infection is the most common sexually transmitted disease.

Factors predisposing to infection

Since close personal contact appears to be required for transmission it is not surprising that the single most important factor in the acquisition of anogenital warts is the frequency with which casual sexual intercourse takes place. Thus, it is estimated that 70% of patients attending clinics for sexually transmitted disease have had anogenital warts. In addition, extrapolation from human inoculation studies suggests that the presence of irritated or traumatised skin greatly enhances the likelihood of infection when one is exposed to the virus in an infected partner. In men lack of circumcision, presumably by providing a warm moist environment, also appears to be a risk factor.

Immunological factors are critical both in the development and in the resolution of human wart virus infection. Depressed cell mediated responsiveness greatly enhances the likelihood of infection as indicated by the increased incidence of warts in immunosuppressed patients (Schneider et al 1983). Of particular interest to the gynaecologist is the increased prevalence and growth rates of anogenital warts in women who are mildly immunosuppressed as a result of pregnancy or use of oral contraceptive pills (Seski et al 1978). Diabetics seem at particular risk for the development of anogenital warts (Skuraton 1978). The reasons for this are unknown but decreased tissue health, increased frequency of irritating vaginal discharge, and systemic factors modifying resistance to infection are probably important.

Association with other sexually transmitted diseases

Statistics obtained from clinics for sexually transmitted diseases suggest that patients with condyloma acuminata are more likely to have other sexually transmitted diseases. For instance, in such clinics, 12–34% of patients with genital warts have concomitant gonorrhoea (Harahap 1979; Jenkens & Riley 1980). Patients seen in standard dermatological practices are much less likely to have gonorrhoea but the incidence of candidiasis and nongonococcal urethritis is appreciable (Fairris et al 1984; Mitchell et al 1985).

Incubation period

The incubation period for anogenital wart virus infection is not known with certainty. In one epidemiological study, wives resuming intercourse with infected husbands recently returned from the Far East developed warts 4–6 weeks later (Barrett et al 1954). Other investigators have estimated the average incubation period at approximately 3 months with a range from 3 weeks to 8 months (Powell 1972). Even longer periods of incubation may occur in cases of HPV-induced laryngeal papillomatosis. Recognition of this long incubation period is important for two reasons. First, in contact tracing, a previous rather than current sexual partner may be the source of the infection. Second, during therapy, new warts (even in the absence of sexual exposure) may well appear for several months following successful eradication of all visible lesions. In fact, many of the warts thought by physician and patient to be recurrent because of treatment failure are in reality entirely new warts arising from nearby incubating virus (Ferenczy et al 1985).

Latency

Latency may be viewed conceptually in a manner similar to the incubation period. In effect it is the presence of HPV DNA in tissues which morphologically show no evidence of HPV infection. Thus, in normal appearing tissues 15 mm distant from laser treated genital warts, HPV DNA could be recognized with hybridisation probes in almost half of patients studied (Ferenczy et al 1985). That this latent DNA has the potential for activation and virion assembly is suggested by the fact that, on follow-up, it was primarily those patients in whom latent DNA was found who developed clinical evidence of new wart formation. It is not known how long HPV DNA can remain latent. However,

based on studies of normal laryngeal tissue in patients who had previously had laryngeal papillomatosis, it is likely to be many months or even many years (Steinberg et al 1983).

Contagion

Contagion between individuals appears to occur mainly as a result of close skin-to-skin contact. The degree of contagiousness for genital HPV infections seems relatively great. At least 25%, and more likely up to 65%, of those having sexual contact with infected partners become infected themselves (Barrett et al 1954; Jenkins & Riley 1980; Levine et al 1984). The recognition of penile warts in the consorts of infected women often requires magnified observation after acetic acid preparation. This recently recognised requirement probably accounts for the lower level of contagiousness found in earlier studies. The situation with anal warts is less clear. A very high proportion (60–80%) of patients with anal and perianal lesions have had anal intercourse but contact tracing has been surprisingly unsuccessful in turning up penile warts in the sexual partners of these women and homosexual men (Oriel 1971; Carr & William 1977).

Most studies have emphasised the sexual nature of the contact necessary for the transmission of warts but non-venereal spread is also possible. This is perhaps most dramatically demonstrated in instances where fully developed warts have been found on the fetus at the time of birth (Tang et al 1978). The source for these infections is not clear but in utero infection appears to occur in some mammals infected with papilloma viruses (Amtmann et al 1984). Anogenital warts are also occasionally found in children who have not been sexually abused (Sait et al 1985; Stringel et al 1985), and warts once present on an individual can be further spread on one's self through the process of scratching and autoinoculation. Finally, and most intriguing, there is the problem of HPV-induced laryngeal papillomatosis. Current evidence indicates that in at least two-thirds of these infected children their mothers had warts present in the birth canal at the time of parturition (Cohen et al 1980; Quick et al 1980; Mounts et al 1982). Because of this, the safety and appropriateness of vaginal delivery for women with vulvovaginal warts is currently receiving considerable attention.

Natural history and immunology

Like most other viral diseases, warts often undergo spontaneous resolution. This spontaneous resolution occurs most dramatically in children with common hand and foot warts but it is also observed, to a lesser degree, in adults with anogenital warts. It is not known why spontaneous resolution occurs readily in some individuals and not at all in others but the type of wart, the duration of the wart, the number of viral particles present within the wart, and the age and immunological status of the patient seem to be important factors.

Both humoral and cell mediated immune responsiveness have been studied in HPV infections (Bender et al 1983; Kienzler et al 1983). Most of these studies have been carried out in patients with non-genital warts, but almost certainly the processes apply to anogenital warts as well. In the case of humoral immune response it can be shown that virus-specific IgM antibodies develop in the majority of those who have been infected. Later, and in a smaller number of individuals, virus-specific complement fixing IgG antibodies are also found. The development of these latter antibodies often correlates temporally with the remission of warts but a cause and effect relationship does not seem likely since firstly, warts are not found more frequently in agammaglobulinaemic patients; secondly, some warts regress in the absence of IgG antibodies; and thirdly, reinfection can occur in the presence of IgG antibodies. By analogy with other types of viral infections it is probable that wart-specific antibodies are related more to the prevention of viral dissemination than they are to the resolution of the disease.

Remission of warts is regularly accompanied by evidence of cell mediated immune responsiveness (Thivolet et al 1982; Bender et al 1983; Tagami et al 1985). Specifically, levels of migration inhibition factor increase and skin test reactivity to wart extract is enhanced in individuals whose warts subsequently resolve. The importance of cell mediated immune responsiveness in the resolution of warts is emphasised by the fact that individuals with even minor depression of cell mediated immune responsiveness are more susceptible to wart virus infection, are less likely to demonstrate spontaneous regression and respond less well to treatment. However, wart virus infection itself may cause reversible depression of cell mediated immune responsiveness through antigenic overload and this in turn may adversely affect regression of the infection (Mohanty & Roy 1984).

Clinical experience suggests that, when compared to common, non-genital warts, condyloma acuminata are less likely to undergo spontaneous resolution and they respond less well to therapy. This relative resistance may be related to immune phenomena. As an example, anogenital warts contain fewer recognisable viral particles and for this reason may offer less antigenic stimulation. Moreover, anogenital warts tend to occur in adults rather than in children and it is recognised that children generally handle all types of viral infections more effectively than do older individuals.

Oncogenic potential of HPV infection

The overwhelming majority of individuals with warts never experience any significant complications as a result of their infection. However, recent studies suggest that under certain circumstances HPV infection can play a role in the induction of malignancy (Lynch 1982; Crum & Levine 1984; Smith & Campo 1985). This appears to be particularly true for genital malignancy which is a problem occurring with ever greater frequency and in younger individuals. The factors suggesting a potential oncogenic role for HPV infection include, first, the recognition that the closely related animal papillomaviruses are both good transforming agents and proven causes of malignant tumours (Amtmann et al 1984). Second, in the rare syndrome epidermodysplasia verruciformis, HPV 5 infection, occurring in the dual setting of depressed cell mediated immune responsiveness and excess sunlight exposure, regularly leads to the appearance of cutaneous squamous cell carcinomas (Ostrow et al 1982; Androphy et al 1985). Third, histological evidence of squamous cell carcinoma has been found within lesions which are otherwise typical of warts (Lynch 1982). The coincidence of these two lesions has been reported for warts on the fingers, tongue, larynx, lung and foot but is particularly notable on the genitalia where this association is present in 5–15% of all vulvar malignancies. Fourth, a very high percentage of women who have colposcopic or cytological evidence of cervical dysplasia (CIN I-III) have associated HPV infection of the cervix

(Reid et al 1984; Binder et al 1985). Fifth, most women with cervical dysplasia have antibodies to HPV and a considerable number have previously had genital warts (Daling et al 1984). Sixth, and most importantly, HPV DNA can be recovered from about 80% of genital epithelial carcinomas when these tumours are studied with monoclonal antibodies or DNA hybridisation probes (Ikenberg et al 1983; Boshart et al 1984; Crum et al 1984; Gross et al 1985; Scholl et al 1985).

A number of factors seem to be important in determining whether a given HPV genital infection will result in malignant transformation. The most significant of these factors appears to be the specific type of HPV virus causing the infection. Thus, infections with HPV 6 and 11 (the most common HPV types found in genital warts) are rarely identified in frank carcinomas (Gissmann et al 1983) whereas HPV 16 and 18 (less commonly found in genital warts) are the types regularly identified within malignant cells (Crum et al 1984; Gross et al 1985; Schwarz et al 1985; Yee et al 1985). Other factors, less well studied, include the presence of immunosuppression (Schneider et al 1985), the availability of tumour promotors such as smoking and other environmental factors (Mabuchi et al 1985; Prakash et al 1985; Sasson et al 1985) and the histological type of tissue infected. In regard to the latter point, infection of transitional tissue such as occurs in the cervix and anus seems to be associated with greater degrees of risk than does infection elsewhere (Buscema & Woodruff 1980; Purola et al 1983).

Absolute proof of an aetiological relationship will require prospective studies in which patients with various types of HPV infection are observed for the development of carcinoma. Limited studies wherein cervical HPV infections have been followed for months to several years certainly seem to support the hypothesis that HPV infection is the single most important factor in the development of cervical carcinoma (Walker et al 1983; Evans & Monaghan 1985; Evans-Jones et al 1985; Wickenden et al 1985).

Therapy

Even though anogenital warts have been historically considered as a trivial problem, our current understanding regarding their high degree of contagiousness and their oncological potential suggests that a rather aggressive approach to therapy is required of all clinicians (Silva et al 1985).

Appropriate therapy includes both non-specific and specific approaches. Non-specific steps include contact tracing to reduce reinfection and general contagiousness, observation of 'hidden' mucosal surfaces (urethra, vagina, cervix, anus) for additional warts, magnified observation of the genitalia to recognise the full extent of the infection, appropriate tests to identify any other concomitant sexually transmitted diseases (Cooper & Singha 1985), reduction in irritative factors through treatment of vaginitis and alleviation of sweat retention, and, where necessary, cessation of oral contraceptive in order to enhance immune responsiveness.

Specific treatment involves two overlapping approaches: destructive measures and immunotherapy. The overlap occurs because destructive techniques may, by way of inducing an inflammatory reaction, also initiate immune responsiveness. The most commonly used and most effective treatment modalities are listed below. In choosing among them it should be remembered that no one approach is 100% effective and that concomitant and sequential combinations may be necessary.

Podophyllin (Miller 1985) made up as a 25% concentration in tincture of benzoin has been the most widely used therapeutic agent for anogenital warts for many years. It is still an excellent choice for moist sessile warts. Correct application requires that the entire surface of the wart be 'painted' but, conversely, care must be taken to avoid application to normal skin in order to minimise subsequent discomfort. Most clinicians advise that the podophyllin be washed off 4–8 hours after application but I have found that if little or no podophyllin has been applied to surrounding normal skin, washing is not necessary. Reapplication of podophyllin to remaining warts is carried out at 7-day intervals. I limit the number of applications to five retreatments both because of diminishing therapeutic returns and also because of a desire to avoid unproductive and possibly tumour promoting chronic irritation of the tissue. Systemic side-effects, especially during pregnancy, can occur as a result of inappropriately generous topical podophyllin therapy (Fisher 1981). Safety can generally be assured if 0.5 ml or less of the 25% solution is applied during any one treatment session. Four recently reported controlled studies have demonstrated eradication rates of 22, 25, 51, and 75% in varying circumstances (Simmons 1981a; Gabriel & Thin 1983; Bashi & Ven 1985; Jensen 1985).

Tri- or bichloroacetic acid prepared as a saturated solution is particularly useful on non-keratotic flat warts. Extreme care must be used during application since both acids are extremely caustic; any spillage on to surrounding tissue will instantly result in tissue destruction. These acids are best applied with a modified cotton tipped applicator. A conventional wooden stick applicator is cracked in half and a very small amount of cotton is twisted on to one of the split ends such that the size of the new tip is one-quarter that of the original. Calcium alginate urethral swabs can also be used although, because of their tight winding, they hold the acid poorly. With either swab, the wetted tip should be brushed against the lip of the bottle so as to dislodge any loose drops. The moistened swab is then touched to each wart. Within 1–3 minutes after application the wart will turn white and the patient will experience a moderate amount of discomfort. This discomfort peaks at about 10–20 minutes and thereafter subsides. Reapplication to remaining warts is carried out at 7-day intervals. No controlled studies regarding the use of these acids have been published but in one instance trichloroacetic acid added to podophyllin resulted in no additional benefit (Gabriel & Thin 1983).

Cryotherapy utilising sprays or probes cooled with nitrous oxide or liquid nitrogen works well on all small warts and is perhaps the treatment of choice for those anogenital warts which have a dry, keratotic surface. Here, too, retreatment at weekly intervals is usually necessary. Cure rates of 70–100% have been published for uncontrolled studies. Reports from two recent controlled studies indicated cure rates of 41 and 80% (Simmons et al 1981b; Bashi & Ven 1985).

Surgical excision (Jensen 1985) and *electrosurgical destruction* (Robinson 1980; Simmons et al 1981) represent the treatment of choice for large anogenital warts. Since only epidermal cells are involved in wart virus infection, surgical removal is best carried out using a shave technique. Haemostasis can be obtained through the application of silver nitrate, ferric chloride or ferric subsulphate (Monsel's) solution. Electrosurgical destruction

avoids problems with haemostasis but, unless a cutting current is used in a shave technique, such treatment does not allow for an adequate biopsy specimen. Cure rates of 80–90% are generally possible with either approach.

Laser destruction has become very popular in recent years (Bellina 1983; Ferenczy 1983, 1984a; Stanhope et al 1983; Grundsell et al 1984; Kruger-Baggesen et al 1984). As is true for most new therapies, initial reports from uncontrolled studies claimed cure rates of close to 100%. However, two controlled studies comparing laser therapy to conventional surgery or electrosurgery have showed little advantage for the laser approach in either cure rates or patient preference (Billingham & Lewis 1982; Duus et al 1985). As for electrosurgical destruction, laser therapy does not provide tissue for histological observation. Nevertheless, there are undoubtedly circumstances where the finely focused laser beam offers certain technical advantages and this approach may well become the treatment of choice for cervical, urethral (Fuselier et al 1980; Ferenczy 1984b) and vaginal warts (Ferenczy 1984c).

Fluorouracil in a 5% cream causes a great deal of irritation to normal tissue surrounding warts and thus has a poor record for patient acceptance. There may, however, be special circumstances (vaginal and urethral warts) where this method is preferable (Wallin 1977; Ferenczy 1984c).

Topically applied or systemically administered *retinoids* (Boyle et al 1983) together with intralesionally injected *bleomycin* (Shumer & O'Keefe 1983; Bunney et al 1984) are best considered experimental with unproven records in the treatment of anogenital warts. Both do have considerable therapeutic potential and it is likely that with better study they will prove useful in the future.

The dawn of immunotherapy for warts several years ago was greeted with considerable enthusiasm. Unfortunately, these approaches have thus far not lived up to the high expectations with which they were introduced. Specifically, controlled studies for the usage of *levamisole* (Saul et al 1980), *transfer factor*, and *autologous vaccines* (Malison et al 1982) have demonstrated results that were no better than placebo response. Sensitisation of the patient to 2% dinitrochlorobenzene (DNCB) followed by subsequent repeated applications of more dilute solutions directly to warts results in 60–85% cure rates for non-genital warts (Johansson & Forstrom 1984; Lee et al 1984). However, no significant studies have been published regarding this approach for anogenital warts. Some excitement currently exists for the use of intralesional or intramuscular injection of one or the other of the interferons but here again, published data to fully support this therapy are not yet available.

It seems likely that total, safe therapy for anogenital warts will require the development of either effective antiviral antibiotics or a vaccine suitable for use in children. However, as regards the former, the presence of non-replicating latent virus in normal appearing tissue adjacent to treated warts warrants considerable pessimism in terms of the possibility of total eradication of virus with antibiotics. As regards the latter, the tremendous number of HPV types greatly complicates the preparation of a vaccine that would be effective against warts of all varieties.

MOLLUSCUM CONTAGIOSUM

The aetiological agent

The putative cause of molluscum contagiosum is a DNA virus which has the electron microscopic characteristics of a poxvirus (Postlethwaite 1970). This virus is a large, brick shaped particle which is located in the cytoplasm of infected epithelial cells. This virus is present in all lesions of molluscum contagiosum but it has never been cultured and even the earlier human-to-human inoculation studies have not recently been successfully repeated. Inoculation of the virus into various cell cultures does result in cellular phagocytosis together with the subsequent development of visible cytopathic effects but replication does not occur because of a block at the protein uncoating step (McFadden et al 1979).

The molluscum contagiosum virus infects only epithelial tissues. Within these cells histological evidence of infection occurs in the form of large cytoplasmic inclusion bodies. Such infection causes an increase in epithelial cell proliferation which is clinically reflected as a small, wart-like papule. The centre of each molluscum lesion contains a cavity

filled with a white globule of dead cells and viral protein (Reed & Parkinson 1977). This globule is known as the Henderson-Patterson, or molluscum, body. Often the cavity communicates with the surface of the skin through a small umbilicated pore. In some cases this communication appears to occur as a result of infection via the ostia of the hair follicle (Uehara & Danno 1980; Ive 1985) but the occurrence of umbilicated lesions on non-hair-bearing skin and mucosae indicates that this is not always the case (Legrain & Pierard 1985).

Clinical features

Epidemiological studies suggest that molluscum contagiosum viral infection is passed from person to person (Brown et al 1981; Felman 1984). Thirty or more years ago the close personal contact necessary for such spread occurred almost entirely among children. In western society today, owing to less crowded childhood living conditions, the first chance for contagion often occurs as a result of sexual activity among young adults (Lynch 1972). As a result currently more than half of all infections occur after the age of puberty. And, like other sexually transmitted viral diseases, the prevalence of molluscum contagiosum is increasing (Chief Medical Officer 1981). The lesions are now frequently encountered in private practices, in student health service clinics and in clinics for sexually transmitted diseases (Wilkin 1977; Dennis et al 1985).

The incubation period for molluscum contagiosum infection is not known with certainty. Estimates based on contagion among children and on older experimental (and somewhat suspect) human-to-human inoculation studies suggest an incubation period averaging 4–8 weeks with a range of 1–25 weeks. Such a long incubation period makes contact tracing difficult and for this reason the lesions of molluscum contagiosum are found in current sexual partners only about 20% of the time.

The clinical lesion of molluscum contagiosum is a smooth surfaced, dome shaped or flat topped papule which is typically 1–5 mm in diameter. Central umbilication (a pathognomonic sign) is present in about 25% of the lesions (Fig. 14.5). The papules vary appreciably in colour. Most are white, reflecting the presence of the central white

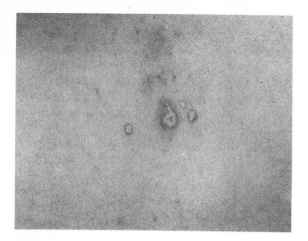

Fig. 14.5 Umbilicated and non-umbilicated papules of molluscum contagiosum occurring on the inner thigh.

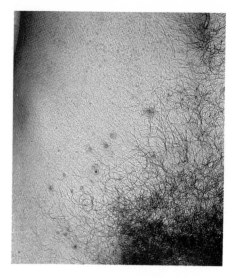

Fig. 14.6 Perilesional inflammatory changes are present around multiple molluscum contagiosum of the pubic area.

molluscum body, but some are skin coloured, a few are pink to red and a few are translucent. These latter lesions appear as small vesicles and have led to the colloquial terminology of 'water warts'. An inflammatory reaction occurs around the lesions of molluscum contagiosum about 10% of the time. This varies clinically from a light pink, surrounding eczematisation (Rockoff 1978) to a bright red, furuncle-like reaction encompassing the wart (Fig. 14.6; Lynfield & Laude 1982). These inflammatory changes probably occur when viral protein is extruded into surrounding connective tissue where it incites a foreign body reaction (Pierard-Franchimont et al 1983). Uncommon and atypical lesions of molluscum contagiosum appear as solid white plaques, pedunculated papules and giant cyst-like lesions (Lynch 1968).

Molluscum contagiosum in children are located most often on the face, trunk and extremities. In adult women they are most likely to occur on the inner thighs, whereas in adult men penile lesions are commonly present. In adults of both sexes the pubic area is often affected. Rarely lesions are found on genital mucous membranes. Most lesions of molluscum contagiosum are asymptomatic and are accidentally discovered by the patient or an examining physician. Occasionally mild pruritus is present.

Typically, 2 to 20 individual lesions of molluscum contagiosum are present but in immunocom-

promised patients, hundreds may develop (Peachey 1977; Pauly et al 1978). Some degree of trauma to the skin is probably required in order to allow successful inoculation. This presumption is supported by the occasional presence of linearly distributed papules occurring at the site of an old scratchmark.

The diagnosis of molluscum contagiosum can usually be made on the basis of clinical observation. Confirmation of a clinical diagnosis, if desired, can be obtained by way of biopsy or through cytological examination of material expressed from the central umbilication (Wada & Masukawa 1977).

Natural history and immunology

In childhood the lesions of molluscum contagiosum resolve spontaneously without scarring or other serious sequelae (Ogino & Ishida 1984). Though less well studied, such resolution presumably also occurs in adults (Steffen & Markman 1980). The time period to spontaneous resolution is highly variable. Individual lesions regress within several months (Steffen & Markman 1980) but continued autoinoculation may lead to the persistence of disease for one or more years. Resolution of the lesions when it does occur is accompanied by a predominantly lymphocytic infiltrate (Steffen & Markman 1980; Ogino & Ishido 1984) which is probably due to the activation of immunological responsiveness.

Antibody formation is recognised in patients with molluscum contagiosum (Shirodaria & Matthews 1977) but the amount of antibody formed, the frequency with which it is present and the time course of its appearance do not correlate well with the resolution of lesions. Cell mediated immune responsiveness has hardly been studied but the frequency and severity of molluscum contagiosum infection in atopic individuals (Ogino & Ishida 1984; Ive 1985) and in those with more severe depression of cell mediated immunity (Katzman et al 1985; Lombardo 1985; Sarma & Weilbaecher 1985) pay testimony to its importance. Immunity conferred by molluscum contagiosum virus infection is probably not permanent, since reinfection is possible.

Therapy

The lesions of molluscum contagiosum are of no known medical importance but, in the interest of decreased contagiousness, therapy is usually carried out. Effective therapy requires the removal or destruction of the virally infected central cells. The white globular molluscum body can be expressed (albeit with some difficulty) with a comedone extractor or the entire lesion can be scraped away with a dermal curette. Cryotherapy utilising a nitrous oxide cooled probe or liquid nitrogen applied by spray or cotton tipped applicator also works well, as does the application of bi- or trichloroacetic acid. Alternatively a 0.7% solution of cantharidin (Cantherone) can be applied. Over a period of 48 hours this creates a blister underneath the lesion and in due time the wart is sloughed off, along with the blister roof. This latter approach is quite painless and is particularly appropriate for infants and infected children. No matter which approach is chosen retreatment is usually necessary, not only for the few lesions which fail to respond, but also for those new lesions which have arisen as a result of the long incubation period.

REFERENCES

Amtmann E, Volm M, Wayss K 1984 Tumour induction in the rodent Mastomys natalensis by activation of endogenous papilloma virus genomes. Nature 308: 291

Ananthakrishnan N, Ravindran R, Veliath A J et al 1981 Lowenstein-Buschke tumor of penis—a carcinomimic. Report of 24 cases with review of the literature. British Journal of Urology 53: 460–465

Androphy E J, Dvoretzky I, Lowy D R 1985 X-linked inheritance of epidermodysplasia verruciformis. Archives of Dermatology 121: 864–868

Barrett T L, Silbar J D, McGinley J P 1954 Genital warts—a venereal disease. Journal of the American Medical Association 154: 333–334

Bashi S A, Ven D 1985 Cryotherapy versus podophyllin in the treatment of genital warts. International Journal of Dermatology 24: 535–536

Bellina J H 1983 The use of the carbon dioxide laser in the management of condyloma acuminatum with eight-year follow-up. American Journal of Obstetrics and Gynecology 147: 375

Bender M E, Ostrow R S, Watts S et al 1983 Immunology of human papillomavirus: warts. Pediatric Dermatology 1: 121–126

Billingham R P, Lewis F G 1982 Laser versus electrical cautery in the treatment of condylomata acuminata of the anus. Surgery, Gynecology and Obstetrics 155: 865–867

Binder M A, Cates G W, Emson H E et al 1985 The changing concepts of condyloma. A retrospective study of colposcopically directed cervical biopsies. American Journal of Obstetrics and Gynecology 151: 213–219

Boshart M, Gissmann L, Ikenberg H et al 1984 A new type of papillomavirus DNA, its presence in genital cancer biopsies and in cell lines derived from cervical cancer. The EMBO Journal 3: 1151–1157

Boyle J, Dick D C, Mackie R M 1983 Treatment of extensive virus warts with etretinate (tigason) in a patient with sarcoidosis. Clinical and Experimental Dermatology 8: 33–36

Brown S T, Nalley J F, Kraus S J 1981 Molluscum contagiosum. Sexually Transmitted Diseases 8: 227–234

Bunney M H, Nolan M W, Buxton P K et al 1984 The treatment of resistant warts with intralesional bleomycin: a controlled clinical trial. British Journal of Dermatology 111: 197–207

Buscema J, Woodruff J D 1980 Progressive histobiologic alterations in the development of vulvar cancer. American Journal of Obstetrics and Gynecology 138: 146

Carr G, William D C 1977 Anal warts in a population of gay men in New York City. Sexually Transmitted Diseases 4: 56

Centers for Disease Control 1983 Condyloma acuminatum—United States, 1966–1981. MMWR 32: 306–308

Chief Medical Officer 1981 Sexually transmitted diseases. British Journal of Venereal Diseases 57: 402–405

Chief Medical Officer 1985 Sexually transmitted diseases. Genitourinary Medicine 61: 204–207

Chuang T -Y, Perry H O, Kurland L T, Ilstrup D M 1984 Condyloma acuminatum in Rochester, Minn, 1950–1978. Archives in Dermatology 120: 469–475

Cohen S R, Seltzer S, Geller K A et al 1980 Papilloma of the larynx and tracheobronchial tree in children. A retrospective study. Annals of Otology 89: 497–503

Cooper C, Singha S K 1985 Condylomata acuminata in women: the effect of concomitant genital infection on response to treatment. Acta Dermato-venereologica (Stockholm) 65: 150–153

Crum C P, Levine R U 1984 Human papillomavirus infection

and cervical neoplasia: new perspectives. International Journal of Gynecology and Pathology 3: 376–388

Crum C P, Ikenberg H, Richart R M, Gissman L 1984 Human papillomavirus type 16 and early cervical neoplasia. New England Journal of Medicine 310: 880–883

Daling J E, Chu J, Weiss N S, Emel L, Tamini H K 1984 The association of condylomata acuminata and squamous carcinoma of the vulva. British Journal of Cancer 50: 533–535

Dennis J, Oshiro L S, Bunter J W 1985 Molluscum contagiosum, another sexually transmitted disease: its impact on the clinical virology laboratory. Journal of Infectious Diseases 151: 376

Duus B R, Philipsen T, Christensen J D et al 1985 Refractory condylomata acuminata: a controlled clinical trial of carbon dioxide laser versus conventional surgical treatment. Genitourinary Medicine 61: 59–61

Evans A S, Monaghan J M 1985 Spontaneous resolution of cervical warty atypia: the relevance of clinical and nuclear DNA features: a prospective study. British Journal of Obstetrics and Gynecology 92: 165–169

Evans-Jones J C, Forbes-Smith P A, Hirschowitz L 1985 Follow-up of women with cervical koilocytosis. Lancet 1: 1445

Fairris G M, Statham B N, Waugh M A 1984 The investigation of patients with genital warts. British Journal of Dermatology 111: 736–738

Felman Y M 1984 Molluscum contagiosum. Cutis 33: 113

Ferenczy A 1983 Using the laser to treat vulvar condylomata acuminata and intraepidermal neoplasia. Canadian Medical Association Journal 128: 135–137

Ferenczy A 1984a Treating genital condyloma during pregnancy with the carbon dioxide laser. American Journal of Obstetrics and Gynecology 148: 9

Ferenczy A 1984b Laser therapy of genital condylomata acuminata. Obstetrics and Gynecology 63: 703

Ferenczy A 1984c Comparison of 5-fluorouracil and CO_2 laser for treatment of vaginal condylomata. Obstetrics and Gynecology 64: 773–778

Ferenczy A, Mitao M, Nagi N et al 1985 Latent papillomavirus and recurring genital warts. New England Journal of Medicine 313: 784–788

Fisher A A 1981 Severe systemic and local reactions to topical podophyllum resin. Cutis 28: 233–266

Fuselier Jr H A, McBurney E I, Brannan W, Randrup E R 1980 Treatment of condylomata acuminata with carbon dioxide laser. Urology 15: 265

Gabriel G, Thin R N T 1983 Treatment of anogenital warts. Comparison of trichloracetic acid and podophyllin versus podophyllin alone. British Journal of Venereal Diseases 59: 124–126

Gissmann L, Wolnik L, Ikenberg H et al 1983 Human papillomavirus types 6 and 11 DNA sequences in genital and laryngeal papillomas and in some cervical cancers. Proceedings of the National Academy of Science of the USA 80: 560–563

Gissmann L, Boshart M, Durst M et al 1984 Presence of human papillomavirus in genital tumors. Journal of Investigative Dermatology 83: 26s–28s

Gross G, Hagedorn M, Ikenberg H et al 1985 Bowenoid papulosis. Presence of human papillomavirus (HPV) structural antigens and of HPV 16-related DNA sequences. Archives of Dermatology 121: 858–863

Grundsell H, Larsson G, Bekassy Z 1984 Treatment of condylomata acuminata with the carbon dioxide laser. British Journal of Obstetrics and Gynaecology 91: 193–196

Harahap M 1979 Asymptomatic gonorrhoea among patients with condylomata acuminata. British Journal of Venereal Diseases 55: 450

Ikenberg H, Gissmann L, Gross G et al 1983 Human papillomavirus type-16-related DNA in genital Bowen's disease and in Bowenoid papulosis. International Journal of Cancer 32: 563–565

Ive F A 1985 Follicular molluscum contagiosum. British Journal of Dermatology 113: 493–495

Jenkins H M L, Riley V C 1980 A review of outpatient management of female genital warts. British Journal of Clinical Practice 34: 273

Jensen S L 1985 Comparison of podophyllin application with simple surgical excision in clearance and recurrence of perianal condylomata acuminata. Lancet ii: 1146

Johansson E, Forstrom L 1984 Dinitrochlorobenzene (DNCB) treatment of viral warts. Acta Dermato-venerealogica (Stockholm) 64: 529–533

Katzman M, Elmets C A, Lederman M M 1985 Molluscum contagiosum and the acquired immunodeficiency syndrome. Annals of Internal Medicine 102: 413–414

Keating M A, Young R H, Carr C P et al 1985 Condyloma acuminatum of the bladder and ureter: case report and review of the literature. Journal of Urology 133: 465

Kienzler J L, Lemoine M T H, Orth G et al 1983 Humoral and cell-mediated immunity to human papillomavirus type I (HPV-I) in human warts. Journal of Dermatology 108: 665–672

Kryger-Baggesen N, Larsen J F, Pedersen P H 1984 CO_2-laser treatment of condylomata acuminata. Acta Obstetrica et Gynecologica Scandinavica 63: 341–343

Lee S, Cho C K, Kim J G, Chun S I 1984 Therapeutic effect of dinitrochlorobenzene (DNCB) on verruca plana and verruca vulgaris. International Journal of Dermatology 23: 624–626

Legrain A, Pierard G E 1985 Molluscum contagiosum may affect primarily the epidermis without involving hair follicles. American Journal of Dermatopathology 7: 131–132

Levine R U, Crum C P, Herman E et al 1984 Cervical papillomavirus infection and intraepithelial neoplasia: a study of male sexual partners. Obstetrics and Gynecology 64: 16

Libby J M, Frankel J M, Scardino P T 1985 Condyloma acuminatum of the bladder and associated urothelial malignancy. Journal of Urology 134: 134

Lombardo P C 1985 Molluscum contagiosum and the acquired immunodeficiency syndrome. Archives of Dermatology 121: 834

Lynch P J 1968 Molluscum contagiosum of the adult. Archives of Dermatology 98: 141–143

Lynch P J 1972 Molluscum contagiosum venereum. Clinical Obstetrics and Gynecology 15: 966–975

Lynch P J 1982 Warts and cancer. American Journal of Dermatopathology 4: 55–60

Lynfield Y L, Laude T A 1982 Molluscum contagiosum: an unusual presentation. Cutis 30: 321

Mabuchi K, Bross D S, Kessler I I 1985 Epidemiology of cancer of the vulva. A case-control study. Cancer 55: 1843–1848

McFadden G, Pace W E, Purres J et al 1979 Biogenesis of poxviruses: transitory expression of molluscum contagiosum early functions. Virology 94: 297–313

Malison M D, Morris R, Jones L W 1982 Autogenous vaccine therapy for condyloma acuminatum. A double-blind controlled study British Journal of Venereal Diseases 58: 62–65

Meisels A, Roy M, Fortier M et al 1981 Human papillomavirus infection of the cervix. The atypical condyloma. Acta Cytologica 25: 7

Miller R A 1985 Podophyllin. International Journal of Dermatology 24: 491–498

Mitchell D M, Kellett J K, Haye K 1985 Investigation of patients with genital warts presenting to dermatological and to genito-urinary departments. British Journal of Dermatology 113: 22

Mohanty K C, Roy R B 1984 Thymus drived lymphocytes (T cells) in patients with genital warts. British Journal of Venereal Diseases 60: 186–188

Mounts P, Shah K V, Kashima H 1982 Viral etiology of juvenile- and adult-onset squamous papilloma of the larynx. Proceedings of the National Academy of Science of the USA 79: 5425–5429

Nyeem R, Wilkinson E J, Grover L J 1982 Condylomata acuminata of the cervix: histopathology and association with cervical neoplasia. International Journal of Gynecology and Pathology 1: 246–257

Ogino A, Ishida H 1984 Spontaneous regression of generalized molluscum contagiosum turning black. Acta Dermatovenerealogica (Stockholm) 64: 83–86

Oriel J D 1971a Natural history of genital warts. British Journal of Venereal Diseases 47: 1–13

Oriel J D 1971b Anal warts and anal coitus. British Journal of Venereal Diseases 47: 373–376

Ostrow R S, Bender M, Niimura M et al 1982 Human papillomavirus DNA in cutaneous primary and metastasized squamous cell carcinomas from patients with epidermodysplasia verruciformis. Proceedings of the National Academy of Science of the USA 79: 1634–1638

Partridge E E, Murad T, Shingleton H M et al 1980 Verrucous lesions of the female genitalia. I. Giant condylomata. American Journal of Obstetrics and Gynecology 137: 412

Pauly C R, Artis W M, Jones H E 1978 Atopic dermatitis, impaired cellular immunity and molluscum contagiosum. Archives of Dermatology 114: 391–393

Peachey R D G 1977 Severe molluscum contagiosum infection with T cell deficiency. British Journal of Dermatology 97: 49

Pierard-Franchimont C, Legrain A Pierard G E 1983 Growth and regression of molluscum contagiosum. Journal of the American Academy of Dermatology 9: 669–672

Postlethwaite R 1970 Molluscum contagiosum: a review. Archives of Environmental Health 21: 432

Powell Jr L C 1972 Condyloma acuminatum. Clinical Obstetrics and Gynecology 15: 948–965

Prakash S S, Reeves W C, Sisson G R et al 1985 Herpes simplex virus type 2 and human papillomavirus type 1 in cervicitis, dysplasia and invasive cervical carcinoma. International Journal of Cancer 35: 51–57

Purola E E, Halila H, Vesterinen E 1983 Condyloma and cervical epithelial atypias in young women. Gynecologic Oncology 16: 34–40

Quick C A, Krzyzek R A, Watts S L et al 1980 Relationship between condylomata and laryngeal papillomata. Annals of Otology 89: 467–471

Reed R J, Parkinson R P 1977 The histogenesis of molluscum contagiosum. American Journal of Surgical Pathology 1: 161–166

Reid R, Crum C P, Herschman B R et al 1984 Genital warts and cervical cancer. III. Subclinical papillomaviral infection and cervical neoplasia are linked by a spectrum of continuous morphologic and biologic change. Cancer 53: 943–953

Robinson J K 1980 Extirpation by electrocautery of massive lesions of condyloma acuminatum in the genito-perineoanal region. Journal of Dermatological Surgery and Oncology 6: 733

Rockoff A S 1978 Molluscum dermatitis. Journal of Pediatrics 92: 945–947

Roy M, Meisels A, Fortier M et al 1981 Vaginal condylomata: a human papillomavirus infection. Clinical Obstetrics and Gynecology 24: 461

Sait M A, Garg B R 1985 Condylomata acuminata in children: report of four cases. Genitourinary Medicine 61: 338–342

Sarma D P, Weilbaecher T G 1985 Molluscum contagiosum in the acquired immunodeficiency syndrome. Journal of the American Academy of Dermatology 13: 682–683

Sasson I M, Haley N J, Hoffman D et al 1985 Cigarette smoking and neoplasia of the uterine cervix: smoke constituents in cervical mucus. New England Journal of Medicine 312: 315–316

Saul A, Sanz R, Gomez M 1980 Treatment of multiple viral warts with levamisole. International Journal of Dermatology 19: 342

Schneider A, Kraus H, Schumann R, Gissman L 1985 Papillomavirus infection of the lower genital tract: detection of viral DNA in gynecological swabs. International Journal of Cancer 35: 443–448

Schneider V, Kay S, Lee H M 1983 Immunosuppression as a high-risk factor in the development of condyloma acuminatum and squamous neoplasia of the cervix. Acta Cytologica 27: 220–224

Scholl S M, Pillers E M K, Robinson R E, Farrell P J 1985 Prevalence of human papillomavirus type 16 DNA in cervical carcinoma samples in East Anglia. International Journal of Cancer 35: 215–218

Schwarz E, Freese U K, Gissmann L et al 1985 Structure and transcription of human papillomavirus sequences in cervical carcinoma cells. Nature 314: 111–114

Seski J C, Reinhalter E R, Silva Jr J 1978 Abnormalities of lymphocyte transformations in women with condylomata acuminata. Obstetrics and Gynecology 51: 188

Shirodaria P V, Matthews R S 1977 Observations on the antibody responses in molluscum contagiosum. British Journal of Dermatology 96: 29–34

Shumer S M, O'Keefe E J 1983 Bleomycin in the treatment of recalcitrant warts. Journal of the American Academy of Dermatology 9: 91–96

Silva P D, Micha J P, Silva D G 1985 Management of condyloma acuminatum. Journal of American Academy of Dermatology 13: 457–463

Simmons P D 1981 Podophyllin 10% and 25% in the treatment of ano-genital warts. A comparative double-blind study. British Journal of Venereal Diseases 57: 208–209

Simmons P D, Langlet F, Thin R N T 1981 Cryotherapy versus electrocautery in the treatment of genital warts. British Journal of Venereal Diseases 57: 273–274

Skuraton L E 1978 Resistant condylomata acuminata in diabetics. Archives of Dermatology 114: 800

Smith K T, Campo M S 1985 The biology of papillomaviruses and their role in oncogenesis. Anticancer Research 5: 31–48

Stanhope C R, Phibbs G D, Stuart G C E, Reid R 1983 Carbon dioxide laser surgery. Obstetrics and Gynecology 61: 624–627

Steffen C, Markman J -A 1980 Spontaneous disappearance of molluscum contagiosum. Report of a case. Archives of Dermatology 116: 923–924

Steinberg B M, Topp W C, Schneider P S, Abramson A L 1983 Laryngeal papillomavirus infection during clinical remission. New England Journal of Medicine 308: 1261–1264

Stringel G, Spence J, Corsini L 1985 Genital warts in children. Canadian Medical Association Journal 132: 1397

Tagami H, Oku T, Iwatsuki K 1985 Primary tissue culture of spontaneously regressing flat warts. In vitro attack by mononuclear cells against wart-derived epidermal cells. Cancer 55: 2437–2441

Tang C-K, Shermeta D W, Wood C 1978 Congenital condylomata acuminata. American Journal of Obstetrics and Genecology 131: 912

Thivolet J, Viac J, Staquet M J 1982 Cell-mediated immunity in wart infection. International Journal of Dermatology 21: 94–98

Uehara M, Danno K 1980 Central pitting of molluscum contagiosum. Journal of Cutaneous Pathology 7: 149–153

Wada Y, Masukawa T 1977 Cytologic diagnosis of molluscum contagiosum of the mons pubis. Acta Cytologica 21: 125

Walker P G, Singer A, Dyson J L, Oriel J D 1983 Natural history of cervical epithelial abnormalities in patients with vulval warts. British Journal of Venereal Diseases 59: 327

Wallin J 1977 5-fluorouracil in the treatment of penile and urethral condylomata acuminata. British Journal of Venereal Diseases 53: 240–243

Wickenden C, Malcolm A D B, Steele A, Coleman D V 1985 Screening for wart virus infection in normal and abnormal cervices by DNA hybridisation of cervical scrapes. Lancet i: 65

Wilkin J K 1977 Molluscum contagiosum venereum in a women's outpatient clinic: a venereally transmitted disease. American Journal of Obstetrics and Gynecology 128: 531–535

Yee C, Krishnan-Hewlett I, Baker C C, Schlegel R, Howley P M 1985 Presence and expression of human papillomavirus sequences in human cervical carcinoma cell lines. American Journal of Pathology 119: 361–366

Gardnerella vaginalis vaginitis
W E Josey and E O Hill

INTRODUCTION AND HISTORICAL BACKGROUND

Gardnerella vaginalis vaginitis is a commonly occurring disease during the reproductive years. The major clinical manifestation is a malodorous, non-purulent leukorrhoea. Some women with the infection are unaware of any problem. Others notice the discharge but regard it as only a minor nuisance and do not seek medical advice. However, many women find the condition to be very unpleasant and therefore are anxious to obtain relief.

G. vaginalis vaginitis is a relative newcomer to the list of known lower genital tract infections, the clinical and laboratory features having first been described in 1954 by Gardner & Dukes. They attributed the disorder to a small bacterial agent with morphological features and growth requirements similar to those characteristic of the genus *Haemophilus*. Previously, organisms believed to be species of *Haemophilus* had been isolated from the genitourinary tracts of both sexes by various workers, but none had specifically associated these organisms with leukorrhoea.

In a more detailed report published in 1955, Gardner & Dukes proposed the name *Haemophilus vaginalis* for the newly discovered bacterium, and advanced the concept that this organism is the aetiological agent in most cases of so-called 'non-specific vaginitis'. They established criteria for clinical diagnosis, emphasising the appearance of the vaginal discharge, the elevated pH of the vagina, and the wet mount finding of squamous epithelial cells coated with myriad tiny, rod-shaped bacteria (clue cells of Gardner). Over the next several years a number of studies were conducted by other investigators, most of whom confirmed the association of the bacterium with a distinctive type of leukorrhoea, unaccompanied by any of the classical signs of inflammation (in the absence of some other concurrent infection).

After the appearance of these early reports, further microbiological studies in various laboratories led to uncertainty regarding the proper classification of the organism, some authorities favoring assignment to the genus *Corynebacterium*. However, as additional microbiological characterisation tests were applied, it became increasingly evident that a totally new genus designation was needed. The recent official adoption of the generic name *Gardnerella* is a fitting tribute to Dr H L Gardner, for it was largely through his investigative efforts that this bacterium has gained acceptance as a significant pathogen in the female genital tract.

TAXONOMY

Determination of the proper taxonomic position of *Gardnerella vaginalis* has been a vexing microbiological problem, only recently resolved. The designation *Haemophilus vaginalis*, as suggested by Gardner & Dukes (1955), was used by most early investigators in reports of both clinical and laboratory studies. However, further study of the organism by various microbiologists raised doubts about the appropriateness of its assignment to the genus *Haemophilus*. In 1963, Zinnemann & Turner, on the basis of certain coryneform features exhibited by the organism, suggested the name *Corynebacterium vaginale*. The latter designation was endorsed by Dunkelberg (1977), as well as some other authorities, and was widely used in the literature on vaginitis throughout the 1970s.

In 1980, Greenwood & Pickett, utilising a variety of test procedures, clarified the taxonomy by demonstrating conclusively that the organism does not belong to either the genus *Haemophilus* or the genus *Corynebacterium*. They proposed the new name, *Gardnerella vaginalis*, which has been accepted as the official terminology in Edition 9 of Bergey's manual.

Although the guanine and cytosine (G+C) content of the DNA of *G. vaginalis* is similar to that of *Haemophilus* species, DNA hybridisation studies show no genetic relationship between these two bacterial types (Greenwood & Pickett 1980). *G. vaginalis* is separated from members of the genus *Corynebacterium* by a number of differences, including the higher G+C content of the latter. Electron microscopy studies by Criswell et al (1971) show that *G. vaginalis* is essentially a gram-negative bacterium, whereas the corynebacteria are gram-positive. Results of biochemical analyses of the cell wall of *G. vaginalis* are also compatible with gram-negativity.

Since it is likely that this bacterium will henceforth be called *Gardnerella vaginalis*, instead of *Haemophilus vaginalis* or *Corynebacterium vaginale*, the authors have chosen to refer to the disease under consideration in this chapter as *Gardnerella vaginalis* vaginitis. Such confusion in taxonomy is by no means unique in the infectious disease literature, a well-known example being the past usage of various synonyms for *Candida albicans*. Nevertheless, the taxonomic problem undoubtedly has been one of the factors contributing to widespread uncertainty among clinicians as to the true significance of the disease.

PATHOGENESIS

Concept of Gardnerella vaginalis as a surface parasite

Gardnerella vaginalis is a small, pleomorphic, gram-variable but predominantly gram-negative, non-motile rod. Like *Neisseria gonorrhoeae*, it is capnophilic and somewhat difficult to cultivate. Gardner & Dukes (1955) described it as a non-invasive pathogen, apparently producing leukorrhoea as a result of its action on desquamated epithelial cells

and vaginal secretions. They concluded that the organism parasitises detached vaginal epithelial cells, a concept supported by studies of Tarlinton & D'Abrera (1967) on the glycogen content of affected cells.

In studies conducted by Gardner & Kaufman (1981), no histopathological changes were identified in vaginal biopsies taken from infected patients, and various staining techniques failed to demonstrate the organism within the tissues. Since the vaginal tissues are not invaded, there is no significant inflammatory response in the host. Thus, *G. vaginalis* may be described as essentially a surface parasite.

Fulfilment of Koch's postulates

In their original description, Gardner & Dukes (1955) presented the results of their studies in fulfilment of Koch's postulates, including the association of the bacterium with the characteristic leukorrhoea, its isolation and growth in pure culture from affected women, and the results of human inoculation experiments. In their early experiments with human volunteers, vaginal insertion of impure material from the vaginas of infected patients produced the disease in 11 of 15 women, but when organisms in pure culture were inoculated, only 1 of 13 women developed the disease. However, in subsequent experiments by Criswell et al (1969), using a 12-hour inoculum instead of a 24-hour inoculum, vaginal instillation of organisms in pure culture produced the disease in 5 of 9 subjects. From these human inoculation experiments the incubation period was set at about 7 days.

As reviewed by Gardner (1980), numerous workers have confirmed the association of *G. vaginalis* with the characteristic leukorrhoea, and have noted disappearance of the discharge upon eradication of the organisms. A small minority have been unable to correlate vaginal colonisation with leukorrhoea. It is probable that the frequent association with other lower genital tract infections has confused some investigators, and that the absence of a true inflammatory response has misled others. Assuming accuracy of bacteriological identification techniques employed, we believe that the high rates of clinically inapparent vaginal colonisation reported by a few investigators can be explained by their lack of appreciation of the abnormal findings, particularly the clue cells of Gardner found in the wet mount preparation.

Superinfection by endogenous bacteria

Chen et al (1979) showed that the vaginal odour associated with the disease (best appreciated when 10% KOH is added to the discharge) is related to an increased amine concentration produced by mixed bacterial organisms. In a companionate study, Spiegel et al (1980) presented evidence of increased growth of anaerobes in women with clinically manifest *G. vaginalis* vaginitis.

It is noteworthy that, similarly, vaginal trichomoniasis is associated with increased numbers of aerobic (Gardner & Kaufman 1981) and anaerobic (Levison et al 1979) organisms in patients with clinically overt disease, but not in women with subclinical infection, at least with respect to aerobic organisms (Gardner & Kaufman 1981). Symptomatic trichomoniasis is also associated with a strong and offensive odour.

We interpret these findings to mean that superinfection by endogenous vaginal organisms, especially anaerobes, may be involved in the clinical manifestations of both *G. vaginalis* vaginitis and trichomoniasis. This concept, while acknowledging a secondary role for endogenous organisms, nevertheless recognises the primary or aetiological role of *G. vaginalis* and *Trichomonas vaginalis* in producing the leukorrhoea with which each agent is associated.

MODE OF ACQUISITION

Significance of reinfection after successful treatment

Gardnerella vaginalis infection, like *Trichomonas vaginalis* infection, is acquired mainly through sexual intercourse. The high rate of reinfection in patients whose sexual partners remain untreated must be regarded as prima facie evidence of venereal transmission. In the study by Pheifer et al (1978) *G. vaginalis* was reisolated from 6 of 11 women with either new or untreated sexual partners following initial eradication of the organisms in these women by antibiotic therapy. We have observed numerous such cases in clinical practice.

Epidemiological features of Gardnerella vaginalis infection

Available epidemiological and demographic data from the literature indicate that women with the infection exhibit certain characteristics similar to those found in venereal disease patients. Of particular significance is the observed association with various other sexually transmitted diseases. Thus, a number of studies have documented the association with trichomoniasis. Josey & Lambe (1976) reported that a variety of sexually transmitted diseases were diagnosed either concurrently or at some other time in 52% of 184 private gynaecological patients infected with *G. vaginalis*. They also noted an increased frequency of cervical neoplastic lesions (dysplasia, carcinoma in situ, and invasive carcinoma) in women with *G. vaginalis* vaginitis, a finding considered to be epidemiologically significant in view of the known association of cervical neoplasia with sexually transmitted diseases.

G. vaginalis vaginitis appears to be more prevalent in venereal disease clinic patients than in the general population. For instance, in a study conducted in the UK by Bhattacharyya & Jones (1980), 24% of 3241 venereal disease clinic patients had positive cultures for *G. vaginalis*, whereas only 5.8% of 1022 women attending gynaecological clinics had positive cultures.

G. vaginalis infection has only rarely been demonstrated in virginal women and premenarchal girls (Dunkelberg 1977; Gardner & Kaufman 1981). Although McCormack et al (1981) reported the recovery of *G. vaginalis* from 16 of 56 college women reputed to be sexually inexperienced (as determined by questionnaire), their study suffers from the lack of confirmation of a virginal state in these women by gynaecological examination. We have recovered *G. vaginalis* from a number of teenage girls as young as age 14, nearly all of whom have admitted participation in sexual intercourse. The occasional identification of *G. vaginalis* in premenarchal girls (Hammerschlag et al 1978) does not constitute evidence of commensal vaginal inhabitation, it being a well-known fact that *Neisseria gonorrhoeae*, *Trichomonas vaginalis* and other sexually transmitted agents are sometimes found in female children.

Sexual contact studies

Several studies have shown high rates of recovery of *G. vaginalis* from the sexual partners of infected women. Gardner & Dukes (1959) demonstrated urethral colonisation in 91 of 101 men whose wives were infected. Pheifer et al (1978) recovered the organisms from 79% of male consorts of infected women. These rates of recovery for *G. vaginalis* are comparable to those that have been reported for *T. vaginalis* in similar studies of male consorts of women with vaginal trichomoniasis. It is generally acknowledged that a high rate of concurrent infection in the sexual partners of individuals with a particular disease entity constitutes the most direct evidence of venereal communicability of that disease; for example, considerable significance was attached to the results of sexual contact studies in establishing the venereal mode of transmission of type 2 herpes simplex virus (Josey et al 1972).

Biological properties of Gardnerella vaginalis

Finally, it is notable that *G. vaginalis* shares certain common biological properties with members of the venereal family of microbial agents. These properties include the rather fastidious requirements of most sexually transmitted organisms for their growth and propagation, their relative instability when removed from their natural environment, and their special affinity for genitourinary sites in both sexes (Josey 1974). The possession of such properties by *G. vaginalis* is congruent with a venereal mode of transmission and argues against its being a component of the normal vaginal flora, as some authors have suggested.

RELATION TO 'NON-SPECIFIC VAGINITIS'

Prior to the recognition of *Gardnerella vaginalis* vaginitis as a specific disease entity it was thought that mixed bacterial infection accounted for many otherwise unexplained vaginal discharges, even though the putative aetiological agents could not be differentiated from bacterial organisms commonly inhabiting the vagina. Such cases were often classified as 'non-specific vaginitis', notwithstanding the fact that no clearly defined clinical pattern for such disease has ever been delineated.

The concept of 'non-specific vaginitis' was discredited by the discovery that *G. vaginalis* infection accounts for the vast majority of cases of infectious leukorrhoea not attributable to candidiasis or trichomoniasis. Recently, however, some authors have resurrected the term, employing it as a synonym for *G. vaginalis* vaginitis (Spiegel et al 1980; Vontver & Eschenbach 1981). The rationale of these authors for their use of this term is their belief that *G. vaginalis* is a component of the normal vaginal microflora, and that the syndrome with which it is associated is inherently polymicrobial in its causation. They suggest that 'non-specific vaginitis' is a synergistic infection, with anaerobic bacteria playing the most important role.

As discussed by Brown et al (1984), the latter hypothesis disregards some of the established facts and misconstrues other data pertaining to the pathogenesis and epidemiology of *G. vaginalis* vaginitis. Anaerobic organisms do not cause infection in the intact, mature vagina. Rather, the overgrowth of anaerobes results from the favourable environment brought about by the primary pathogen, in this case *G. vaginalis*. Hence, employment of the term 'non-specific vaginitis' is inappropriate and confusing. We likewise decry the advocacy by various authors of other similar designations for the disease such as 'anaerobic vaginosis' and 'bacterial vaginosis'.

PREVALENCE

Gardnerella vaginalis vaginitis is one of the most frequently encountered infections in gynaecological practice. An estimated 10–20% of adult women in the general population of the United States harbour the organism. For instance, Lewis et al (1972) obtained positive cultures in 18.75% of 1008 women attending a county health department clinic in North Carolina.

The organism is recovered with less frequency in postmenopausal women than in women of reproductive age, and only rarely in premenarchal girls. In the study by Josey & Lambe (1976), the age range of 184 gynaecological patients with positive cultures was 14–57 years (average age 28 years). Rodgers et al (1978) reported an age range of 18–52 years (mean 25 years) in a study of 150 infected women attending a California venereal disease clinic.

As would be expected, the prevalence of *G. vaginalis* infection varies in different population groups, being higher in groups with increased rates of sexual promiscuity. Dunkelberg et al (1970a) obtained positive cultures in 31% of 200 women attending a venereal disease clinic in Atlanta, Georgia. As noted previously, Bhattacharyya & Jones (1980) obtained positive cultures in 24% of 3241 venereal disease clinic patients in the UK, but in only 5.8% of 1022 women attending regular gynaecological clinics.

Current data indicate that *G. vaginalis* infection accounts wholly or in part for one-third to one-half of all cases of vaginitis observed in urban gynaecological practice in the United States. In 20 000 consecutive cases of leukorrhoea managed by Fleury (1981), *G. vaginalis* vaginitis was diagnosed in 33%, candidiasis in 20.5% and trichomoniasis in 9.5%. Gardner & Kaufman (1981) diagnosed *G. vaginalis* infection, either alone or concurrently with candidiasis or trichomoniasis, in 45.2% of patients with vaginitis.

In a series of 100 patients with leukorrhoea studied by Josey et al (1976), 35 had *G. vaginalis* vaginitis, 53 had candidiasis, and 15 had trichomoniasis. *G. vaginalis* was identified alone in 22 patients, in association with *Candida* in 6, in association with *Trichomonas vaginalis* in 5, and with both *Candida* and *T. vaginalis* in 2.

SYMPTOMS

Vaginal discharge and odour are the only two complaints commonly voiced by the patient. Some women with the infection are unaware of the problem. Others notice the discharge but do not consider it to be medically significant. Many women, however, find the condition to be very unpleasant, with constant staining of the underclothing. Undoubtedly, the prevalence of the disease is one of the reasons why so many women feel compelled to use a vaginal douche regularly.

In the study by Josey et al (1976), approximately 20% of 164 patients with positive cultures volunteered the complaint of a vaginal odour. Others acknowledged the presence of an odour when questioned about this symptom. A vague irritation was experienced by some patients, but itching was unusual in the absence of associated candidiasis.

SIGNS

The discharge is usually described as grey or white, thin, and homogeneous. In about 15% of cases the discharge contains gas bubbles, as also seen in some cases of trichomoniasis. The gas is probably produced as a product of the metabolism of superinfecting anaerobic bacteria.

As observed in vaginal trichomoniasis, there is a broad clinical spectrum of the disease. Josey et al (1976) evaluated the gross appearance of the discharge in a group of patients in whom no other infection was evident. They noted that the amount of the discharge varied considerably, from very slight to copious. The character of the discharge was also variable, most often having the appearance of a thin paste. In the more severe cases it was milky and could be identified externally as it flowed on to the vulva.

The characteristic odour of the discharge is caused by amines released as byproducts of the metabolism of associated bacterial organisms (Chen et al 1979). It is described as 'fishy', and becomes very strong when 10% KOH is added to the discharge on a glass slide.

The pH of the discharge is usually 5.0 or above. However, the pH determination is of limited value in differential diagnosis, as it is also elevated in patients with trichomoniasis.

METHODS FOR RAPID DIAGNOSIS

Wet mount preparations

Although the experienced examiner will often strongly suspect *Gardnerella vaginalis* vaginitis on the basis of the appearance and odour of the vaginal discharge, *a positive diagnosis can be made only by demonstrating the presence of the organisms*. The identification of clue cells of Gardner in the wet mount

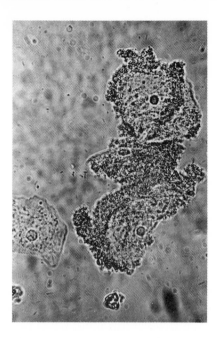

Fig. 15.1 Clue cells of Gardner in wet mount preparation (courtesy of Drs R H Kaufman and H L Gardner).

preparation may be regarded as a confirmatory finding by virtue of the fact that clue cells, by definition, are epithelial cells parasitised by *G. vaginalis*. As illustrated in Fig. 15.1, the affected squamous epithelial cells will be seen to be coated with the tiny bacilli, obscuring the normal outline of the cell wall and giving the cell a granular appearance. Pus cells are few in the absence of some other concurrent infection, and there is also a paucity of lactobacilli on the slide. Frequently, separate clumps of *G. vaginalis* may be seen floating in the surrounding fluid.

In their extensive screening studies for *G. vaginalis* infection, Bhattacharyya & Jones (1980) demonstrated that clue cells are almost always perceptible in wet smears obtained from women harbouring the organisms, even in the absence of a distinctly abnormal discharge. However, considerable experience is required to become proficient in recognising clue cells and differentiating between normal epithelial cells. We are of the opinion that a high degree of proficiency can only be acquired through practice in correlating wet smear findings with bacteriological cultures for *G. vaginalis* in a large number of both infected and uninfected women.

Stained smears

Dunkelberg (1977), as well as Bhattacharyya & Jones (1980), reported the Gram stained vaginal smear to be a highly reliable method of confirming the diagnosis. However, their results were not duplicated by others, such as Smith et al (1977). Gram stained smears are characterised by the presence of many small, Gram-negative bacilli, frequently forming solid fields outside the epithelial elements.

The Papanicolaou stained smear has also been utilised for diagnosis (Lewis & O'Brien 1969) but in our experience has not proved sufficiently reliable for clinical usage.

Although fluorescent antibody procedures for detection of *G. vaginalis* in direct smears have been described (Vice & Smaron 1973), the antisera have not been made readily available.

ISOLATION AND IDENTIFICATION OF GARDNERELLA VAGINALIS

Transport media

Vaginal swabs may be inoculated directly on to primary plating media or held in a transport medium until delivered to the laboratory. A variety of transport media have been used, including 1% proteose peptone no. 3 in distilled water, heart infusion broth (Difco) with 1% proteose peptone no. 3, thioglycolate broth, modified Stuart's medium, Amies transport medium, and the culturette (Marion Scientific) (Gardner & Dukes 1955; Dunkelberg et al 1970b; Akerlund & Mardh 1974; Smith 1975; Golberg & Washington 1976; Bailey et al 1979). Akerlund & Mardh (1974) reported that modified Stuart's medium and 1% proteose peptone no. 3 in distilled water gave the same results with specimens cultured within 4 hours. Bailey et al (1979) reported that heart infusion broth with 1% proteose peptone no. 3 held for 6 hours gave the same results as direct plating. No parallel comparisons of other transport systems, nor definitive studies to determine the maximum time that specimens may be held, appear in the literature. Most authors report plating of transport specimens within 4–6 hours; many authors do not indicate the time the specimen was held in transport before plating. One must assume, therefore, that any of the above transport media or systems may be used, and that delay in transport should not exceed 6 hours.

Cultivation

Basically, three differential characteristics have been utilised to detect *Gardnerella vaginalis* on primary plating media: colonial morphology on peptone-starch-dextrose (PSD) agar; fermentation or hydrolysis of starch, and haemolysis of human blood.

The method described by Dunkelberg et al (1970), using a PSD agar as a primary isolation and differential medium, has been commonly employed. After 48 hours of incubation in a candle jar or CO_2 incubator, colonies appear dull white, 0.5–2.0 mm in diameter, with an entire border, convex and domed. Under a dissecting microscope (40×) with transmitted light, the colonies appear as characteristic 'button colonies' with a dense centre.

A modified form of PSD agar (starch agar) using 1% corn starch and 1.5% agar in purple broth base was described by Smith (1975). This medium offers the differential characteristic of the fermentation of starch resulting in an acid reaction of the indicator surrounding colonies of *G. vaginalis*.

Michelsen et al (1977) described the use of an opaque (1% corn starch) GC agar base (Baltimore Biological Laboratory) upon which *G. vaginalis* is detected by a clear halo surrounding the colonies resulting from starch hydrolysis. These authors added colistin and nalidixic acid to provide a degree of selectivity.

Vaginalis (V) agar was described by Greenwood et al (1977). Human blood (5%) is included in a Columbia agar-proteose peptone no. 3 base. Colonies of *G. vaginalis* show a unique, diffuse zone of beta haemolysis as a differentiating feature. Smith (1979) reported starch agar and V agar to give comparable results for isolation of *G. vaginalis* from clinical specimens.

The use of a human blood bilayer agar medium with Tween 80 (HBT agar) was recently described by Totten et al (1982). The authors suggest that the differential characteristic of colonial morphology and haemolysis is so specific that the experienced microbiologist may need only to use the Gram stain for presumptive identification.

Other media that have been used include choco-late agar, sheep blood–beef infusion agar, and Columbia-colistin-nalidixic acid (CNA) agar; none of these media, however, provide the very useful, presumptive differential characteristics of the starch and human blood agars.

All primary plating media should be incubated in a 2–10% CO_2 environment, which can be accomplished with a candle extinction jar or CO_2 incubator. Although obligately anaerobic strains of *G. vaginalis* have been reported (Malone et al 1975), there is little evidence that an anaerobic environment should be used routinely (Bailey et al 1979).

Identification

Presumptive identification of *G. vaginalis* can readily be made from Gram stains of the suspect 'button' colonies on PSD agar (Dunkelberg et al 1970b), or of colonies that ferment or hydrolyse starch on the starch agars (Smith 1975; Michelson et al 1977), or from Gram stains of the characteristic colonies producing a diffuse zone of beta haemolysis on V (Lewis & O'Brien 1969) or HBT agars (Totten et al 1982). On primary plates, the organisms usually appear as small, pleomorphic, gram-variable but predominantly gram-negative rods, some of which are beaded. With experience, presumptive identification can be made with a high degree of confidence on the basis of the colony morphology and Gram stain.

Several schemes for the further identification of suspect colonies have been proposed. The scheme of Dunkelberg et al (1970b) has commonly been used in clinical laboratories. Organisms fitting the above colonial and cellular morphology that are oxidase- and catalase-negative, and that ferment dextrose, maltose, and starch (but not mannitol), can be identified as *G. vaginalis*. Greenwood & Pickett (1979) recommend that colonies showing diffuse beta haemolysis on V agar, with characteristic cellular morphology and no haemolysis on sheep blood agar, and which are catalase- and oxidase-negative and hydrolyse hippurate, are adequately differentiated as *G. vaginalis*. Piot et al (1982) recommend that characteristic colonies showing diffuse beta haemolysis on HBT agar can be identified by Gram stain in 90–97% of the cases. Additional tests for alpha and beta glucosidase, hippurate and starch hydrolysis provided a discriminative value of up to 99%.

TREATMENT

Treatment of *Gardnerella vaginalis* vaginitis should be directed toward eradication of the organisms from the vagina and prevention of reinfection. Currently, we prefer one of the cephalosporin antibiotics, such as cephradine, given orally to both the patient and her husband or sexual partner in a dosage of 500 mg four times daily for 5 days. In our experience, as well as that of Brown et al (1984), cephradine has proved to be highly efficacious, contradicting suggestions in the literature that successful treatment must be directed toward the anaerobic organisms associated with the infection. As in trichomoniasis, treatment of male consorts is essential for successful therapy. It is prudent to advise the patient of the possible occurrence of *Candida* overgrowth in the vagina during broad-spectrum antibiotic treatment, and to consider providing her with a topical antifungal preparation to use in the event of resultant pruritus vulvae.

Metronidazole is also effective (Pheifer et al 1978; Fleury 1981; Brown et al 1984) but the optimum dosage has not been established at this writing. Our experience with metronidazole suggests that successful treatment requires 1–1.5 g daily for 7 days.

Ampicillin is an alternate antibiotic choice (Rodgers et al 1978) but is less effective than either cephradine or metronidazole. The suggested dosage of ampicillin is 500 mg four times daily for 7 days.

Other antibacterial drugs and topical medications are largely ineffective. Douching may relieve the malodorous discharge temporarily but does not cure the infection.

REFERENCES

Akerlund M, Mardh P A 1974 Isolation and identification of Corynebacterium vaginale (Haemophilus vaginalis) in women with infections of the lower genital tract. Acta Obstetrica et Gynecologica Scandinavica 53: 85–90

Bailey R K, Voss J L, Smith R F 1979 Factors affecting isolation and identification of Haemophilus vaginalis (Corynebacterium vaginale). Journal of Clinical Microbiology 9: 65–71

Bhattacharyya M B, Jones B M 1980 Haemophilus vaginalis infection. Diagnosis and treatment. Journal of Reproductive Medicine 24: 71–75

Brown D B Jr, Kaufman R H, Gardner H L 1984 Gardnerella vaginalis vaginitis: the current opinion. Journal of Reproductive Medicine 29: 300–306

Chen K C S, Forsyth P S, Buchanan T M, Holmes K K 1979 Amine content of vaginal fluid from untreated and treated patients with nonspecific vaginitis. Journal of Clinical Investigation 63: 828–835

Criswell B S, Ladwig C L, Gardner H L, Dukes C D 1969 Haemophilus vaginalis vaginitis by inoculation from culture. Obstetrics and Gynecology 33: 195–199

Criswell B S, Marston J H, Stenback W A, Black S H, Gardner H L 1971 Haemophilus vaginalis 594, a gram-negative organism? Canadian Journal of Microbiology 17: 865–869

Dunkelberg W E 1977 Corynebacterium vaginale. Sexually Transmitted Diseases 4: 69–75

Dunkelberg W E Jr, Skaggs R, Kellogg D S Jr, Domescik G K 1970a Relative incidence of Corynebacterium vaginale (Haemophilus vaginalis), Neisseria gonorrhoeae, and Trichomonas spp. among women attending a venereal disease clinic. British Journal of Venereal Diseases 46: 187–190

Dunkelberg W E Jr, Skaggs R, Kellogg D S Jr 1970b Method for isolation and identification of Corynebacterium vaginale (Haemophilus vaginalis). Applied Microbiology 19: 47–52

Fleury F J 1981 Adult vaginitis. Clinical Obstetrics and Gynecology 24: 407–438

Gardner H L 1980 Haemophilus vaginalis vaginitis after 25 years. American Journal of Obstetrics and Gynecology 137: 385–391

Gardner H L, Dukes C D 1954 New etiologic agent in nonspecific bacterial vaginitis. Science 120: 853

Gardner H L, Dukes C D 1955 Haemophilus vaginalis vaginitis. A newly defined specific infection previously classified 'nonspecific vaginitis'. American Journal of Obstetrics and Gynecology 69: 962–976

Gardner H L, Dukes C D 1959 Haemophilus vaginalis vaginitis. Annals of the New York Academy of Sciences 83: 280–289

Gardner H L, Kaufman R H 1981 Benign diseases of the vulva and vagina, 2nd edn. GK Hall Medical Publishers, Boston

Golberg R L, Washington J A 1976 Comparison of isolation of Haemophilus vaginalis (Corynebacterium vaginale) from peptone-starch-dextrose agar and Columbia colistin-nalidixic acid agar. Journal of Clinical Microbiology 4: 245–247

Greenwood J R, Pickett M J 1979 Salient features of Haemophilus vaginalis. Journal of Clinical Microbiology 9: 200–204

Greenwood J R, Pickett M J 1980 Transfer of Haemophilus vaginalis Gardner and Dukes to a new genus, Gardnerella: G vaginalis (Gardner and Dukes) comb. nov. International Journal of Systemic Bacteriology 30: 170–178

Greenwood J R, Pickett M J, Martin W J, Mack E G 1977 Haemophilus vaginalis (Corynebacterium vaginale): methods for isolation and rapid biochemical identification. Health Laboratory Science 14: 102–106

Hammerschlag M R, Alpert S, Rosner I et al 1978 Microbiology of the vagina in children: normal and potentially pathogenic organism. Pediatrics 62: 57–62

Josey W E 1974 The sexually transmitted infections. Obstetrics and Gynecology 43: 465–470

Josey W E, Lambe D W Jr 1976 Epidemiologic characteristics of women infected with Corynebacterium vaginale (Haemophilus vaginalis). Journal of the American Venereal Disease Association 3: 9–13

Josey W E, Nahmias A J, Naib Z M 1972 The epidemiology of

type 2 (genital) herpes simplex virus infection. Obstetrical and Gynecological Survey 27: 295–302

Josey W E, McKenzie W J, Lambe D W Jr 1976 Corynebacterium vaginale (Haemophilus vaginalis) in women with leukorrhea. American Journal of Obstetrics and Gynecology 126: 574–578

Levison M E, Trestman I, Quach R, Sladowski C, Floro C N 1979 Quantitative bacteriology of the vaginal flora in vaginitis. American Journal of Obstetrics and Gynecology 133: 139–144

Lewis J F, O'Brien S O 1969 Diagnosis of Haemophilus vaginalis by Papanicolaou smears. American Journal of Clinical Pathology 51: 412–415

Lewis J F, O'Brien S M, Ural U M, Burke T 1972 Corynebacterium vaginale vaginitis. American Journal of Obstetrics and Gynecology 112: 87–90

McCormack W M, Evrard J R, Laughlin C F et al 1981 Sexually transmitted conditions among women college students. American Journal of Obstetrics and Gynecology 139: 130–133

Malone B H, Schreiber M, Schneider N J, Holdeman L V 1975 Obligately anaerobic strains of Corynebacterium vaginale (Haemophilus vaginalis). Journal of Clinical Microbiology 2: 272–275

Michelson P A, McCarthy L R, Mangum M E 1977 New differential medium for the isolation of Corynebacterium vaginale. Journal of Clinical Microbiology 5: 488–489

Pheifer T A, Forsyth P S, Durfee M A, Pollock H M, Holmes K K 1978 Nonspecific vaginitis: role of Haemophilus vaginalis and treatment with metronidazole. New England Journal of Medicine 298: 1429–1434

Piot P, Van Dyck E, Totten P A, Holmes K K 1982 Identification of Gardnerella (Haemophilus) vaginalis. Journal of Clinical Microbiology 15: 19–24

Rodgers H A, Hesse F E, Pulley H C, Hines P A, Smith R F 1978 Haemophilus vaginalis (Corynebacterium vaginale) vaginitis in women attending public health clinics: response to treatment with ampicillin. Sexually Transmitted Diseases 5: 18–21

Smith R F 1975 New medium for isolation of Corynebacterium vaginale from genital specimens. Health Laboratory Science 12: 219–224

Smith R F 1979 Comparison of two media for isolation of Haemophilus vaginalis. Journal of Clinical Microbiology 9: 729–730

Smith R F, Rodgers H A, Hines P A, Ray R M 1977 Comparisons between direct microscopic and cultural methods for recognition of Corynebacterium vaginale in women with vaginitis. Journal of Clinical Microbiology 5: 268–272

Spiegel C A, Amsel R, Eschenbach D A, Schoennecht F, Holmes K K 1980 Anaerobic bacteria in nonspecific vaginitis. New England Journal of Medicine 303: 601–607

Tarlinton M N, D'Abrera V S E 1967 Identity of a disputed, Haemophilus-like organism in non-specific vaginitis. Journal of Pathology and Bacteriology 93: 109–118

Totten P A, Amsel R, Hale J, Piot P, Holmes K K 1982 Selective human blood bilayer media for isolation of Gardnerella (Haemophilus) vaginalis. Journal of Clinical Microbiology 15: 141–147

Vice J L, Smaron M F 1973 Indirect fluorescent antibody method for the identification of Corynebacterium vaginale. Applied Microbiology 25: 908–916

Vontver L A, Eschenbach D A 1981 The role of Gardnerella vaginalis in nonspecific vaginitis. Clinical Obstetrics and Gynecology 24: 439–460

Zinnemann K, Turner G C 1963 The taxonomic position of Haemophilus vaginalis (Corynebacterium vaginale). Journal of Pathology and Bacteriology 85: 213–219

PART IV

Special circumstances and conditions

Vulvovaginal infection in young and old
C P Douglas

Oestrogen lack is about the only factor, apart from being female, which is common to genital tracts of the young and the old. The vagina is the main element in the difference from the point of view of infection. As far as the vulva goes, the skin is little affected by the hormones but the underlying tissues are. In the child the deeper tissues are not developed and so the labia do not give the protective effect of the labia of reproductive ages. In the old lady shrinkage of the introitus may protect a little but loss of fatty tissue and the relative lack of involution in the vestibule and urethra permit infection in a manner similar to that in the child. The two states therefore require quite separate considerations except in regard to the urethra.

PREMENARCHAL CHILD

Early days and weeks

A mucus discharge, sometimes blood stained, may be seen coming from the apparently oedematous introitus. This is essentially an increased cervical mucus discharge and vaginal transudate which results from the transfer of maternal oestrogen to the fetus. Of no clinical significance as a rule, it may be a means of protection to the genital tract in passage through the mother's vagina, especially if the presentation is breech. Both chlamydia and gonococci can affect the conjunctiva and produce pathological changes—also perhaps producing pneumonia. Nonetheless, there is no evidence that there is genital tract damage by these organisms. Indeed chlamydia has been isolated from the vagina in children whose mothers have been found puerperally to have chlamydia in the genital tract (Lumicae & Heggie 1979) but no infant effect has been seen. Thus no significance need be attached to the neonatal discharge.

'Nappy rash'—an irritation and redness vulvally and over the buttocks which is usually infected from the bowel content—results from ammonia under the napkin which is hot and wet, allowing maceration and infection, a process accelerated by the transparent covering of disposable units, although not unknown with the use of towelling napkins. The napkins (diapers) should be changed frequently, the skin washed after every bowel motion, and the skin allowed to dry fully in warm air before recovering. If purulent, erythromycin cream can be applied but in general good hygiene is enough to cure the condition. If the skin is very sensitive dimethicone 10% cream should be massaged into the whole area five times a day for a week then once or twice daily to waterproof the skin.

Later changes

Until the oestrogen surge, which comes a year or so before the menarche, the vaginal mucosa is thin and has no glycogen, has no lactobacilli and so no acidity, and the pH is about 7.2. The labia are small and not protruding since the deep fat has not been deposited and the 'protective wall' has not yet developed. In theory therefore the vagina should be very susceptible to infection but in practice this is not so: the lack of oestrogen means that the vestibule and clitoral area are the prominent features and the vaginal orifice is barely seen or felt and so is not really prone to infection.

It may be said therefore that there are two modes of infection in the child (Altchek 1981):

Vulvitis leading to secondary vaginitis. Easily the most common form of infection; when there is a primary vulvitis there is always a slight spill over into the lower end of the vagina. Infection taking this route is generally that associated with poor hygiene, and education of the mother about giving the child regular bathing, especially after bowel movements and, more particularly, meticulous drying thereafter will usually clear the conditon. Loose fitting cotton pants will help to reduce the incidence, if they are clean every day.

Vaginitis leading to secondary vulvitis. Much less common and may be difficult to investigate. It should be remembered that odd congenital anomalies, such as ectopic ureter, may be the cause of a 'discharge', but this is most uncommon before puberty; for some reason the ureter seldom leaks until the development of the genital tract is complete and so it is more of a problem in early menstrual years.

The presentation of vulvovaginal discharge is very variable, generally being noticed by the child's mother who notes the child's irritability, scratching, staining of the underclothes, etc. The child may complain of burning on micturition or just soreness.

There are many factors involved in this vaginal mode of presentation and these can be listed under the following headings:

General infection
   Non-specific
   Specific (napkin (diaper) rash)
Foreign bodies
Trauma
Skin diseases
Allergies
Sexually transmitted diseases

Non-specific infection. Usually from bowel organisms, this is the most common but really has to be diagnosed by exclusion since there are many reasons for coliform organisms being found in the vagina. They are more often a symptom than a cause, however. Simple vaginal swabs may give a result which is confusing rather than helpful in this context—a considerable literature has grown up about an organism now called *Gardnerella vaginalis* but previously called *Haemophilus vaginalis*—but this appears to be an endemic organism in certain areas rather than a general organism. In the absence of foreign bodies it does seem, however, to be

a significant organism causing considerable tenderness and it is probably best treated by the local instillation of lactic acid 5% by an eye dropper, followed by the use of a sulphonamide-containing cream, such as Sultrin. This can be applied by the mother through a small nozzle gently so as not to damage the hymeneal ring.

Probably the most common source of nonspecific infection is the presence of a *'foreign body'* in the vagina. Small children have enquiring minds and often use objects like pencils to investigate themselves. The pencil is usually used with the pointed end first and the lead point breaks off in the vagina. Coins or other precious baubles, such as marbles or beads, may be popped into place to hide them; indeed, in certain tribes in northern Nigeria the vagina is actually used as a purse by maidens. More commonly, however, softer accidental foreign bodies cause discharge, frequently material from toilet paper used a little too enthusiastically in cleaning; fragments from the edge of the paper gradually accumulate and become irritant foreign bodies. Although rectal examination can detect the more solid bodies and perhaps milk the paper masses towards the introitus so that they present, a small paediatric speculum (or simple nasal speculum) should be used to look carefully at the vagina for impalpable objects and then the foreign body can be removed with a pair of nasal forceps.

In summer time children playing naked on the sands may well get sand in the vulva, and this can be very irritating and sometimes infected. It is then necessary to wash out the vagina with a small syringe using saline or lactic acid.

Specific infections. The three most important but not necessarily the most common are gonorrhoea chlamydia and *Enterobius vermicularis*. The worm is common and its eggs can be transmitted across the perineum and get into the lower end of the vagina. They carry coliform organisms with them—hence confusing vaginal swabs being found. The worms and ova can be seen on vaginal smears or by the 'Sellotape method' on the perineum.

Gonorrhoea is the most important organism, often suspected and not commonly found, but very important when it is. Below the age of 12 it is rare and its presence is almost always the result of sexual contact of some sort. If found or seriously suspected it is best to admit the child to hospital for the four purposes of getting a better history, a better diagnosis, checking of contacts, and the certainty of proper treatment (Farrell et al 1982). The contacts are usually family members (mother or female sibling) with the disease, or teenage or adult males—the most common group. Sex play (with peers) is a transmitter and assault by the family males or 'friendly' visitors complete the sources.

All that has been said about gonorrhoea is equally relevant to chlamydia infection, which is probably much more common (Bump 1985).

Candidiasis is uncommon in young children, perhaps because the glycogen content of the vaginal skin is the favourite medium of the yeast and this has not, as yet, developed. So uncommon is it that a search for a medical reason must be made. The two situations in which it is usually found are in children who have been given antibiotics for a fairly long time, and children who are diabetic—it may indeed be the first indication of that condition. The treatment is to instil drops of nystatin suspension into the vagina and use an antifungal cream on the perineum. In the younger child, more effective is a 0.5% or 1% gentian violet solution applied with an eye dropper to the vagina. This is quite practicable if the child is still using disposable napkins but in the older child the colour is less acceptable because of stained clothing and so the nystatin, although less effective, is preferred.

Trichomonas is a most uncommon infection—coital transmission is the rule and so it affects only older children, but occasionally it may be personal contact, not necessarily of a sexual nature. Nonetheless, the rest of the family should be treated, and recurrence is likely. Age related metronidazole dosage is curative if reinfection does not occur.

Amoebiasis is a common vulvar and vaginal infection in children in areas where the condition is endemic and it requires full treatment for the condition, currently metronidazole (Gardner & Kaufman 1981).

In the past diphtheria could affect the vagina but it is not seen now. Other such organisms include *Shigella*, chickenpox, smallpox, and occasional upper respiratory tract infections.

Confusion may arise with the finding of organisms in the genital tract which are of no significance and which only reflect some irritation, possibly from allergic or chemical agents which cause vulvitis. Such must be looked for and superfatted soap and drying with no other additions, such as bubble baths which for children are particularly inappropriate, and other toiletries are excluded.

Viruses. Two viruses which affect the vulva of infants are that of condylomata acuminata and of herpes simplex. Condylomata do present occasionally on the labia minora or even on the vestibule. Owing to the fact that one cannot sensibly restrict movement in a child, cryocautery is the most appropriate form of treatment for condylomata and treatment with podophyllin should be avoided because the immature skin ulcerates easily. Herpes simplex rarely occurs in infants. Occasional reports are present of acute type 2 herpes which seem to be usually related to sexual assault (Hare & Mowla 1977). Avoidance of superimposed infection is most important in these conditions; possibly the use of Betadine solution, which is the most easily applied and effective way of preventing that, and in addition povidone iodine may have some antiviral effect.

There is no doubt that herpes simplex type 2 can be found in the vagina of the neonate if the mother is an excretor. The significance of this is not certain and its incidence unclear but there is no doubt that an infection with the virus in general carries high mortality to the fetus and infected mothers are best delivered by Caesarean section when the membranes are unruptured. Herpes type 1 can also occur on the vulva and may be very painful. Fortunately, a preparation of acyclovir is now available for parenteral therapy of the neonate, which is more effective in preventing the long-term effects of the virus than it is in the adult.

It must not be forgotten that if sexual transmission (associated with males) of gonorrhoea is probable, then other sexually transmitted diseases must be looked for, particularly syphilis, rare through that event is.

Another infective manifestation on the vulva is an 'undiagnosable' ulcer. A round ulcer with a granular base from which no organism can be cultured and in which histopathology simply shows granulation tissue, may occur at any age: the eponym Lipschutz ulcer is often used because the original description in 1913 was of such an ulcer occurring in children and young women (Lipschutz 1927). It still occurs, and generally disappears spontaneously after a very variable length of time. Meticulous hygiene is the best treatment as there is no evidence that antibiotic therapy makes any difference and it only encourages an overgrowth of candidiasis.

Another mysterious affliction which appears to have an infective origin, but from which no organism can be found, is a form of acute vulvitis (Huffman 1981). This is sudden in onset and self-limiting in a few days but has its counterpart in adults in whom a similar angry painful red vulvitis occurs which is clinically indistinguishable from candidiasis of the vulva, but from which no organism can be isolated. Again, hygiene and perhaps sedation help but the use of a corticosteroid cream of 0.5% hydrocortisone may ease the discomfort; a stronger cream may ulcerate.

Another lesion about which there is argument as to whether it is infective in origin or not is labial adhesion. No respecter of social class, it seems unlikely that infection plays a significant part in its development but such adhesions are more common in overweight babies than thin ones. Presumably activity in the legs of the plump baby rubs the tender epithelium of the labiae against each other, abrading them and allowing slender adhesions to form. The condition is most common between 4 months and 2 years of life. Ignorance of aetiology has led to many therapies. The use of oestrogen cream, progesterone cream, or even simple ointment massaged to the area has been recommended. It is unlikely that endocrine creams benefit from the hormone content since vulvar skin is little affected by hormones and almost certainly it is the firm massage which gradually separates the area of adhesion. There is much literature condemning simple separation in one attempt, but there is no evidence to substantiate this condemnation. Pressure outward with the thumbs placed firmly on the labia will separate the adhesions in most cases, and a little Vaseline, cold cream or lanolin gently smoothed into the skin for 2 or 3 days prevents recurrence of the adhesions. If the separation does not prove possible in that manner a sound passed into the introitus and held firm so that pressure over it can be maintained for a few minutes will almost always succeed: the immediate treatment is much more reassuring to the mother and less traumatic to the child in the long run.

A condition known as prolapse of the urethral mucosa is quite often seen in 4- to 6-year-old children. The oestrogen mediated growth of the deep tissue has not yet occurred and the urethra is still prominent, so that poor hygiene, together with trauma from such garments as tight underclothes which are not as clean they could be, results in the emergence of a red, friable, tumour from the urethra easily made to bleed. Diagnosis is easily made by passing a catheter which is clearly surrounded by the whole tissue and this is pathognomonic. Two forms of treatment are usual. The best, unfortunately requiring an anaesthetic, is to pass two sutures through the urethra above the lesion in a 90° different direction. The tumour is then excised and the point of crossing of the sutures pulled out of the meatus, cut, and used to make four sutures: this method prevents retraction of the urethral mucosa, and allows quick healing; no catheter is necessary, and the child can go straight home. The other method, without anaesthesia, is to insert a catheter and tie a tight suture around it above the lesion. The catheter will fall out after 3 days or so. With this method there is a high risk of urinary tract infection with all its damaging sequelae developing and it seems therefore the less appropriate treatment.

POSTMENOPAUSAL INFECTION

Diseases of the vulva in this group of women very frequently have multiple causes, ranging from specific infection to psychological disorders, complicated by the fact that the vulvar skin is one of the body's two most popular sites for bacterial populations. Coliform and faecal organisms predominate and their pathogenicity can depend very much on the well-being of the host; if she suffers from chronic illness or is neglected in old age they may gain easy access to the tissues and produce active infection.

There is therefore a need for oestrogen support of the tissue for protection of the vagina as well as treatment. Pessaries and creams are many, and although at first the epithelium is very thin the absorption into the circulation is easy. It reduces as the skin thickens, and so the risk of hyperstimulation of endometrium is very slender. It must be remembered however that there is an intensely individual response to oestrogen therapy. In some, hormone needs to be applied nearly every month; in others it may only need a 'refresher' about once a year.

Perhaps the simplest of such infections is folliculitis. Easy to diagnose and to treat, all it requires is to shave the hair from the affected areas (usually labia majora and pubis) and then to use a bacitracin cream three times a day, or erythromycin orally if it proves resistant to the cream for chronic reactive vulvitis.

Ammoniacal dermatitis is a pest in the care of the very old. The superficial organisms which are usually involved are *Bacteroides* and *Staphylococcus aureus*. They act on urea and produce ammonia which, together with dampness and the falling together of slack ageing tissues, gives an irritating affection. Hygiene principally, a simple bactericidal cream, and the occasional use of a very mild steroidal cream will help.

Chronic reactive vulvitis is another disorder on the borderline of infection. A characteristic of overweight women with psychological anxieties, it really does not affect the genital tract as a rule, being much more obvious on the inner thigh. Nevertheless, the labia majora may be involved as there is a sebaceous element to the lesion (Friedrich 1976). Cure is difficult as the cause is obscure in most patients but letting the patient talk her troubles out and the careful and infrequent use of a mild hydrocortisone/antibiotic cream is helpful. Intertrigo must not be forgotten as a differential diagnosis, but this does not affect the vulva per se.

Candidiasis is less common than in reproductive age. Nevertheless it does occur and sometimes poses a problem of diagnosis since it may coexist with more sinister conditions. Diabetes is a common associated factor and must be looked for. Very often the vagina is also affected and the treatment must include vaginal therapy, but in this age group a cutaneous origin is not uncommon. The vulva is red and the only obvious 'white' element is a sort of ridged appearance, unlike the vagina which usually has discrete white plaques. Occasionally the ridging is patchy with clear red skin showing in the gaps and therefore a diagnosis of Paget's disease must be entertained, even though the presence of candidiasis is substantiated, and unless the condition clears up very quickly and completely with antifungal agents, biopsy should be made. There are plenty of new antifungal drugs from which to choose but in the elderly econazole nitrate lotion is the least irritant and is as effective as any. The new persistent creams and pessaries with a triglyceride and polygel base may be more effective, giving a reduced need for application.

Bacteriological diagnosis is absolutely essential because the symptoms can be the same with a wide range of organisms. For example, the incidence of curved rod organisms (e.g. mobiluncus) is in direct negative correlation with the incidence of candidiasis, and the treatment of course is quite different but the symptoms in the older lady are very similar.

Granulomatous lesions. While granulomatous lesions of the vulva are mainly found in the reproductive age, the sequelae, particularly of lymphogranuloma venereum (caused by *Chlamydia trachomatis*, serotypes L1–3) may be in evidence from the destructive changes which have occurred. Evidence of such destructive lesions on the vulva in postmenopausal women should alert the physician to the possibility of rectal stricture, which is frequently associated with vulvar destruction by this organism. In addition if surgery, either cosmetic or reparative, is required it is absolutely essential to give the patient a 3-week course of tetracycline prior to surgery or else the wound will not heal.

Granuloma inguinale (Donovanosis) is most unlikely to occur in the elderly but on occasion it may be seen as a raised ulcer with a granular pavement-like base and diagnosis can be made either by finding the causative organism in a smear from biopsy tissue stained with a silver stain, or by histological examination. The histological study of ulcers in such patients requires very careful assessment as there is often confusion between squamous cell carcinoma and the pseudoepitheliomatous hyperplasia of granuloma inguinale.

Very rarely a tuberculous ulcer will be found on the vulva, clinically similar to carcinoma but only a histological diagnosis can make the position clear.

Pus in the vagina is a rare finding in the postmenopausal woman and is virtually never associated with a true diagnosis of atrophic vaginitis, which is a misnomer as there is seldom pathological infection in such cases. Where pus is found it invariably stems from the uterus with implications of pyometra and adenocarcinoma, and as swabs almost always grow nothing, the presence of pus in the vagina makes mandatory the investigation of the uterine cavity. In fact, chronic endometritis is relatively common in old women and at postmortem small intrauterine abscesses are often found. This infection may go on to cause low grade salpingitis. Nonetheless, in the absence of carcinoma carefully proved by thorough curettage, to prevent a continuing modest purulent discharge giving vulvovaginitis, it may become necessary to give the patient a month's treatment of a relatively high dose of oestrogen, such as Premarin 0.625, together with a general antibiotic to reinforce the uterine blood supply and initially cause endometrial growth which successfully reduces infection in the ageing tissue.

Occasionally a membranous appearance of the lower vagina, sometimes with pus, is seen in undernourished women who may squat or sit on stones, threshing corn or breaking stones. The organism seen is a fusospirochaete and it is best to remove the membrane, if necessary under anaesthesia, and then give a course of a penicillin with attention to hygiene and nutrition.

REFERENCES

Altchek A 1981 Paediatric vulvovaginitis. Pediatric Clinics of North America 28: 397

Bump R C 1985 Chlamydia trachomatis as a cause of prepubertal vaginitis. American Journal of Obstetrics and Gynecology 65: 384–385

Farrell M K, Billmire E, Sharmoy J A, Hammond J 1982 Prepubertal gonorrhoea—a multidisciplinary approach. Pediatrics 67: 151

Friedrich E G Jr 1976 Vulvar disease. W B Saunders, Philadelphia, p 104

Gardner H L, Kaufman R H 1981 Miscellaneous vaginitides. In: Benign diseases of the vulva and vagina, 2nd edn. G H Hall, Boston, p 390

Hare M J, Mowla A 1977 Genital herpes virus infection in a prepubertal girl. British Journal of Obstetrics and Gynaecology 84: 147

Huffman J W 1981 Dermatologic disorders of perineum and vulva. In: Huffman J W, Dewhurst C J, Capraro V J (eds) The gynaecology of childhood and adolescence. W B Saunders, Philadelphia, p 115

Lumicae G G, Heggie A D 1979 Chlamydia infections. Pediatric Clinics of North America 26: 269

Tropical infections
I Mc L Brown, A S Latif and N F Lyons

INTRODUCTION

Geographical, climatic and other factors influence the increase in the number of micro-organisms causing lower genital tract infection in tropical areas. The relative lack of development of health services in many emerging countries and the associated lack of sophistication of the population are contributory causes. Many other factors may be involved, including a reduced awareness of the need for personal hygiene, and many traditional forms of treatment which involve the insertion of vegetable and other foreign material into the vagina.

Studies of the normal vaginal flora in developing countries are rare and conflicting. Mason et al (1983) in a survey of microbial flora of pregnant women found a similar range of organisms compared with those found in developed countries. They found however that faecal streptococci were isolated more frequently (59% of patients) from their patients than from women in Europe (Corbishley 1977) although other faecal organisms were not more common. Lactobacilli were isolated in only 41% of their patients, which is much lower than that reported from developed countries.

Variations in the prevalence of potentially pathogenic organisms may mean that infections common in the developed world may be found even more frequently in developing countries. An example of this is infection with *Trichomonas vaginalis*. Studies from Central Africa (McCallum 1973; Mason et al 1983) have suggested that *T. vaginalis* occurs in 31.47% of women and this rate is higher than that generally reported for Europe and the United States.

Those infections which occur commonly in developed countries are considered elsewhere in this book.

Only those infections which are primarily confined to tropical countries will be described in detail. The infections to be considered are:

1. Amoebiasis;
2. Chancroid;
3. Granuloma inguinale;
4. Lymphogranuloma venereum;
5. Schistosomiasis;
6. Tuberculosis.

AMOEBIASIS

Epidemiology

Amoebiasis occurs throughout the world but is most prevalent in tropical regions, particularly where sanitation and living conditions are poor. A recent survey in Nigeria (Oyerinde et al 1978) showed an overall prevalence rate of 11.2%, with infection being particularly common in patients from the lower end of the socioeconomic spectrum. The highest percentage of infection occurred in those using well water (23.4%).

Although amoebiasis usually produces symptoms of intestinal and hepatic involvement, infection can be found in the lower genital tract. This usually occurs as a result of spread from the anus (Cohen 1973), but direct venereal infection may also occur (Mylius & Ten Seldam 1962).

The presence of a rectovaginal fistula may facilitate infection (Cohen 1973) and if the continuity of the epithelium of the vagina or the cervix is broken, this leaves an ideal site for implantation of the parasite. Another factor which may facilitate the growth of the parasite is pH of the vagina, as growth is optimal in the pH range of 7.2–7.8. McClatchie & Sambhi (1971), who reported three cases of amoebiasis of the genital tract in postmenopausal women, suggest that the change in vaginal pH after the menopause may have been a factor.

Involvement of the genital tract appears to be very unusual and by 1973 Cohen was able to report less than 100 cases in the world literature. This is probably an underrepresentation, however, as it is likely that only the more severe cases are reported. This is supported by the fact that in a cytological survey of the cervix, Munguia et al (1966) found 24 cases of genital amoebiasis of 100 000 women during a 5-year period. Further evidence suggesting a higher incidence of genital tract amoebiasis comes from the work of Bhaduri (1957) in India where he found the presence of *Entamoeba histolytica* in 11.4% of women with a vaginal discharge and in 7.7% of excised fallopian tubes.

Although the lesions usually occur in adults, Wynne (1980) reports the case of a 14-month-old girl with invasive perineal amoebiasis where there was destruction of the anus, the rectovaginal septum, the pelvic floor and the perineum. The lesion appeared to be particularly rapidly invasive and he suggests that young children still in nappies may be particularly susceptible to the disease.

Clinical presentation

The most common presentation of amoebiasis of the lower genital tract is with serosanguineous or purulent discharge. There is often severe pain and tenderness and the patient may complain of dyspareunia. Although there may be a recent history of diarrhoea, this is not always the case.

The clinical appearance is of ulceration on the cervix or the vagina. The vulva may be involved, but this is very rare. The ulcers can vary in size from a few millimetres to several centimetres in diameter and occasionally the ulceration may be extensive. The ulcers usually have a grey sloughy base with irregular overhanging margins. They bleed easily and are surrounded by an area of induration. Extensive sloughing without ulceration has been described (van Coeverden de Groot 1963).

Diagnosis

The diagnosis may be confirmed by cytology, by histological examination of biopsy material, by

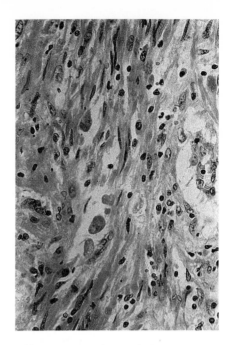

Fig. 17.1 Haematophagous *Entamoeba histolytica* trophozoites in smooth muscle.

direct microscopy of the discharge, or scrapings from the ulcer (Fig. 17.1).

Munguia et al (1966) have shown that the trophozoite forms of *E. histolytica* can be recognised on Papanicolaou smears from the cervix and asymptomatic cases may be picked up in this way. The most reliable method of diagnosis is to prepare wet smear preparations of material from the infected site when trophozoites with typical motile pseudopodia may be seen. Often the diagnosis will be confirmed histologically where a biopsy has been taken for an ulcerated lesion of the cervix or vagina. There is a chronic inflammatory response with tissue destruction, ulceration and autolysis. *E. histolytica* can usually be seen within the affected areas.

Treatment

Usually no specific local surgical treatment is required and patients can be managed on anti-amoebic therapy alone. Metronidazole has now largely replaced emetine hydrochloride as it is less toxic but equally effective.

CHANCROID

Chancroid is a sexually transmissible infection which is found more often in men than in women. Chancroid usually occurs in the lower socio-economic group in tropical and subtropical areas of the world. When the infection is encountered in temperate climates it has usually been imported by itinerants.

Epidemiology

In the United Kingdom the incidence of chancroid has been reported as being less than 0.1 per 100 000 each year from 1973 to 1980 (Chief Medical Officer 1979, 1980, 1981). In the western world, sporadic cases and minor outbreaks have been reported from time to time. In 1973 55 cases were diagnosed in Paris (Morel 1974) and a small outbreak was reported from Winnipeg, Canada (Hammond et al 1978a). In most developing countries the incidence of chancroid is much higher, although in Swaziland (Burney 1976) and Nigeria (Sogbetun et al 1977) chancroid is rarely seen. In India chancroid is reported to account for 10% of all sexually transmitted diseases (STD) (Nair et al 1973). In Zimbabwe chancroid was found to be the commonest form of STD at one clinic in Harare (Latif 1981). Of 695 men seen at this clinic, 38.4% had chancroid, while 15.4% of the 234 women seen had the infection. In 1981, 4391 women were seen at the four STD clinics in Harare; of these 12.7% had chancroid (City Health Department 1981). Over the same period of time, 43 529 men attended these clinics and 37.9% of these had chancroid. In Singapore, the incidence of chancroid was 25 per 100 000 each year over a period of 10 years (Rajan & Pang 1979). In Riyadh, Saudi Arabia, chancroid was found in 1.3% of men attending an STD clinic (Pareek & Chowdhury 1981).

Chancroid is diagnosed more often in men than in women (Rajan & Sng 1981). The reason for this bias is still unclear. The male to female ratio has been reported as being from 20:1 to 50:1.

Aetiology and pathology

Chancroid is caused by *Haemophilus ducreyi*. This is a gram-negative coccobacillus which may be found in the undermined edge of the ulcer. When material from this site is examined microscopically the organisms will be found in small clusters or chains typically described as the 'school of fish' arrangement. The organism is difficult to culture in the laboratory and requires specialised facilities. In areas where chancroid is prevalent these facilities are usually lacking and hence the diagnosis is made on the typical clinical characteristics. A presumptive diagnosis may be made by identifying the organisms microscopically after Gram staining material obtained from the edge of the ulcer. Borchardt & Hoke (1970) described a method of cultivating *H. ducreyi* from ulcer material inoculated into the patient's own inactivated serum. The organism may be cultured on Mueller-Hinton medium and other solid media containing haemin chloride (Hammand et al 1978b). The cultured colony of *H. ducreyi* remains adherent and sticky, and if pushed across the surface of the medium the colony will remain intact. The cultured organisms may be identified by biochemical tests. They give negative results to all tests except those for nitrate reduction and alkaline phosphatase production.

It is now believed that the typical ulcers of chancroid need not necessarily be due to *H. ducreyi*. Up to 60 different bacteria have been implicated in the causation of genital ulcers which clinically resemble chancroid. Amongst these are *Neisseria gonorrhoeae*, *Corynebacterium* species, staphylococci, streptococci and herpes simplex virus. Whether these organisms play a primary aetiological role or are secondary invaders following trauma or herpetic ulceration is not clear. Fourteen different microorganisms were isolated from genital ulcers of 49 men who attended an STD clinic in Harare, Zimbabwe in 1981 (Table 17.1). The majority of men had more than one bacterium.

Clinical presentation

The incubation period is normally 5–10 days but it may be as short as 1 day or as long as 15 days. Multiple lesions are usually found. In women the lesions are commonly found on the labia majora, the clitoris and the perivulval skin (Fig. 17.2). Lesions are often seen at the perianal margin and at the posterior fourchette. Rarely lesions are seen in the vault of the vagina and the cervix. Half the patients

Table 17.1 Micro-organisms isolated from the genital ulcers of 49 men attending a sexually transmitted disease clinic in Harare, Zimbabwe in 1981

Organism	Number of times isolated
Coagulase-negative staphylococcus	27
Staphylococcus pyogenes	7
Streptococci	
alpha haemolytic	8
group B	4
group D	11
anaerobic	5
Klebsiella species	7
Non-lactose fermenting coliform	5
Lactose fermenting coliform	2
Neisseria gonorrhoeae	4
Diphtheroids	4
Candida species	2
Micrococcus species	1
Pseudomonas aeruginosa	1
Total number of isolates	88

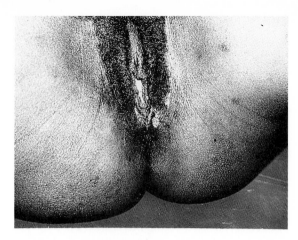

Fig. 17.2 Typical ulcerative lesion of chancroid at the fourchette. The patient presented 10 days after the onset of symptoms.

with chancroid have inguinal lymphadenitis which is usually unilateral but can be bilateral. The lymph nodes become inflamed and matted together to form a unilocular mass which is known as a bubo. Within 5 to 7 days of the development of the bubo, suppuration occurs and the mass becomes fluctuant. If the abscess ruptures it will discharge its contents through a single sinus. The ulcerative process will continue at the site. The skin rather than the mucosa is the site of predilection for chancroid ulcers in females. Invariably the ulcers are painful. The base of the ulcer is of irregular necrotic material covered in pus. The ulcer edge undermines normal skin. Palpation of the ulcer will produce excruciating pain and will reveal the non-indurated nature of the lesion, hence the pseudonym 'soft sore'. The ulcer, which has an irregular margin, is about 7–10 mm in diameter. Occasionally multiple small lesions or '*dwarf chancroid*' may be seen. Patients often complain of dysuria and painful defaecation will occur if the lesion is on the anal margin. Signs of other STDs such as gonorrhoea, genital herpes and syphilis may be found in some patients.

Diagnosis

The accurate diagnosis of chancroid depends on a thorough history and clinical examination. A pre-sumptive diagnosis is made by identifying *H. ducreyi*-like organisms in smears of ulcer exudates. The diagnosis is confirmed by culture isolation of the organism. Dark ground microscopic examination of ulcer material should be carried out to exclude syphilis. It may be necessary to repeat this examination daily for 3 days if treponemes are not found initially.

Smear examination

A painful non-indurated ulcer is always suggestive of chancroid. Search must then be made for *H. ducreyi*. A cotton wool tipped applicator stick is used to collect material from beneath the undermined edge of the ulcer. This procedure is extremely painful and should be carried out with care. Material collected should then be rolled out on to a glass slide. After staining by Gram's or Giemsa method the smear is examined microscopically under high power. Search is made for polymorphonuclear leucocytes and for gram-negative coccobacilli which appear in short chains or clusters mimicking a school of fish or parallel lines of bacilli. Occasionally these gram-negative bacilli are found within the cytoplasm of the polymorphonuclear leucocytes. In our own experience (Latif 1982) we found *H. ducreyi*-like organisms in only 50% of patients who had ulcers which were clinically typical of chancroid. Bacteria such as streptococci and *Bacterium melaninogenicus* may give rise to similar microscopic appearances.

Culture

Whenever possible attempts should be made to culture the organism and to identify it by biochemical tests. Blood or blood products are necessary for the cultivation of the organisms. Initially defibrinated rabbit serum was used and later fresh whole clotted blood was tried. Subsequently, Borchardt & Hoke (1970) described a method using the patient's own inactivated serum. Cultured organisms were found to be gram-negative coccobacilli which appeared in parallel lines. However, using liquid media numerous contaminants also grew. A selective solid medium containing 1% isovitalex and 3 μg/ml vancomycin has been used successfully (Hammond et al 1978b). Using this medium contamination with other micro-organisms was much less. Organisms may be cultured readily on Mueller-Hinton medium.

The colony of *H. ducreyi* is adherent and can be pushed across the surface of the medium intact. Gram stained smears of the colony show long parallel rows of gram-negative bacilli. All biochemical tests are negative except those for nitrate reduction and alkaline phosphatase.

Skin test

The intradermal injection of killed *H. ducreyi* into one forearm and the injection of normal saline as a control in the other forearm is the basis of the Ito-Reenstierna test. The development of a papule 7–10 mm in diameter after 48 hours at the site of injection of the killed micro-organisms is suggestive of chancroid of at least 14 days' duration, or that the patient may have had chancroid or this intradermal test in the past. This test is no longer routinely performed.

Serological tests

Recently an immunofluorescent test for the detection of antibody has been described. This test has not yet been fully evaluated (Denis et al 1978). The rapid identification of *H. ducreyi* using monoclonal antibody staining techniques is at present being evaluated.

Treatment

It can never be overemphasised that all sexual contacts of the patients should be thoroughly examined and investigated. It is also important that in all patients with an STD syphilis should be excluded. In patients with genital ulcers repeated dark ground microscopic examinations should be performed on material obtained from ulcers. At the first visit patients should also have blood taken for serological tests for syphilis. The non-specific venereal disease research laboratory test and a specific test such as the absorbed fluorescent treponemal antibody test or *Treponema pallidum* haemagglutination assay should be performed initially, and each month for 3 months before the diagnosis of syphilis is discarded.

Sulphonamides

These have been the drugs of choice for chancroid for almost half a century. We have found increasing resistance to sulphonamides especially in patients who have developed buboes. However cotrimoxazole in a dose of 960 mg twice a day for 7 days orally is effective. A single oral dose of trimethoprim 1000 mg/sulphamethopyrazine 800 mg is effective.

Tetracycline

Tetracycline in a dose of 2 g daily was found to be effective by some workers. However, others have cultured tetracycline resistant *H. ducreyi*. Tetracycline will mask a syphilitic infection.

Streptomycin

Streptomycin given in a dose of 1 g intramuscularly daily for 10 days is effective.

Kanamycin

In the event of treatment failure, kanamycin in a dose of 500 mg twice daily for 7 days is effective.

Thiamphenicol

In view of the fact that patients requiring injections need either hospitalisation or daily attendance we decided to use thiamphenicol in a dose of 2.5 g orally initially and 1.25 g 7 days later. This regime of treatment cured 92% of patients (Latif 1982). No side-effects were encountered.

It is suggested that thiamphenicol in such doses would also cure syphilis during the incubation period (Petzoldt 1971).

GRANULOMA INGUINALE

This is one of the three traditional tropical STDs, the other two being chancroid and lymphogranuloma venereum. This infection is found more often in men than in women and occurs almost exclusively in the coloured races (King et al 1980). In the United Kingdom patients suffering from granuloma inguinale are usually immigrants.

Epidemiology

Granuloma inguinale was first described in India by McLeod in 1882 (see King et al 1980).

In the United Kingdom the incidence of granuloma inguinale per 100 000 of population has been recorded as 0.01 to 0.04 each year from 1973 to 1979 (Chief Medical Officer 1979, 1980, 1981). This infection is thought to occur commonly in tropical and subtropical areas of the world. Reports from workers in Africa suggest that it is rare amongst STD patients (Sogbetun et al 1977; Latif 1981; Nsanze et al 1981). This disease is endemic in southern India, especially along the eastern coast (Lal & Nicholas 1970; Willcox 1974). In 1925 it was reported that 25% of the 20 000 inhabitants of Papua New Guinea had granuloma inguinale and in 1973 in the Central District of Papua New Guinea its incidence was 175 per 100 000 (Willcox 1980). In Sabah and Sarawak all of the tropical STDs are rare (Catterall 1981). In Zimbabwe granuloma inguinale is uncommon (Willcox 1949; Latif 1981). In the United States 2403 cases were seen in 1947 and 103 cases in 1971. Granuloma inguinale occurs mainly in men (Lal & Nicholas 1970) and is associated with poor hygiene, promiscuity and low socioeconomic status.

Whether this infection is sexually transmissible has been questioned. It has been believed that the causative agent is an inhabitant of the intestinal tract and can cause ulcers by autoinoculation of the faecal material on injuried skin (Goldberg 1964).

Often the infection is not transmitted to sexual partners of infected patients. Factors indicating the venereal nature of the disease are that lesions usually occur on the genitalia, they occur in promiscuous persons, and they are often associated with other forms of STD.

Aetiology and pathology

Granuloma inguinale is caused by *Calymmatobacterium granulomatis*. This is a gram-negative, nonsporing, encapsulated bacillus and was first discovered by Donovan in India in 1905. These encapsulated rods are found in the cytoplasm of large mononuclear cells in material obtained from ulcers. These structures are called 'Donovan bodies' and when stained by the Romanovsky method, the capsule is pink and the body shows bipolar condensation of chromatin—the so-called closed safety pin appearance.

The capsule of *C. granulomatis* has antigenic properties immunologically similar to those found in the capsule of *Klebsiella pneumoniae*. Histologically the lesions show increased vascularity, considerable cellular infiltration with polymorphonuclear leucocytes and monocytes and in tissue stained by a Romanovsky method the typical intra- and extracellular Donovan bodies.

Clinical presentation

The incubation period is 7–30 days but may be as short as 1 day or as long as 6 months. In women lesions may be found on the mons pubis, labia majora, fourchette and perianal skin. Occasionally lesions are found on the buttocks, abdomen, breasts, inguinal region and the mouth. Lesions may also be found on the cervix or inside the vagina.

The initial lesion is a papule or a subcutaneous nodule which may be pruritic. It enlarges and initially it is firm but with time softens. In the inguinal region this lesion is known as a pseudobubo. Within a few days ulceration occurs, which is of variable size, irregular in shape and is painless. The ulcer may be indurated and is velvety and bright pink or red in colour. It has rolled up edges and is covered with a serosanguineous exudate. The skin around the ulcer becomes thickened and grey, and the ulcer spreads by continuity along skin folds. The lesions tend to spread posteriorly to the perineum and anal region. In female patients there is a tendency to extensive fibrous tissue formation which can lead to deformity. Regional lymphadenopathy is unusual but the lymphatics may become involved in the fibrous process when gross lymphoedema of the labia and clitoris can occur. This can mimic the appearance of lymphogranuloma venereum. Secondary bacterial involvement may also cause lymphadenitis. In pregnant women extensive ulceration may occur.

Occasionally in patients with long-standing disease, acute inflammation occurs together with severe tissue necrosis which can be complicated by septicaemia and be fatal. Systemic infection from the primary site rarely occurs but may lead to osteitis, arthritis or lesions in the liver and spleen. In the sclerotis form of granuloma inguinale there may be stenosis of the introitus and anus.

Malignancy has been reported in association with granuloma inguinale (Goldberg & Annamunthodo 1966; Davis 1970). A basal cell or squamous cell carcinoma may occur. Care is required in interpreting histological reports as pseudoepitheliomatous hyperplasia, which is a benign condition in granuloma inguinale, may be difficult to differentiate from carcinoma. *C. granulomatis* has also been implicated in the causation of carcinoma of the vulva and carcinoma of the penis. In 9 out of 62 cases of cancer of the penis, antibodies to *C. granulomatis* were found (Garg et al 1978).

Diagnosis

The diagnosis of granuloma inguinale should be confirmed by microbiological studies. Syphilis should be excluded by performing repeated dark ground microscopic examinations of ulcer material and by performing serial serological tests for syphilis. The lesions of granuloma inguinale can mimic condylomata and a number of cases of granuloma inguinale have a concomitant syphilitic infection.

Examination of smears

Granulomatous material obtained by punch biopsy or scrapings of ulcer edges should be stained by a

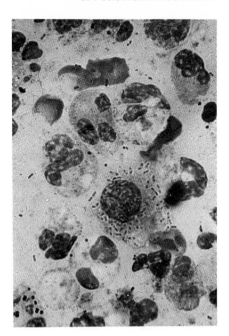

Fig. 17.3 *Calymmatobacterium granulomatis* organisms within the cytoplasm of a monocyte.

Romanovsky method and examined microscopically (Fig. 17.3). Donovan bodies with intense bipolar staining will be found inside large mononuclear cells.

Culture

Cultivation of *C. granulomatis* on artificial media is difficult. The organism can be cultured on the yolk sac of a developing chick embryo or a liquid medium containing a hydrolysate of lactalbumin or an enzymatic digest of soya meal.

Biopsy

Microscopic examination of appropriately stained preparations of material obtained from the ulcer edge may show the typical Donovan bodies.

Intradermal test

An intradermal test has been devised but the high incidence of false positive results has precluded its use.

Serological tests

A complement fixation test has also been reported (Goldberg & Annamunthodo 1966) but scarcity of antigen has limited its use.

Treatment

The drug of choice for the treatment of granuloma inguinale is streptomycin. This is given in a dose of 1 g daily intramuscularly for 3 weeks. Penicillin and sulphonamides have not been found to be effective in treating this condition. However, co-trimoxazole 960 mg twice daily for 10 days was found to be effective in India (Garg et al 1978). Tetracycline 2 g daily given with streptomycin 1 g daily over a period of 14 days is also effective. Other drugs which have been used in the management of granuloma inguinale are chloramphenicol, ampicillin, gentamicin and lincomycin. In the United States, ampicillin is now the recommended drug of choice. It is given in a dose of 1 g daily for 1 to 3 months.

Follow-up is important as relapses may occur after apparently successful treatment. If the condition relapses retreatment with the same antibiotic is usually effective.

LYMPHOGRANULOMA VENEREUM

This is a sexually transmissible infection which has a predilection for the lymphatic system. It was noted to occur in the 15th and 16th centuries among Spaniards in America (Willcox 1980). Lymphogranuloma venereum was proved to be a distinct venereal disease in 1913, and in 1925 Frei described a specific skin test (see Osoba 1981a). The infection can have a devastating effect on the body and can cause gross distortion of the vulva, elephantiasis of the male genitalia and rectal stricture.

Epidemiology

Lymphogranuloma venereum occurs throughout the world. It is frequently seen in patients attending STD clinics in Africa, South America, the West Indies, India and South-East Asia. In Ibadan, Nigeria (Sogbetun et al 1977), of 578 patients seen at STD clinics over a period of 30 months, 2.5% had this infection. In Uganda it was found in 1.5% of STD patients (Osoba 1981b). In Ghana 13.7% of STD patients had lymphogranuloma venereum and in Sudan 2.7% of STD patients had this infection (Osoba 1981b).

In India over a 10-year period 6% of patients with STD had lymphogranuloma venereum (Sowmini 1978) and 2.5% of STD patients in Lusaka, Zambia were found to have lymphogranuloma venereum (Osoba 1981a). In Zimbabwe in 1980 it was found that 4.3% of men attending an STD clinic in Harare had lymphogranuloma venereum and of 4391 women seen at all STD clinics in Harare in 1981, 3.2% had lymphogranuloma venereum (City Health Department 1981). In the United Kingdom the incidence of lymphogranuloma venereum was reported as being between 0.14 per 100 000 in 1973 and 0.06 per 100 000 in 1980 (Chief Medical Officer 1979, 1980, 1981). Lymphogranuloma venereum is uncommon in Sabah and Sarawak (Catterall 1981), the Pacific Islands (Willcox 1980) and Saudi Arabia (Pareek & Chowdhury 1981).

Aetiology

The lymphogranuloma venereum agent was at one time thought to be a filtrable virus. The infection can be transferred experimentally to animals and back to man from animals thus infected. It is now known that the causal agent is of the genus *Chlamydia* within the order Rickettsiales. Chlamydiae are not viruses and contain both DNA and RNA. The infectious particle is 400 nm in diameter. The organism has a rigid cell wall which contains muramic acid and has the ability to produce glycogen-containing inclusion bodies within invaded cells. Chlamydiae divide by binary fission.

The infectious form of the chlamydial agent is the elementary body, which is a rigid walled particle 0.3 μm in diameter. This is known as the reticulate body, which is non-infectious but metabolically active. The reticulate body multiplies within eukaryotic cells to form a microcolony within a cytoplasmic vacuole. Finally the cell ruptures, liberating a new generation of infectious metabolically inactive elementary bodies.

Classification of chlamydiae

Chlamydiae are divided into two large groups on the basis of their ability to produce glycogen-containing inclusion bodies. Those that produce glycogen-containing inclusions are members of Group A. Those which do not have the ability to produce glycogen are Group B.

Chlamydia trachomatis belongs to Group A and *C. psittaci* belongs to Group B. There are 14 serotypes of the Group A chlamydia. The serotypes A, Ba, B and C are the causal agents of hyperendemic trachoma. The serotypes D, E, F, G, H, I and K cause non-gonococcal urethritis, non-specific genital infection, inclusion conjunctivitis and non-specific ophthalmia neonatorum. The serotypes L1, L2 and L3 cause lymphogranuloma venereum.

It is possible that a particular strain may be responsible for a particular syndrome, for instance rectal stricture, or genital ulceration. However this has not yet been proved.

Pathology

The base of the primary genital lesion consists of granulation tissue surrounded by necrotic tissue. Microscopic findings are not specific for lymphogranuloma venereum. The epithelium at the edge of the ulcer may show pseudoepitheliomatous hyperplasia.

There is infiltration with lymphocytes and plasma cells. Within the lymph nodes multiple necrotic foci are seen. There is infiltration with polymorphonuclear leucocytes, plasma cells and there is a marked hyperplasia of the germinal centres. Abscesses will develop with time and the inflammatory process continues and extends into perinodal tissue and skin.

Abscesses drain through multiple sinuses. In both sexes obstruction to lymphatics occurs due to fibrosis at the site of the primary lesion or in the lymph node. In females this can lead to giant lymphoedema of the labia producing irregular swelling and distortion known as an esthiomene. If obstruction to the lymphatics is permanent, this gross distortion remains and results in depigmentation and recurrent ulceration. The primary lesion may heal very quickly so that the patient presents with lymphatic involvement only.

In women the initial site of inoculation may be in the upper two-thirds of the vagina or on the cervix. The lymphatic drainage from these areas is to the internal and external iliac nodes. In homosexual males and females the primary site may be inside the rectum where lymphatic involvement again occurs and there may be fibrous strictures.

Clinical presentation

The primary lesion. The interval between exposure to the infection and the appearance of the primary lesion is usually about 2–5 days but an incubation period of up to 5 weeks has been described. The primary lesion may be a small transient painful lesion which can be confused with herpetic ulceration. This is noticed in 25–30% of males but in the majority of females may not be noticed at all. It usually heals spontaneously. The inguinal lymph nodes become enlarged and painful 1–6 weeks after the primary lesion appears. If the condition is untreated the disease will run a course of 6 to 8 weeks and may then resolve completely. Intermittent relapses of lymphadenitis however are likely to occur. In 70% of untreated patients there will be persisting lymphatic obstruction.

Inguinal syndrome. This is the most common presentation in males. In females this syndrome occurs if the primary site of infection is on the external genitalia or in the lower third of the vagina. Inguinal lymphadenitis occurs 1–4 weeks after the appearance of the primary lesion. The lymph node enlargement is unilateral in most cases. The glands are painful, tender and become matted together as a result of periadenitis. The bubo that results is multiloculated. If untreated the bubo may resolve spontaneously within 2 weeks. Alternatively abscesses may rupture through the skin via multiple sinuses. Enlargement of lymph nodes above and below the inguinal ligament may give the bubo a grooved appearance and this sign is highly suggestive of lymphogranuloma venereum (Fig. 17.4). During this acute phase of lymphadenitis there is poor drainage of lymph from the area of primary infection. This results in lymphoedema of the labia on the affected side. With early treatment, the lymphoedema is shortlived and resolves completely. If fibrosis occurs in the lymph nodes and lymphatic channels permanent lymphoedema results. Healing

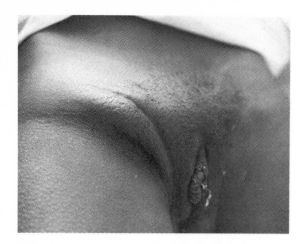

Fig. 17.4 The groove sign of lymphogranuloma venereum. A small ulcer present on the right labium minor.

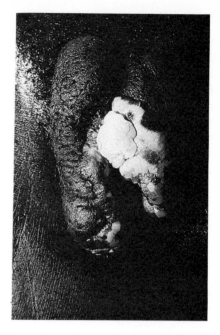

Fig. 17.5 Lymphogranuloma venereum showing bilateral chronic lymphoedema of the vulva—esthiomene.

occurs in the inguinal region with scarring, and occasionally recurrent sinus formation occurs.

If primary infection occurs in the upper two-thirds of the vagina or on the cervix, the internal iliac lymph nodes become involved. This can lead to low backache or symptoms and signs of peritonitis.

Anorectal syndrome. Women with primary infection in the posterior wall of the vagina may develop inflammation and lymphadenitis in the rectovaginal septum. The patient may complain of rectal bleeding and later a purulent anal discharge occurs. Proctoscopy reveals ulceration and inflammation of the rectal mucosa with multiple punctate haemorrhages and a mucopurulent discharge.

System involvement. There may be extensive involvement of the lymphatic system even though the patient may appear to have only localised disease (Osoba & Beetlestone 1976). Generalised lymphadenopathy with evidence of supraclavicular and axillary lymph node enlargement may occur.

Late manifestations. Infiltration and fibrosis of the inguinal lymph glands can lead to total destruction and replacement by scar tissue. The area drained by the affected lymph nodes becomes lymphoedematous so that the labia on the affected side may appear as a large, firm polypoidal mass (Fig. 17.5). Over a period of months or years these areas become depigmented and malignant change can occur. Perirectal involvement with fibrosis and scarring results in a tubular stricture of the rectum. This is associated with constipation and abdominal

distension. Although the early inflammation is usually restricted to the rectum a more extensive proctocolitis simulating ulcerative colitis may occur. Perirectal abscesses may rupture into the vagina or bladder and rectovaginal, rectovesical or vesicovaginal fistulae may occur.

Diagnosis

The diagnosis is based on history, clinical findings, an intradermal skin test and chlamydial culture and serology.

Frei test

The Frei test is now obsolete and should not be relied upon for diagnosis. Intradermal injection of 0.5 ml of a suspension of killed chlamydia (available commercially as Lygranum) is carried out in the forearm and 0.5 ml of saline injected as a control into the opposite arm. The development of a papule with a diameter greater than 7 mm at the site of injection indicates a positive test. The test becomes positive 2 weeks after the initial infection. The test, however, is non-specific and the commercially prepared antigen is no longer available.

Chlamydial culture

Giemsa stained smears taken from scrapings of the suspected ulcer or pus aspirated from buboes may be scanned microscopically for the presence of inclusion bodies, but the sensitivity of tests for inclusions is low and attempts should be made wherever possible to culture the organisms. Chlamydia may be cultured in the yolk sac of fertile hens' eggs but this is a time-consuming and laborious method and now chlamydiae are usually cultured on living cell lines. This requires specialised laboratory facilities however and these are usually not available in developing countries. Chlamydia may be isolated after inoculation on to inactivated McCoy cells (Darougar et al 1971). After inoculation and incubation of the McCoy cells, Giemsa stained monolayers are scanned for inclusions. *C. trachomatis* may be identified in ulcer exudates and bubo aspirates using monoclonal, antibody staining techniques.

Serology

The complement fixation test has been widely used for the diagnosis of lymphogranuloma venereum. The test measures group reactive antibody and cannot be used to distinguish between different chlamydial infections. The rapid isotope precipitation test also detects group reactive antibody but is more sensitive than the complement fixation test.

The microimmunofluorescent test is used to detect specific chlamydial serotype antigens. It is a highly specific and sensitive test for the detection of different immunoglobulin classes of type-specific chlamydial antibody (Treharne et al 1973). At present there are 14 distinct serotypes of *Chlamydia trachomatis*. By using the microimmunofluorescent test, titres of specific IgG, IgA and IgM may be measured. A high titre of IgG antibody in serum indicates an acute infection. In lymphogranuloma venereum serum, titres of greater than 1 in 256 are very suggestive of acute infection.

Treatment

C. trachomatis is still highly susceptible to erythromycin and tetracycline. It is also sensitive to rifampicin, spiramycin and chloramphenicol.

The drug of choice is tetracycline given in a dose of 500 mg four times a day for 14 days. Erythromycin in similar doses is just as effective and is preferred in pregnant women. Occasionally surgery will be indicated for cosmetic reasons or where rectal strictures have become malignant.

Syphilis should be excluded by dark field microscopy and serological tests.

SCHISTOSOMIASIS

Schistosomiasis (bilharziasis) is relatively unknown in temperate climates but provides one of the most important public health problems in tropical and subtropical areas. Its effects can be wide-ranging and involvement of the lower genital tract is fairly common in areas where the disease is endemic.

Epidemiology and pathogenesis

Man is host to three species of schistosomiasis fluke but may on occasion carry others which normally parasitise other animals.

Schistosoma japonicum infection is confined to areas in the Far East including China, Japan and the Philippines. *S. mansoni* occurs throughout tropical Africa with an endemic focus in the Nile river delta and also along the eastern belt of the South American continent. Small foci are found in other regions. *S. haematobium* is restricted mainly to Africa and adjacent areas of the Middle East.

Infection is acquired following penetration of the skin by the larval cercariae which emerge in large numbers from parasitised fresh water molluscs. These snail vectors are species-specific. The genus *Oncomelania* is the intermediate host of *S. japonicum*, *Biomphalaria* and *Australorbis* are parasitised by *S. mansoni* and *Bulinus* and *Physopsis* by *S. haematobium*.

Following maturation in the liver of the human host, the maturing flukes migrate to their final site, mate and produce eggs within 46 weeks. *S. japonicum* and *S. mansoni* normally lodge in the mesenteric venules and *S. haematobium* lives primarily in the vesicular circulation. Eggs of the two former species pass through the gut wall and of the latter into the bladder. These eggs contain ciliated miracidial larvae which, when liberated into fresh water, parasitise suitable snail hosts.

The major pathology caused by infection with

schistosomes is caused by passage of eggs through tissue. Initial inflammatory response is followed by fibrotic change and dead eggs trapped in the tissue often calcify.

Because of the final site of lodgement of *S. haematobium* this species is the most likely to be involved in pathology and symptomatology of the lower genital tract, although ectopic distribution of the other species may occur.

The frequency of lower genital tract involvement in schistosomiasis is difficult to estimate, since many cases are not diagnosed clinically as they may be asymptomatic. Bland & Gelfand (1970) found that 12 patients out of 55 where the cervix had been removed showed evidence of bilharziasis. They also report that 17% of the local female population in Harare, Zimbabwe have evidence of bilharziasis on cervical cytological screening. The frequency with which schistosomiasis involves different genital organs also varies. Youssef et al (1970) reported that, in a survey of 397 cases of genital tract schistosomiasis, the cervix was shown to be involved in 30.5%, the vagina in 26% and the vulva in 17%.

Clinical presentation

Vulva. Lesions of the vulva present most commonly before puberty. The earliest symptom is often irritation which may be accompanied by an area of inflammation but this often passes unnoticed. The usual presenting feature is a papillomatous lesion developing on the labia majora. The growth is usually sessile and can become very large. Bilharzial caruncles appearing at the urethral meatus are also common, particularly in very young girls. Ulceration of bilharzial lesions of the vulva is very uncommon.

Vagina. Very often vaginal bilharziasis is asymptomatic but the patient may complain of a vaginal discharge, bleeding, pain, dyspareunia and the presence of a mass. The vaginal wall may show firm nodules of varying sizes or papillomatous masses similar to those found at the vulva. In very recent infection the vagina may be diffusely inflamed and tender. Ulceration is rare but can occur.

Cervix. This is the site most commonly involved in genital tract schistosomiasis and, unlike involvement of the vulva and vagina, often presents with an ulcerative lesion. The ulcers are usually fairly large with a granulating surface. Polypoidal lesions

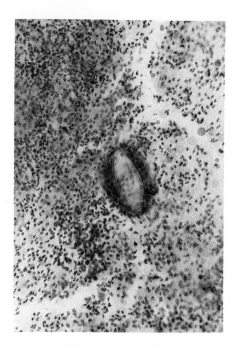

Fig. 17.6 Ovum of *Schistosoma haematobium* in a cervical smear.

are also common and sometimes hard nodules resembling chronic nabothian follicles may be found (Charlewood et al 1949). Polypoidal growths are usually friable and bleed readily.

If the lesions are symptomatic there is usually bleeding and a purulent discharge. These symptoms, together with the clinical findings, will often simulate malignant disease of the cervix.

Diagnosis

The diagnosis of all forms of lower genital tract schistosomiasis should be confirmed by histology. Biopsies will show a typical concentric arrangement of histiocytes surrounding granulomas with schistosome ova at the centre. Cervical cytology has been suggested as a method for diagnosing involvement of the cervix when ova can be readily demonstrated (Fig. 17.6). A search can be made for evidence of schistosomiasis elsewhere but this does not of course confirm that the genital tract lesion is of the same aetiology.

Treatment

The treatment of genital tract schistosomiasis is essentially medical, although large papillomatous growths may have to be removed surgically.

There have been several new drugs introduced for the treatment of bilharziasis which are less toxic and more effective than the older regimes (Gilles 1981). For the treatment of *S. haematobium*, which is the most common form found in the genital tract, metrifonate is the drug of choice. It is given in a dose of 10 mg/kg on three occasions at intervals of 2 weeks. It has a low incidence of side-effects and is relatively cheap. Other drugs which can be used are niridazole (Ambilhar), hycanthone and praziquantel. Oxamniquine is effective against *S. mansoni* although the drug of choice for this parasite and also *S. japonicum* is praziquantel.

TUBERCULOSIS

Tuberculosis is still a common disease in many parts of the developing world although it is now seen infrequently in developed countries. Genital tract tuberculosis was first described by Morgagni in the mid 18th century (see Schaefer 1970).

Incidence

The frequency of genital tract tuberculosis in the general population is difficult to assess accurately. Figures depend on notification of the disease and with large numbers of symptomless patients it tends to be under-reported. This is particularly so for developing countries. The estimates of the frequency of genital tract tuberculosis have varied widely but all have shown a decreasing incidence from upper to lower genital tract.

Kohler (1975) found 21 cases of tuberculous cervicitis from 1969–1973. These cases presented in a city where approximately 3500 cases of tuberculosis were notified annually at the time. Stallworthy (1952) however found no cases of cervical involvement in 78 cases of genital tuberculosis. Most reports from developed countries report an incidence of less than 1% (Sutherland 1956; Israel et al 1963) but in countries where tuberculosis is rampant figures as high as 10% for involvement of the cervix have been reported (Kirloskar et al 1968).

Tuberculosis of the vagina and the vulva are less common than involvement of the cervix. By 1949, for example, only 100 cases of vulval involvement had been reported in the literature (Brenner 1976).

Pathology

It is generally accepted that primary infection of the female genital organs occurs very rarely. Infection of the vulva or the vagina without any evidence of tuberculosis in the upper genital tract or of extragenital involvement is reported, but may reflect lack of full investigation, or that the primary lesion has already healed. Some workers do feel however that tuberculosis can be acquired during sexual contact with an infected male. In this event the lesion will develop at the site of a coital injury on the fourchette or in the posterior fornix of the vagina (Stewart 1967). Usually female genital tract tuberculosis occurs secondarily to tuberculosis elsewhere in the body, with the primary infection most commonly being the lungs. The mode of spread to the genital organs is usually haematogenous although there may be direct spread from abdominal organs or spread by lymphatics. The fallopian tubes are infected initially with spread to the uterus and ovaries by direct extension. The cervix may be involved by haematogenous spread but more often by spread from the endometrium.

The gross appearance of cervical tuberculosis can take many forms. There may be an ulcer or a papillomatous lesion but the most common is a granulomatous mass. The microscopic appearance is similar to that found elsewhere in the body, with concentric arrangement of histiocytes and the presence of multinucleated Langhans' giant cells. Caseation is often seen at the centre of the lesions.

Vaginal and vulval lesions present initially as nodules which transform early into ulcers with soft ragged edges. Marked vaginal stenosis can occur (Coetzee 1972), presumably following scarring and fibrosis. Vulval tuberculosis in particular often mimics carcinoma of the vulva.

The microscopical findings are similar to those of tuberculosis elsewhere.

Clinical presentation

The presenting complaints for all three sites may be of an offensive vaginal discharge, abnormal uterine bleeding, pain or dyspareunia, or the presence of a mass. As the lesions may be ulcerative or papillomatous the diagnosis must always be considered in such cases where tuberculosis is common. Frequently the initial diagnosis will be of malignancy.

Table 17.2 Summary of main features of infections discussed

Infection	Presenting features in lower genital tract		Investigation	Treatment
Amoebiasis	Symptoms:	Discharge, pain and tenderness, dyspareunia	Microscopy of discharge, cytology or histology	Metronidazole
	Appearance:	Ulceration and sloughing		
Chancroid	Symptoms:	Painful ulceration, inguinal lymphadenitis	Gram stain of ulcer exudate Isolate organism on Mueller-Hinton medium	Cotrimoxazole, tetracycline Where drug resistance is encountered: streptomycin thiamphenicol erythromycin
	Appearance:	Multiple ulcers with irregular margins and a soft base containing necrotic material and pus. Grossly inflamed and matted inguinal lymph glands with suppuration, unilocular bubo		
Granuloma inguinale	Symptoms:	Pruritic papule or subcutaneous nodule	Romanovsky stain of material from edge of ulcer	Streptomycin and tetracycline, cotrimoxazole
	Appearance:	Enlarging nodules which break down revealing indurated, beefy-red ulceration		
Lymphogranuloma venereum	Symptoms:	The primary lesion is a small transient painful ulcer which is followed by painful enlargement of the inguinal lymph glands	Giemsa stained smears of ulcer material or pus from buboea Culture and serology and monoclonal antibody staining	Tetracycline, erythromycin
	Appearance:	The initial lesion resembles herpetic ulceration. The lymph glands are matted together and development of a multilocular bubo is common		
Schistosomiasis	Symptoms:	Irritation and inflammation, discharge	Cervical smears Histology	*S. haematobium* Metrifonate, praziquantel, niridazole, hycanthone *S. mansoni* praziquantel, oxamniquine *S. japonicum* praziquantel
	Appearance:	Papillomatous lesions, firm nodules and caruncles. Cervical ulcers with granulating surface		
Tuberculosis	Symptoms:	Offensive discharge, abnormal bleeding, pain or dyspareunia and the presence of a mass	Histology	Standard antituberculosis regimes. Surgery if required
	Appearance:	Granulomatous mass, papilloma or ulceration		

The patient may also have symptoms and signs of upper genital tract tuberculosis such as infertility, pelvic pain and menstrual disturbances.

Diagnosis

Any lesion of the lower genital tract where tuberculosis is suspected should be biopsied. Typical tubercles may be seen with giant cells, epithelioid cells, caseation and peripheral lymphocytosis. The histological appearance is not always clearcut however, particularly if there is a superimposed pyogenic infection. The identification of tubercle bacilli confirms the histological diagnosis. All patients should have a chest X-ray, but it is important to note that a pulmonary lesion will not always be recognised, particularly if the primary complex has healed. Tkachuk et al (1967) recommend that all patients with genital tract tuberculosis should have a full urological examination, as 30% of 184 patients in their series had infection of the urinary tract.

Treatment

Before the introduction of antituberculous drugs surgery was the main form of treatment for genital tract tuberculosis and was accompanied by a high incidence of postoperative complications and even mortality. Surgery is now confined to cases which fail to respond to chemotherapy.

The choice of antituberculous agents in developing countries will be dictated not only by effectiveness and complications but by availability and cost. As treatment will be continued for a prolonged period of time it is also important for the regime to be simple to ensure patient compliance. In Harare, Zimbabwe, two treatment regimes are used depending on the results of examination of specimens for acid-fast bacilli (AFB). Regime A (AFB negative) is streptomycin, pyrazinamide, isoniazid and thiacetazone (HT3) daily for 2 months followed by daily HT3 for a further 10 months. Regime B (AFB positive) is streptomycin, pyrazinamide, rifampicin and HT3 daily for 2 months followed by daily HT3 for a further 6 months. If side-effects do occur our second-line treatment is that recommended by Sutherland (1979). This is a combination of isoniazid, ethionamide and rifampicin.

SUMMARY

The diagnosis and management of lower genital tract infections in developing countries can be difficult and confusing. Many of the infections present with similar signs and symptoms and often there will not be adequate laboratory facilities to aid in the confirmation of clinical diagnoses. Table 17.2 outlines the main features of the infections discussed.

REFERENCES

Bhaduri K P 1957 Entamoeba histolytica in leukorrhea and salpingitis. American Journal of Obstetrics and Gynecology 74: 434

Bland K G, Gelfand M 1970 The effects of schistosomiasis on the cervix uteri in the African female. Journal of Obstetrics and Gynaecology of the British Commonwealth 77: 1127–1131

Borchardt K A, Hoke A W 1970 Simplified laboratory technique for diagnosis of chancroid. Archives of Dermatology 102: 188–192

Brenner B N 1976 Tuberculosis of the vulva. South African Medical Journal 50: 1798–1800

Burney P 1976 Some aspects of sexually transmitted disease in Swaziland. British Journal of Venereal Diseases 52: 412–414

Catterall R S 1981 Sexually transmitted diseases in Sabah and Sarawak. British Journal of Venereal Diseases 57: 363–366

Charlewood G P, Shippel S, Renton H 1949 Schistosomiasis in gynaecology. Journal of Obstetrics and Gynaecology of the British Empire 56: 367–385

Chief Medical Officer 1979 Extract from the annual report for the year 1977. British Journal of Venereal Diseases 55: 225–229

Chief Medical Officer 1980 Extract from the annual report for the year 1978. British Journal of Venereal Diseases 56: 178-181

Chief Medical Officer 1981 Extract from the annual report for the year 1979. British Journal of Venereal Diseases 57: 402–405

City Health Department 1981 Sexually transmitted disease patterns in the municipal STD clinics. In: City of Harare, Zimbabwe annual report, p 61

Coetzee L F 1972 Tuberculous vaginitis. South African Medical Journal 46: 1225–1226

Cohen C 1973 Three cases of amoebiasis of the cervix uteri. Journal of Obstetrics and Gynaecology of the British Empire 80: 476–479

Corbishley C M 1977 Microbial flora of the vagina and cervix. Journal of Clinical Pathology 30: 745–748

Darougar S, Treharne J D, Dwyer R St C, Kinnison J R, Jones B R 1971 Isolation of TRIC agent (chlamydia) in irradiated McCoy cell culture from endemic trachoma in field studies in Iran. British Journal of Ophthalmology 55: 591–599

Davis C M: Granuloma inguinale—a clinical, histological and ultrastructural study. Journal of the American Medical Association 211: 632–636

Denis G A, Chapel T A, Jeffries C D 1978 An indirect fluorescent antibody technique for Haemophilus ducreyi. Health Laboratory Science 15: 128–132

Garg B R, Lal S, Sivamani S 1978 Efficacy of co-trimoxazole in Donovanosis. British Journal of Venereal Diseases 54: 348–349

Gilles H M 1981 The treatment of schistosomiasis. Journal of Antimicrobial Chemotherapy 7: 113–114

Goldberg J 1964 Studies on granuloma inguinale. VII. Some epidemiological considerations of the disease. British Journal of Venereal Diseases 40: 140–145

Goldberg J, Annamunthodo H 1966 Studies on granuloma inguinale. VIII. Serological reactivity of sera from patients with carcinoma of penis when tested with Donovania antigens. British Journal of Venereal Diseases 42: 205–209

Hammond G W, Chang J L, Wilt J C, Ronald A R 1978a Antimicrobial susceptibility of Haemophilus ducreyi. Antimicrobial Agents and Chemotherapy 13: 608–612

Hammond G W, Chang J L, Wilt J C, Albritton W L, Ronald

A R 1978b Determination of the haem requirement of Haemophilus ducreyi. Journal of Clinical Microbiology 7: 243–246

Israel S L, Roitman H B, Clancy C 1963 Infrequency of unsuspected endometrial tuberculosis. Journal of the American Medical Association 183: 63–65

King A, Nicol C, Rodin P (eds) 1980 Venereal diseases. Balliere Tindall, London

Kirloskar J, Tucasi P, Vasancua C C 1968 Tuberculosis of the cervix. Journal of Obstetrics and Gynaecology of India 18: 709–712

Koller A B 1975 Granulomatous lesions of the cervix uteri in black patients. South African Medical Journal 49: 1228–1232

Lal S, Nicholas C 1970 Epidemiological and clinical features in 165 cases of granuloma inguinale. British Journal of Venereal Diseases 46: 461–463

Latif A S 1981 Sexually transmitted disease in clinic patients in Salisbury, Zimbabwe. British Journal of Venereal Diseases 57: 181–183

Latif A S 1982 Thiamphenicol in the treatment of chancroid in men. British Journal of Venereal Diseases 58: 54–55

McCallum M 1973 A survey of selected vaginal flora in Malawian women. Central African Journal of Medicine 19: 176–178

McClatchie S, Sambhi J S 1971 Amoebiasis of the cervix uteri. Annals of Tropical Medicine and Parasitology 65: 207–210

Mason P R, MacCallum M-S, Patterson B, Latif A S 1983 The vaginal flora of pregnant women in Zimbabwe. Journal of Obstetrics and Gynecology East Central Africa 2: 102–104

Morel P 1974 The soft chancre. Nouvelle Presse Médicale 3: 2104–2106

Munguia H, Franco E, Valenzuela P: Diagnosis of genital amoebiasis in women by the standard Papanicolaou technique. American Journal of Obstetrics and Gynecology 94: 181–188

Mylius R E, Ten Seldam R E J 1962 Venereal infection by Entamoeba histolytica in a New Guinea native couple. Tropical and Geographical Medicine 14: 20–26

Nair B K H, Viswam M P, Venugopal B S, Nair P S 1973 An epidemiological study of venereal disease. Indian Journal of Medical Research 61: 1697–1707

Nsanze H, Fast M V, D'Costa L J D, Curran J, Ronald A 1981 Genital ulcers in Kenya. Clinical and laboratory study. British Journal of Venereal Diseases 57: 378–381

Osoba A O 1981a Lymphogranuloma venereum. In: Harris J R W (ed) Recent advances in sexually transmitted diseases. Churchill Livingstone, London, pp 211–216

Osoba A O 1981b Sexually transmitted diseases in tropical Africa. British Journal of Venereal Diseases 57: 89–94

Osoba A O, Beetlestone C A 1976 Lymphographic studies in acute lymphogranuloma venereum infection. British Journal of Venereal Diseases 52: 399–403

Oyerinde J P O, Alonge A A, Adegbite-Hollist A F, Ogunbi O 1978 The epidemiology of Entamoeba histolytica in a Nigerian urban population. International Journal of Epidemiology 8: 55–59

Pareek S S, Chowdhury M N H 1981 Sexually transmitted diseases in Riyadh, Saudi Arabia. A study of patients attending a teaching hospital clinic. British Journal of Venereal Diseases 57: 343–345

Petzoldt D 1971 Single dose treatment of gonorrhoea with penicillin or thiamphenicol and the effect on Treponema pallidum in experimental syphilis. British Journal of Venereal Diseases 47: 377

Rajan V S, Pang R 1979 Treatment of chancroid with Bactrim. Annals of the Academy of Medicine of Singapore 8: 63–66

Rajan V S, Sng E H 1981 Chancroid. In: Harris J R W (ed) Recent advances in sexually transmitted diseases. Churchill Livingstone, London

Schaefer G 1970 Tuberculosis of the female genital tract. Clinics in Obstetrics and Gynaecology 13: 965–998

Sogbetun A O, Alausa K O, Osoba A O 1977 Sexually transmitted diseases in Ibadan, Nigeria. British Journal of Venereal Diseases 53: 155–160

Sowmini C N 1978 Late manifestations of lymphogranuloma venereum. Paper presented at the 29th General Assembly of the International Union against Venereal Diseases and Treponematoses, Leeds

Stallworthy J 1952 Genital tuberculosis in the female. Journal of Obstetrics and Gynaecology of the British Empire 59: 729–736

Stewart D B 1967 Tuberculosis of the female genital tract. In: Lawson J B, Stewart D B (eds) Obstetrics and gynaecology in the tropics and developing countries. Edward Arnold, London, pp 451–460

Sutherland A M 1956 Tuberculosis of the endometrium. Journal of Obstetrics and Gynaecology of the British Empire 63: 161–172

Sutherland A M 1979 Gynaecological tuberculosis. British Journal of Hospital Medicine 22: 569–576

Treharne J D, Darougar S, Jones B R 1973 Characterization of a further micro-immunofluorescence serotype of chlamydia: TRIC type G. British Journal of Venereal Diseases 49: 295–300

Tkachuk V N, Volovish L Y, Skylarchik A K 1967 Combined tuberculous infection of the reproductive and urinary tracts in women. Akusherstvo i Ginekologia 2: 40–44 (reviewed in English in Journal of Obstetrics and Gynaecology of the British Commonwealth 74: 635, 1967)

van Coeverden de Groot H A 1963 Amoebic vaginitis. South African Medical Journal 37: 246–247

Willcox R R 1949 A venereal disease survey of the African in Southern Rhodesia. Southern Rhodesian Government, Salisbury

Willcox R R 1974 Granuloma inguinale. In: Morton R S, Harris J R W (eds) Recent advances in sexually transmitted diseases. Churchill Livingstone, Edinburgh

Willcox R R 1980 Venereal diseases in the Pacific Islands. Papua New Guinea. British Journal of Venereal Diseases 56: 277–281

Wynne J M 1980 Perineal amoebiasis. Archives of Disease in Childhood 55: 234–236

Youssef A F, Fayad M M, Shafeek M A 1970 Bilharziasis of the cervix uteri. Journal of Obstetrics and Gynaecology of the British Commonwealth 77: 847–851

Parasitic, fungal and bacterial infections of the outer genitals and perigenital sites
D Petzoldt and R Schroeter

PERIGENITAL PARASITIC INFECTIONS

Scabies

Definition and pathogenesis

The causative organism is the mite *Sarcoptes scabiei*. The female mite measures 0.4 mm and can just be detected by the naked eye. It burrows in the stratum corneum, where 10–25 eggs are deposited. Afterwards the female dies. The larvae hatch after 3 or 4 days and leave the burrow. On the surface of the skin they search for new burrowing sites on the same or a new host. After about 2 weeks they reach maturity. The male mite dies soon after copulation. The whole mite population on an infested individual is, therefore, rather small, not exceeding 20 mites. Skin areas with little or no sebaceous glands are preferred: interdigital webs, wrists, elbows, anterior axillary folds, areolae of female breasts, paraumbilical region, buttocks and genitalia. Face and scalp are spared except in the infant.

Transmission is brought about mainly by close body contact, but shared clothing, bed linen, towels etc. can also be responsible for infestation. In the young adult the mites are often transmitted during sexual intercourse with the result that symptoms start and may be heaviest at the perigenital region, and other sexually transmitted diseases may coexist.

Clinical features and diagnosis

A papular eruption in typical distribution as mentioned above, intense pruritus and excoriations are the most common clinical signs of scabies. Urticae and eczematous changes are also met with. Second-ary bacterial infection in the form of impetiginisation is a quite common complication especially in children. The characteristic burrows of the mite, thin greyish ridges of 5–20 mm length, are quite diagnostic but only very seldom seen.

The very troublesome pruritus is worst at night and not restricted to the sites of infestation. It is probably caused by a sensitisation to mite antigenes, because it starts only 4–8 weeks after a first infection, but almost immediately when a reinfection occurs. It is also present in minimal scabies, which is seen in very clean persons whose other clinical signs are very inconspicuous.

In nodular scabies pruritic nodules can reach the size of a pea and are quite often situated at the perigenital region (Plate 53).

The diagnosis of scabies is made by identification of a mite, ova or faecal pellets: a drop of oil is placed on a burrow or a papule, the skin over the lesion scraped off and the scrapings placed on a microscope slide, covered with a coverslip, cleared by a drop of xylole and examined by 10 × magnification (figs 18.1, 18.2). Success depends on experience, persistence and luck. If the patient has already used antiparasitic topical agents, the search will almost always be unsuccessful. Similar symptoms in other family members, in close friends and sexual contacts are very suggestive for the diagnosis scabies.

Therapy and control

The treatment of choice is the pesticide gamma benzene hexachloride (GBH) = lindane (Gamene, Kwell, Kwellada). For an adult, 30–60 mg or 60–120 ml GBH cream or lotion are needed. After an

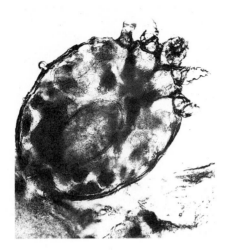

Fig. 18.1 Scabies mite on skin scrapings with egg inside.

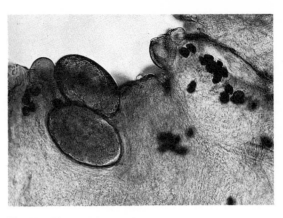

Fig. 18.2 Eggs and faecal pellets of scabies mite from papular lesion.

initial bath it must be applied to all parts of the body from the neck downwards and special care must be given to all body folds. After 24 hours it is washed off and fresh clothing and bed linen put on. The used clothes are either washed in hot water and ironed, or drycleaned, or aired for 5 days in fresh air. A second application after another week ensures the destruction of all freshly hatched larvae.

After specific treatment pruritus, eczematisation and secondary bacterial infection do not subside immediately. Topical steroids and antipruritic agents, especially in nodular scabies, are often needed for some considerable time and patients must be instructed accordingly. Otherwise they will repeat the GBH treatment over and over again, which results in generalised eczematisation of the skin.

About 10% of GBH is absorbed percutaneously and should therefore not be used in the treatment of pregnant women, nursing mothers, small children and infants. They should be treated with 6–10% precipitated sulphur in a cream or lotion base, applied nightly for 3 nights.

If mites appear resistant to GBH, alternate treatment is possible with 10% crotamiton (Eurax) for 2 nights. As described above, 24 hours after the second application clothes and bed linen are changed and treated. Sexual contacts, roommates and family members should all be considered for treatment.

Pediculosis pubis

Definition and pathogenesis

Lice infestation of the pubic hair is caused by the crab louse (*Phthirus pubis*), which favours hairy skin areas with apocrine glands. Sites of infestation in the adult are therefore the pubic region and the axillae. In heavily infested individuals the hair of the thighs and lower abdomen and also the eyelashes are involved as well.

In children before puberty only the eyelashes are infested.

Pubic lice are broader than head or body lice. With their claw-like second and third pair of legs they attach themselves firmly to the base of the hair and the adjacent skin. While feeding they inject digestive juices into the skin which causes pruritus and bluish-grey macules (taches bleues). The female lays up to 10 eggs (nits) each day, which are fastened to the hair shafts. Transmission usually occurs during sexual contact, but sometimes shared clothes, linen or towels can be responsible.

Clinical features and diagnosis

If infestation is very slight, pruritus of the affected sites will be the only symptom. In advanced cases there may be excoriations, eczematisation and secondary bacterial infection as well. Itching as a rule is not very intent and quite often the infestation is discovered by chance while an examination is carried out for some other sexually transmitted disease.

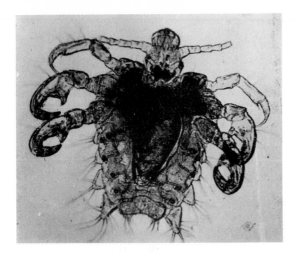

Fig. 18.3 Crab louse (*Phthirus pubis*).

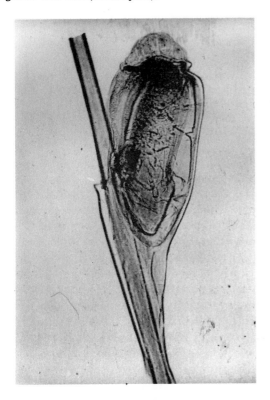

Fig. 18.4 Crab louse nit on hair shaft.

The opaque greyish lice are not easy to detect. They appear as immobile dots at the base of pubic or axillary hair (Plate 54). With the help of a magnifying glass they can be identified (Fig. 18.3). For identification of the usually quite numerous nits a hair with a nit fastened to it is examined under the microscope (Fig. 18.4). The bluish bite marks can be seen on the inside of the thighs, on the abdomen and at the side of the trunk towards the axillae.

Therapy and control

Lindane (GBH) lotion or shampoo is applied to the pubic hair area, to the perineal region and to the axillae including liberally adjacent skin areas. The lotion is washed off after 24 hours, and then fresh underwear is put on and bed linen and towels are changed. Soiled garments and linen are washed in hot water or drycleaned. Treatment should be repeated after a week. After successful treatment the lice and nits do not fall off spontaneously. The patient must be instructed to remove them with forceps or a special lice comb.

Sexual contacts must be treated as well. If there are children they must be carefully examined for infestation of the eyelashes, which need special treatment with ophthalmic ointments and mechanical removal of the lice.

Ticks

Ticks are large bloodsucking mites that live in trees and bushes. They let themselves drop on anything that moves underneath. When they happen to fall on the smooth, almost hairless human skin they usually crawl about for a while till they have found some soft skin fold or a hairy area where they can attach themselves securely. It is therefore not seldom that ticks are found inside the pubic hair region, in the umbilicus or in the groin. They are greyish-brown with a smooth surface. The fully engorged tick reaches the size of a pea (Plate 55).

When removing a tick, it is important to remove it complete with head and mouth, using forceps. It can be induced to loosen its grip when touched with a hot instrument or if suffocated by a drop of oil or some vaseline.

Ticks can transmit Rocky Mountain fever and early summer encephalitis. If a tick bite occurs in an epidemic area the appropriate passive immunisation must be considered. Ticks are also vectors of *Borrelia burgdorferi*, the causative agent of Lyme disease.

FUNGAL INFECTIONS OF THE PERIGENITAL REGION

Tinea cruris

Definition and pathogenesis

Tinea cruris is a dermatophyte infection of the groins. The species implicated are the same that cause foot ringworm disease, i.e. different species of *Trichophyton* and *Epidermophyton floccosum*. They invade only glabrous skin and do not involve the mucosa. They proliferate in the stratum corneum and may affect the terminal hairs as well. In temperate climate tinea cruris is mostly seen during hot weather and in obese persons who also suffer from tinea pedis, from where the infection of the groins takes its origin.

Clinical features and diagnosis

The lesions consist of sharply marginated areas with papules, pustules and scales along the margin, while the centre shows only slight erythema and scaling. The process usually starts at the groin and spreads slowly peripherically, eventually involving the insides of the thighs, the great labia, the gluteal folds, the rima ani and the buttocks. Patients complain of a feeling of discomfort and of more or less severe pruritus. Quite often topical steroids have been applied over long periods. In such cases itching and the inflammatory reaction are suppressed but the spread of the infection is facilitated and lesions may involve great parts of the trunk (Plate 56).

The diagnosis is made by direct and cultural examination of scales. The material is taken from the edges of the lesions after cleansing the site with surgical spirit. For microscopic examination thin pieces of scales are mounted with 10–20% potassium hydroxide (KOH) on microscope slides, covered with a coverslip and pressed gently. After a few minutes the preparation will have cleared and hyphae and arthrospores can be detected, although the differentiation from artefacts may be difficult for the inexperienced. Further material should always be sent to a mycological laboratory for cultural diagnosis.

Therapy and control

If only small areas are involved, topical measures alone will be sufficient. Regular washing of the groin with an antiseptic soap is essential. Afterwards the skin is dried carefully and an antimycotic agent applied, preferably in a liquid or powder vehicle. Preparations containing imidazole derivates (miconazole and clotrimazole) or ciclopiroloxamine have a broad range of antimycotic activity. Tolnaftate is effective against dermatophytes only. In hospitalised patients Castellani's paint can be used with good effect. The treatment must be carried out regularly till all lesions have cleared. Coexisting tinea pedis and/or unguium must be treated likewise to avoid reinfection from this focus. If large areas are involved, the systemic application of ketoconazole or griseofulvin for a few weeks will be advisable.

Prophylactic measures include improvement of personal hygiene, avoidance of synthetic undergarments and the liberal application of talcum powder to the intertrigines several times a day.

Candida intertrigo

Definition and pathogenesis

Of pathogenic yeasts the genus *Candida* and the species *Candida albicans* are the most ubiquitous. In many otherwise healthy individuals saprophytic *Candida* can be cultured from the mucous surfaces of the mouth, gastrointestinal tract and from the vagina. Under favourable conditions (broadspectrum antibiotic or systemic steroid treatment, oral contraceptives, diabetes, low general resistance etc.) parasitic growth of *Candida albicans* causes problems. A frequent complication is vaginal thrush, which is dealt with in Chapter 10. Here only the invasion of glabrous skin will be mentioned.

Glabrous skin becomes susceptible to *Candida* infection when maceration due to occlusive conditions in intertriginous areas provides the hot moisture which yeast cells prefer. Especially in the obese diabetic, vaginal thrush will tend to spread to the outer genitals involving the labia majora, the perineum, perianal region and the groin. Submammary folds, abdominal folds and axillae may also be affected.

Clinical features and diagnosis

Candida-infected intertriginous areas of glabrous skin are intensly red, erosive and oozing. Outside the more or less sharp margin to normal skin there are satellite red papules, white pustules or dried-up small lesions with a characteristic scaly fringe (Plate 57).

Diagnosis is confirmed by a Gram or methylene blue stained smear revealing the oval or round yeast cells and pseudohyphae, as well as by cultural examination. The material for the culture is taken by swab from the exudative areas and from the vagina. The faeces must also be examined by culture.

Therapy and control

Treatment starts with a hip-bath or careful washing of the intertriginous areas. Moist compresses with some disinfective agent will quickly stop the oozing. This is followed by daily application of eosin paint or aqueous gentian violet (0.5%). If paints provide problems with bed linen or undergarments, a cream or lotion containing nystatin, amphotericin or some broad-spectrum antimycotic agent (miconazole, clotrimazole) is indicated. After application clean pieces of linen are inserted between skin folds to reduce further occlusive effect and mechanical irritation of contacting skin surfaces. The coexisting vaginal and intestinal *Candida* infection must be treated appropriately. Control of diabetes must be achieved and a reduction of body weight aimed at. Systemic application of ketoconazole (Nizorale) will be helpful in controlling the infection, but the described topical measures cannot be dispensed with.

BACTERIAL INFECTIONS OF THE PERIGENITAL REGION

Folliculitis and furuncles

Definition and pathogenesis

Both conditions are staphylogenic pustular infections of hair follicles. The causative agent is coagulase-positive *Staphylococcus aureus*. The infection often takes its origin from foci in the anterior nares and the perineum.

In folliculitis only the follicle and the sebaceous gland are affected and necrosis does not occur. It is quite common in young people of seborrhoic state who may also suffer from acne vulgaris. Thighs and buttocks are predominantly involved. In furuncles the inflammation involves the perifollicular tissue with necrosis and destruction of the follicle. Obesity, warm climates, poor hygienic conditions, friction of clothes, underlying disorders such as diabetes, immunodeficiency states or malignancies may all combine to give rise to furuncles, which, however, can also occur in otherwise healthy individuals. The buttocks, groin and anogenital region are the most affected sites (Plate 58). Recurrent furunculosis poses therapeutic problems, but there is no proof that a special immunological state or phage type is implicated.

Typical carbuncles with suppuration from several follicular orifices are hardly ever seen at the perigenital region, but deep staphylogenic abscesses may develop at the buttocks or along the gluteal folds.

Deep, irregular, fistulating and extremely chronic abscesses at the groin, perineum and along the rima ani, from which a variety of pathogenic organisms can be cultured, are a symptom of acne conglobata. They are extremely rare in female patients.

Clinical features and diagnosis

Folliculitis consists of pustular nodules at the site of a hair follicle. *Staphylococcus aureus* can be cultured from the pus. The nodules heal without a scar. Furuncles start as small inflammatory dome-shaped dark red and quite painful nodules, sometimes singly but more often in crops, and develop into large perifollicular abscesses, which fluctuate, point, break and then discharge necrotic material and pus. They are always very painful and heal with a scar.

Therapy and control

Superficial folliculitis and small follicular abscesses can be controlled by improved hygienic measures and some topical antibiotic or antiseptic spiritus or lotion (Betadine). Large fluctuating boils should be incised and drained. The antibiotic sensitivity of the bacterial strain should always be assessed and in large abscesses and recurrent furunculosis systemic antibiotic treatment administered. Daily antiseptic baths and daily change of underwear and towels are indicated. Antibiotic cream should be applied to the anterior nares and the perineum to prevent reinfection from foci.

Erysipelas

Definition and pathogenesis

Erysipelas is an infection of the dermis, caused by group A streptococci, in rare exceptions by *Staphylococcus aureus*. Lymphatic vessels and lymph nodes are always involved. The organisms enter the dermis through small breaks in the skin, the reservoir of the streptococci being quite often the pharynx. In adults the most frequently involved site is the lower leg, especially if oedematous. The germs enter through lesions of foot ringworm or ulcus cruris. The outer genitals are very seldom the site of infection, but in obese diabetic women with intertrigo erysipelas develops in the adipose abdominal skin fold (Plate 59).

Clinical features and diagnosis

The disease starts abruptly with high fever, often associated with rigor and headache. The involved skin may at this time still have a normal aspect, but within hours becomes hot, painful to touch, oedematous and bright red. The erythema is irregular but sharply marginated. Small erythematous patches may appear along the lymphatic vessels; the regional lymph nodes are swollen and painful. If the outer genitals are the seat of the erysipelas the labia majora may become grossly oedematous. Vesicles and bullae can develop inside the erythematous area, which may become haemorrhagous. From the content of the bullae streptococci can be cultured, otherwise it is difficult to arrive at a cultural diagnosis.

Therapy

Erysipelas always requires systemic administration of an antibiotic. In most cases penicillin will be sufficient. Erythromycin and tetracycline are also effective. The antibiotic treatment should be carried out for at least 3 weeks to avoid recurrence. The local pain can be eased by wet compresses. The patient must stay in bed till the temperature is normalised.

A possible underlying skin condition providing the entrance site for streptococci must be attended to.

Erythrasma

Definition and pathogenesis

The causative agent is *Corynebacterium minutissimum*, that lives normally in intertriginous areas. Under favourable conditions it can change into a superficial parasite.

Clinical features

Clinical features consist in almost symptomless reddish-brown or light brown, sharply marginated and slightly scaling plaques. The groin and axillae are predominantly involved (Plate 60). When viewed under Wood's light the lesions show a characteristic scarlet fluorescence. Culture of the organisms is rather difficult and normally not necessary for diagnosis.

Treatment

Keratolytic ointments, spirits containing sulphur and acetyl salicylic acid or an ointment containing erythromycin will clear the lesions quickly. If large areas are affected, erythromycin or tetracycline may be given systemically for 2 weeks.

Intertrigo

Definition and pathogenesis

Intertrigo is primarily a non-infectious dermatitis of large body folds, where skin surfaces rub together. Predisposing factors are obesity, hot weather and poor personal hygiene. Permanent friction, moist heat and the retention of cutaneous excretions cause inflammation, maceration and later bacterial and mycotic secondary infection. Inguinal, abdominal and submammary folds are principally involved.

Clinical features

The process starts as a pruritic irritation in intertriginous areas. When fully developed intertrigo presents as a sharply marginated, erosive and oozing erythema, which may be covered by crusts and vegetating masses. The lesions are restricted to the areas where skin surfaces touch (Plate 61). If they spread beyond or if satellite lesions on non-intertriginous skin develop, secondary fungal or bacterial infections must be taken into consideration.

Therapy and control

The intertrigines must be washed or bathed twice daily with some mild antiseptic, such as Betadine (Povidone Iodine). Afterwards careful drying, preferably with an electric fan, is essential. On oozing areas tap water soaks are applied several times daily for a few days, and later treated with some antiseptic lotion gel or spray. Non-erosive areas are powdered freely. Pieces of linen are put between the folds to prevent further friction.

For prophylaxis the patient should be instructed to wear wide and comfortable clothes which are not made of synthetic fibres or wool. Hygienic measures must be improved and body weight reduced.

Simple intertrigo must be differentiated from Candida intertrigo, tinea cruris and erythrasma, as well as from other non-infectious dermatoses that may at times involve body folds, such as seborrhoic dermatitis, psoriasis, atopic dermatitis, contact dermatitis and pemphigus.

REFERENCES

Arndt K A 1978 Manual of dermatologic therapeutics with essentials of diagnosis, 2nd edn. Little, Brown, Boston

Behrman H T, Labow T A, Rozen J H 1978 Common skin diseases, diagnoses and treatment, 3rd edn. Grune & Stratton, New York

Maddin S 1982 Current dermatologic therapy. W B Saunders, Philadelphia

Rook A, Wilkinson D S, Ebling F J G 1979 Textbook of dermatology, 3rd edn. Blackwell Scientific Publications, Oxford

PART V

Effects and consequences of genital infection

Psychological aspects of female genital tract infections
P Slade

INTRODUCTION

All physical conditions occur within a psychosocial context and emotional distress may operate as a contributory aetiological factor, concomitant and/or consequence of infectious disease. In genital tract infections the involvement of psychological factors may be highly significant because of the recurrent nature of many of these conditions, their implications for psychological adjustment, self-esteem and sexual functioning. The possibility of serious long-term consequences, such as infertility or chronic abdominal pain, also arises. Optimal care of the patient with genital tract infection requires recognition of the importance of these considerations and their implications for treatment.

PSYCHOSOCIAL FACTORS IN SUSCEPTIBILITY TO INFECTIOUS DISEASE

It is now recognised that the development of an infection is not the inevitable consequence of exposure to a pathogen. Although the particular bacterial and viral agents causing genital tract infection have not been the main focus of study in this area, results indicate that only a percentage of individuals exposed to a pathogen show evidence of colonisation and only a percentage of those colonised subsequently become ill. Cornfeld & Hubbard (1961), for example, indicated that only 20–40% of individuals colonised with streptococci subsequently became ill. Similarly, Totman & Kiff (1979) reported that the development of cold symptoms was not the inevitable consequence of the experimental inoculation of volunteers with two rhinoviruses. Considerable individual differences exist in suscep-

tibility to infection and it is likely that this variability also applies to the range of pathognomonic agents causing female genital tract infection.

This variability is presumed to be mediated by the effectiveness of the individual's immune system. Jemmott & Locke (1984) and many previous authors have indicated that the functioning of the immune system is influenced by psychosocial variable. Although research in this complex area is still in its infancy, the impact of several factors which are presumed to be associated with stress has been subject to specific scrutiny. These factors have included the effects of bereavement, life changes, examinations and psychological vulnerability. Most studies in this area have not focused on genital tract infections and a general review is beyond the scope of this chapter. The limited evidence specific to genital tract infection will be described in detail.

Aetiological factors in the development and recurrence of the herpes simplex virus and other genital tract infections

Herpes simplex virus occurs in two variant forms—type I, which generally produces lesions on facial sites, and type II which usually affects genital sites (Nahmias & Roizman 1973). After the initial infection a phase of latency occurs when no symptoms are apparent. The active phase generally recurs but the frequency of recurrence varies considerably in different individuals. Luby & Klinge (1985) reported a range of 0 to 35 recurrences of genital herpes in a 12-month period. The factors which trigger recurrence are still unclear but it is of interest that more than 50% of a group of sufferers viewed emotional stress as an important precipitant in their own cases (Guinan et al 1981).

Watson (1983) studied the relationship between

undesirable life stress and recurrence of herpes symptoms. The Life Experiences Survey—a list of events including items such as deaths or illness in family or friends, employment changes, financial and relationship difficulties—was used to assess events occurring in the year preceding interview. A significant correlation was found between this measure and the number of recurrences in the previous 6 months.

In this study a measure of locus of control was also considered. This concept, developed by Rotter (1966), suggests that individuals can be assessed on the degree to which they perceive themselves as exerting control over their own lives. Individuals who view their lives as controlled by others or by fortune are considered to show external locus of control, while those who view themselves as the main architect of their experience are considered to show internal locus of control. The latter category is generally considered to be associated with better psychological adjustment. Watson reported that an internal locus of control moderated the effects of undesirable life stress on recurrence rates. Those individuals with high levels of life stress and external locus of control showed higher frequencies of recurrence than individuals experiencing similar life stress with internal locus of control. Unfortunately, the direction of causation is unclear, as high recurrence rates could theoretically increase the probability that sufferers viewed themselves as lacking in control over their own lives. Finally, high levels of social support were also associated with lower recurrence rates and may therefore operate as a protective factor.

In evaluating this study it is important to recognise that a correlation coefficient of 0.32 between life events and recurrence rate indicates that only 9% of the variance in the latter is accounted for by this factor. The use of self-report techniques as opposed to structured interviewing in order to obtain a reliable measure of life change has been criticised on the grounds of lack of objectivity, as the individual concerned decides whether an event has occurred (Paykel 1983). Guinan et al (1981) reported that herpes sufferers believed emotional stress was often an important precipitating factor in their recurrences. When this is the case self-report measures are likely to be subject to artificial elevation through the process of 'effort after meaning'

(Brown & Harris 1978). This suggests that individuals who are suffering from some unpleasant condition or state will seek explanations for their difficulties and hence may report higher frequencies of stresses.

Williams & Deffenbacher (1983) considered the relationship between yeast infections as diagnosed in routine gynaecological screenings and life events. The Life Experiences Survey and a questionnaire concerning experiences with yeast infections were completed. Negative life change, while not related to the current presence or absence of infection at the time of assessment, was positively correlated with the reported number of yeast infections in the previous year, level of concern about these infections and the number of visits made to a physician on account of this complaint. These differences could not be accounted for by differential use of antibiotics or oral contraceptives.

One final study of stress and infection is reported by McGuire et al (1980). Groups with and without evidence of non-specific vaginitis who were symptomatic and asymptomatic were compared using a life stress scale. No differences were found between the groups. However, in this study only an absolute categorisation of presence or absence of infection was made with no estimate of frequency of recurrence. Where significant effects have been reported the association appears to be with the latter type of measure.

The role of personality variables in predicting frequency of recurrence of genital tract infections has received scant attention. However, Stout (1984) reported that sufferers from genital herpes showing high recurrence rates differed from those with low recurrence on several dimensions of the Minnesota Multiphasic Personality Inventory. This is a scale which assesses a range of different features of personality. Stout suggests that the pattern shown by the high recurrers is one which is consistent with a state of increased autonomic arousal, which may imply that an individual was functioning under a high level of stress.

Although these studies are all clearly limited in scope and suffer from methodological weaknesses, particularly in the assessment of life events, there are some suggestions that psychological factors may play some aetiological role, particularly in rate of recurrence of infections. The fact that recurrence rate rather than specific occurrence appears to be a more sensitive measure in this context may suggest that it is the cumulative effect of life changes that is important rather than a recurrence occurring as a specific response to a stressful experience. Such issues await prospective longitudinal studies for resolution.

REACTIONS TO GENITAL HERPES AND OTHER GENITAL TRACT INFECTIONS

Most studies concerning reactions to genital tract infections have focused on the specific condition of genital herpes.

Individuals suffering with genital herpes are required to cope not only with the physical discomfort of the condition but also with the knowledge that they are an infected individual, that recurrence is likely, unpredictable and beyond their control and that their sexual relationships now carry the potential for infecting others. These factors may carry negative implications for an individual's self-esteem, sexual adjustment and personal relationships. The fact that initial infection often occurs in late adolescence or early adulthood when psychological development is still progressing and relationships are formative and vulnerable may increase the potential negative impact of this condition on the individual.

At an anecdotal level, Luby & Gillespie (1981) have described a sequence of responses to herpes which sometimes occurs.

1. Initial shock and emotional numbing.
2. A frantic search for an immediate cure.
3. A sense of isolation and loneliness as the person becomes aware of the chronicity of the disease.
4. Anger directed at the person who is the source of the infection.
5. Fear about the consequences of the disease upon sexuality.
6. A leper effect with feelings of ugliness.
7. Feelings of depression.
8. Reactivation of underlying psychopathology in rare cases.

This model at present remains unsubstantiated and the few systematic studies of reactions to herpes tend to indicate a less detrimental effect on psychological, social and sexual functioning than has generally been predicted.

Knowlton (1984) studied levels of anger in herpes sufferers. There were no differences between sufferers and a control group on a trait measure of anger. This is considered to be a stable measure of personality which does not alter with time. However, the herpetic group showed an elevation of 'state' anger: a measure of the current level of anger. It is likely that although the groups may not differ in their general tendency to become angry, anger may be a common reaction to this diagnosis.

Shaw (1984) compared women with recurrent (defined as in excess of 6 months) genital herpes with *Haemophilus* and trichomoniasis patients and a non-infected control group. Using the Minnesota Multiphasic Personality Inventory the groups did not differ on levels of depression, anxiety or social withdrawal. However, the herpetic group reported a significantly lower level of sexual satisfaction. Unfortunately, sample sizes in this study were small.

Luby & Klinge (1985) reported results from 74 genital herpes sufferers who completed an extensive questionnaire concerning the impact of this infection on their lives. Herpes had not interfered greatly with work performance, with relationships with colleagues or social situations with friends or new acquaintances of the same sex. Satisfaction and enjoyment of work were slightly impaired. The effect of herpes was felt most acutely in the area of sexual relationships, with more than half the subjects reporting significantly reduced sexual pleasure and inhibited sexual freedom. Two-thirds reported fears of transmitting herpes to others. There was general pessimism about ever establishing normal relationships and many individuals reported considerable worry about future rejections when prospective partners learned of their herpes. Psychological distress, when it was reported, was clearly linked to specific sexual concerns; the development of specific sexual functioning difficulties; reductions in feelings of sexual pleasure and a feeling of undesirability. Psychological distress was also particularly related to feelings of lack of control over herpes symptoms and uncertainty about when an individual is contagious. It is of interest that there were no significant sex differences in the perceived effects of herpes. While this is the most extensive psychological study of herpes sufferers presently available, it must be noted that the sample was primarily drawn from a self-help centre. This group may differ significantly in many ways from the typical sufferer. Only 17% of the sample believed their adjustment to their disease was poor and it is possible that individuals who are clearly making active attempts to cope with their difficulties may show lower levels of distress and dysfunction than other sufferers.

Herpes is already the second most common sexually transmitted disease (STD) (Schwab 1982) and is said to be rapidly becoming the first. The limited data available indicate the infection exerts a specific negative impact on sexual adjustment and that psychological distress is often linked to a perceived lack of control. The former finding confirms results reported from studies of patients attending STD clinics. Catalan et al (1981) interviewed new attenders at an STD clinic and one-third of women reported they had recently experienced at least one form of sexual dysfunction which they considered to be a problem. This most commonly took the form of coital orgasmic dysfunction but loss of libido and dyspareunia were also reported. Almost all women who felt their sexual dysfunction constituted a problem wanted professional help to deal with their difficulty. It is of interest that females reporting sexual dysfunction were particularly likely to be categorised as psychiatric cases, with the most common symptoms being anxiety and depression. Many of the females studied had attended the clinic because they had been traced as contacts and on testing half were given no clinical diagnosis. Those without diagnoses did not show reduced levels of sexual dysfunction and indeed records by the venereologist were significantly more likely to note sexual or psychological problems for this group. It is unclear whether a population at risk of STD is essentially one with high levels of sexual dysfunction or whether the knowledge of the possibility of infection acted as a precipitant. As details of the timing of the onset of dysfunction are not provided this is impossible to evaluate. If the latter hypothesis is correct then the knowledge of absence of infection may resolve sexual difficulties spontaneously. Certainly a higher frequency of sexual difficulty was reported by this clinic sample than in

a general gynaecological outpatient clinic (Levine & Yost 1976) or in a family planning clinic (Begg et al 1976).

McGuire et al (1980) have suggested that presentation at a gynaecology clinic or STD clinic with symptoms of vaginitis without evidence of infection may be indicative of dissatisfaction with sexual functioning. Physical causes may be being utilised as an explanation of poor sexual relationships. Women complaining of abnormal vaginal discharge, vulval irritation or introital dyspareunia were compared with other attenders who did not report these complaints. Subjects were categorised as clinically normal or abnormal on the basis of vaginal and cervical examination. Women who were complaining of vaginitis symptoms but who showed no clinical abnormality reported more problems in sexual relationships than their symptomatic but clinically abnormal counterparts. They also indicated that their vaginitis symptoms tended to interfere more with their sexual frequency, lead to shorter duration of intercourse and reduced libido more commonly than the clinically abnormal group. In addition, symptomatic groups as a whole showed poorer marital adjustment than the asymptomatic groups. One incongruous finding was that the symptomatic but clinically normal groups reported the greatest ease of obtaining orgasm. In general this report would tentatively support suggestions by Catalan et al (1981) that absence of clinical findings in women presenting for treatment of infections may be associated with increased levels of sexual problems in women. However, it also appears that, in general, those women in whom there is clear clinical evidence of some form of genital tract infection also show an elevated frequency of sexual problems, probably as a response to their condition. Psychological methods of coping with the problem of infection may influence the frequency of such reactions and influence psychological adjustment.

Coping with genital herpes

Coping can be defined as 'any and all responses made by an individual who encounters a potentially harmful outcome'. Two major functions of coping have been identified; coping that is directed at managing or changing the source of stress, which is known as problem-focused coping; and coping that is directed towards managing the emotional response to the problem, known as emotion-focused coping (Folkman & Lazarus 1980). It has been suggested that emotion rather than problem-focused coping may be more relevant in health problems, as attempting to change the disease process through action may often be unrealistic and lead to repeated experience of failure. Specifically, disease management strategies such as seeking numerous different medical and non-medical opinions and using a variety of different medications and treatments would be included in this category. When a disease is essentially incurable, as in the case of genital herpes, such attempts may lead to repeated patterns of raised hope followed by disillusion and a gradual development of feelings of helplessness.

There are a wide variety of additional coping strategies which individuals may use when faced with difficulties. These include wishful thinking, which usually involves unrealistic assessments such as hoping that the infection will magically disappear, or daydreaming that in reality one is infection-free. Eliciting social support is another common strategy. This involves finding situations in which it is possible to talk over intimate problems in an accepting non-critical atmosphere and can involve either friends or family.

The use of blame can also be a reaction to adversity. Individuals may show internal or external patterns of causal attribution. External attribution would be exemplified by blaming the individual from whom the infection had been contracted. Self-blame or internal attribution is more complex. It can take the form of 'characterological self-blame' where individuals view themselves as responsible as a result of some global, constitutional, unmodifiable trait of character, as exemplified by the statement 'I have herpes because I am loose and promiscuous'. Alternatively, self-blame can be characterised as 'behavioural self-blame', in which case the responsibility is seen as due to some specific modifiable behavioural deficit which does not imply pervasive self-criticism. An example in this context would be 'I have caught herpes because I acted impulsively on that occasion'. The former type of self-blame is all encompassing, while the latter relates shortcomings to a specific negligent behaviour.

Finally, individuals often develop specific patterns of thinking about their illness involving a high frequency of stressful cognitions focusing upon the negative aspects of a situation. Alternatively positive thoughts which attempt to generate a more optimistic view can be utilised. The latter differ from wishful thinking in being located in reality rather than incorporating a daydream-like escapist quality.

Manne & Sandler (1984) have systematically investigated how herpes sufferers attempt to cope with their infection and how the different strategies may be associated with psychological adjustment. The majority of the sample of 152 subjects studied were drawn from self-help groups. It is likely that this feature of sample selection limits the general applicability of the results to all sufferers. The authors assessed the usage of all the methods of coping previously detailed, together with measures of self-esteem, sexual problems, depression and the degree to which the subject was bothered by having herpes. A single overall adjustment measure was created by summing these last four variables. The severity of the physical condition was assessed using measures of number of recurrences per year, durations of outbreaks and length of infection in years.

Psychological adjustment was not associated with the severity of the condition in terms of number or duration of outbreaks. In addition, the longer the subjects had suffered with herpes the lower the level of depression and the less bothered they were by herpes. Those who perceived themselves as having high levels of social support from others showed higher self-esteem. Perceived helpfulness of others was associated with fewer sexual problems and better overall adjustment.

High levels of depression were associated with perceiving others as holding negative attitudes towards oneself, using frequent disease management strategies and characterological self-blame. Wishful thinking, high levels of stressful thoughts, blame directed to the person who had caused the infection were all associated with psychological maladjustment. Behavioural self-blame was not associated with negative psychological variables. The authors also confirmed other research which suggests that females are not more adversely affected psychologically than males.

It is of interest that the coping variables accounted for 51% of the variation in psychological adjustment, with the use of stressful thoughts being the most powerful predictor of negative outcome. Wishful thinking and the absence of social support also made significant contributions. In contrast the severity and length of infection accounted for under 2% of the variance in overall adjustment.

Implication for treatment

Although Manne & Sandler (1984) have highlighted particular strategies which are associated with poor psychological adjustment, the direction of causation in unclear. It is premature to state categorically that modification of certain coping strategies and the encouragement of alternatives may enhance adjustment and treatment studies are awaited.

However Manne & Sandler's study raises potential intervention strategies for serious consideration. High frequencies of stressful thoughts or wishful thinking appear to be maladaptive. A clinical psychologist might initially assist the sufferer to identify these particular thought patterns through the self-monitoring of cognitions. This could be followed by the development of distraction techniques or the practice of substitution by alternative positive thoughts. Characterological self-blame or external attributions could be highlighted and converted to behavioural self-blame, which may be less self-destructive. Further use of disease management strategies could be discouraged by highlighting the destructive repeating cycle of hope and disillusion and the futility of attempting to control an outcome which is essentially uncontrollable at our present level of knowledge.

Levels of social support could be enhanced by the development of more self-help groups in which mutual support and a reduction in any sense of isolation could be effected. Woddis (1983) recently provided a descriptive report on the workings of such a group. The association between perceiving others as cold or blaming and depression may im-

ply the need for staff to evaluate their own attitudes and non-verbal behaviour in the care of these patients. A warm non-critical atmosphere is clearly important. Perception of attitudes of others is subjective and no objective ratings of behaviour have yet substantiated the relationship between these measures.

The PLISSIT model (Annon 1976) may also be of value for herpes sufferers. This treatment involves the provision of Permission, Limited Information, Specific Suggestions and if necessary referral for Intensive Therapy. Permission is given to ventilate anger, guilt, depression or frustration. Discussion of feelings is encouraged and acceptance of these as a normal consequence is made explicit. The limited information consists of providing details of the incidence, signs and symptoms of genital herpes and information about when an individual is likely to be infectious. Details of the association with cervical cancer and the possibility of obstetric complications in future pregnancy would also be provided. The importance of adequate information has been highlighted by several studies. Luby & Klinge (1985) particularly noted that fear of transmitting herpes was a very common anxiety. However Guinan et al (1981), when studying the course of untreated cases, have clearly shown that infectiousness in the absence of visible lesions is extremely rare. This information would provide useful reassurance to sufferers.

Specific suggestions consist of advising the patient to make frequent observations of the genital area for detection of recurrence, the avoidance of sexual activity during recurrence, the need for regular cervical smears and the necessity of informing obstetricians about the history of the condition. The importance of communication about the condition with current and future partners would also be stressed. Methods of achieving this, with the possibility of role-playing alternative strategies, could also be considered.

Again the efficacy of this model in reducing psychological distress and sexual dysfunction remains to be assessed. The models presented are not mutually exclusive and combinations of elements may be most effective. Psychological intervention may offer considerable potential for improving psychological adjustment to this condition.

BEHAVIOURAL PATTERNS IN THE AETIOLOGY OF GENITAL TRACT INFECTIONS AND METHODS OF MODIFICATION

Behavioural patterns in aetiology

Sweet & Gibbs (1985) suggest there is currently an epidemic of STDs. They suggest that this primary epidemic is resulting in a secondary epidemic of pelvic inflammatory disease with its common consequence of chronic abdominal pain and a tertiary epidemic of infertility due to tubal factors. These long-term sequelae may lead to adverse psychological reactions and these, together with implications for intervention, will be considered in detail in subsequent sections.

Women with multiple sexual partners have been shown to experience a 4.6 times increased risk of developing acute salpingitis, compared to those in monogamous relationships (Eschenbach 1980). The same author reported that women who have a previous episode of pelvic inflammatory disease are more likely to suffer subsequent infections. Contraceptive methods used also influence risk, with oral contraceptives, diaphragms and condoms providing some protection, while the use of intrauterine devices increases the risk of infection up to 13-fold dependent upon type of construction (Sweet & Gibbs 1985).

The high level of risk in adolescents is of particular concern, with Weström (1980) reporting that 70% of salpingitis cases were younger than 25 years of age; 33% experienced their first episode before the age of 19 years. In view of implications for fertility, the fact that 75% were nulliparous must lead to anxiety. The risk of a sexually active adolescent developing acute pelvic inflammatory disease was estimated as one in eight.

Weström (1975) conducted a longitudinal study of women with laparascope-confirmed salpingitis. Despite antibiotic therapy, patients with at least one episode showed a 21% rate of infertility compared with 3% in a control group. With a single episode, risk to fertility was 11% rising to 34% for two episodes and 54% after three or more episodes.

While Sweet & Gibbs (1985) justifiably state: 'In order to prevent the significant economic and medical sequelae of pelvic inflammatory disease methods of prevention and treatment must be developed which are based upon the microbiologic aetiology of the disease', methods which would promote behavioural changes to reduce risk factors would also be worthy of attention. The behavioural changes to be promoted would focus on minimising numbers of sexual partners and encouraging the use of contraceptive techniques which afford protection against infection. The main target population would be the adolescent female who is at present jeopardising her future fertility.

Preventive behaviour and the health belief model

Physicians are in contact with the at-risk population in general practice, at family planning clinics and in school health settings. Given the substantial rise in risk to fertility with more than one episode of infection, promotion of behavioural change within the gynaecology clinic at first infection is also of value.

The factors which determine preventive health care behaviour have been encompassed in the Health Belief Model (Becker & Maiman 1975). Readiness to take action is postulated to be determined by: an individual's perceived vulnerability to a particular condition; the perceived severity of that condition; her evaluation of the feasibility, effectiveness and benefits of the proposed action weighed against her perception of its physical, psychological and financial costs. Finally, some 'cue to action' must occur.

Application of the model in reducing the risk of pelvic inflammatory disease

In order for a women to perceive her vulnerability she must be aware of the link between multiple sexual partners, certain contraceptive practices and pelvic infection and infertility. She must then view herself as 'at risk'. The links could be made more routinely explicit in health care settings in general and in specific clinical contacts for contraceptive advice, abortion counselling or when general minor gynaecological or urinary symptoms are reported. Easy-to-recall figures of relative risks concerning numbers of sexual partners over defined durations of time would help individuals to assess their vulnerability. Unfortunately the latter is not a simple process and mechanisms such as denial can operate even where adequate information has been provided.

The woman must also perceive the possibility of infertility as a serious consequence for her. Most women in late adolescence do ultimately foresee themselves having children but the importance of this factor at that stage will vary considerably. However, outlining the difficulties in conception which can result from tubal blockage together with the complex and painful treatments which many women choose to endure and the psychological distress that infertility can cause may influence an individual's perception of the severity of such an outcome. It is important at this stage that levels of anxiety induced are carefully visually monitored. While low levels of perceived severity provide insufficient motivation for change there is evidence to suggest that very high levels of perceived seriousness are inhibitory and are also associated with a low likelihood of taking preventive health care action (Leventhal et al 1965).

The feasibility, effectiveness, benefits and costs of the behavioural changes required will depend upon many factors. The feasibility of reducing the number of sexual partners would depend on the individual's powers of self-control, assertiveness and ability to recognise precipitating factors leading to casual sexual encounters. The feasibility of using contraceptive methods reliably may depend on her readiness to accept herself as a sexually active female, as lack of preparedness can be related to denial of this reality. Medical practitioners could provide information concerning the effectiveness of these behavioural changes in reducing relative risk of infection and subsequence infertility.

The benefits and the costs to the individual could depend upon a wide range of issues which may include a woman's own satisfaction with her sexual lifestyle, whether she wished to alter this for other reasons, the importance of frequent sexual contact for the relief of sexual tension and the fear of rejection from potential partners if a relationship were established on a non-sexual basis during its initial phase. Compliance with contraceptive recommendations may require greater organisation, planning and a decrease in spontaneity and even in some cases decreased reliability if an intrauterine device was being replaced by other methods.

Finally, the 'cue to action' could be a stimulus provided by a medical practitioner stating concern about risks involved.

While it is important that new methods for control of infection are developed, the potential role of the medical practitioner as educator and as a valuable resource in the generation of behavioural changes leading to more adequate preventive health care by patients should not be underestimated.

INFERTILITY

Infertility, defined as failure to conceive within a year of unprotected sexual intercourse, is well recognised as a potential consequence of pelvic inflammatory disease. Collins et al (1984) reported that tubal dysfunction was one of the best indicators of poor prognosis in an infertility sample. The introduction of in vitro fertilisation techniques have generated new hopes for these couples but with its limited availability and low success rates many couples must learn to cope with this limitation of their natural functioning.

Infertility can affect the psychological adjustment of the individual and also have impact on the marital and sexual relationship of the couple. Psychological studies, in a search for aetiological factors, have often focused upon infertile groups where there is no clear physical cause. These studies are beyond the scope of this chapter. Only rarely have couples with a specific type of physical abnormality been studied. In general all attenders at infertility clinics are sampled regardless of type and presence or absence of diagnosis. Where differences can be shown between infertile and control groups it is often impossible to assess whether these antecede the problem of infertility and may be considered as contributory aetiological factors or whether they occur as reactions to infertility.

The emotional impact of infertility

There are numerous anecdotal reports concerning reactions to infertility. Unfortunately few provide substantive evidence for their models and their hypotheses will therefore be considered with brevity.

Anecdotal studies have tended to view infertility

within the framework of a life crisis requiring adjustment to several different experiences of loss. These have included the loss of a child never conceived, the loss of control over the course of life, the loss of a particularly socially acceptable role (Kraft et al 1980; McCormick 1980; Daniels et al 1984; Leader et al 1984; Mahlstedt 1985). Reactions are conceptualised to occur within a grieving process with detectable sequential stages of adjustment characterised by different emotions. Mazor (1979) and Menning (1982) both indicate an initial reaction of shock, surprise, disbelief and even denial. This may be accompanied by a lowering of self-confidence and a feeling of defectiveness. Menning suggests this phase is often followed by one of grieving which is likely to involve the experience of anger, isolation, guilt and depression. A third phase of resolution is said to occur when the couple are ready to consider constructively alternative courses of action such as child-free living, adoption or fostering. No indications of the expected time scale of this process nor the potential for differential effects on the sexes are suggested. It must be noted that the proponents of this theoretical framework provide only anecdotal evidence in support of this model of adaptation.

Wilson (1979) reports one of the few studies which have used a longitudinal design to consider the psychological effects of infertility. Prior to first clinic attendance, patients were asked to report on emotional problems caused by their infertility and were then reassessed 4 months later. Although information from 41 patients was obtained and Wilson claims to have delineated a typical pattern of response, actual data are not presented and it is difficult to assess the validity of the findings. Wilson claims that from the time of first recognising a fertility problem to the time, following initial investigation and treatment, when it becomes clear to the patient that a pregnancy is not forthcoming, the following sequence occurs: stage 1—disbelief and denial; stage 2—depression, anger and altered self-image; stage 3—optimism, often at the stage of consulting a physician; stage 4—desperation when after initial investigation attempts to become pregnant have not been successful; stage 5— depression when absolute causes for infertility are encountered, and stage 6—acceptance which is aided by knowing the cause for infertility and that

attempts to correct the cause have been made.

It is unfortunate that data are not presented to substantiate this model and it is unclear how the later stages were derived if follow-ups occurred only over 4 months. No natural time scale is indicated by the author, nor is consideration given to factors which may influence levels of distress or speed resolution. According to this model, women suffering from tubal dysfunction would be likely to be focused in stage 5 of depression when an absolute cause for infertility had been established. Progress to stage 6 would be hypothesised to occur fairly rapidly if acceptance and resolution are aided by knowing the cause rather than coping with uncertainty.

These hypotheses were not substantiated by Lalos et al (1985) who monitored the emotional status of 24 infertile couples before and 2 years after unsuccessful surgical treatment of tubal infertility. Female partners reported more emotional effects than men both prior to surgery and after 2 years but there was no significant change in overall symptomatology in either sex over that time. Specific feelings of grief were reported in 90% of women pre- and postsurgery. However, there was a dramatic rise in feelings of grief in male partners from 50% presurgery to more than 90% at follow-up. Even 2 years after the operation a considerable proportion of the women were experiencing symptoms of irritability, fatigue, depression and restlessness. The most notable feature of the study is the stability of the complaints and the lack of any evidence of resolution. This must question the concept of a natural sequential process and raise the spectre that the experience of psychological symptoms resulting from infertility may not be time-limited but induce a chronic state of emotional distress.

Raval (1986), utilising a cross-sectional design, reported that duration of infertility, duration of treatment and duration of time since diagnosis did not predict emotional distress in either males or females. However, the mean treatment period was again 4 months and possibly this is too short a time to demonstrate phasic effects. It is of interest that both sexes reported an increase in negative emotions when they recognised the presence of a fertility problem but in general a positive change occurred as a result of treatment. These changes were more pronounced in females. These findings would tentatively support Wilson's early stages of depression followed by initial optimism during treatment.

Experimental studies suggest that infertility may adversely affect an individual's sense of control over his or her life (Platt et al 1973; Sklar 1984). There are also suggestions from comparisons between infertile and control groups that self-esteem may be adversely affected (Freeman et al 1983; Platt et al 1973) although this is not invariably supported (Adler & Boxley 1985).

Although high levels of emotional distress have been reported in infertile couples it is unclear whether factors such as anxiety and depression are significantly elevated when compared with control groups of fertile individuals (Freeman et al 1983; Adler & Boxley 1985).

In summary, the hypothesis that infertile couples progress through predictable stages of adjustment still requires experimental verification through longitudinal studies. At present the limited evidence available may indicate that adequate resolution is not necessarily achieved, even after a 2-year duration. Although there is evidence that infertile couples feel less in control of their lives, that self-esteem can be adversely affected and that symptoms of anxiety and depression are common, it is unclear which factors may be useful predictors of adverse psychological reactions. There have been tentative suggestions that women may be more affected than their partners (Sklar 1984; Lalos et al 1985), that psychological dysfunction may reside more commonly with the partner free from organic pathology (Bell 1981) and that personal qualities characterised as more feminine and emotional as opposed to masculine and assertive may be associated with poorer adjustment in both sexes (Adler & Boxley 1985). The value of these variables as predictors remains to be substantiated.

Impact of infertility on the marital relationship

The infertile couple are confronted with a difficulty in achieving an important life goal. As a result of this it has been suggested that the quality of the marital relationship may be affected. Shapiro (1982) suggests that feelings of guilt can often cause serious marital rifts and there may even be subtle

encouragement from the infertile partner for the fertile spouse to seek other relationships. Mahlstedt (1985) indicates that couples may become polarised because of differences in their methods of coping with crisis, with a tendency for emotional outbursts in the female paralleled by repression of reactions in the male. She suggests these differential patterns can result in marital stress.

Systematic studies of the impact of infertility on the marriage are rare. Carr (1963) reported that marital adjustment did not differ between infertile and control groups. However, Bell (1981) indicated that 7 of 20 couples reported that the crisis of infertility was associated with a deterioration in the marital relationship. As half the subjects in this study were interviewed at the initiation of treatment and half during its progression it was not clear at which stage these negative changes prevailed. Lalos et al (1985) compared couples prior to surgical treatment for tubal dysfunction and 2 years later. They indicated that, in general, partners' feelings for each other had worsened over that time and their views on the marriage were also less favourable. All women prior to the operation reported they 'loved their partner very much' whereas 2 years later fewer than two-thirds affirmed that statement. The majority of participants also reported feeling they could not show their sadness and disappointment openly before their partners.

While infertility may cause stress within the marital relationship, it is likely that different couples respond in different ways. It is possible that some couples may become closer as they face this adversity together while other relationships may disintegrate. Again it is important that future research should try to identify couples most at risk of adverse reactions so that therapeutic help could be offered at an early stage.

The impact of infertility on sexual functioning

There are many anecdotal reports (Elstein 1975; Keye 1984) and case studies (Bullock 1974) which indicate that the experience of infertility can adversely affect sexual functioning both in satisfaction and performance. Keye (1984) suggests the effects can be divided into those mediated by psychological responses to infertility and those which are the function of treatment procedures.

The former may involve feelings of defectiveness and inadequacy which may lead to feelings of being sexually unattractive and undesirable. These reactions may cause decreased libido and decreased capacity to respond sexually.

Aspects of treatment such as coital charting and recording of basal body temperatures can lead to pressure for 'sex on schedule'. The process may become very mechanical, purely oriented towards procreation with the result that the function of mutual pleasuring is lost. Husbands may become irritated by their wives' wishes for intercourse around ovulation and their subsequent phases of lack of interest. The postcoital test is perhaps the most extreme example of a normally pleasant and private function being performed on schedule for scrutiny and evaluation by a third party.

While these observations have obvious face validity as reactions to infertility and to some treatment procedures, their occurrence is not always well established by systematic study. Keye & Deneris (1983) reported that although many couples attributed many of their sexual dissatisfactions to their infertility, the actual prevalence of sexual dysfunction (inhibited sexual desire, anorgasmia, impotence, premature or delayed ejaculation) was not significantly affected by infertility. Similarly, Raval (1986) reported no greater prevalence of sexual dysfunction in an infertile group than in a group of general practice attenders.

However, many patients, particularly the female partners, believe infertility has an adverse effect on their sexual functioning. Bell (1981) found that 4 of 20 female partners and 1 of 20 males reported the development of secondary sexual problems, Lalos et al (1985), in their longitudinal study of tubal dysfunction patients, found female partners were significantly less satisfied with their sexual relationships 2 years after surgical intervention, whereas male partners showed no equivalent change.

The specific impact of the postcoital test has been subject to scrutiny and 10% of males were found to suffer from impotence or ejaculatory failure as a response to this specific situational stress (Drake & Grunert 1979). There was also a tendency in this group for similar dysfunction to occur around ovulation, while sexual functioning at other stages of the cycle was generally normal. De Vries et al (1984) reported reduced foreplay in intercourse conducted for postcoital testing and reduced frequency of orgasm in women under those circumstances. There was no clear evidence to indicate that this reaction generalised beyond this specific situation but it is of interest that there was a positive association between the woman's feeling of closeness to her partner and the adequacy of the postcoital test. Possibly, the creation of any artificiality within a sexual relationship may eventually prove to be detrimental to fertility in physiological terms.

In summary, while infertile groups in general may not experience higher rates of specific sexual dysfunctioning some couples are likely to develop difficulties which they attribute to their condition. Aspects of current treatment may increase the frequency of adverse effects.

Implications for the care of the infertile couple

Keye (1984) reports suggestions for care derived from a survey of infertility patients. These ideas can be roughly divided into those assisting general psychological adaptation to the crisis of infertility and those specifically directed towards minimising adverse marital and sexual reactions.

In the former category, suggestions included the routine discussion of common psychological, sexual and social problems which may accompany infertility. This would enable couples to recognise and accept some difficulties as normal reactions. When people view their responses as unusual or abnormal this itself can increase anxiety and feelings of isolation. It was recommended that evaluation and treatment should proceed at a rate with which the couple felt comfortable rather than adhering to a standardised schedule. In addition, it was recommended that each step should be discussed in detail with the couple before implementation. There was strong feeling that one partner should never be specifically blamed for infertility and that any abnormal findings should be described in objective and non-judgmental ways.

Specific suggestions aimed at reducing marital and sexual sequelae included the limiting of basal body temperature recording and the avoidance of very specific advice regarding the timing and techniques of intercourse. In addition it was suggested that the couple should be encouraged to explore their expectations, feelings and motives concerning their infertility. A particularly useful idea was for couples to plan for sexual activities purely oriented towards pleasure rather than procreation. These might include sexual activities which did not include intercourse.

Where these simple modifications of care prove inadequate in assisting psychological adjustment the options of self-help groups and specific infertility counselling remain. Mahlstedt (1985) reviews some issues that may usefully be addressed in such settings. Couples often need help to grieve for the losses they have encountered and this process can be facilitated by encouraging discussion, in an accepting atmosphere, of many of the negative feelings that arise. Difficulties may be encountered, particularly when reactions are perceived as socially undesirable, for example in the case of feelings of hostility to pregnant women. There is also a need to appreciate that a variety of methods of coping exist and that individuals are likely to vary in the methods they use. It is important that where partners exhibit very different patterns each should accept and respect the other's method rather than allow this difference to stimulate the development of hostility and anger. It is of value to encourage each person to take time to listen and to try to understand how his or her partner is feeling rather than to focus only upon his or her own distress. Couples can also be encouraged to recognise their assets and to take positive steps to maximise their pleasure within their marriage rather than to focus their lives purely on the disappointment of infertility.

It is also important that couples should learn to cope with the harsh facts of reality. Women they know will always accidently become pregnant. There will be cases of child abuse and neglect in the media and they themselves will be subject from time to time to unthinking insensitive comments or advice. By recognising the inevitability of such events, by planning and practising methods of coping with these in advance, episodes of distress can be significantly reduced. There will also be occasions when it may be prudent to suggest a 'holiday' from infertility treatments so that a couple can reestablish a more normal pattern of values and existence for a period of time. This would be appropriate where a couple's life has become dominated by the quest for fertility and where significant sexual

problems appear to be developing as a response to the stress of the situation.

While all these suggestions would appear to show good face validity the actual efficacy of intervention in modifying levels of psychological distress and sexual dysfunction is unclear. Certainly, a demand exists for this type of help. Lalos et al (1985) reported that one-half of the women in their study would have welcomed psychosocial help and support. There are a very limited number of treatment studies. Bresnick & Taymor (1979) found significant improvements in emotional functioning after both long-term and short-term counselling. However, Cooper (1979) was unable to find any substantial positive changes on standardised assessments after a 15-week counselling intervention. In this case sample sizes were very small and the author claimed positive changes at an anecdotal level. Other authors have made similarly poorly substantiated claims for the efficacy of both individual and group treatments (Wilchins 1974; Rosenfeld & Mitchell 1979). It is unfortunately necessary to conclude that the potential positive effects of counselling interventions on adjustment to infertility are at present still relatively unsubstantiated.

ABDOMINAL PAIN

Abdominal pain is a common symptom in women diagnosed as suffering from pelvic inflammatory disease. Jacobson & Weström (1969) reported that 94% of women with this condition, confirmed by laparoscopy, complained of lower abdominal pain. When infection is recurrent a chronic pain condition can develop.

The problem of diagnosis and the prevalence of chronic pelvic pain patients without organic pathology

The diagnosis of pelvic inflammatory disease without resort to laparoscopy has been reported to be unreliable. Kleinhaus et al (1979) found that clinical diagnoses of pelvic inflammatory disease were confirmed at laparoscopy in only 53% of cases. Murphy & Fliegner (1981) reported similar patterns of discrepancy. The suggestion that pathology is absent in a high percentage of cases of abdominal pain has led to a widely expressed view that in many cases such pain is of psychogenic origin (McFadyen 1981). It is commonly implied that a clear dichotomy exists, with psychological factors being important in this latter group, but not where there is evidence of pathology. However other studies, particularly more recently, have questioned whether a large pool of patients without abnormality does exist. Goldstein et al (1979) reported on the laparoscopic results of 109 adolescents with pain of 3 months' to 3 years' duration. Initially 23% had been diagnosed as having no pathology on pelvic examination but this figure decreased to 9% following laparoscopy. Kresch et al (1984) found an 83% rate of pathology at laparoscopy. A similar study by Rosenthal et al (1984) showed a 75% rate of pathology in chronic pelvic pain patients. This recent evidence questions the validity of the view that a high percentage of chronic pelvic pain patients show no organic aetiology. However this does not imply that psychological factors are without importance.

Psychological factors in chronic pelvic pain groups with and without organic pathology

Attempts to establish systematic psychological differences between abdominal pain patients with and without pathology have been unrewarding. Castelnuovo-Tedesco & Krout (1970) assessed psychiatric diagnoses in women with and without organic causes for their abdominal pain. There was no difference in the prevalence of psychiatric disorder. Similarly, attempts to assess psychological profiles have failed to find consistent differences (Rosenthal et al 1984; Renaer et al 1979). However, although it is difficult to discriminate between pain groups with and without pathology, both groups tend to show significantly more psychological distress than control groups suffering no pain.

A small number of studies have indicated differences but these may be explained by methodological factors. Beard et al (1977) compared 18 women with pain in the absence of pathology detected at laparoscopy with 17 women for whom an organic basis for pain had been identified. Although there were no differences in psychopathology as measured by the Middlesex Hospital Questionnaire, the non-organic group showed higher neuroticism scores. There were also suggestions that this group suffered from higher levels of sexual anxiety. However the durations of pain were not matched in

this study and it is therefore possible that differences could be due to the effects of suffering for a longer time period.

The view that sexual anxieties may play a role has been echoed by Gross et al (1980) who found that approximately one-third of an undiagnosed pelvic pain group had experiences of incest as children. However Pearce & Beard (1984), when reviewing the literature on this area of sexual attitudes and difficulties in chronic pelvic pain, concluded that there was still disagreement about the extent of sexual problems or anxiety in this patient group and more systematic investigation was required before concluding that sexual anxiety plays an aetiological role in chronic pelvic pain.

There is a growing body of evidence to suggest that psychological problems where they occur in conjunction with chronic pain are reactive rather than aetiological. This confirms findings from other categories of pain patients where presence or absence of pathology has proved an equally poor predictor of psychological distress (Cox et al 1978). This view is further supported by Sternbach & Timmermans (1975) who found that abnormal scores on the Minnesota Multiphasic Personality Inventory returned to near normal when chronic pain patients were successfully cured.

Sternback (1981) has emphasised the need to differentiate between acute pain, which he states often induces anxiety, and chronic pain which is more often associated with depressive-type symptoms. Many of the effects of chronic pain can erroneously be interpreted as symptoms of primary psychological disturbance. Individuals may be affected by sleep disturbance and irritability. The presence of chronic pain may lead to feelings of exhaustion and consequent apathy. Sternbach cautions against these symptoms being interpreted too readily as evidence of aetiological psychological factors. It is also important to note, as highlighted by Bonica (1979), that not all chronic pain patients show depressive-type symptoms.

Pain as a multidimensional phenomenon

There is evidence to suggest that the experience of pain is not purely a function of nociceptive impulses. Chapman (1984) provides a recent review of this work. The pain experience, particularly when chronic, involves the integration of pain sensation, affective and motivational reactions to the pain, cognitive evaluation of the pain and patterns of communication of pain to others (Renaer 1984).

Individuals with the same degree of pathology do not necessarily report equivalent levels of pain. In many cases discomfort appears disproportionate to tissue damage. A variety of factors, including anxiety, depression, personality and social and cultural variables can affect both the apparent intensity and expression of pain experience. As the impact of these influences has been recognised a variety of psychological interventions have been developed to assist in the management of the chronic pain patient.

It is important to note that these techniques are applicable in the presence or absence of organic pathology and are not restricted to use with the latter group. Indeed where an organic basis for pain is well established but routine pain control techniques are proving ineffective or where pain complaints appear disproportionate to pathology psychological management techniques may be of particular value. In the case of pelvic inflammatory disease where the infection is recurrent and pain poorly controlled or where the infection is presently inactive but pain remains such interventions may be indicated.

Psychological methods of treatment

These can be divided into three categories: physiological, cognitive/behavioural and operant techniques. Unfortunately few treatment studies have focused on abdominal pain patients. In view of this, only a brief description of the types of procedures involved will be provided, rather than an extensive review of the literature.

Physiological techniques

These methods are generally aimed at modifying some of the aetiological factors involved in the genesis of pain. In the case of relaxation techniques, muscular tension or vascular functioning is usually the target for modification. Unfortunately, in the case of abdominal pain, in the presence of organic pathology there is little evidence to suggest that muscular tension or vascular congestion is involved. The latter has been implicated in patients

where no pathology is evident (Duncan & Taylor 1952). Where deep internal structures are involved it is difficult to assess the role of these factors in pain or the impact of techniques such as relaxation on these variables. When pain occurs muscle tension can arise as a secondary phenomenon as a result of a rigid postural stance often adopted as a protective mechanism. It is certainly feasible that relaxation may be appropriate in these circumstances. A study by Pearce et al (1982) indicated the usefulness of relaxation training in women with chronic abdominal pain in the absence of pathology.

Biofeedback training can also be considered as a physiological technique. Unfortunately there is little substantive evidence that pelvic infection is associated with elevations of functioning in any of the systems which can potentially be modified. In the absence of any adequate theoretical rationale for use, the value of biofeedback at present must be restricted to producing a general relaxation response.

Turner & Chapman (1982) provide a detailed review of the usefulness of relaxation and biofeedback in chronic pain populations.

Cognitive/behavioural techniques

These techniques aim to modify attentional, attitudinal and evaluative processes. These procedures are reviewed by Tan (1982), McCaul & Malott (1984) and Trifiletti (1984). Patients may be taught specific skills to cope with pain. These might involve distraction techniques, the use of pleasant imagery or calming self-statements. Patterns of thoughts which aggravate discomfort, such as catastrophising, in which the pain experienced elicits a chain of negative thoughts of increasing intensity which lead to a rise in anxiety and subsequently exacerbation of pain, would be identified. The patient would be taught to substitute more rational and reality-based cognitions. Patients might be taught to relabel their pain sensations in less emotive terms such as tingling or the experience of heat. A variety of techniques have been developed and generally several may be utilised in concert. Unfortunately their efficacy in chronic abdominal pain patients remains unsubstantiated and studies are still awaited.

Operant techniques

This type of intervention is based on the premise that pain experience leads to pain behaviour, such as grimacing, making verbal statements of suffering or decreasing activities to rest. Fordyce (1978) suggests that environmental contingencies operate on these behaviours, in many cases increasing their frequency. As a result, the chronic pain patient may become extremely disabled and show a very low level of activity. Operant techniques are used in a process of rehabilitation to increase the individual's adaptive functioning rather than necessarily affect the experience of pain. As part of an intensive inpatient programme, pain behaviours are systematically ignored while positive active behaviours are systematically reinforced. Fordyce et al (1985) have recently reviewed this area. It is of limited applicability in the case of patients with chronic pelvic infection, as most maintain high levels of activity in their roles as mothers, wives and employees. In rare cases where the pain has led to gross restriction in activity such an approach could be considered.

CONCLUSIONS

Psychological factors have been shown to be of importance in many aspects of genital tract infection. It is important that professional staff should become more aware of common psychological consequences of conditions such as genital herpes, infertility and chronic abdominal pain. Through enhanced awareness and sensitivity to patients' emotional needs it may be possible to prevent the occurrence of some negative reactions. In addition, those which do occur may be identified at an early stage and referral for psychological help could be implemented. Unfortunately, while most of the psychological interventions described in this chapter appear to hold promise, their efficacy has not always been systematically evaluated and further research studies are awaited.

REFERENCES

Adler J D, Boxley R L 1985 The psychological reactions to infertility: sex roles and coping styles. Sex Roles 12: 271–279

Annon J 1976 The behavioural treatment of sexual problems: brief therapy. Harper and Row, Hagerstown

Beard R W, Belsey E M, Lieberman B A, Wilkinson J C M 1977 Pelvic pain in women. American Journal of Obstetrics and Gynecology 128: 566–570

Becker M H, Maiman L A 1975 Sociobehavioural determinants of compliance with health and medical care recommendations. Medical Care 13: 10–24

Begg A, Dickerson M, London N B 1976 Frequency of self reported sexual problems in a family planning clinic. Journal of Family Planning Doctors 2: 41–48

Bell J S 1981 Psychological problems among patients attending an infertility clinic. Journal of Psychosomatic Research 25: 1–3

Bonica J J 1979 The relation of injury to pain. Pain 7: 203–207

Bresnick E, Taymor M C 1979 The role of counselling in infertility. Fertility and Sterility 32: 154–156

Brown G W, Harris T O 1978 Social origins of depression. Tavistock, London

Bullock J L 1974 Iatrogenic impotence in an infertility clinic: illustrative case. American Journal of Obstetrics and Gynecology 120: 476–478

Carr G D 1963 A psychosocial study of fertile and infertile marriages. Unpublished Ph.D. Thesis, University of Southern California

Castelnuovo-Tedesco P, Krout B M 1970 Psychosomatic aspects of chronic pelvic pain. International Journal of Psychiatric Medicine 1: 109–126

Catalan J, Bradley M, Gallwey J, Hawton K 1981 Sexual dysfunction and psychiatric morbidity in patients attending a clinic for sexually transmitted disease. British Journal of Psychiatry 138: 292–296

Chapman C R 1984 New directions in the understanding and management of pain. Social Science and Medicine 19: 1261–1277

Collins J A, Garner J B, Wilson E H, Wrixon W, Casper R F 1984 A proportional hazards analysis of the clinical characteristics of infertile couples. American Journal of Obstetrics and Gynecology 148: 527–532

Cooper S L 1979 Female infertility: its effect on self esteem, body image, locus of control and behaviour. Unpublished Thesis, Boston University School of Education

Cornfeld D, Hubbard J P 1961 A four year study of the occurrence of beta-hemolytic streptococci in 64 school children. New England Journal of Medicine 264: 211–215

Cox G B, Chapman C R, Black R G 1978 The MMPI and chronic pain: the diagnosis of psychogenic pain. Journal of Behavioral Medicine 1: 437–443

Daniels K R, Gunby J, Legge M, Williams T H, Wynn-Williams D B 1984 Issues and problems for the infertile couple. New Zealand Medical Journal 97: 185–187

De Vries K, Degani S, Eibschitz I, Oettinger M, Zilberman A, Sharf M 1984 The influence of the postcoital test on the sexual function of infertile women. Journal of Psychosomatic Obstetrics and Gynaecology 3: 101–106

Drake T S, Grunert G M 1979 A cyclic pattern of sexual dysfunction in the infertility investigation. Fertility and Sterility 32: 542–545

Duncan C H, Taylor H C 1952 A psychosomatic study of pelvic congestion. American Journal of Obstetrics and Gynecology 64: 1–12

Elstein M 1975 Effect of infertility on psychosexual function. British Medical Journal 3: 296–299

Eschenbach D A 1980 Epidemiology and diagnosis of acute pelvic inflammatory disease. Obstetrics and Gynecology 55: 142S–152S

Folkman S, Lazarus R 1980 An analysis of coping in a middle-aged community sample. Journal of Health and Social Behaviour 21: 219–239

Fordyce W E 1978 Learning processes in pain. In: Sternbach R A (ed) The psychology of pain. Raven Press, New York, pp 49–72

Fordyce W E, Roberts A H, Sternbach R A 1985 The behavioural management of chronic pain: a response to critics. Pain 22: 113–125

Freeman E W, Garcia C S, Rickels K 1983 Behavioural and emotional factors: comparisons of anovulatory infertile women with fertile and other infertile women. Fertility and Sterility 40: 195–201

Goldstein D P, de Cholnoky C, Leventhal J M, Emans S J 1979 New insights into the old problem of chronic pelvic pain. Journal of Pediatric Surgery 14: 675–679

Gross R J, Doer H, Galdirola D, Guzinski G, Ripley H S 1980 Borderline syndrome and incest in chronic pain patients. International Journal of Psychiatry in Medicine 10: 79–86

Guinan H E, MacCalman J, Kern E R, Overall Jr J B, Spruance S L 1981 The course of untreated recurrent genital herpes simplex infection in 27 women. New England Journal of Medicine 304: 759–763

Jacobson L, Weström L 1969 Objectivized diagnosis of acute pelvic inflammatory disease. American Journal of Obstetrics and Gynecology 105: 1088–1098

Jemmott III J B, Locke S E 1984 Psychosocial factors, immunologic mediation and human susceptibility to infectious diseases: how much do we know? Psychological Bulletin 95: 78–108

Keye W R 1984 Psychosexual responses to infertility. Clinical Obstetrics and Gynecology 27: 760–766

Keye W R, Deneris A 1983 Female sexual activity, satisfaction and function in infertile women. Infertility 5: 275–285

Kleinhaus S, Hein K, Sheran M, Doely S J 1979 Laparoscopy for the diagnosis and treatment of abdominal pain in adolescent girls. Archives of Surgery 112: 1778–1779

Knowlton K C 1984 Health locus of control and level of anger response to a clinical diagnosis of genital herpes in a selected sample of women. Unpublished Ph.D. thesis, University of Alabama

Kraft A D, Palombo J, Mitchell D, Dean C, Meyers S, Schmidt A W 1980 The psychological dimensions of infertility. American Journal of Orthopsychiatry 50: 618–628

Kresch A J, Seifer D B, Sachs L B, Barrese I 1984 Laparoscopy in 100 women with chronic pelvic pain. Obstetrics and Gynecology 64: 672–674

Lalos A, Lalos O, Jacobsson L, von Schoultz B 1985 The psychosocial impact of infertility two years after completed surgical treatment. Acta Obstetrica Scandinavica 64: 599–604

Leader A, Taylor P J, Daniluk J 1984 Infertility: clinical and psychological aspects. Psychiatric Annals 14: 461–467

Leventhal H, Singer R, Jones S 1965 The effects of fear and specificity of recommendations. Journal of Personality and Social Psychology 2: 20–29

Levine S B, Yost M A 1976 Frequency of sexual dysfunction in a general gynecology clinic: an epidemiological approach. Archives of Sexual Behavior 5: 229–238

Luby E, Gillespie O 1981 Psychological responses to genital herpes. The Helper 3: 2–3

Luby E D, Klinge V 1985 Genital herpes. A pervasive psychosocial disorder. Archives of Dermatology 121: 494–497

McCaul K D, Malott J M 1984 Distraction and coping with pain. Psychological Bulletin 95: 516–533

McCormick T M 1980 Out of control: one aspect of infertility. Journal of General Nursing 9: 205–206

McFadyen I R 1981 Gynaecological pain in the lower abdomen. Clinics in Obstetrics and Gynaecology 8: 33–47

McGuire L S, Guzinski G M, Holmes K K 1980 Psychosexual functioning in symptomatic and asymptomatic women with and without signs of vaginitis. American Journal of Obstetrics and Gynecology 137: 600–603

Mahlstedt P P 1985 The psychological component of infertility. Fertility and Sterility 43: 335–346

Manne S, Sandler I 1984 Coping and adjustment to genital herpes. Journal of Behavioral Medicine 7: 391–410

Mazor M D 1979 Barren couples. Psychology Today 22 (May): 10–12

Menning B E 1982 THe psychosocial impact of infertility. Nursing Clinics of North America 17: 155–163

Murphy A, Fliegner J 1981 Diagnostic laparoscopy: its role in the management of acute pelvic pain. Medical Journal of Australia 1: 571–573

Nahmias A J, Roizman B 1973 Infection with herpes-simplex viruses 1 and 2. New England Journal of Medicine 289: 667–674

Paykel E S 1983 Methodological aspects of life events research. Journal of Psychosomatic Research 27: 341–352

Pearce S, Beard R W 1984 Chronic pelvic pain. In: Broome A, Wallace L W (eds) Psychology and gynaecological problems. Tavistock, London, pp 95–116

Pearce S, Knight C, Beard R W 1982 Pelvic pain—a common gynaecological problem. Journal of Psychosomatic Obstetrics and Gynaecology 1: 12–17

Platt J J, Ficher I, Silver M J 1973 Infertile couples: personality traits and self ideal concept discrepancies. Fertility and Sterility 24: 972–976

Raval H 1986 The inapct of infertility on emotional state and the marital and sexual relationships. Unpublished M. Sc. thesis, Manchester University

Renaer M 1984 Reflections on chronic pain in gynaecologic practice. European Journal of Obstetrics, Gynecology and Reproductive Biology 18: 245–254

Renaer H, Vertommen H, Nijs P, Wagemans L, Van Hemelrijck T 1979 Psychological aspects of chronic pain in women. American Journal of Obstetrics and Gynecology 134: 75–80

Rosenfeld D L, Mitchell E 1979 Treating the emotional aspects of infertility: counselling services in an infertility clinic. American Journal of Obstetrics and Gynecology 135: 177–180

Rosenthal R H, Lung F W, Rosenthal T L, McNeeley S G 1984 Chronic pelvic pain: psychological features and laparoscopic findings. Psychosomatics 25: 833–844

Rotter J B 1966 Generalized expectancies for internal versus external control of reinforcement. Psychological Monographs 80 (no 609): 1–28

Schwab J J 1982 Psychiatric aspects of infectious diseases. Current Psychiatric Therapies 21: 225–239

Shapiro C H 1982 The impact of infertility on the marital relationship. Social Casework 63: 387–393

Shaw J A 1984 Psychological and sexual aspects of genital herpes in women. Unpublished Ph.D. thesis, Texas Technical University

Sklar B 1984 Infertility: its effect on self esteem, marital satisfaction and locus of control orientation among men, women and marital dyads. Unpublished Ph.D. thesis, United States International University

Sternbach R A 1981 Chronic pain as a disease entity. Triangle 20: 27–32

Sternbach R A, Timmermans G 1975 Personality changes associated with reduction of pain. Pain 1: 177–181

Stout C W 1984 Genital herpes and personality. Unpublished Ph.D. thesis, Colorado State University

Sweet R L, Gibbs R S 1985 Infectious diseases of the female genital tract. Williams and Wilkins, Baltimore

Tan S Y 1982 Cognitive and cognitive-behavioural methods for pain control: a selective review. Pain 12: 201–228

Totman R G, Kiff J 1979 Life stress and susceptibility to colds. In: Oborne D J, Gruneberg M M, Eiser J R (eds) Research in psychology and medicine, vol I. Academic Press, New York, pp 141–149

Trifiletti R J 1984 The psychological effectiveness of pain management procedures in the context of behavioural medicine. Genetic Psychology Monographs 109: 251–278

Turner J A, Chapman C R 1982 Psychological interventions for chronic pain: a critical review I. Relaxation training and biofeedback. Pain 12: 1–21

Watson D B 1983 The relationship of genital herpes and life stress as moderated by locus of control and social support. Unpublished thesis, University of Southern California

Weström L 1975 Effect of acute pelvic inflammatory disease on fertility. American Journal of Obstetrics and Gynecology 121: 707–713

Weström L 1980 Incidence, prevalence and trends of acute pelvic inflammatory disease and its consequences in industrialized countries. American Journal of Obstetrics and Gynecology 138: 880–892

Wilchins S A 1974 Use of group 'rap sessions' in the adjunctive treatment of five infertile females. Journal of the Medical Society of New Jersey 71: 951–953

Williams N A, Deffenbacher J L 1983 Life stress and chronic yeast infections. Journal of Human Stress 9: 26–31

Wilson E A 1979 Sequence of emotional responses induced by infertility. Kentucky Medical Association 77: 229–233

Woddis C 1983 Herpes genitalis. The benefits of self help groups for sufferers. The Practitioner 227: 865–866

The evidence for a role for infection in the pathogenesis of lower genital tract cancer
G D Wilbanks and M Turyk

INTRDOUCTION

Cervical cancer was one of the earliest malignancies to be linked with infectious organisms as a possible causative agent. Rigoni-Stern (1842) and Gagnon (1950) related cervical cancer to some factor involved with sexual intercourse, suggesting a venereal or infectious nature to the disease. Virtually all the agents 'infecting' the lower genital tract— bacteria, viruses, and intermediate organisms— have been implicated as a potential causative agent in epithelial cancer of the lower genital tract. Recently, the male has been implicated as contributing the 'infectious agent', sperm, to this list. Since the epidemiology of the various infectious agents has been discussed in detail in Chapter 4, this chapter will concentrate on the mechanisms by which the infectious agents might initiate the carcinogenic process and the data supporting the potential in-

volvement of each (Wilbanks & Turyk 1986). Since most data relate to the cervix, cervical cancer will be the primary cancer discussed. Other cancers of the genital tract will be considered individually or as they relate to the specific organism. If one wishes to evaluate the possible carcinogenicity of these agents, first there must be serial transmission studies; then the cancer association can be evaluated by clinical parameters using epidemiological, serological and pathological data, and by basic parameters usually related to experimental or natural carcinogenesis studies in animals, other human tumours, and in vitro transformation studies. Modern techniques also allow one to assay any 'footprints' of the same agents in the tumours themselves. Table 20.1 lists the potential carcinogens and summarises these observations.

Table 20.1 Potential infectious carcinogens and associated factors

	Venereal transmission	Cancer association			Footprints found in cancer
		Clinical	Basic carcinogenesis		
			Animal	In vitro	
Syphilis	+	±	−	?	−
Gonorrhoea	+	±	−	?	−
Trichomoniasis	+	±	−	?	−
Sperm	+	±	±	±	?
Chlamydia	+	±	−	−	?
Mycoplasma	+	−	?	?	?
Virus					
Adenovirus	?	−	+	+	?
Cytomegalovirus	±	±	−	+	?
Herpes	+	+	+	+	±
Papilloma	+	+	+	+	+

+ Consistent; ± inconsistent or infrequent; − negative; ? no data.

CLASSIC VENEREAL PATHOGENESIS

Syphilis

Levin et al (1942) report one of the earlier scientific analyses of syphilis and cervical cancer showing an association; Wynder et al (1954) did not confirm this is careful studies from the USA and India. Adam et al (1983) in a recent study from Taiwan did note a correlation between those women who had positive serology and cervical cancer in contrast to the control women. However, all studies indicate that syphilis is probably just a non-related disease associated with other venereal factors, such as early onset of coitus and more likely causative agents (Wynder et al 1954). Syphilis does not cause any type of chronic cervical infection likely to be related to a carcinogenic process, and there are no basic animal or in vitro studies indicating a carcinogenic effect.

Gonorrhoea

Gonorrhoea per se seems also to be an unlikely candidate to play a causative role in cervical cancer. Wynder et al (1954) found no correlation in their studies without early coitus as the major variable. All studies involving gonorrhoea are hampered by the lack of a serological test to document prior disease, history alone being relatively inaccurate. There are no animal or basic studies showing a carcinogenic effect.

Beral (1974) drew an interesting correlation between the incidence of gonorrhoea among women in England and Wales and the standard cohort mortality from cervical cancer among women born 20 years earlier. The curves of the two plots have an amazing similarity. But again, the fluctuations of both may be due to changing sexual practices rather than to an effect of gonorrhoea 20 years later. Subsequent analysis of data from the United States failed to show this association. Gardner & Lyon (1974) and James (1974) then questioned the use of cervical cancer mortality rather than mortality data which they suggested made both studies open to question. Recently, two Scandinavian studies by Furgyik (1985) and Lynge and Jensen (1985) again suggest the venereal nature of cervical cancer and that gonorrhoea in the male and female may be re-lated directly or may simply be an indicator of sexual activity. Each study points out the pitfalls of such long-term epidemiological studies.

Gonorrhoea, however, has been noted to be commonly associated with both chlamydia and herpes (Wentworth et al 1973). Also, it has been suggested that gonorrhoeal infection may activate latent herpes infections (Beilby et al 1968). These findings are of interest since it seems likely that more than one factor is likely involved in the carcinogenic process. There are no basic studies or animal experiments implicating the gonococcus as a carcinogen.

Trichomoniasis

Trichomoniasis has several factors indicating a possible association with cervical cancer. As with the other venereal diseases, it is more common in sexually promiscuous persons. Unlike those organisms mentioned previously, chronic infection may result in atypical epithelial changes resembling cervical intraepithelial neoplasia (CIN), but these changes are apparently reversible by treatment of the infection. The classic study of Bechhold & Reichter (1952) seemed to give the definitive answer negating any correlation between trichomoniasis and cervical cancer; more recent studies indicate that further serious evaluations should be made of this agent in association with other potential factors (Alexander 1973). The difficulty of not having an animal model and the problems of maintaining the organism in pure culture make basic carcinogenesis studies difficult. However, the recent in vitro study of Heath (1981), showing that the *Trichomonas* adhered to the rabbit kidney tubule epithelial cells in culture, opens an avenue to further investigations with cultured cervical cells.

Sperm

If indeed cervical cancer and its precursors are a venereal disease, sperm is the most common venereal 'infectious agent' that could have oncogenic potential. In 1965, Reid proposed sperm, and specifically the basic proteins, histones and protamines, as a potentially carcinogenic agent in cervical cancer.

In the early 1970s, a series of experiments using calf thymus histones resulted in the observation that basic proteins were able to transform malignantly BHK21 cells in vitro as reported by Latner & Longstaff (1971, 1979) and Latner et al (1971). In addition, these authors reported a marked increase in invasiveness which was reproducible in vivo (Latner et al 1973). Other workers have shown that these basic proteins, histones and protamines have a high affinity for DNA (Vendrely et al 1960) and, when added to cells in culture, cause inhibition of respiration (Fischer & Brandis 1954), arrest of protein synthesis (Becker & Green 1980), enhanced uptake of RNA (Amos & Kearns 1963) and of albumin (Ryser & Hancock 1965) and a reduction in DNA synthesis (Levine et al 1968).

One of the richest sources of histones and protamines is spermatozoa, where the major function of these proteins appears to be to maintain the DNA in the sperm head in a compact, stable and transportable form (Felix et al 1956). In the human sperm head, the DNA is locked in a sponge-like matrix of chromatin threads composed of arginine-rich proteins. This matrix transports the DNA in a highly protected state.

Reid (1976) proposed that these basic proteins, when released on to the cervix following intercourse, could alter target cells on the cervix in such a way that would begin the process of neoplastic transformation. He suggested that the proteins which are more basic, and thus have a higher avidity for molecular DNA in vitro, would have an increased carcinogenic effect (Reid & Blackwell 1974). Reid and his colleagues (1978) and Singer & Reid (1979) showed that there are individual differences in the composition of basic proteins in the human population, giving further weight to the 'high-risk male' concept of the aetiology of cervical carcinogenesis. Others have speculated on the presence of a male factor in cervical carcinoma: Furgyik (1985) in conjunction with a study of gonorrhoea in the husbands of women with cervical cancer and Skegg et al (1982) in a more general epidemiological study. Certainly some males seem to carry a carcinogenic factor and sperm are common to all.

Early work on the short-term effects of basic proteins from human sperm on cultured cells has shown behavioural and cytoskeletal alterations (French 1980). French et al (personal communication) have recently extended this work to quantitate the metabolic, morphological, and locomotory effects of sperm basic proteins on BHK21 cells in vitro. Preliminary results by French (personal communication) using these basic proteins for in vitro transformation of human cervical organ cultures are too early to provide definitive answers, but should shed some light on the problem.

The concept that the sperm or certain sperm products may be carcinogenic to the human genital tract is intriguing, and must be considered in a review of potential 'infectious agents' and genital tract malignancies, but is far from proven.

Chlamydia

The rapid increase in the knowledge of the epidemiology and pathogenesis of genital infections by *Chlamydia trachomatis* has revealed a possible association with cervical cancer. Chlamydia seems a reasonable candidate, since it does appear to be a common venereal pathogen, and it causes a chronic infection. If there is an analogy with the common chronic chlamydial infection in the eye, trachoma, one might expect a high rate of neoplasia in the unfortunate individuals who suffer from this disease. However, the physiology, pathology, and bacteriology/virology of the eye are quite different from those of the cervix. As mentioned earlier, there is probably more than one factor responsible for genital carcinogenesis, so this difference may not be unexpected.

The main associations have been reported in several studies which have found that patients with early cervical lesions (i.e. CIN) had a higher prevalence of positive chlamydial cultures or serum antibodies to chlamydia than control patients (Hare et al 1981, 1982; Kalimo et al 1981). Allerding et al (1985) and Schachter et al (1982) noted a higher incidence of both chlamydial and human papilloma virus (HPV) changes in Papanicolaou smears of women who developed CIN than control women. Harnekar et al (1985) noted a higher percentage of progression to CIN III in a group of women with chlamydia-associated changes in Pap smears than in the control women. They suggested that chlamydia may act as a carcinogen or potentiating agent in the progression of CIN and invasive cancers.

Kalimo et al (1981) found local IgA antibodies to chlamydia in 24 of 35 (69%) cervical cancer patients with premalignant or malignant clinical changes, in 11 of 28 (39%) patients with cervicitis, and in 3 of 26 (12%) controls. Interestingly, in this same study, IgA antibodies to herpes simplex virus (HSV) were found in 10 of 35 (38%) patients with 'malignant atypia or dysplasia', but in none of the controls or the women with cervicitis. No IgA antibodies to either chlamydia or HSV were found in the serum of any patient.

Chlamydia can apparently cause chronic cervicitis, and in some instances follicular cervicitis (Hare et al 1981). It is also related to infection of the fallopian tubes, so it could be a potential carcinogenic stimulant. However, there are no known malignant diseases caused by chlamydia in animals, and no in vitro transformation has been reported.

One interesting study in progress may shed some light on the possible cervical changes. Since chlamydia, unlike the herpes virus, readily responds to common antibiotics, Hare & Thin (1983) have treated patients with proven CIN prospectively, in a double-blind fashion, prior to definitive therapy. The results of this study may clarify some of the relationships between chlamydial infections and CIN.

Mycoplasma

Mycoplasma hominis and T mycoplasma are common venereal pathogens in women and men. In Seattle venereal disease clinics, the cervical prevalence of T mycoplasma was 93% and that of *M. hominis* 54%. Mycoplasmas are commonly found in association with other venereal pathogens (Alexander 1973).

Gregory & Payne (1970) did not find a correlation between abnormal Pap smears and the presence of mycoplasma in 150 women from a venereal disease clinic and 150 women from a family planning clinic in Michigan. There was a higher number of women with mycoplasma in the venereal disease clinic: 138 versus 57. Interestingly, more women from the family planning clinic had abnor-

mal smears: 7 versus 3. All 3 women with abnormal smears in the venereal disease clinic were positive for mycoplasma, while only 4 of 11 with abnormal smears in the family planning clinic had mycoplasma. There was no histological verification of the abnormal smears or follow-up of these women. The conclusion was that mycoplasma did not significantly influence the occurrence of cellular abnormalities in either population.

Recently, there has been a preliminary report of mycoplasma's association with cervical dysplasia. Averna et al (1980) studied 395 women, of whom 213 had cervical dysplasia: 133 'slight', 53 'intermediate', and 27 'advanced'. These patients with dysplasia were noted to have a decrease in pH and *Lactobacillus acidophilus* in the vaginal cultures with a concomitant increase in *Trichomonas* and mycoplasma. These were commonly found together in patients with dysplasia. There was a negative corelation with *Candida albicans* and dysplasia.

Mycoplasmas are also closely allied with sexual activity, as noted in Chapter 4 and 12. Again it is difficult to separate any venereally transmitted organism and a possible correlation with cervical malignancies. Gregory & Payne (1970) were the first to note a correlation between mycoplasma and mild dysplasia. Alexander (1973) found only an association with 'cervical atypia' but not with 'more significant dysplasias'. The data have been correlated with isolations, not serological data.

There are no animal models or basic studies linking mycoplasma and cancers of the genital tract. Animal infection has mainly been related to salpingitis (Moller & Freundi 1979), as have in vitro studies (Stalheim et al 1976). Mycoplasma seems to be an unlikely candidate as a major factor in genital malignancies.

Virus

Viral infections cause various malignancies in animals, and thus are probably the most likely candidates for an aetiological connection in the infectious pathogenesis of lower genital tract cancer. Rotkin (1967b) postulated a DNA virus as a possible agent in cervical cancer, and Naib et al (1966) observed a correlation between viral and dysplastic changes in Pap smears from a group of clinic patients. From these early simple beginnings, a tremedous amount of clinical, epidemiological, and biological data has been generated in an attempt to relate herpes virus infections and cervical cancer. The American Cancer Society sponsored comprehensive symposia in 1972 and 1980 (Symposium 1973, 1981). These reports will give the interested reader a detailed background of these data.

More recently, another common viral inhabitant of the lower genital tract, the condyloma virus and its relatives, has been implicated in cervical cancer (zur Hausen 1976). This relationship is not a new speculation as 'transformation' of condylomata to cancer was reported early in the century by MacDonald (1921) and Siegel (1962). The association of the condyloma virus and cervical cancer has been hampered by the fact that the virus has only been identified in the lesions since the 1960s, and there is still no method of growing the virus in culture. Therefore, it has been difficult to obtain virus for antigen–antibody studies and transformation experiments. Now that zur Hausen et al (1984) have made monoclonal probes and these are now available to researchers around the world, the association of HPV with specific types of cervical and vulvar neoplasia is becoming very strong. The in vivo transformation studies of Kreider et al (1986) add significant data to this correlation.

Two other viruses have been suggested as possible agents in cervical cancer: cytomegalovirus (Vesterinen et al 1975), and adenovirus (Laverty et al 1977). However, the data on these viruses are preliminary and the associations are not as obvious. Again, time may confirm or reject these associations.

Vulvar cancer is the only other genital cancer to have a serious correlation with a viral infectious aetiology. Kaufman et al (1981) have found a herpes-related RNA in vulvar cancer. The anecdotal inference of a possible correlation between condyloma acuminata and vulvar cancer has been strengthened by the correlation of the presence of HPV structural antigen in vulvar intraepithelial neoplasia (VIN) by Kaufman et al (1981) and Crum et al (1982).

Choriocarcinoma has been speculated to have an infectious aetiology, perhaps viral, because of its high prevalence in certain regions, but no organism

has been identified. Ovarian carcinoma has been found to be less frequent in women who have had mumps, but no explanation for this observation seems related to a virus infectious aetiology. There has been no speculation of an infectious aetiology for endometrial or uterine malignancies.

Adenovirus

Some adenoviruses are known to possess oncogenic properties (Davis et al 1973), but type 19, isolated from the female genital tract by Laverty et al (1977) is not known to induce malignancies. This group and Naib et al (1966) had shown some intranuclear inclusion bodies on Pap smear from patients with adenovirus infections. No correlation with cervical atypia or malignancy has been shown.

Vestergaard et al (1972) noted no correlation between the presence of antibodies to adenovirus and the occurrence of cervical carcinoma. Vesterinen et al (1978) were able to grow the organism in human cervical cultures, but did not observe any changes suggestive of neoplastic transformation.

Although some adenoviruses have malignant potential, the type isolated from the human genital tract does not. Adenovirus infection seems an unlikely cause of genital tract malignancies.

Cytomegalovirus

Cytomegalovirus (CMV) is not clearly a sexually transmitted organism, but is a common inhabitant of the lower genital tract. It does, however, seem to be related to chronic cervicitis (Alexander 1973) and is found in sexually transmitted disease clinic patients in isolation studies (Wertheim et al 1985).

In regard to an association with cervical neoplasia, Fuccillo et al (1971) found no association in patients between haemagglutinating antibodies and the occurrence of carcinoma in situ, but another study (Vesterinen et al 1975) did show a weak association. CMV has been found in semen (Lang & Kummer 1972).

In vitro, human ectocervical cells were resistant to infection, but the endocervical cells showed alterations (Vesterinen et al 1975). The authors postulated that the endocervix was probably the source of the virus in chronic infections. Albrecht & Rapp (1973) were able to induce malignant transformation of hamster cells with ultraviolet-irradiated CMV. This is the strongest possible correlation with postulated human malignancy; however, it has been noted by Marczynska et al (1980) that this system is very sensitive to transformation with many substances and is a long way from human carcinogenesis. Serological data indicated that 80–90% of women have been infected with CMV (Leinikki et al 1972) so that specific correlation with human neoplasia is difficult.

Although CMV is important in obstetrics, it does not seem to be a strong candidate for carcinogenesis in the female genital tract.

Herpes simplex virus type II

The chance observation of a correlation of viral changes and dysplasia in the Pap smear of a group of patients reported by Naib et al (1966) seemed a boon to confirmation of the infectious concept of the aetiology of cervical cancer. This cytological correlation was supported by a prospective study from the same group (Nahmias et al 1973). This study followed 871 women who had genital herpes detected serologically, cytologically, or virologically and compared them with 562 women from the same populace who were negative for serologic antibodies to HSV-2. The rate of dysplasia in the HSV-2 group was twofold that of the control group, and that of carcinoma in situ was eightfold higher. The rate was higher in the recurrent group compared to those whose infection was primary.

A similar study, though not truly prospective, reviewed blood samples drawn years earlier in an obstetric co-operative study, and compared these findings to the occurrence of carcinoma in situ. Catalano & Johnson (1971) reported that 5 of 14 women with antibodies to HSV-2 developed carcinoma in situ in 1 to 8 years, while only 2 to 20 controls developed the lesion.

These observations, coupled with the venereal nature of the epidemiology of cervical cancer (Rotkin 1967a, 1967b; Keesler 1974) and the identification of two types of herpes virus (type I and type II), with type II primarily infecting the genitalia, led to seroepidemiological studies involving many nationalities and populations. Taking into account the various methods of antibody determination and selection of the 'control' population, the correlation

betwen a herpes type II antibody titre and all stages of cervical neoplasia, i.e. preinvasive (dysplasia and carcinoma in situ or CIN) and invasive cancer, has been strong (Rawls et al 1980). However, a recent long-term prospective epidemiological study from Vonka et al (1984) does not support some of the previous data implicating HSV-2. In any case, cervical cancer is not limited to patients with prior genital herpes infections; HSV-2 may be only one of a number of agents which may independently cause this disease (Rawls et al 1980).

The next logical steps in proving a connection between an agent and a malignancy is an in vitro transformation model. Duff & Rapp (1973) were able to transform hamster cells with ultraviolet-irradiated herpes virus. MacNab (1974) was able to produce transformation with a temperature-sensitive mutant live virus. Comacho & Spear (1978), Reyes et al (1979), and Jariwalla et al (1980), among others, have been able to transform rodent cells with herpes type II DNA fragments. Darai & Munk (1973) initially reported some morphological changes in human embryonic lung cell cultures following infection with temperature-sensitive mutants, but the cells did not satisfy the usual characteristic transformation. Marczynska et al (1980) were unable to transform primate or human cervical cells using several types of virus modification. To date, no human cells have been transformed in vitro.

These results strongly suggest that HSV-induced cell transformation does not involve a stable acquisition of specific viral transforming genes or viral proteins. It has been proposed that HSV acts on cells by a 'hit and run' mechanism (Hampar and Ellison 1963; Skinner 1976; Galloway & McDougall 1983). Such mechanisms could include the expression of cellular oncogenes by the insertion of short herpes virus sequences, active HSV recombination into the cellular genome with subsequent excision or rearrangement of the viral genome, and molecular mutagenesis by virus particles (Galloway & McDougall 1983; zur Hausen et al 1984).

HSV has been shown to have mutagenic activity (Schlohofer et al 1983), induce chromosomal abberations (Stich et al 1976; Hampar 1981), initiate cellular DNA repair and replication (Yamanishi et al 1975; Lorentz et al 1976), mediate gene amplification in simian virus 40-transformed cells (Schlohofer & zur Hausen 1982; Matz et al 1984), and induce endogenous retroviruses in murine cells (Hampar et al 1976). A study by Burns & Murray (1981) attempting to induce oral tumours in mice by HSV infection, ultraviolet irradiation, and application of tumour promoter 12-O-tetradecanoyl-phorbol-13-acetate (TPA), found that combinations of HSV + UV + TPA and HSV + TPA formed the most tumours. An in vitro study of weakly tumourigenic HSV-2 transformed cells showed enhancement of neoplastic properties following treatment with TPA (Kucera et al 1983). Such observations form the hypothesis that HSV infections lead to initiating events (zur Hausen 1982; zur Hausen et al 1984). Recurrent cervical infections would lead to a higher frequency of initiating events and increased risk of neoplastic promotion by additional carcinogenic stimulation, such as other venereal infections. Hamper & Ellison (1963) recently published a comprehensive review of herpes transformation studies.

Recent reports of animal studies of carcinogenesis have been rewarding. Wentz et al (1983) have produced cervical cancers and preinvasive changes in guinea pigs following inoculation of ultraviolet- and formalin-inactivated herpes virus. Chen & Swen (1982) reproduced these studies in mice. Most interesting are the recent reports from both these groups in which they were able to prevent the formation of cancer by prior vaccination. Wentz et al (1983) used an ultraviolet-inactivated whole HSV-2 preparation with Freund's adjuvant. Chen et al (1984) used a coat protein vaccine prepared from HSV-1.

London et al (1974) did not observe any cancers in Cebus monkeys which were chronically infected vaginally with HSV-2, although some changes described as dysplasia were reported. This study was discontinued short of the planned time for follow-up.

One obvious clue to the relation of a virus to a tumour would be the discovery of the virus in the tumour. Aurelian et al (1981) have been the only investigators to grow a live herpes virus from a culture of cells from carcinoma in situ. Numerous studies have attempted to detect HSV-specific antigens, RNA and DNA in cervical carcinoma tissues. AG-4 and ICSP 11/12 have been found in both cer-

vical carcinoma tissues and in HSV-2 transformed cells (Aurelian et al 1971; Flannery et al 1977; Dreesman et al 1980; Green et al 1982). HSV-2 RNA transcripts have been detected in up to 60% of cervical carcinoma specimens, although the data vary greatly with probes from different parts of the genome (McDougall et al 1980, 1982; Eglin et al 1981, 1984). However, it is possible that the probes detected non-specific mammalian cell RNA (Peden et al 1982). These results need to be substantiated by demonstrating HSV RNA by more sensitive techniques (i.e. northern blotting). HSV-2 DNA sequences have occasionally been detected in cervical cancers (Frenkel et al 1972; Park et al 1983). It remains to be determined if these DNA sequences correlate with detection of viral antigens and transcripts.

Many viral diseases have been eliminated by vaccination programmes; measles, polio, etc., and even a herpes virus-induced lymphoma in chickens (Mareck's disease) have been controlled by vaccine (Symposium 1973). The animal studies of Wentz et al (1981) and Chen et al (1984) suggest that a herpes vaccine is effective in preventing cervical cancer in these models. It would seem logical, even though highly speculative, that one method of 'proving' the viral aetiology of cervical cancer would be to prevent the infection by vaccination in a group of high risk young women, and follow them and a control cohort to see if the development of neoplastic changes was indeed eliminated or significantly reduced by preventing the disease (Skinner 1980). Until recently, however, this was not possible, since there was no effective herpes vaccine; but there does now appear to be an effective human herpes vaccine (Skinner 1980). In these studies an 'antigenoid' vaccine, $AcNFU_1(S^-)MRC$ has been used toward prevention or modification of herpes genitalis. The vaccine contains a number of important viral coat polypeptides and glycoproteins whose antigenicity survived the preparative procedure as adjudged by antibody identification on polyacrylamide gels and Ouchterlony gel diffusion.

In a recent report (Skinner et al 1982), a group of 42 sexual consorts of patients with recurrent genital herpes was vaccinated, and after an average follow-up of 1 year, none developed genital herpes. It would have been expected that 12 of 35 (34%) such consorts would have developed herpes in that time period. These results remain true in later reports with more patients and longer observation time (Skinner 1986 personal communication). These patients now total 404 consorts at risk with an average follow-up of 24 months. Only 2 (0.5%) have become infected with HSV after receiving two vaccinations, and each had only one mild infection with no recurrence at additional follow-up after 8 and 16 months.

A significant neutralising antibody response was obtained in 90% of seronegative consorts receiving the high vaccine dosage, and in 77% of seronegative consorts receiving the lower dosage.

In the group of 70 patients vaccinated following a 'primary' genital infection, 19 of these patients have experienced 28 recurrences during the first year following vaccination. Twenty primary HSV patients from the same clinic were not vaccinated. During the first year of follow-up 17 of the 20 patients experienced 51 recurrences. In the group of 24 patients with severe recurrent disease, 70% reported improvement, although the average follow-up was only 4 months. About half of these patients had rise in antibody titre.

The pieces of the puzzle linking herpes virus to cervical cancer are being discovered in many laboratories. With the extent of work being done using a variety of sophisticated techniques, the connection may be confirmed or refuted in the next few years.

Kaufman et al (1981) have found antigens of HSV-2 in squamous cell carcinoma of the vulva. This would not be unexpected as the herpes virus also infects the vulva and there have been anecdotal suggestions that squamous cell carcinomas of the lip may follow herpes virus type I infections (Kaufman et al 1981). This finding also gave additional support to the speculation by Schwartz & Naftolin (1981) that perhaps the HSV-2 virus latent in the neurological ganglia may feed recurrences in the vulva and vagina. These recurrences would be the source of carcinogen involved in these cancers.

The correlation between herpes infections and these genital cancers is not as well supported as in the cervix, but is probably worth further study. Interestingly, there seems to be an increase in intra-epithelial vulvar cancers and these are occurring in younger women (Schwartz & Naftolin 1981).

Papilloma virus

There are growing indications that HPV is involved in cervical dysplasia and/or may play a major role in converting that condition to invasive cancer (Syrjanen et al 1984; zur Hausen et al 1984). A circumstantial association of condyloma acuminata and genital cancers, both vulvar and cervical, has been noted for many years. However, HPV was not even mentioned as a possible aetiological agent in a 1973 review of cervical cancer (Symposium 1973). Only recently have there been sufficient data about HPV to warrant more than speculation about a causal role of HPV in genital cancers. The problem in studying this organism is the difficulty in detecting the viral particles in the genital lesions and the inability to grow the virus in vitro. It was only with the classic study of Goldschmidt & Kligman (1958) that the infectious, viral nature of these lesions was demonstrated through experimental inoculation of human volunteers with filtered venereal wart products. The description of the 'flat condyloma' by Meisels et al (1977) has caused a re-evaluation of the diagnostic criteria, both cytological and histological, of the early neoplastic lesions of the cervix. At least some of the lesions previously diagnosed as dysplasia (CIN I–II) or even carcinoma in situ (CIN III) are now considered 'flat condylomas'. The concepts of an 'atypical' condyloma (Meisels et al 1977), CIN adjacent to typical condylomas, and CIN with condylomatous features are currently confusing the picture of these early neoplastic lesions of the cervix (Rubinstein 1980; Syrjanen 1984). Similar re-evaluations of the relation of condylomas to neoplastic lesions of the vulva and vagina are also being reappraised. There seems to be an increase in the occurrence of condyloma and genital epithelial neoplasia in immunodeficient women (Shokri-Tabibzadeh et al 1981; Schneider et al 1983).

Genital infections with HPV are more common than HSV-2, but until suitable DNA probes were available no strong correlations between cervical cancer and HPV infections could be made. Now that several investigators have made cloned DNA probes, many specific types of HPV have been identified. Four have been associated with cervical involvement—HPV-6, 11, 16, 18—and two—HPV-16 and 18—are found in a high percentage of cervical cancers (de Villers et al 1981; Durst et al 1983; Boshart et al 1984; Gissman 1984). Lancaster et al (1986), in studying metastatic lesion from 18 invasive squamous carcinoma and adenocarcinoma of the cervix found the same HPV type in the metastases of all the four squamous and one adeno-carcinoma in which tumour was identified histolo-gically in the metastases. HPV-18 has been found in approximately 25% of cervical tumours and in three cervical tumour cell lines (Boshart et al 1984), while HPV-16 has been found in 61–68% of cervic-al tumours and severe dysplasias (CIN III; Durst et al 1983; Wagner et al 1984). Only 6–32% of con-dylomas and mild dysplasia contained HPV-16 or 18; most also contained HPV-6 or 11, suggesting that those containing HPV-16 or 18 are more likely to progress to invasive cancer (Durst et al 1983; Wagner et al 1984). The molecular virology of HPV is moving at an amazingly rapid rate. This has been nicely summarised for the clinician by McCance (1986).

As many as 70% of the cervical lesions initially thought to be early neoplastic lesions (CIN I/mild dysplasia) are now identified as HPV infections (Meisels et al 1977). The differentiating factor be-tween HPV infections and CIN is aneuploidy (Reid et al 1984). There are also intermediate lesions with features of HPV infection and CIN: koilocytosis is found in 25–50% of dysplasias (Syrjanen 1980; Meisels & Morin 1981) and nuclear atypia and dys-plasia in 50% of condylomas (Ludwig et al 1981). Over a period of 14 months, 5% of women with condyloma and 10% of women with atypia and dys-plasia developed more severe lesions (Meisels & Morin 1981). Abnormal mitotic figures are strongly associated with aneuploidity (Reid et al 1984); 70% of condyloma with abnormal mitoses contained HPV-16 compared to only 8% of condyloma with normal mitoses (Crum et al 1984).

Cervical dysplasias have been shown to contain morphological changes associated with HPV infec-tions (Grunebaum et al 1983). This association has been confirmed by the detection of HPV structural antigens in 43% of CIN I, 15% of CIN II, 4% of CIN III, and in tissues adjacent to 13% of CIN III and 10% of carcinoma in situ lesions (Kurman et al 1983).

The patient's age has been associated with the severity of cervical lesions: condyloma—27.47

years; CIN—30.8 years, carcinoma in situ—36.75 years, invasive carcinoma—39.81 years (Meisels & Morin 1981). Patients who had HPV associated with CIN, carcinoma in situ or invasive carcinoma lesions were significantly younger than those who did not have HPV (Meisels & Morin 1981; Crum et al 1983; Grunebaum et al 1983).

The precise relationship between these HPV in-fections and cervical neoplasia, i.e. causative or casual, must be delineated, for as high as 1% of Pap smears from some screening programmes indicate HPV infections (Meisels & Morin 1981). This rises to 3% in the under-30 age group. In a college gynaecological clinic, 47% of 425 asymptomatic young women had colposcopic evidence of HPV cervical lesions (Summerlin 1985).

Several types of papilloma viruses form papillo-mas which often transform to squamous cell carcinomas in the presence of a mutagen, i.e. epidermodysplasia verruciformis following expo-sure to sunlight, juvenile multifocal laryngeal papillomas after X-irradiation (Gardner & Lyon 1974; Pfister 1979). Thus, cervical papillomas or dysplasias may serve a promoting function, which in the presence of an initiator, i.e. HSV-2 or smok-ing, leads to cervical neoplasia (zur Hausen 1982; zur Hausen et al 1984). Recently it has been documented that 10% of women with cervical HPV infections might be concomitantly exposed to HSV infections (Syrjanen et al 1984).

Vulvar carcinoma and its precursors, VIN, would also seem likely candidates to be related to HPV infections, since condylomas commonly occur on the vulva. HPV DNA has been detected in invasive carcinoma of the vulva by several in-vestigators (Green et al 1982; Zachow et al 1982; Gissman et al 1983). The recent studies of Crum and his associates (1982) found the reverse correla-tion in that they identified HPV structural antigen in only 4 of 68 vulvar intraepithelial lesions (5.9%). When they correlated the presence of HPV antigen and DNA content of 39 of these lesions, only 2.8% (1/35) of the aneuploid lesions stained positive for HPV while 50% (2/4) of the polyploid lesions were positive. They felt that the finding of HPV antigen was useful in distinguishing VIN from simple con-dyloma. This is in keeping with the concept that epithelial maturation is required for virion assem-bly and thus by definition the less differentiated lesions of VIN would not contain the HPV antigen. Whether the HPV genome exists in a non-replicating state within the aneuploid cell population of VIN is unknown at this time. Pilotti et al (1984) examined 21 patients with VIN and found 14 cases with histological evidence of HPV in both neoplastic and adjacent areas of non-neoplastic cells: 64% of these cases contained HPV-specific antigens, 44% contained intranuclear viral particles, and 37% of the women demonstrated simultaneous carcinoma in situ of the cervix and/or perineum. As in cervical neoplasias, the age of those women with HPV-associated lesions was significantly younger than the age of women with lesions that did not contain HPV. In all cases, HPV was found in lesions with features similar to bowenoid carcinoma and different from verrucous carcinoma, suggesting an aetiological role of HPV in bowenoid carcinoma.

The papilloma virus has long been known to cause tumours in animals. Perhaps it has a major part to play in the occurrence of human genital tract neoplasias. Certainly this bears further study now that techniques for such correlations have been developed.

CONCLUSIONS

It is likely that cervical neoplasia results from the interaction of a number of factors over a period of time. Many studies have documented that the most important epidemiological risk factors for the development of cervical cancer are early age at first intercourse and the number of sexual partners (Fenoglio & Ferenczy 1982; Singer & French 1984). It seems that exposure to the causative agent at the time when the cervix, specifically the metaplastic epithelium, is immature and thus sensitive to the agent's effects is the most important epidemiological risk factor for cervical cancer.

If indeed genital malignancies are the result of outside carcinogens, 'infectious agents' are strong candidates for initiators and/or promoters of cancers of the cervix and vulva. Both areas are exposed to a variety of infectious agents, many of which, particularly some of the viruses, cause tumours in animals and malignant transformation of cells in vitro. Although Aurelian et al (1973) feel that Koch's postulations have been fulfilled by HSV-2 in cervical cancer, others do not share this conclusion. HPV is now almost equal to the fulfilment of these postulates (zur Hausen et al 1984). Certainly the relationship of HSV-2 and HPV to cervical cancer is the closest to a definitive association. The relation of HSV-2 and HPV to vulvar cancer is more tentative. There are no other genital cancers that have a proposed infectious basis.

It is important to keep in mind, however, the many other infectious agents common to the genital tract may be related to the neoplastic process. Recently smoking has been found to be a major variable in the occurrence of cervical cancer (Clarke et al 1982). With newer techniques in epidemiology, immunology, and culture methods, other organisms or factors may be identified as primary or associated carcinogens. The conclusions of this chapter may be quite different 10 years hence.

REFERENCES

Adam E, Kaufman R H, Melnick R H, Levy A H, Rawls W E 1983 Seroepidemiological studies of herpes virus type 2 and carcinoma of the cervix. American Journal of Epidemiology 98: 77–87

Albrecht T, Rapp F 1973 Malignant transformation of hamster embryo fibroblasts following exposure to ultraviolet irradiated human cytomegalovirus. Virology 55: 53–61

Alexander E R 1973 Possible etiologies of cancer of the cervix other than herpesvirus. Cancer Research 33: 1485–1496

Allerding T J, Jordan S W, Boardman R E 1985 Association of human papillomavirus and chlamydia infections with incidence of cervical neoplasia. Acta Cytologica 29: 653–660

Amos H, Kearns K E 1963 Influence of bacterial ribonucleic acid on animal cells in culture II. Protamine enhancement of RNA uptake. Experimental Cell Research 32: 14–25

Aurelian L, Strandberg J D, Melendez L V, Johnson L A 1971 Herpesvirus type 2 isolated from cervical tumor cells grown in tissue culture. Science 174: 704–707

Aurelian L, Davis H J K, Julian C G 1973 Herpesvirus type 2 induced tumor specific antigens in cervical carcinoma. American Journal of Epidemiology 98: 1–9

Aurelian L, Manak M M, McKinlay M, Smith C C, Klacsmann K T, Gupta P K 1981 The herpesvirus hypothesis—are Koch's postulates satisfied? Gynecologic Oncology 12: S56–S87

Averna R, Martelli D, Migliorini D, Sandelli M 1980 Mycoplasia and dysplasia of the uterine cervix. Bollettino dell' Istituto Sieroterapico Milanese 59:348–358

Bechhold E, Reichter N B 1952 The relationship of trichomonas infections to false diagnosis of squamous carcinoma of the cervix. Cancer 5: 442–457

Becker F F, Green H 1960 The effects of protamines and histones on the nucleic acids of ascites tumor cells. Experimental Cell Research 19: 361–375

Beilby J O W, Cameron C H, Catterall R D, Davidson D 1968 Herpesvirus hominis infection of the cervix associated with gonorrhea. Lancet i: 1065–1066

Beral V 1974 Cancer of the cervix: a sexually transmitted infection? Lancet i: 1037–1040

Boshart M, Gissmann L, Ikenberg H, Kleinheina A, Scheurlen W, zur Hausen H 1984 A new type of papillomavirus DNA, its presence in genital cancer biopsies and in cell lines derived from cervical cancer. EMBO Journal 3: 1151–1157

Burns J C, Murray B K 1981 Conversion of herpetic lesions to malignancy by ultraviolet exposure and promoter application. Journal of General Virology 55: 305–313

Catalano L W, Johnson L D 1971 Herpesvirus antibody and carcinoma in situ of the cervix. Journal of the American Medical Association 217: 447–450

Chen M, Swen Y 1982 Experimental studies on induction of cervical carcinoma in mice by genital herpes simplex virus. In: Shiota H, Chen Y-C, Prusoff W H (eds) Herpesvirus; clinical, pharmacological and basic aspects Excerpta Medica, Amsterdam, pp 358–364

Chen M H, Wu J G, Chen B P et al 1984 Prevention of HSV-2 latent infection with subunit vaccine prepared from HSV-1. In: Rapp F (ed) Herpesvirus Alan R. Liss, New York, pp 651–661

Clarke E A, Morgan R W, Newman A M 1982 Smoking as a risk factor in cancer of the cervix: additional evidence from a case-control study. American Journal of Epidemiology 115: 59–66

Comacho A, Spear P G 1978 Transformation of hamster embryo fibroblasts by a specific fragment of the herpes simplex virus genome. Cell 15: 993–1002

Crum C P, Braun L A, Shah K V et al 1982 Vulvar intraepithelial neoplasia: correlations of nuclear DNA content and the presence of a human papilloma virus (HPV) structural antigen. Cancer 49: 468–471

Crum C P, Egawa K, Barron B, Fenoglio C M, Levine R, Richart R M 1983 Human papilloma virus infection (condyloma) of the cervix and cervical intraepithelial neoplasia: a histopathologic and statistical analysis. Gynecologic Oncology 15: 88–94

Crum C P, Ikenberg H, Richart R M, Gissmann L 1984 Human papillomavirus type 6 and early cervical neoplasia. New England Journal of Medicine 310: 880–883

Darai G, Munk K 1973 Human embryonic lung cells abortively infected with herpes virus hominis type 2 show some properties of cell transformation. Nature 241: 268

Davis D B, Culbecco R, Eisen H N, Ginsberg H S, Wood W B 1973 Microbiology, 2nd edn. Harper and Row, New York, pp 1232–1234

de Villers E M, Gissmann L, zur Hausen H 1981 Molecular cloning of viral DNA from human genital warts. Journal of Virology 40: 932–935

Dreesman G R, Burek J, Adam E et al 1980 Expression of herpes-induced antigens in human cervical cancer. Nature 283: 591–593

Duff R, Raff F 1973 Oncogenic transformation of hamster embryo cells after exposure to inactivated herpes simplex virus type 1. Journal of Virology 12: 209–217

Durst M, Gissmann L, Ikenberg H, zur Hausen H 1983 A papillomavirus DNA from cervical carcinoma and its preva-

lence in cancer biopsy samples from different geographical regions. Proceedings of the National Academy of Science of the USA 80: 3812–3815

Eglin R P, Sharp F, MacLean A B, MacNab J C M, Clements J B, Wilkie N M 1981 Detection of RNA complementary to herpes simplex virus DNA in human cervical squamous cell neoplasms. Cancer Research 41: 3597–3603

Eglin R P, Kitchner H C, MacLean A B, Denholm R B, Cordiner J W, Sharp F 1984 The presence of RNA complementary to HSV-2 (herpes simplex virus) DNA in cervical intraepithelial neoplasia after laser therapy. British Journal of Obstetrics and Gynaecology 91: 265–269

Felix K, Fischer H, Krekels A 1956 Protamines and nucleoprotamines. Progress in Biophysical Chemistry 6: 1–23

Fenoglio C M, Ferenczy A 1982 Etiologic factors in cervical neoplasia. Seminars in Oncology 9: 349–372

Fischer H, Brandis H 1954 Effects of histones on animal cells. Naturwissenschaften 41: 533

Flannery V L, Cortney R J, Schaffer P A 1977 Expression of an early, non-structural antigen of herpes simplex virus in cells transformed in vitro by herpes simplex virus. Journal of Virology 21: 284–291

French P 1980 The effects of sperm basic proteins added to human squamous epithelial cells in culture. Micron 11: 467–468

French P Personal communication

French P, Potter C W, Wilbanks G D 1986 Behavior, morphologic and metabolic effects of human sperm basic proteins on BHK 21 cells. Australian Journal of Medical Science (in press).

Frenkel N, Roizman B, Cassai E, Nahmias A J 1972 A DNA fragment of herpes simplex 2 and its transcripts in human cervical cancer tissue. Proceedings of the National Academy of Science of the USA 69: 3786–3789

Fuccillo D A, Sever J L, Moder F L, Chen T C, Catalano L W, Johnson L D 1971 Cytomegalovirus antibody in patients with carcinoma of the uterine cervix. Obstetrics and Gynecology 38: 599–601

Furgyik S 1985 Increased frequency of carcinoma of the uterine cervix in women married to men with previous gonorrheal infection. Acta Obstetrica et Gynecologica Scandinavica 64: 245–249

Gagnon F 1950 Contributions to the study of the etiology and prevention of cancer of the cervix of the uterus. American Journal of Obstetrics and Gynecology 60: 516–522

Galloway D A, McDougall J K 1983 The oncogenic potential of herpes simplex viruses: evidence for a 'hit-and-run' mechanism. Nature 302: 21–24

Gardner J W, Lyon J L 1974 Cancer of the cervix: a sexually transmitted infection: Lancet 2: 470–471

Gissmann L 1984 Papillomaviruses and their association with cancer in animals and in man. Cancer Surveys 3: 161–181

Gissmann L, Wolnik L, Ikenberg H, Koldovsky V, Schnurch H G, zur Hausen H 1983 Human papillomavirus type 6 and 11 DNA sequences in genital and laryngeal papillomas and in some cervical cancers. Proceedings of the National Academy of Science of the USA 80: 560–563

Goldschmidt H, Kligman A M 1958 Experimental inoculation of humans with ectodermotrophic viruses. Journal of Investigative Dermatology 31: 175–182

Green M, Brackmann K H, Sanders P R et al 1982 Isolation of a human papillomavirus from a patient with epidermodysplasia verruciformis: presence of related viral DNA genomes in human urogenital tumors. Proceedings of the National Academy of Science of the USA 79: 4437–4441

Gregory J E, Payne F E 1970 Cervical cytology and mycoplasma in two populations. Acta Cytologica 14: 434–438

Grunebaum A N, Sedlis A, Silman F, Fruchter R, Stanek A, Boyce J 1983 Association of human papillomavirus infection with cervical intraepithelial neoplasia. Obstetrics and Gynecology 62: 448–455

Hampar B 1981 Transformation induced by herpes simplex virus: a potentially novel type of virus-cell interaction. Advances in Cancer Research 35: 27–41

Hampar B, Ellison S A 1963 Cellular alterations in the MCH line of Chinese hamster cells following infection with herpes simplex virus. Nature 192: 145–147

Hampar B, Aaronson S A, Derge J G, Chakrebarty M, Showalter S D, Dunn C Y 1976 Activation of an endogenous mouse type c virus by ultraviolet-irradiated herpes simplex virus types 1 and 2. Proceedings of the National Academy of Science of the USA 73: 646–650

Hare M J, Thin R N 1983 Chlamydial infection of the lower genital tract of women. British Medical Bulletin 39: 138–144

Hare M J, Toone E, Taylor-Robinson D et al 1981 Follicular cervicitis—colposcopic appearances and association with chlamydia trachomatis. British Journal of Obstetrics and Gynaecology 88: 174–180

Hare M J, Taylor-Robinson D, Cooper P 1982 Evidence for an association between chlamydia trachomatis and cervical intraepithelial neoplasia. British Journal of Obstetrics and Gynaecology 89: 489–492

Harnekar A B, Leiman G Markowitz S, 1985 Cytologically detected chlamydial changes and progression of cervical intraepithelial neoplasias. Acta Cytologica 29: 661–664

Heath J P 1981 Behavior and pathogenecity of trichomonas vaginalis in epithelial cell cultures: a study by light and scanning electron microscopy. British Journal of Venereal Diseases 57: 106–117

James W 1974 Cervical cancers and sexual behaviour. Lancet 2: 657

Jariwalla R J, Aurelian L, Paul O P T 1980 Tumorigenic transformation induced by a specific fragment of DNA from herpes simplex virus type 2. Proceedings of the National Academy of Science of the USA 77: 2279–2283

Kalimo K, Terho P, Homkonen E, Gronroos M, Halonen P 1981 Chlamydia trachomatis and herpes simplex virus IgA antibodies in cervical secretions of patients with cervical atypia. British Journal of Obstetrics and Gynaecology 88: 1130–1134

Kaufman R H, Dreesman G R, Burek J et al 1981 Herpesvirus-induced antigens in squamous cell carcinoma of the vulva. New England Journal of Medicine 305: 483–488

Keesler I I 1974 Perspectives on the epidemiology of cervical cancer with special reference to the herpes virus hypothesis. Cancer Research 34: 1091–1110

Kreider J W, Howlett M K, Lill N L et al 1986 In vivo transformation of human skin with human papillomavirus type II from condylomata accuminata. Journal of Virology 59: 369–376

Kucera L S, Daniel L W, Waite M 1983 12-O-tetradecanoyl-13-acetate enhancement of the tumorigenic potential of herpes simplex virus type 2 transformed cells. Oncology 40: 357–362

Kurman R J, Jenson A B, Lancaster W D 1983 Papillomavirus infection of the cervix: II. Relationship to intraepithelial neoplasia based on the presence of specific viral structural proteins. American Journal of Surgery and Pathology 7: 39–52

Lancaster W D, Castellano C, Santos C, Delgado G, Kurman R J, Jenson B 1986 Human papillomavirus deoxyribonucleic acid in cervical carcinoma from primary and metastatic sites. American Journal of Obstetrics and Gynecology 154: 115–119

Lang D J, Kummer J F 1972 Demonstrations of cytomegalovirus in semen. New England Journal of Medicine 287: 756–758

Latner A L, Longstaff E 1971 Transformation of mammalian cells by crude histones. British Journal of Cancer 25: 280–283

Latner A L, Longstaff E 1979 Modification by crude histones of gene activity for lactate dehydrogenase. Nature 224: 71–73

Latner A L, Longstaff E, Lunn J M 1971 Invasive properties of histone transformed cells. British Journal of Cancer 25: 568–573

Latner A L, Longstaff E, Turner G A 1973 Enhanced malignant behavior of cells treated with crude rat liver histone. British Journal of Cancer 27: 218–229

Laverty C R, Russell P, Black J, Kappagoda N, Benn R A V, Booth N 1977 Adenovirus infection of the cervix. Acta Cytologica 2: 114–117

Leinikki P, Heinonen K, Pettay O 1972 Incidence of cytomegalovirus infection in early childhood. Scandinavian Journal of Infectious Diseases 4: 1–5

Levin M, Kress L C, Goldstein H, 1942 Syphillis and cancer: reported prevalence among 7761 cancer patients. New York State Journal of Medicine 42: 1737–1745

Levine A S, Nesbit M E, White J G, Yarbro J W 1968 Effects of fractionated histones on nucleic acid synthesis in 6C3HED mouse ascites tumor cells and in normal spleen cells. Cancer Research 28: 831–837

London W T, Nahmias A J, Naib Z M, Fuccillo D A, Ellenberg J H, Sever J L 1974 A non-human primate model for the study of the cervical oncogenic potential of herpes simplex virus type 2. Cancer Research 34: 1118–1121

Lorentz A K, Munk K, Daria G 1976 DNA repair replication in human embryonic lung cells infected with herpes simplex virus. Virology 82: 401–408

Ludwig M E, Lowell D M, LiVolsi V A 1981 Cervical condylomatous atypia and its relationship to cervical neoplasia. American Journal of Clinical Pathology 76: 255–262

Lynge E, Jensen O M 1985 Cohort trends in incidence of cervical cancer in Denmark in relation to gonorrheal infection. Acta Obstetrica et Gynecologica Scandinavica 64: 291–296

McCance D J 1986 Genital papillomavirus infections: virology. In: Oriel J D, Harris J R W (eds) Recent advances in sexually transmitted diseases. Churchill Livingstone, Edinburgh, pp 200–210

MacDonald C 1921 Venereal wart converted into a carcinoma by cauterization. Illinois Medical Journal 40: 233

McDougall J K, Galloway D A, Fenoglio C M 1980 Cervical carcinoma: detection of herpes simplex virus RNA in cells undergoing neoplastic change. International Journal of Cancer 25: 1–8

McDougall J K, Crum C P, Fenoglio C M, Goldstein L C, Galloway D A 1982 Herpesvirus-specific RNA and protein in carcinoma of the uterine cervix. Proceedings of the National Academy of Science of the USA 79: 3853–3857

MacNab J C M 1974 Transformation of rat embryo cells by temperature sensitive mutants of herpes simplex virus. Journal of General Virology 24: 143–153

Marczynska B, McPheron L, Wilbanks G D, Tsurumoto D M, Deinhardt F 1980 Attempts to transform primate cells in vitro by herpes simplex virus. Cell Biology 48: 114–125

Matz B, Schlenhofer J R, zur Hausen H 1984 Identification of a gene function of herpes simplex virus type 1 essential for amplification of simian virus 40 DNA sequences in transformed hamster cells. Virology 134: 328–337

Meisels A, Morin C 1981 Human papillomavirus and cancer of the uterine cervix. Gynecologic Oncology 12: S111–S123

Meisels A, Fortin R, Roy M 1977 Condylomatous lesions of the cervix: II. Cytologic, colposcopic and histopathologic study. Acta Cytologica 21: 379–390

Moller B R, Freundi E A 1979 Experimental infection of the genital tract of female Grivet monkeys by mycoplasma hominis: effects of different route of infection. Infection and Immunity 26: 1123–1128

Nahmias A J, Naib Z M, Josey W E, Franklin E, Jenkins R 1973 Prospective studies of the association of genital herpes simplex infection and cervical anaplasia. Cancer Research 33: 1491–1497

Naib Z M, Nahmias A J, Josey W E 1966 Cytology and histopathology of cervical herpes simplex infection. Cancer 19: 1026–1031

Park M, Kitchener H C, Macnab J C M 1983 Detection of herpes simplex virus type 2 DNA restriction fragments in human cervical carcinoma tissue. EMBO J 2: 1029–1034

Peden K, Mounts P, Hayward G S D 1982 Homology between mammalian cell DNA sequences and human herpesvirus genomes detected by a hybridization procedure with high complexity probe. Cell 31: 71–80

Pister H 1979 Biology and biochemistry of papillomaviruses. Reviews of Physiology, Biochemistry and Pharmacology 99: 111–181

Pilotti S, Rilke F, Shah K V, Delle Torre G, De Palo G 1984 Immunohistochemical and ultrastructural evidence of papilloma virus infection associated with in situ and microinvasive squamous cell carcinoma of the vulva. American Journal of Surgery and Pathology 8: 751–761

Rawls W E, Clarke A, Smith K O, Docherty J J, Gilman S C, Graham S 1980 Specific antibodies to herpes simplex virus 2 among women with cervical cancer. Cold Spring Harbor Conferences on Cell Proliferation 7: 717–733

Reid B L 1965 Cancer of the cervix uteri: review of causal factors with an hypothesis as to its origin. Medical Journal of Australia 1: 375–383

Reid R 1976 Current and future experimental approaches to etiology. In: J A Jordan, A Singer (eds) The cervix. W B Saunders, Philadelphia, pp 442–450

Reid B L, Blackwell P M 1974 Histone and polyaminoacid DNA interactions at molecular and cellular levels. Eighth International Congress on Electron Microscopy, Canberra, vol. II, pp 270–271

Reid B L, French P W, Singer A, Hagan B, Coppleson M 1978 Sperm basic proteins: correlation with socioeconomic class. Lancet ii: 60

Reid R, Fu Y S, Herschman B R et al 1984 Genital warts and cervical cancer: IV. The relationship between aneuploid and polyploid cervical lesions. American Journal of Obstetrics and Gynecology 150: 189–199

Reyes G R, LaFemina R, Hayward D, Hayward G S 1979 Morphological transformation by DNA fragments of human herpesviruses: evidence for two distinct transforming regions in herpes simplex virus types 1 and 2 and lack of correlation with biochemical transformation of the thymidine kinase gene. Cold Spring Harbor Symposium on Quantitative Biology 44: 629–641

Rigoni-Stern D 1842 Fatti statistici relativi alle mallatie cancrose che servirono di base alle poche cose dette dal Dottore G. Servire. Pragg Path Therap 2: 507

Rotkin I D 1967a Sexual characteristics of a cervical cancer population. American Journal of Public Health 57: 815–829

Rotkin I D 1967b Adolescent coitus and cervical cancer: associations of related events. Cancer Research 27: 603–617

Rubinstein E 1980 Probably virus-induced epithelial lesions in pre-invasive cervical cancer. Acta Obstetrica et Gynecologica Scandinavica 59: 529–534

Ryser H J P, Hancock R 1965 Histones and basic polyamino acids stimulate the uptake of albumin by tumor cells in culture. Science 150: 501–503

Schachter J, Hill I C, King E B et al 1982 Chlamydia fractionates and cervical neoplasia. Journal of the American Medical Association 248: 2134–2138

Schlohofer J R, zur Hausen H 1982 Induction of mutations within the host cell genome by partially inactivated herpes simplex virus type I. Virology 122: 471–475

Schlohofer J R, Gissmann L, zur Hausen H 1983 Herpes simplex virus-induced amplification of SV40 sequences in transformed Chinese hamster embryo cells. International Journal of Cancer 32: 99–103

Schneider V, Kay S, Lee H M 1983 Immunosuppression as a high-risk factor in the development of condyloma acuminatum and squamous neoplasia of the cervix. Acta Cytologica 27: 220–224

Schwartz P, Naftolin F 1981 Type 2 herpes simplex virus and vulvar carcinoma in situ. New England Journal of Medicine 305: 517–518

Shokri-Tabibzadeh S, Koss L G, Molnar J, Romney S 1981 Human papillomavirus and neoplasia of the genital tract in immunodeficient women. Gynecologic Oncology 12: S129–S140

Siegel A 1962 Malignant transformation of condyloma acuminata. American Journal of Surgery 103: 613–617

Singer A, French P 1984 Natural history and epidemiology of cervical carcinoma. In: McBrien D C H, Slater T F (eds) Cancer of the uterine cervix. Academic Press, London, pp 6–30

Singer A, Reid B L 1979 Does the male transmit cervical cancer? Contemporary Obstetrics and Gynecology 13(4): 173–180

Skegg D C G, Corwin P A, Paul C, Doll R 1982 Importance of the male factor in cancer of the cervix. Lancet ii: 581–583

Skinner G R B 1976 Transformation of primary hamster embryo fibroblasts by type 2 herpes simplex virus: evidence for a 'hit and run' mechanism. British Journal of Experimental Pathology 57: 361–376

Skinner G R B 1980 Pre-pubertal vaccination against herpes simplex virus infection towards prevention of cervical carcinoma. Blair Bell Memorial Lecture, Royal College of Obstetricians and Gynaecologists, London

Skinner G R B, Woodman C, Hartley C et al 1982 Early experience with vaccine AcNFU$_1$(S-)MRC towards prevention or modification of herpes genitalis. Developments in Biological Standardization 52: 333–344

Skinner G R B 1986 Personal communication

Stalheim O H V, Proctor S J, Gallagher J E 1976 Growth and effects of ureaplasmas (T. mycoplasmas) in bovine oviductal organ culture. Infection and Immunity 13: 915–125

Stich H F, Hsu T C, Rapp R 1976 Virus and mammalian chromosomes. I. Localization of chromosomal aberrations after infection with herpes simplex virus. Virology 22: 439–445

Summerlin W 1985 Cervicitis in college students. Journal of the American Medical Association 254(3): 360–361

Symposium 1973 Herpes virus and cervical cancer. Cancer Research 33: 1345–1563

Symposium 1981 Herpes virus and cervical cancer (condyloma). American Cancer Society, St Petersburg, Florida

Syrjanen K J 1980 Condylomatous lesions in dysplastic and neoplastic epithelium of the uterine cervix. Surgery in Obstetrics and Gynecology 150: 372–386

Syrjanen K J 1984 Current concepts of human papillomavirus infections and their relationship to intraepithelial neoplasia and squamous cell cancer. Obstetrical and Gynecological Survery 39: 252–265

Syrjanen K, Mantyjarvi R, Vayrynen M 1984 Herpes simplex virus infection of females with human papilloma virus lesions in the uterine cervix. Cervix 2: 25–32

Vendrely R, Knoblock-Mazen A, Vendrely C 1960 A comparative biochemical study of nucleohistones and nucleoprotamines in the cell. In: J S Mitchell (ed) The cell nucleus. Butterworth, London, pp 200–205

Vestergaard B F, Hornsleth A, Pedersen S N 1972 Occurrence of herpes and adenovirus antibodies in patients with carcinoma of the cervix uteri. Cancer 30: 68–74

Vesterinen E, Leinikki P, Sakstela E 1975 Cytopathogenicity of cytomegalovirus to human ecto- and endocervical epithelial cells in vitro. Acta Cytologica 19: 473–481

Vesterinen E, Vaheri A, Paavonen J, Saksela E 1978 Adenovirus infection and cytopathic alterations of human cervical epithelial cells in vitro. Acta Cytologica 22: 566–569

Vonka V, Kanka J, Hirsch I et al 1984 Prospective study on the relationship between cervical neoplasia and herpes simplex type-2 virus: II. herpes simplex type-2 antibody presence in sera taken at enrollment. International Journal of Cancer 33: 61–66

Wagner D, Ikenberg H, Boehm N, Gissmann L 1984 Identification of human papillomavirus in cervical swabs by deoxyribonucleic acid in situ hybridization. Obstetrics and Gynecology 64: 767–772

Wentworth B B, Bonin P, Homes K K, Gutman L, Wiesner P, Alexander E R 1973 Isolation of viruses, bacteria and other organisms from VD clinic patients: methodology and problems associated with multiple isolations. Health Laboratory Science 10: 75–81

Wentz W, Reagan J, Heggie A, Fu Y, Anthony D 1981 Induction of uterine cancer with inactivated herpes simplex virus types 1 and 2. Cancer 48: 1783–1790

Wentz B E, Heggie A D, Anthony D D, Reagan J W 1983 Effect of prior immunization on induction of cervical cancer in mice by herpes simplex virus type 2. Science 222: 1128–1129

Wertheim P, Galama J, Geelen J, Buurman C, Van der Kjoordaa J 1985 Epidemiology of infections with cytomegalovirus (CMV) and herpes simplex virus in promiscuous women: absence of exogenous reinfection with CMV. Genitourinary Medicine 61: 383–386

Wilbanks G D, Turyk M E 1986 Cervical and vulva neoplasia: past and present concepts. In: De Palo G, Rilke F, zur Hausen H (eds) Herpes and papilloma virus. Raven Press, New York, pp 115–132

Wynder E L, Cornfield J, Schroff P D, Doraiswami K R 1954 A study of environmental factors in carcinoma of the cervix. American Journal of Obstetrics and Gynecology 68: 1016–1052

Yamanishi K, Ogino T, Takahashi M 1975 Induction of cellular DNA synthesis by a temperature sensitive mutant of herpes simplex virus type 2. Virology 67: 450

Zachow K R, Ostrow R S, Bender M et al 1982 Detection of human papillomavirus DNA in anogenital neoplasias. Nature 300: 771–771

zur Hausen H 1976 Condylomata acuminata and human genital cancer. Cancer Research 36: 530

zur Hausen H 1982 Human genital cancer: synergism between two virus infections or synergism between a virus infection and initiating events? Lancet ii: 1370–1372

zur Hausen H, Gissmann L, Schlohofer J R 1984 Viruses in the etiology of human genital cancer. Progress in Medicine and Virology 30: 170–186

Long-term consequences of pelvic inflammatory disease
L Weström

INTRODUCTION

From a clinical point of view, the majority of women suffering from pelvic infections recover completely. This was true even before the advent of chemotherapy (Heynemann 1953). However, pelvic infections can cause persisting morphological damage to different structures in the genital tract. A sequela of the infection might therefore be decreased or abolished reproductive capability—in many cases not becoming apparent until years after the disease episode. Around the turn of the century, only a small percentage of women who had had acute salpingitis ever conceived after their infection (Forssner 1907).

During the past decades, progress in microbiology (Mårdh 1980) as well as improved diagnostic methods in clinical gynaecology (Frangenheim 1959; Jacobson & Weström 1969) have increased our knowledge of pelvic inflammatory disease (PID). An ever increasing armamentarium of therapeutic agents has become available for its treatment. Logically, therefore, the long-term sequelae of pelvic infections should decrease. In fact, the *proportion* of women having had PID and suffering from its sequelae seems to be smaller today than in the preantibiotic era (see below).

On the other hand, since the mid-1960s we have seen sexually transmitted genital infections become pandemic (Aral & Holmes 1984; Sweet & Gibbs 1985b), accompanied by a concomitant, but smaller, epidemic of complications such as PID (Adler 1980; CDC 1980; St John et al 1981a, 1981b; WHO 1981). This secondary epidemic of PID must have claimed its proportional toll of sequelae in an increasing *number* of women. Thus, in spite of progress in clinical gynaecology, the proportion of women suffering sequelae to PID in the total

population might be larger today than half a century ago. Indeed, recent observations of significant increases during the past decade of both non-surgical female sterility (Ford 1978a, 1978b; Mosher 1982; Mosher & Pratt 1982; Belsey 1983; Mosher & Aral 1985) and of ectopic pregnancy (Urquhart 1979, 1984; Weström et al 1981; CDC 1982b; Rubin et al 1983) could be facets of the hitherto concealed epidemic of sequelae trailing after the PID epidemic.

The current 'state of the art' as to the long-term effects of PID is discussed below.

PELVIC INFLAMMATORY DISEASE

Definition

PID is defined as the acute clinical syndrome associated with ascending spread of micro-organisms (unrelated to pregnancy and surgery) from the vagina and the cervix to the endometrium, fallopian tubes, and/or contiguous structures (CDC 1982a).

It should be observed that this definition excludes infections such as tuberculosis, as well as pelvic peritonitis with origin in the gastrointestinal tract. The latter type of pelvic infection was, however, often included in earlier reports on PID. Many such reports also included puerperal salpingitis as well as 'chronic or unqualified' PID (Heynemann 1953; Weström 1980b). This is one factor which precludes direct comparisons between studies on PID.

Aetiology and epidemiology

By definition, the micro-organisms causing the infection of the upper genital tract in PID should also be demonstrable in the lower genital tract. Two main groups of aetiological agents can be identified in PID: firstly, endogenous micro-organisms, i.e. organisms (normally) colonising the lower genital tract of the female (Eschenbach et al 1975; Mårdh 1980), and secondly, exogenous organisms, the majority of which are transmitted during sexual intercourse, such as *Neisseria gonorrhoeae* (Runge 1953), *Chlamydia trachomatis* (Eilard et al 1976; Mårdh et al 1977) and *Mycoplasma hominis* (Mårdh & Weström 1970).

In a community, the prevalence of sexually transmitted diseases (STDs) is influenced by religious and sexual attitudes and traditions as well as by socioeconomic, demographic, and perhaps racial factors. Consequently, complications with the STDs, such as PID, are influenced by the same factors. Therefore, both the total incidence of PID and the proportion of PIDs caused by STD-agents vary from region to region as well as from time to time.

From about 1960 up to the late 1970s, the prevalence of gonorrhoea showed a two- to fourfold increase in most parts of the world (Aral & Holmes 1984; Sweet & Gibbs 1985b). Of women with gonorrhoea, 10–19% develop symptoms of PID (Weström et al 1982). In most regions, the incidence of gonorrhoea-associated PID has increased roughly in proportion to the increase in gonorrhoea (CDC 1980; WHO 1981).

C. trachomatis is now established as an important cause of PID—in some regions even more so than the gonococcus (Bowie & Jones 1981; Weström & Mårdh 1983a). In young women with a cervical chlamydial infection, some 8–10% develop salpingitis (Weström et al 1982). In recent studies from Europe, *C. trachomatis* has accounted for about half of all PID cases in women under the age of 25 (Weström & Mårdh, 1983a). In the USA, the corresponding proportion in hospital-treated cases of PID has been estimated to be 20–40% (Sweet et al 1983). If non-gonococcal urethritis in the male (which is most often caused by chlamydia) is taken as a marker of chlamydial genital infections in a society, then a fourfold increase of such infections has been observed since the mid-1950s (Catterall 1975; Aral & Holmes 1984)—at least in England and Wales.

The role of *M. hominis* in the epidemiology of PID has been less extensively studied. Recent publications (Möller 1983) indicate a significant role of *M. hominis* in 15–30% of cases of PID.

Taken together, the sexually transmitted PID-causing organisms have accounted for up to 75% of PID cases in women in the fertile ages during the 1970s and early 1980s in western industrialised countries (Mårdh 1980; Weström 1980b).

Facultative and strictly anaerobic bacteria as well as aerobic bacterial species normally found in the endogenous flora of the lower female genital tract have been isolated from the upper genital tract in a proportion of women with PID (Eschenbach et al 1975; Mårdh 1980). This has also been the case in a fraction of STD-associated cases of PID.

Isolates of endogenous micro-organisms have been proportionally more common in: (1) somewhat older women (Weström & Mårdh 1984a); (2) women using intrauterine contraceptive devices (IUCDs) (Weström et al 1976); (3) severe disease (Eschenbach et al 1975); (4) recurrent PID (Sweet et al 1981), and (5) after surgical procedures such as legal abortions, curettage and IUCD-insertions (Weström & Mårdh 1983b).

Roughly proportional to the increase of the STDs in general, the *total* incidence of PID in women under the age of 44 has shown a 5–10% annual increase since the mid-1960s in Europe, the USA, and Canada (Adler 1980; CDC 1980; St John et al 1981a, 1981b; WHO 1981; Aral & Holmes 1984). From the industrialised countries, several studies (Wright & Laemmle 1968; Eschenbach et al 1977; CDC 1980; Weström 1980b; WHO 1981) agree on a total annual incidence of PID during the 1960s and 1970s of 10 to 13 per 1000 women in the age group 15–44, with a peak incidence close to 20/1000 women/year in the high risk age group 15–24 years. In the birth cohorts from 1945 to 1954, one can calculate a cumulative proportion of 15% of women who have ever had PID by their 30th birthday (Weström 1980b).

Considering a rate of up to 75% of STD-associated PID, the impact of the 30-year STD epidemic on the incidence of PID becomes obvious. Likewise, given a rate of PID of 1/7 30-year-old women, even a low rate of post-PID sequelae must have had a significant impact on the total disease pattern and reproductive capability of the generations of young women who passed through the STD epidemic of the 1960s and 1970s.

PATHOPHYSIOLOGICAL BACKGROUND TO THE SEQUELAE OF PID

The acute phase

The spread of micro-organisms from the cervix to the upper genital tract is mainly canalicular, i.e. via the endometrial cavity (Falk 1946; Weström & Mardh 1984a). Accordingly, the tubal infection starts in the mucosa. The oedema of the inflammatory reaction causes a volume increase in the mucosa and the submucosal layers of the tubal wall. Because of the folding of the mucosa, the volume increase becomes most apparent in the ampullary portion of the tube. The increase in volume and pressure causes the serosa to give way along the margin of the mesosalpinx. This results in a swelling of the entire organ as well as in a shortening of the mesosalpinx. In most women, the very distal part of the fallopian tube, close to its fimbriated end, lacks mesosalpinx. Here the serosa cannot yield to the volume increase. The result will be a functional fibrous ring through which the tube's outermost part is drawn following the longitudinal stretching of the mucosa. This brings the fimbriae in close proximity to one another (Rees & Annels 1969). During the combined processes of inflammation and repair, the fimbriae 'heal' together, thereby sealing off the infectious process in the uterine tube from the pelvic cavity (Heynemann 1953; Rees & Annels 1969; Weström & Mårdh 1984a). During the initial stages of the mucosal infection, infectious exudate, including viable micro-organisms, leaks through the abdominal orifice of the tube into the pelvic cavity. There the infectious process might continue on adjacent peritoneal surfaces as well as in the ovaries. Continuing spread of the infection to the appendix (periappendicitis) has been reported (Wölner-Hanssen & Mårdh 1985) as well as a paracolic spread to the liver capsule (perihepatitis; Fitz-Hugh 1934; Wölner-Hanssen et al 1980).

The inflammation causes more or less extensive cell death and tissue damage in the mucosal, muscular, interstitial and serosal layers of the tubal wall (Heynemann 1953; Weström & Mårdh 1984a) as well as of the serosal and subserosal layers of the pelvic peritoneum. Disappearance of the cilia from the tubal surface has been reported (Vasquez et al 1983). The fibrinous inflammatory exudate covering the serosal surfaces may become organised and 'glue' adjacent surfaces to one another.

During the course of acute salpingitis, the combined processes of inflammation and repair—as seen down a laparoscope—begin with a reddening and swelling of the tubal mucosa seen in the funnel-shaped abdominal end and on the fimbriae. A purulent or seropurulent exudate covers the mucosal surfaces and leaks through the tubal orifice. The tubes may be slightly swollen, but their morphology and mobility remain normal. This is designated mild disease (Weström 1975; Weström & Mårdh 1984a). Later, the entire tube becomes reddened and swollen. The fimbriae begin to creep through the functional fibrous ring, giving the distal end of the tube a 'paraphimotic' appearance. The mesosalpinx is swollen and shortened. This leads to a restricted mobility of the tube. Fibrin deposits appear on the serosal surfaces. The close proximity of the inflamed and swollen surfaces to one another leads to the formation of sticky 'wet' adhesions between the tubes, ovaries, and adjacent peritoneal surfaces. The inflammatory exudate is usually scant. The inflammatory reactions and restricted mobility of the organs make a full and detailed view down the laparoscope difficult. This is characteristic of moderately severe disease (Weström 1975; Weström & Mårdh 1984a).

Later still, the peritoneal surfaces of the entire pelvis become inflamed. At this stage, the swollen organs, adhesions, inflammatory reactions, and exudate impair vision down the laparoscope to such an extent that only parts of the uterine fundus and proximal uterine tubes are identifiable. In this inflammatory tumour, the infectious process may lead to extensive tissue destruction with abscess formation, and these stages are typical of severe disease (Weström 1975; Weström & Mårdh 1984a).

Obviously, the infectious process may halt at any stage—spontaneously or as a result of treatment.

In the preantibiotic era, reports were given on frequent flare-ups of acute salpingitis after apparent clinical recovery (Curtis 1921; Holtz 1930; Studdiford et al 1938; Haffner 1939; Hundley et al 1950). Micro-organisms—particularly gonococci—could be demonstrated in the fallopian tubes long after the acute episode (Curtis 1921; Studdiford et al 1938). This led clinicians and researchers to accept the concept of persisting tubal infection—or chronic salpingitis—inevitably leading to sterility.

Since the advent of chemotherapy, the possibility of a persisting tubal infection has by and large been denied. Interestingly, however, during the last few years, French researchers (Henry-Suchet et al 1981) have reported on the isolation of *Chlamydia trachomatis* from the fallopian tubes of women subjected to tubal reconstructive surgery because of sterility many years after the initial episode. It is also a well known and accepted fact that postinfection tubal lesions can be diagnosed in many women who have never had an episode of clinically overt PID. In many such cases of tubal obstruction, high titres of specific serum antibody to *C. trachomatis* have been demonstrated (Punnonen et al 1979; Cevenini et al 1982; Jones et al 1982; Moore et al 1982). Therefore, we can no longer completely deny the possibility of sublinical long-lasting or persisting tubal infections (probably in most cases chlamydial) eventually leading to sterility.

On the other hand, the very nature of the STDs makes double infections as well as reinfections common. Previously, it was uncommon for gynaecologists to perform epidemiological follow-up of the sexual partners of their patients with PID—even in STD-associated cases. In many cases, therefore, the women were sent back to the source of infection after treatment in hospital. In our clinic, we began routine examinations for *C. trachomatis* in 1976. In chlamydia-positive patients, we also examined and treated their sexual partners. This was followed by a significant drop in the rate of second infections—from 20% to less than 12% (Weström 1985b). Thus, a 'persistent' infection may equally well be a series of repeated infections.

Repair and end-result

As mentioned, the process of repair goes on simultaneously with the infectious process. When the infection has been overcome, the inflammatory reaction gradually subsides along with continuing repair. The end-result will be either a complete restitution or more or less extensive scarring and/or functional impairment.

A functional restitution is the end-result in the majority of antibiotic-treated non-tuberculous tubal infections. After one episode of mild disease

Table 21.1 Percentage of women who were infertile after salpingitis related to severity of inflammatory changes seen at laparoscopy. Patients had had only one infection

Inflammatory changes*	Percent infertile in age group		Total
	15–24 years	25–34 years	
Mild	5.8	7.8	6.1
Moderately severe	10.8	22.0	13.4
Severe	27.3	40.0	30.0

*See text.
From Weström 1985b.

(treated with antibiotics), such restitution was seen in up to 94% of the cases, after moderately severe infection in up to 89%, and after severe disease in up to 70% of the cases (Weström 1980a, 1985b; Table 21.1).

The persisting morphological damage seen in some cases after a pelvic infection can be divided into three types—each appearing alone or in various combinations with one another on one or both sides of the pelvis.

1. Damage to the tubal wall
2. Tubal occlusion
   a. distal
   b. proximal
3. Peritubal damage
   a. restricted mobility
   b. adhesions

The tubal wall is first and most severely affected by the infectious process. In the mucosal epithelium, the process of repair seems to cause comparatively little damage. Intratubal mucosa to mucosa adhesions may be formed (Nordenskjöld & Ahlgren 1983). Such adhesions may interfere with egg-transport. Deciliation of the tubal epithelium has been reported after salpingitis (Vasquez et al 1983). However, such an end-result in itself should not cause any functional impairment because women with Kartagener's syndrome have been known to conceive. In liquid-filled closed fallopian tubes (hydrosalpinx), the tubal mucosa becomes atrophic and its folds flattened (Heynemann 1953; Weström & Mårdh 1984a). This might, however, be a result of an increased intraluminal pressure rather than of the infectious process per se. After PID, the subserosal interstitial tissue of the tubes may become infiltrated by fibrocytes. The end-result will be a macroscopically normal but rigid tube, often with a 'paraphimotic' abdominal ostium. The rigidity and the shortening of the mesosalpinx lead to decreased motility. The functional capacity of such tubes has been little studied. Although such tubes are often patent, it is logical to assume that restricted mobility, tubal rigidity, paraphimotic ostium, and intraluminal adhesions result in an impaired ovum pick-up mechanism as well as decreased ability of ovum and blastocyst transport. Overall decreased fecundity as well as proportionally increased risk of a tubal pregnancy should follow (see below).

The best-documented post-PID end-result with respect to fertility is an occlusion of the distal end of the fallopian tubes (Heynemann 1953). The process leading to such an occlusion has been described above. The end-result is a more or less distended, club- or retort-shaped tube, closed in its distal end—a sactosalpinx. In some cases the glued-together fimbriae can be identified as a star-shaped scar on the serosal surface.

In a proportion of cases of tubal infertility there is diagnosis of an occlusion of the proximal part of the fallopian tube, i.e. close to its uterine portion. In the majority of such instances the remaining part of the tube seems completely normal. The aetiology of such a proximal occlusion has been disputed. Endometriosis is probably one important factor. In a proportion of cases with a proximal occlusion, however, it seems reasonable to assume an infectious aetiology—especially in cases also presenting with other stigmata of postinfection damage.

The inflammatory reactions of the peritoneal surfaces of the tubes, uterus, broad ligament, bowel, adjacent intestines, and pelvic walls cause fibrin deposits which may 'glue' the organs to one another. Such deposits may become organised with ingrowing fibroblasts and eventually result in more or less extensive and more or less dense adhesions. Such adhesions are most often seen between the tubes and adjacent surfaces of the uterus and the broad ligament. Often, the ovaries are involved. The adhesions as well as serosal and interstitial scar tissue lead to decreased mobility of the organs. With regard to the ovaries, intra- and periovarian scar tissue may interfere with the cycle-induced volume changes of the organ as well as with follicle growth and ovulation. In such cases, cycle-related or continuous pelvic pain may be elicited (Falk

1965; Weström 1975)—a not uncommon complaint after PID.

The morphological end-results after PID described above may appear in all possible combinations and may be more or less extensive in one or both sides of the pelvis. Attempts have been made to correlate the various end-results of PID with different aetiological factors, such as microbial aetiology of the infection, use of IUCDs etc. By and large, no such correlations have been proven or agreed upon. For the woman afflicted with these end-results of PID, fecundity may be decreased in the range of absolute sterility to insignificant impairment. Defective tubal function is documented in a 7- to 10-fold increased risk of a tubal pregnancy after PID as compared with women who have never had the disease (Urquhart 1979; Weström et al 1981). The woman who is debilitated by chronic pelvic post-PID pain is well known to any gynaecologist.

Thus, we must consider three sequelae after PID—in(sub)fertility, tubal pregnancy, and chronic pelvic pain.

METHODS OF DIAGNOSING POST-PID DAMAGE

An unequivocal proof of the preserved function of the reproductive tract after PID is, of course, an intrauterine pregnancy. Unfortunately, this seems to be the only functional test available. Because in most cases (75%) pelvic infections afflict women below the age of 25 (WHO 1981) and most women today postpone their childbearing until after that age, there is often a considerable time-span between the PID episode and pregnancy planning. In our studies (Weström 1975, 1980a, 1985b) over half the women protected themselves against risk of pregnancy for more than 3 years after the disease episode. Accordingly, follow-up studies with respect to fertility after PID must be extended over long periods of time—preferably 5 years or more.

Examinations of tubal patency

Because of the significant correlation between infertility and post-PID tubal occlusion, the first and most often used methods for short-term follow-up of women after PID were examinations of the patency of the fallopian tubes. A number of such methods are described (Thomas 1962).

Gas-insufflation (Rubin 1920) through the genital tract is one such method. At gas-insufflation—or pertubation—of the genital tract, a device is fitted to the uterine portio and gas (air, carbon dioxide, nitrous oxide or oxygen) is insufflated under slight pressure into the genital tract. The passage of gas through the tubes into the abdominal cavity can be evaluated on a pressure recorder, by auscultation through the abdominal wall of the bubbling of gas through the abdominal orifices of the tubes, and indirectly by the patient's report of shoulder pain caused by the collection of gas under the diaphragm in the erect position. Previously, gas-insufflation was used both in studies on tubal physiology and after PID (Bret & Legros 1959).

Gas-insufflation has the advantage of being a cheap method. It does not need any extra equipment—not even electricity—and can therefore be used as a clinic procedure and under primitive conditions such as in rural areas in developing countries. The method has the disadvantage of being a 'blind' procedure. The results are often difficult to interpret. Gas leaking from the device is a common problem.

Hysterosalpingography is the method most often used for the evaluation of the interior of the female genital tract (see Falk 1965). It has the advantage of giving a good view of the interior parts of the cavities—cervix, endometrial cavity, and fallopian tubes. The mucosal lining, the width of the passages, their patency, as well as uterine malformations can be evaluated in detail. Hysterosalpingography has the disadvantage of giving the woman a more than negligible dose of X-rays directly over the gonads. Intraperitoneal adhesions and tubal rigidity cannot be evaluated. Sometimes, spasmic contractions at the uterotubal junction prevent the escape of contrast agent into the tubes—thereby giving a false diagnosis of proximal occlusion (Mendel 1964).

Both gas-insufflation and hysterosalpingography have the disadvantage of increased risk of unintentional spread of a cervical infection upwards in the genital tract. Thus, a 0.25–2% 'flare-up' of PID has been reported after hysterosalpingography (Bang 1950).

During the last few years, *second-look laparoscopy* has been used in small series after PID (Wölner-Hanssen & Weström 1983; Teisala et al 1987). During a second-look laparoscopy a full and detailed view is obtained of the internal genitalia and pertubation of the tubes can be performed using coloured dyes. Using this method, minor lesions—such as adhesions and tubal rigidity—can also be diagnosed. However, the procedure is too expensive for routine use and also carries a certain—albeit small—risk to the patient. Comparisons between the findings at a second-look laparoscopy and the future fertility of the woman in question have not yet been performed.

Second-look laparoscopy should be restricted to series of research patients. In such studies it may be useful for the evaluations of differences in treatment results between different antibiotic regimens.

STUDIES ON THE SEQUELAE OF PID

General remarks

During the first 20 years of this century, surgery was the rule for treatment of PID (Heynemann 1953). Such a treatment, of course, left the woman with no possibility of ever becoming pregnant after her disease episode. Beginning just after the First World War, conservative treatment was suggested in an attempt to preserve fertility in some cases (Ahlström 1919). Non-surgical therapy gained more and more acceptance. Yet, as late as 1939, 30% of women treated for PID in Norway were directly subjected to surgery (Haffner 1939). After the advent of chemotherapy, conservative treatment of PID has been the rule and surgery the exception.

Over the years, many attempts have been made to evaluate the long-term results of conservative treatment of PID. When reviewing the literature, it becomes obvious that comparisons between the results presented must be made with the utmost care. There are many reasons for this:

1. The terminology. The currently used definition of PID (CDC 1980) was not given and accepted until 1982. In many earlier publications terms such as adnexitis, salpingitis, salpingo-oophoritis, salpingitis/parametritis and pelvic peritonitis were used (Heynemann 1953). Although the majority of patients in such earlier studies obviously had PID in the 'modern' sense, many studies included 'subchronic', 'unqualified', 'chronic' and puerperal cases as well.

2. The diagnosis of PID. In the published series, different criteria have been used for the diagnosis of PID. Generally, the criteria chosen have been such as to select only moderately severe or severely ill patients. It has been shown that a clinical diagnosis of PID has a low accuracy, especially in mild disease. In one large series (Jacobson & Weström 1969) the clinical diagnosis of PID was verified by laparoscopy in only 65% of the cases. Thus, in clinically diagnosed cases in series on PID—especially those also including mild cases—up to one diagnosis in three might be wrong.

3. The selection of patients. All series published present results from hospital treated cases. Women who need hospital treatment for PID represent only the 'tip of the iceberg' in PID. With few exceptions, the patients in the studies reported have been really ill—in some series severely ill. In view of our current knowledge (Jacobson & Weström 1969; Weström & Mårdh 1983a, 1983b, 1984a, 1984b) we can estimate that the patients followed after PID in earlier series represent only about half of all symptomatic PID cases in society—and generally those who were most severely ill. Previously, only women from the lowest socioeconomic strata of society were offered free hospital care—another bias in the selection of patients. Not until the early 1960s did free hospital treatment become available for most people—and then only in a few countries.

4. The follow-up. As mentioned, many years must pass before any reliable results can be obtained on fertility after PID. Most women afflicted with PID have their disease episode many years before a pregnancy is planned (Weström 1980a; Sweet et al 1983). In our series (Weström 1975, 1980a, 1985b) over half the patients protected themselves against pregnancy during the first 3 years after the disease episode(s). Because a diagnosis of infertility is not given until after at least 2 years of pregnancy exposure (WHO 1975), the women rendered infertile by PID do not appear in the follow-up series until after a further couple of years. In some of the older series, only married

women were followed with respect to fertility after PID. Finally, because of the increasing geographical mobility of young people today, the tracing of a person many years after a disease episode becomes increasingly difficult. In this respect, the computed person identification registers used in some countries (e.g. Sweden) have been of good help in the follow-up.

5. Confounding variables. During the long periods of time necessary when studying fertility after PID, a number of factors might appear which influence the fertility of the women. Such variables include intra-abdominal pelvic surgery and endometriosis as well as—at one and of the spectrum—decreased fecundity with increasing age (Fédération Cecos: Schwartz & Mayaux 1982). Furthermore, before claiming that infertility is caused by PID we must—apart from having diagnosed a tubal pathology—have found normal cervical factors, ovulatory mechanism and endometrial factors in the female as well as a normal sperm count in the male.

All these limiting factors must be borne in mind when reading the literature and comparing the results between different series from different countries and different time periods.

Mortality

The prognosis of PID quo ad vitam is good. In the preantibiotic era, Holtz (1930) reported a mortality of 1.3% in a series of 1262 patients with PID. Haffner (1939) reported two deaths (both postoperative) in a series of 484 women. After the advent of chemotherapy, only occasional deaths have been reported. In Sweden, six cases of fatal PID were reported in about 100 000 disease episodes in women under the age of 40 from 1970 up to and including 1980 (OSS 1970–1980). In our series of about 2500 cases since 1960 the mortality was nil. Nowadays, death from PID is most often due to rupture of a tubo-ovarian abscess with generalised peritonitis (see Sweet & Gibbs, 1985a). In such instances, mortality rates are from 6 to 8%.

Repeated infections

The differentiation between a repeated infection and a recurrence of a recently treated PID is sometimes difficult. In our series (Weström 1975), we regarded the reappearance of signs and symptoms of acute PID within 6 weeks of the end of treatment as a manifestation of recurrence of the infection; after 6 weeks it was considered to be the manifestation of a new infection.

As mentioned, the very nature of the STDs as well as the reluctance among many gynaecologists to perform epidemiological follow-up in patients with STD-associated PID have made repeated infections common.

In the preantibiotic era, Holtz in 1930 and Haffner in 1939 reported repeated episodes of PID in 19 and 22% respectively of their conservatively treated patients. After the advent of chemotherapy, Hedberg & Spetz (1958) and Falk (1965) gave reports of 12 and 13% respectively of repeated PID in their patients. In our 1960–1967 series (Jacobson & Weström 1969; Weström 1975), 22.7% of patients had more than one episode of PID. After 1977, when we began epidemiological follow-up of chlamydial PID, the reinfection rate dropped to 12% (Weström 1985b). In an ongoing series, less than 4% of young women with their first episode of laparoscopically verified PID had a new infection within 1 year of the first occurrence (Weström unpublished observations). This seems to be a significant decrease, because most repeated PIDs appear within 1 year of the first episode (Weström 1976)— a fact that also strengthens the assumption that neglected follow-up of the sexual partners of PID patients is one important factor for repeated PID.

On the other hand, it has been claimed (Hundley et al 1950; Sweet et al 1981) that fallopian tubes damaged by one episode of infection should comprise a locus minoris resistentieae and more readily be infected by opportunistic bacteria ascending from the lower genital tract. This theory is supported by observations that repeated episodes of PID are less often STD-associated than primary episodes (Sweet et al 1981) and also by the fact that a non-gonococcal first episode of PID is equally often followed by new infections as is gonorrhoea-associated PID (Weström 1976; WHO 1981). In our studies, we have seen no significant differences in the rates of repeated infections after first episodes that have been mild, moderately severe, or severe, or between non-gonococcal and gonococcal first episodes of PID (Weström 1976, 1980b; Weström & Mårdh 1983b).

Women who have had one episode of PID carry a

Table 21.2 Percentage of infertile patients and controls among those who exposed themselves to the risk of pregnancy and either conceived or had a diagnosed tubal occlusion

Number of infections	Percentage infertile in age group		Total
	15–24 years	25–34 years	
None (controls)	0	0	0.0
One	9.4	19.2	11.4
Two	20.9	31.0	23.1
Three or more	51.6	60.0	54.3

From Weström 1985b.

6- to 10-fold risk increase of having a new episode as compared with women who have never had PID (Weström 1976; WHO 1981). Among other things, this probably also reflects the fact that other risk factors of PID such as young age, educational background, socioeconomic status, and exposure to STDs rarely change after the first PID episode.

Whatever the reason, the increased risk of PID in women who have had their first episode must be borne in mind, because each new episode of PID just about doubles the risk of infertility (Weström 1980a, 1985b; Table 21.2). Therefore, the (young) woman who has had her first episode of PID should be carefully educated about risk factors (IUCD usage, exposure to STDs, too liberal sexual relations) (Weström 1980b), as well as factors to protect against PID (use of condom and/or contraceptive pills (Svensson et al 1984), monogamous sexual relations).

If we could decrease the rate of repeated infections from 20 to 5%, then the subsequent infertility rate can be calculated to drop from 17% to about 10%.

Infertility

Infertility is defined as the inability of a couple to conceive after 2 years of regular unprotected sexual intercourse (WHO 1975). Infertility should be separated from sterility, which is the permanent inability of a person to achieve a pregnancy with any partner. Childlessness, on the other hand, also includes couples who can conceive, but in whom pregnancy wastage and/or perinatal mortality leave them with no living offspring.

Infertility can be caused by factors in the male, by factors in the female, or by a combination of male/female factors. In any population there is a low number of persons with congenital sterility (chromosomal aberrations, genital malformations etc.). These persons contribute to a low—and probably constant—rate of 'core sterility'. To this might be added a proportion of persons with inborn or acquired endogenous diseases leading to in(sub)fertility. In the female, such defects include polycystic ovary syndrome, endometriosis, abnormalities of hypothalamic or pituitary functions, hyperprolactinaemia and other endocrine disorders. Unlike 'core sterility' these defects are possible to treat, but like 'core sterility' they comprise a rather constant proportion of persons in a society. Thus, from an epidemiological point of view, it is reasonable to assume that the different birth cohorts of the last few generations should have just about equal proportions of persons in the 'core sterility' and 'endogenous in(sub)fertility' groups.

To these two groups can be added a varying proportion of persons rendered involuntarily (or voluntarily) sterile from different acquired exogenous factors. Such varying aetiological factors for infertility include postinfection damage to the genital tract, iatrogenic factors (surgery and irradiation), and possibly (largely unknown) toxic factors. From an epidemiological point of view, we must also consider the impact of delayed childbearing, which might bring a proportion of women over the peak fecundity age into the ages of decreasing fecundity (Fédération Cecos: Schwartz & Mayaux 1982). Significant changes in any of those aetiological factors for infertility would influence the total ratio of infertile couples in a society.

Estimates of the current 'crude infertility rate' in Europe and the USA have shown that by the end of 1 year of unprotected sexual intercourse, 10–15% of married or cohabiting couples will fail to conceive (Lenton et al 1977).

If infertility as a sequel to the PID epidemic has been of significance, then an increase in the total infertility rate should be demonstrable. In the USA several surveys have shown an increase in non-surgical infertility since 1965. Mosher (1982) and Mosher & Pratt (1982) showed statistically significant increases between 1965 and 1976 of non-surgical infertility among couples where the wife was 25–29 years old. Ford (1978a, 1978b) showed that between 1973 and 1976 non-surgical sterility

doubled among married women of reproductive age in the USA and also increased significantly among widowed, divorced or separated women. However, from these studies, the cause of the increase could not be determined. On the other hand, using a multivariate analysis, Mosher & Aral (1985) reported that 'available evidence shows a strong association between sexually transmitted diseases, pelvic inflammatory disease, and infertility trends. Our projections indicate that STDs operating through PID account for . . . . one-half to one-third of the increase'.

In our follow-up of infertility after PID (Weström 1980a; 1985b), we found a rate of infertility not attributable to PID of about 4% in both patients and controls, and post-PID infertility due to tubal occlusion after one infection in 11% of the patients but in none of the controls (Table 21.2).

In studies on infertility, the proportion of couples in whom post-PID tubal damage was diagnosed in the women varies from a few per cent up to 90% (Belsey 1983). The differing results obtained in such studies probably reflect varying biases in patient selection (Cates et al 1985) economic factors, interest of the study group in question etc., rather than the true proportions of the reasons for infertility in the society. However, in most reports on tubal reconstructive surgery (Siegler 1979) there is agreement on 30–60% of women with postinfection tubal damage denying any prior episode of PID. Such figures indicate that 'silent' PID may account for between one-third and two-thirds of post-PID infertility (Henry-Suchet et al 1982; Sweet et al 1983). Accordingly, 'silent asymptomatic PID' may be at least as common as clinically overt disease episodes.

In follow-up studies after PID, a number of authors have used different methods for evaluating tubal patency. Thus, Bret & Legros (1959), using insufflation, found patent fallopian tubes in 20 out of 50 women treated during the acute episode with prednisolone and penicillin. Fifteen of those women eventually got pregnant. Viberg (1964) used the recovery from the vagina of intra-abdominally injected radiolabelled gold as a test of tubal patency. He found a good correlation between Au[198] passage through the genital tract and later pregnancy, whereas none of the women with a negative test conceived.

Hysterosalpingography for the evaluation of tubal patency after PID was used by Hüter & Hartmann (1959). They found patent tubes in 21 out of 36 patients treated with tetracycline. Hedberg (1959) and later Hedberg and Ånberg (1965) reported tubal patency in 80% of women treated with penicillin for a first episode of gonorrhoea-associated PID. Falk (1965) found normal hysterosalpingograms in 87% of 235 patients followed after PID episodes who had been treated with streptomycin plus penicillin with or without added prednisolone. Abnormal findings on one or both sides of the pelvis were found in 61/235 women (13%). Of these 61 women, 16 eventually conceived.

Wölner-Hanssen & Weström (1983) used a second-look laparoscopy 16 to 33 weeks after treatment to evaluate the end-results. In 13 patients, they found 2 with bilaterally occluded tubes: a preliminary infertility rate of 15%. In 8 patients, the second-look laparoscopy revealed previously inflamed and adhered adnexa to be perfectly normal. Teisala et al (1987) used second-look laparoscopy in 20 patients. In 9 of these they found pelvic adhesions or tubal occlusion at the second-look. The method of second-look laparoscopy seems promising, but needs further evaluation and its results should be correlated to later conceptions.

As mentioned, prospective studies on fertility/infertility rates after PID are difficult to perform. Nevertheless, quite a few such studies have been published—mainly from Europe and up to 1965. A selection of such studies is tabulated in Table 21.3. For reasons mentioned earlier, comparisons between the different studies should be made with care.

In the preantibiotic era, two large Scandinavian series (Holtz 1930; Haffner 1939) which were followed for more than 4 years, gave pregnancy rates of at most 27% of the total material. After correction for voluntary infertility the figures were at best 43% (Haffner 1939). It should be observed, however, that Holtz (1930) followed fertility only in married women, and also that 30% of the women in Haffner's (1939) original series were operated on. The diagnostic criteria of PID in those two series were such as to include hospital treated febrile women with an elevated erythrocyte sedimentation rate (ESR) and palpable adnexal masses. If from our antibiotic treated series (Weström 1985b) we select women with severe disease, we

find a corrected pregnancy rate of 70% (Table 21.1).

Two studies (Hedberg & Spetz 1958; Viberg 1964) in which only patients with gonorrhoea-associated PID received antibiotic treatment (penicillin) presented a corrected pregnancy rate in a total of 324 women of 60–70%. In some smaller series (Bret & Legros 1959; Hüter & Hartmann 1959; Hurtig 1963) the pregnancy rates in the total material varied between 22% and 60%. These patients were treated with different antibiotics with or without added corticosteroids. The follow-up times were short (2 years) or not given. In the studies mentioned so far, the diagnosis of PID was based on clinical criteria alone.

In one series of patients with laparoscopically verified PID, Sundén (1959) found an uncorrected pregnancy rate of 58% in 52 patients after 3 years. In 1965, Falk presented his series of follow-up in 283 women treated for laparoscopically verified PID with a combination of streptomycin and penicillin with or without added prednisolone. He found a corrected pregnancy rate of 81%. There was no difference between those who had and those who had not been given prednisolone. However, in his series the observation period was rather short (2–5 years) and of his total material of 283 evaluable patients, 113—i.e. close to one-third—were voluntarily childless during the observation period. In our 1960–1967 series (Weström 1975), 415 patients and 184 controls were followed after one or more episodes of laparoscopically verified PID for 4 to 15 years (mean 9 years). We found a corrected pregnancy rate of 79%. Like Falk (1965), we found a better prognosis for fertility in younger women as compared to those of somewhat older age. We also found a significant impact of repeated infections—each new episode of PID just about doubled the rate of post-PID infertility. Detailed analyses of the extended series from Lund are given in Table 21.1, 21.2 and 21.4–21.6. Thus, without considering the objections to comparisons given above, we find that after the advent of chemotherapy, the proportion of women becoming pregnant after one or more episodes of conservatively treated PID roughly doubled.

In the series presented above, attempts were made to correlate the final outcome after PID with findings during the acute episode. In the preantibiotic era, most authors agreed on a lower pregnancy rate after gonorrhoea-associated PID than after PID caused by other agents ('Wundkeime'; Holtz 1930; Heynemann 1953; Runge 1953). In most series treated with antibiotics, the fertility prognosis after gonorrhoea-associated PID was significantly better than after non-gonococcal PID (Hedberg & Spetz 1958; Falk 1965; Weström 1975). An explanation of this might be that the antibiotics given in most series were optimal with regard to *Neisseria gonorrhoeae*, but might be suboptimal with regard to, for example, anaerobic bacteria, mycoplasmas, and *Chlamydia trachomatis* (Weström 1975).

The fertility prognosis after chlamydia-associated PID was studied by Svensson et al (1983), who followed 299 patients and 82 controls over 2.5 to 7.5 years. Of the women who exposed themselves to a chance of pregnancy, 25.3% of the patients and 6.7% of the controls did not conceive during a period extending for 1 year. After one episode of acute PID, there were no differences in fertility/infertility rates between women who harboured *C. trachomatis*, *N. gonorrhoeae*, both, or neither organism in the lower genital tract at the acute episode. A chlamydial aetiology to PIDs followed by tubal occlusion is also suggested by seroepidemiological studies of infertile women. Thus, Punnonen et al (1979), Cevenini et al (1982), Gump et al (1983), Henry-Suchet et al (1982), Jones et al (1982), Conway et al (1984), and Kane et al (1984) have all found similar results, i.e. that in infertile women with a diagnosed tubal occlusion the proportions of women having serum antibody to *C. trachomatis* were significantly larger than in infertile women with normal hysterosalpingograms. In women with occluded tubes, the geometrical mean titres of antichlamydial antibody in serum were significantly higher than in women with normal hysterosalpingograms. Like the women subjected to tubal reconstructive surgery mentioned earlier, 30 to 60% of the women with tubal obstruction as revealed by hysterosalpingogram had no history of clinically overt PID.

Again, the data suggest a large proportion of 'silent' asymptomatic PID—this time correlated to *C. trachomatis* infection. On the other hand, high and persisting titres of antichlamydial antibody might also indicate a recent challenge—or repeated challenges—of the serovar in question.

Most authors have found a positive correlation between later infertility and long periods of pelvic pain, palpable adnexal masses, and elevated ESR at the acute episode (Holtz 1930; Haffner 1939; Falk 1965). In our studies (Table 21.1) women followed after one episode of laparoscopically verified acute PID had a lower infertility rate (6.1%) if the episode was laparoscopically mild (see above) than if it was moderately severe (13.4%) or severe (30.0%).

Several authors have pointed to an increased risk of PID in women using IUCDs (Faulkner & Ory 1976; Weström et al 1976; Senanayake & Kramer 1980; Edelman et al 1982; Gray & Campbell 1985) and the protective effect of use of hormonal contraception against the risk of ascending infection (Senanayake & Kramer 1980; Editorial 1981; Svensson et al 1984; Wölner-Hanssen et al 1985) as compared to using no contraception. In women using oral contraceptive pills, PID—as seen down the laparoscope—was mild significantly more often than in women using other contraceptive methods or those not using contraception (Svensson 1983). This finding argues for a better fertility prognosis in women using pills at the time of their disease episode than in other women. A better fertility prognosis in pill-users is also suggested by Svensson et al (1983). The risk of subsequent infertility in women who had used an IUCD was determined by Cramer et al (1985) and by DaLing et al (1985). These groups found increased relative risks of tubal infertility in IUCD-users of 2.0 and 2.6 respectively, as compared with women who had never used an IUCD. These findings are in accordance with reports (Gump et al 1983; Gibson et al 1984) on correlation between IUCD usage, chlamydial infections and infertility.

It is therefore not impossible that a fraction of the 'silent' PIDs referred to might be asymptomatic (chlamydial?) tubal infections in IUCD-using women.

The most extensive long-term follow-up after PID is the (still ongoing) studies from Lund, Sweden (Weström 1975, 1976, 1980a, 1985b; Weström et al 1979; Svensson 1983; Svensson et al 1983). A summary of the results so far obtained is given below. The study population analysed included 1204 women aged between 15 and 34 years who were treated for one or more episodes of laparoscopically verified PID at the Department of

Table 21.3 Rates of women who become pregnant after conservatively treated acute pelvic inflammatory disease

Year	Author(s)	Follow-up time (years)	No. of women	Diagnosis	Chemotherapy (+/−)	Percentage of women who became pregnant	
						Total	Corrected
1907	Forssner	NG	66	Clin	−	6	−
1930	Holtz	4	800	Clin	−	17	25
1939	Haffner	3–9	284	Clin	−	27	43
1958	Hedberg & Spetz	4	216	Clin	78 + 138 −	30	60
1958	Hüter & Hartmann	2	36	Clin	+	22	−
1959	Bret & Legros	NG	50	Clin	+	30	−
1959	Sundén	3	52	Lap	+	58	−
1963	Hurtig	5	50	Clin	+	60	−
1964	Viberg	3–5	108	Clin	+	−	60–70
1965	Falk	2–5	283	Lap	+	47	82
1975	Weström	4–15	415	Lap	+	63.4	79

NG = not given; Clin = clinical; Lap = laparoscopy. In the corrected figures, voluntarily infertile women were excluded.

Table 21.4 Reproductive events after pelvic inflammatory disease in 1204 patients and after laparoscopy in 150 controls treated at the Department of Obstetrics and Gynaecology, Lund, Sweden, 1960–1979

Event	Patients		Controls	
	n	%	n	%
Pregnant				
Total	746	62.0	112	74.7
Uterine	699		111	
Ectopic	47		1	
Not pregnant				
Total	458		38	
Voluntarily	259	21.5	32	21.3
Involuntarily				
Post-PID★	150	12.4	0	0.0
Other★	49	4.1	6	4.0
Total	1204		150	

★See text.
From Weström 1985b.

Table 21.5 Percentage of infertility due to tubal occlusion after gonococcal and non-gonococcal PID in women who had one infection and taking no precautions against pregnancy

Aetiology	Percentage post-PID infertility		Total
	15–24 years	25–34 years	
Gonococcal	6.5	5/13	9.0
Non-gonococcal	11.1	16.5	12.5

From Weström 1980b.

Obstetrics and Gynaecology, University Hospital, Lund, Sweden, between 1960 and 1979. All patients had a normal menstrual pattern and none had any known abnormality capable of impairing infertility at the time of their infection. A total of 150 women, comparable to the patients in age, parity, and socioeconomic status, were given a laparoscopy because of clinically assumed PID. In all these subjects, laparoscopy revealed entirely normal intrapelvic conditions. These women served as controls and had, like the patients, no fertility-reducing factor at the time of the laparoscopy. The criteria for a laparoscopic diagnosis of PID were those given above. The patients were treated in hospital with bed-rest and different antibiotic regimens. All women were followed after the laparoscopy until their first pregnancy. Those not becoming pregnant were followed until December 1984.

In the follow-up (Table 21.4), the women were classified as pregnant or not pregnant. Pregnancies were subdivided into intrauterine or ectopic. The women not becoming pregnant were divided into voluntarily infertile, i.e. women who had protected themselves against pregnancy throughout the follow-up period, and those who were involuntarily not pregnant. The latter category was further divided into women with proven tubal obstruction, i.e. those with post-PID infertility, and women (couples) with other causes for infertility or incompletely examined couples.

Details of the results are given in Tables 21.1, 21.2, and 21.4–21.6.

Four trends are easily deducible from the results.

Table 21.6 Percentage of infertility after pelvic inflammatory disease in women who had had only one episode of the disease, related to different antibiotic treatment regimens

Regimen (daily dose)	Period	Infertile (%)
Streptomycin (1 g) + penicillin (800 000 iu)	1960–1965	12.5
Chloramphenicol* (1 g) + penicillin* (2.4 g)	1963–1971	11.2
Ampicillin* (2–4 g)	1968–1974	12.9
Doxycycline* (200 mg + 100 mg)	1971–1979	10.0

*Oral treatment
From Weström et al 1979.

Table 21.7 Calculated cumulative rate of post-pelvic inflammatory disease infertility in a hypothetical cohort of 100 000 women born in 1950 using available data on sexually transmitted diseases, pelvic inflammatory disease and post-pelvic inflammatory disease infertility

Year	Birthday	Cumulative total number of women infertile from PID
1970	20th	849
1975	25th	1656
1980	30th	2431
1985	35th	2689

From Weström 1985b.

First. The younger the woman at her (first) PID episode, the better the fertility prognosis (Tables 21.2, 21.2, 21.5).

Second. Each new PID episode just about doubled the rate of women rendered infertile by PID (Table 21.2).

Third. A mild infection had a significantly better fertility prognosis than moderately severe or severe disease (Table 21.1).

Fourth. Gonorrhoea-associated PID had a better fertility prognosis than non-gonococcal PID with the treatment regimens used. (We did not know of chlamydia until the very last years of these studies; Table 21.5).

Comparisons between different treatment regimens in women who had had only one PID episode did not reveal any significant differences in infertility rates after the disease (Table 21.6). This was regardless of whether the treatment had or had not been theoretically optimal with regard to gonococci and/or chlamydia.

If we now put together the various known data on the epidemiology, aetiology and prognosis of PID, we can estimate the impact of PID on the fecundity of a given birth cohort of women by computing the different variables and calculate the cumulative number of women in that cohort who were rendered infertile by clinically overt PID (Table 21.7). The table gives details of birth cohort of 100 000 women who were born in 1950. That cohort was chosen because those women reached the risk age for PID at the approximate time when we began to obtain detailed data on its epidemiology. Furthermore, that birth cohort 'passed through' the STD epidemic of the 1960s, 1970s and 1980s. As seen in Table 21.7, by their 30th birthday, just over 2400 women out of the 100 000 were calculated to be infertile after PID. If we assume an epidemic of 'silent' PID as large as that of overt PID, we could perhaps double that sum.

Ectopic pregnancy

In any population the number of ectopic pregnancies is related to the prevalence of fertile women exposed to the chance of pregnancy and to the distribution of risk factors for ectopic pregnancy among such women. Commonly accepted risk factors include increased age, postinfection and postoperative tubal damage, and other tubal lesions. The immediate effects of such risk factors are often concealed by the use of contraceptives. Furthermore, contraceptive use in itself might influence the epidemiology of ectopic pregnancy.

In a comprehensive review on retrospective studies of the ratios of ectopic to intrauterine pregnancies, Urquhart (1979) found an overall ratio of ectopic to intrauterine pregnancy of 1:182. His review covered a total of 30 388 ectopic pregnancies from the literature between 1937 and 1974. By and large, the incidences of ectopic pregnancy seem to have been rather constant up to the mid 1950s.

After that, significant increases have been reported from almost all countries in the industrial western hemisphere (Beral 1975; Weström et al 1981; CDC 1982b). In Europe, the ectopic:uterine pregnancy ratio has roughly doubled each decade since 1955 (see Weström et al 1981). In Lund, Sweden, the ectopic:uterine pregnancy ratio remained at a constant 5:1000 level from 1944 to 1964. During the 5-year periods 1965–1969, 1970–1974 and 1975–1979 the ratios were 6.8:1000, 7.5:1000, and 11.1:1000 (Weström et al 1981). In the USA Urquhart (1984), again reviewing available data, reported an increase from 17 800 ectopic pregnancies in 1970 to 62 000 in 1982, giving an ectopic:intrauterine pregnancy ratio of 4.5:1000 in 1970 and 11.8:1000 in 1982.

These significant increases in the ectopic:uterine pregnancy ratios must have an explanation in some changes in the distribution of risk factors for ectopic pregnancy in the female population. Before discussing the risk factors, we must, however, consider one important factor, viz. better diagnostic methods. Some decades ago, almost all ectopic pregnancies were diagnosed first after tubal rupture or tubal abortion with massive intraperitoneal haemorrhage. Today, sensitive pregnancy tests such as determination in serum of the beta subunit of the chorionic gonadotropin molecule, ultrasonography, and laparoscopy give possibilities for the diagnosis of an ectopic pregnancy at an early stage —before rupture. Indeed, today we diagnose tubal pregnancies that might 'heal' spontaneously. It is not known how large a proportion of the increase in ectopics is accounted for by such pregnancies.

Among the accepted risk factors postinfection tubal damage seems to be the most common—at least as judged from specimens removed at operation. In most series, 38–52% of tubes removed at an operation for ectopic pregnancy showed signs of earlier inflammation (Krohn & al 1952). Some 30–60% of women operated on for ectopic pregnancy gave a history of previous PID (Weström et al 1981). In prospective studies on ectopic pregnancy after PID from the preantibiotic era, Holtz (1930) reported that 2 out of 279 women followed for more than 4 years were subjected to operation because of ectopic pregnancy. Hübscher (1933) reported ectopics in 2 out of 133 women. Haffner (1939) reported 1 ectopic per 169 uterine pregnancies after

conservatively treated PID. In our 1960–1979 follow-up study, 38 out of 544 first pregnancies were ectopic (Weström 1980a), giving a converted ratio of 4.6 ectopic per 1000 diagnosed conceptions.

In his 1979 review, Urquhart calculated an index of 0.27 ectopic pregnancies per 100 woman years of non-contraception among low risk women, i.e. women with no known risk factor for ectopic pregnancy. Using the same method, we (Weström et al 1981) calculated a corresponding figure of 2.7 ectopics per 100 woman years in women who had at some time had PID. In his review, Urquhart found 3.0 ectopics per 100 woman years in women who had had PID at some time. These figures indicate a 7- to 10-fold increased risk of ectopic pregnancy in women who have had PID as compared to women who have never had PID.

A contributing—albeit small—factor to the increase in the total incidence of ectopic pregnancy is the use of conservative surgery for ectopic pregnancy, i.e. leaving the (damaged) fallopian tube behind after having removed the pregnancy. Frotzler & Ahlgren (1981) found that 6% of the ectopics appeared in a tube which had previously carried a pregnancy.

Another factor that might contribute to some of the increase is, again, increasing age of the pregnancy-seeking women. In our series (Weström et al 1981) ectopic pregnancy was twice as common (12.9/1000 conceptions) in women in the 30–39 year age group as in the age group 20–29 (6.9/1000 conceptions). An important contributing factor to the increase in ectopic pregnancy is use of IUCDs. In their recently published series, Frotzler & Ahlgren (1981) reported that 30–50% of women operated on because of ectopic pregnancy were using an IUCD at the time of conception.

In our series (Weström et al 1981), we found an ectopic pregnancy rate of 0.3 per 100 woman years among 'low risk' IUCD-using women in the age group 20–29 years. The corresponding risk in 'low-risk' women in the same age group not using IUCD's was again 0.3. This means that in a population of women protecting themselves against a chance of pregnancy by using an IUCD, the risk of an ectopic pregnancy is as high (or low) as among pregnancy-seeking women. Therefore, the larger the proportion of IUCD-using women in a population, the higher the number who are 'unprotected' against an ectopic pregnancy.

In the observed increase of ectopic pregnancy, we do not know the proportions accounted for by better diagnosis, conservative surgery, increasing pregnancy-seeking age, IUCD usage, and post-PID damage. A careful estimate calculates that one-quarter to one-third of the increase in ectopic pregnancy during the last two decades might be accounted for by the PID epidemic. Assuming an equally large epidemic of 'silent' PID, the proportion might be doubled.

Chronic pelvic pain

The woman suffering from chronic pelvic pain as a sequela to pelvic infection is well known to every gynaecologist. The pathophysiology of such pain is discussed earlier in this chapter. The theory of inflammatory reactions caused by peritoneal fluid prostaglandins and prostanoids as a source of such pain no longer seems valid (Dawood et al 1984). In the literature, this sequela has raised little interest. In his follow-up after PID, Falk (1965) reported that 17% of his patients complained of such pain. If we define chronic pelvic pain as a period of pain exceeding 6 months and having caused the woman to seek medical aid, then 18% in our 1960–1967 series (Weström 1975) suffered from this sequela after PID. The corresponding figure in the group of controls was 5%. The pain is described as dull, continuing, most often cycle-related with worsening around the time of ovulation and postovulation. Sometimes the pain is one-sided. Severe dyspareunia is the rule—often leading to conflicts with the sexual partner. Some women suffer so severely that they ask for operative treatment, despite knowing that an operation reduces their chances of ever becoming pregnant to nil.

We have found that many of these women can be relieved from their pain with medical treatment similar to the treatment of endometriosis, i.e. continuous danazol or progresterone therapy. Also combined contraceptive pills could have some effect.

In our series, there was a strong correlation between chronic pelvic pain and infertility, i.e. the majority of women suffering from pelvic pain were infertile as well.

CONCLUSION

Summing up, then, we can now depict an epidemic of sequelae trailing after the PID epidemic which in its turn reflects the STD epidemic of the past 30 years.

Of the women afflicted with PID during those years, a total of one-quarter (Weström 1976; Weström & Mårdh 1984a, 1984b) suffered from one or more of the following: infertility, ectopic pregnancy or chronic pain. With a cumulative rate of 15% of women who have had PID by their 30th birthday in birth cohorts around 1950 (Weström 1980b) and basing calculations only on the clinically overt cases, we find that 1 woman out of 25 from those cohorts suffered from one or more sequelae of PID. Indeed, a profound impact has been noted on the health and fecundity of generations of women. Yet there are some rays of hope.

In the Scandinavian countries, the annual incidences of gonorrhoea showed all-time highs in the early 1970s and thereafter decreased significantly (OSS 1979). Along with this, the proportions as well as incidences of gonorrhoea-associated PID have decreased (Weström 1980b, 1985a). In England and Wales and in the USA, the incidences of gonorrhoea have levelled out and shown slight decreases during the last few years (Adler 1980; Aral & Holmes 1984). In England, decreasing numbers of adolescent girls with STDs have been observed (Robinson et al 1985). In Sweden the annual incidences of PID in women in the under 30 age groups has shown a significant decrease since 1977 (Weström 1985a). We do not yet know whether these observations are the first signs that the PID epidemic may have peaked.

Notwithstanding, for many years to come we must harvest the seeds of the PID epidemic of the 1960s, 1970s and 1980s in terms of an increasing number of women seeking help for childlessness, potentially life-threatening ectopic pregnancy, and chronic pain. A decreasing rate of such sequelae of PID can only be achieved by continuing research, education, and day to day efforts in our fight against STDs.

REFERENCES

Adler A 1980 Trends for gonorrhoea and pelvic inflammatory disease in England and Wales and for gonorrhoea in a defined population. American Journal of Obstetrics and Gynecology 138: 901–904

Ahlström E 1919 Die Behandlung nicht tuberkulöser Adnexentzündungen. Acta Obstetrica et Gynecologica Scandinavica 5: 765–774

Aral S O, Holmes K K 1984 Epidemiology of sexually transmitted disease. In: Holmes K K, Mårdh P-A, Sparling P F, Wiesner P J (eds) Sexually transmitted diseases. McGraw Hill Book Company, New York, pp 127–141

Bang J 1950 Complications of hysterosalpingography. Acta Obstetrica et Gynecologica Scandinavica 29: 383–388

Belsey M A 1983 Epidemiologic aspects of infertility. In: Holmes K K, Mårdh P-A (eds) International aspects on neglected sexually transmitted diseases. Western Hemisphere Publishing, Washington DC, pp 269–299

Beral V 1975 An epidemiological study of recent trends in ectopic pregnancy. British Journal of Obstetrics and Gyneacology 82: 775–782

Bowie W R, Jones H 1981 Acute pelvic inflammatory disease in out-patients: association with Chlamydia trachomatis and Neisseria gonorrhoea. Annals of Internal Medicine 95: 686–688

Bret A J, Legros R 1959 Corticothérapie générale et local et récupération fonctionelle tubaire. Gynécologie et Obstétrique (Paris) 58: 522–526

Cates W, Farley T M M, Rowe P J 1985 Worldwide patterns of infertility: is Africa different? Lancet ii: 596–598

Catterall R D 1975 The situation of gonococcal and nongonococcal infections in the United Kingdom. In: Danielsson D, Juhlin L, Mårdh P-A (eds) Genital infections and their complications. Almqvist & Wiksell, Stockholm, pp 5–13

CDC 1980 Pelvic inflammatory disease: United States. MMWR 28: 605–607

CDC 1982a Sexually transmitted diseases treatment. Guidelines. MMWR 31: 43–45

CDC 1982b Ectopic pregnancy surveillance 1970–1978. Center for Disease Control, Atlanta, GA (July)

Cevenini R, Possati G, La Placa M 1982 Chlamydia trachomatis infection in infertile women. In: Mårdh P-A, Holmes K K, Oriel J D, Piot P, Schachter J (eds) Chlamydial infections. Elsevier Biomedical Press, Amsterdam, pp 189–192

Conway D, Glazener C M A, Caul E O et al 1984 Chlamydial serology in fertile and infertile women. Lancet i: 191–193

Cramer D W, Schiff I, Schoenbaum S C et al 1985 Tubal infertility and the intra-uterine device. New England Journal of Medicine 312: 941–947

Curtis A H 1921 Bacteriology and pathology of fallopian tubes removed at operation. Surgery, Gynecology and Obstetrics 33: 621–631

DaLing J R, Weiss N S, Metch D J et al 1985 Primary tubal infertility in relation to the use of an intra-uterine device. New England Journal of Medicine 312: 937–941

Dawood Y, Khan-Dawood F S, Wilson L J 1984 Peritoneal fluid prostaglandins and prostanoids in women with endometriosis, chronic pelvic inflammatory disease, and pelvic pain. American Journal of Obstetrics and Gynecology 148: 391–395

Edelman D A, Berger G S, Keith L 1982 The use of IUDs and their relationship to pelvic inflammatory disease: a review of epidemiologic and clinical studies. In: Leventhal J M, Hoffman J J, Keith L, Taylor P J (eds) Current problems in obstetrics and gynecology, vol 5. Medical Publishers, Chicago, pp 5–62

Editorial 1981 Contraception and pelvic inflammatory disease. Sexually Transmitted Diseases 8: 89–91

Eilard T, Brorsson J-E, Hamark B, Forssman L 1976 Isolation of chlamydia in acute salpingitis. Scandinavian Journal of Infectious Diseases 9: 82–84S

Eschenbach D A, Buchanan T M, Pollock H et al 1975 Polymicrobial etiology of acute pelvic inflammatory disease. New England Journal of Medicine 293: 166–171

Eschenbach D A, Harnisch J P, Holmes K K 1977 Pathogenesis of acute pelvic inflammatory disease: role of contraception and other risk factors. American Journal of Obstetrics and Gynecology 128: 838–850

Falk H C 1946 Interpretation of the pathogenesis of pelvic infections as determined by cornual resection. American Journal of Obstetrics and Gynecology 52: 66–73

Falk V 1965 Treatment of acute non-tuberculous salpingitis with antibiotics alone and in combination with glucocorticoids. Acta Obstetrica et Gynecologica Scandinavica 44 (suppl 6)

Faulkner W L, Ory H W 1976 Intra-uterine devices and acute pelvic inflammatory disease. Journal of the American Medical Association 235: 1851–1853

Fédération Cecos: Schwartz D, Mayaux M J 1982 Female fecundity as a function of age. New England Journal of Medicine 306: 404–406

Fitz-Hugh T 1934 Acute gonococcal peritonitis of the right upper quadrant in women. Journal of the American Medical Association 102: 2094–2096

Ford K 1978a Contraceptive efficacy among married women 15–44 years of age in the United States 1970–1973. Advanced Data 26 (6 April), Vital and Health Statistics of the National Center for Health Statistics/DHEWS (PHS) 78–1250

Ford K 1978b Contraceptive utilization in the United States. 1973 and 1976. Advanced Data 36 (18 August), Vital and Health Statistics of the National Center for Health Statistics/DHEW (PHS) 78–1250

Forssner H 1907 Adnexitis gonorrhoica. Archiv für Gynaekologie 83: 447–451

Frangenheim H 1959 Die Laparascopie und die Kuldoscopie in der Gynäkologie, 1st edn. Georg Thieme Verlag, Stuttgart

Frotzler G, Ahlgren M 1981 Diagnos och behandling av 503 fall av extra-uterin graviditet. Hygiea, Stockholm 90: 385

Gibson M, Gump D, Ashikaga T, Hall B 1984 Patterns of adnexal inflammatory damage, chlamydia, the intra-uterine device, and history of pelvic inflammatory disease. Fertility and Sterility 41: 47–51

Gray R H, Campbell O M 1985 Epidemiologic trends of PID in contraceptive use. In: Zatuchni G, Goldsmith A, Sciarra J (eds) Intrauterine contraception. Harper & Row, Philadelphia, pp 398–411

Gump D W, Gibson M, Ashikaga T 1983 Evidence of prior pelvic inflammatory disease and its relationship to Chlamydia trachomatis antibody and intra-uterine device use in infertile women. American Journal of Obstetrics and Gynecology 146: 153–159

Haffner J 1939 Resultatene av den konservative og operative salpingitt behandling. Nordisk Medicin III: 2255–2260

Hedberg E 1959 Den gonorrhoiska salpingitis prognos. Läkartidningen 56: 2184–2189

Hedberg E, Anberg A 1965 Gonorrhoeal salpingitis. Views on treatment and prognosis. Fertility and Sterility 16: 125–129

Hedberg E, Spetz S 1958 Acute salpingitis. View on prognosis and treatment. Acta Obstetrica et Gynecologica Scandinavica 37: 131–154

Henry-Suchet J, Catalan F, Loffredo V et al 1981 Chlamydia trachomatis associated with chronic inflammation in abdominal specimens from women selected for tuboplasty. Fertility and Sterility 36: 599–605

Henry-Suchet J, Catalan F, Loffre D O V 1982 Antibody titer to Chlamydia trachomatis in acute salpingitis and obstructive sterilitis. In: Mårdh P-A, Holmes K K, Oriel J D, Piot P, Schachter J (eds) Chlamydial infections. Elsevier Biomedical Press, Amsterdam, pp 183–187

Heynemann T 1953 Entzündungen der Adnexe. In: Seitz L, Amreich A (eds) Biologie und Pathologie des Weibes, vol. V. Urban & Schwarzenberg, Berlin, p 19–107

Holtz F 1930 Klinische Studien über die nicht tuberculöse Salpingo-oophoritis. Acta Obstetrica et Gynecologica Scandinavica 10 (suppl 1)

Hübscher K 1933 Über die Häufigkeit von Konzeptionen nach konservierend und konservativer Behandlung von Adnexentzündungen. Zentralblatt fur Gynaekologie 57: 2061–2065

Hundley Jr J M, Diehl W K, Baggot J W 1950 Bacteriological studies in salpingitis with special reference to gonococcal viability. American Journal of Obstetrics and Gynecology 60: 977–983

Hurtig A 1963 Cortisone in obstetrics and gynecology. In: Greenhill J P (ed) Year book of obstetrics and gynecology 1963–1964. Year Book Medical Publishers, Chicago, pp 369–375

Hüter K A, Hartmann P 1959 Antiphlogistische Kortikosteroide in Kombination mit Tetracyclin in der Behandlung entzündlicher Genitalerkrankungen der Frau. Geburtshilfe und Frauenheilkunde 18: 1221–1239

Jacobson L, Weström L 1969 Objectivized diagnosis of acute pelvic inflammatory disease. American Journal of Obstetrics and Gynecology 105: 1088–1098

Jones R B, Arery B R, Hui S L, Cleary R E 1982 Correlation between serum anti-chlamydial antibodies and tubal factors as a cause of infertility. Fertility and Sterility 38: 553–558

Kane J L, Woodland R M, Forsey T, Darougar S, Elder M G 1984 Evidence of chlamydial infection in infertile women with and without fallopian tube obstruction. Fertility and Sterility 42: 843–848

Krohn L, Priver M S, Goltlib M H 1952 New etiological factor in ectopic pregnancy. Journal of the American Medical Association 150: 1291–1292

Lenton E A, Weston G A, Cook I D 1977 Long-term follow-up of the apparently normal couple with a complaint of infertility. Fertility and Sterility 28: 913–919

Mårdh P-A 1980 An overview of infectious agents of salpingitis, their biology and recent advances in methods of detection. American Journal of Obstetrics and Gynecology 138: 933–951

Mårdh P-A, Weström L 1970 Tubal and cervical cultures in acute salpingitis with special reference to Mycoplasma hominis and T-strain mycoplasmas. British Journal of Venereal Diseases 46: 179–186

Mårdh P-A, Ripa T, Svensson L, Weström L 1977 Chlamydia trachomatis infection in patients with acute salpingitis. New England Journal of Medicine 296: 1377–1379

Mendel E B 1964 Chronic tubal spasm. International Journal of Fertility 9: 383–385

Möller R B 1983 The role of mycoplasmas in the upper genital tract of women. Sexually Transmitted Diseases 10(S): 281–284

Moore D E, Foy H, Daling J R et al 1982 Increased frequency of

serum antibodies to Chlamydia trachomatis in infertility due to tubal disease. Lancet ii: 574–577

Mosher W D 1982 Infertility trends among US couples 1965–1976. Family Planning Perspectives 14: 22

Mosher W D, Aral S O 1985 Factors related to infertility in the United States 1965–1976. Sexually Transmitted Diseases 12: 117–123

Mosher W D, Pratt W F 1982 Reproductive impairments among married couples. United States National Center for Health Statistics, Vital Health Statistics

Nordenskjöld F, Ahlgren M 1983 Laparoscopy in female infertility. Acta Obstetrica et Gynecologica Scandinavica 62: 609–615

OSS 1970–1980 Official statistics of Sweden, National Bureau of statistics. Liber Förlag/Allmänna Förlaget, Stockholm

OSS 1979 Aktuell information från socialstyrelsens nämnd för hälsoupplysning. VS-nytt 1: 15

Punnonen R, Terho P, Nikkanen V, Meurman O 1979 Chlamydial serology in infertile women by immunofluorescence. Fertility and Sterility 31: 656–659

Rees E, Annels E H 1969 Gonococcal salpingitis. British Journal of Venereal Diseases 45: 205–215

Robinson G E, Forster G E, Munday P E 1985 The changing pattern of sexually transmitted diseases in adolescent girls. Genitourinary Medicine 61: 130–132

Rubin G L, Peterson H B, Dorfman S T et al 1983 Ectopic pregnancy in the United States: 1970 through 1978. Journal of the American Medical Association 249: 1725–1729

Rubin I C 1920 Nonoperative determination of patency of fallopian tubes in sterility. Intra-uterine inflation with oxygen and production of an artificial pneumo-peritoneum: preliminary report. Journal of the American Medical Association 74: 1017–1019

Runge H 1953 Gonorrhoe der weiblichen Geschlechtsorgane. In: Seitz L, Amreich A (eds) Biologie und Pathologie des Weibes, vol. V. Urban & Schwarzenberg, Berlin, p 413–490

St John R K, Blount J, Jones S-O 1981a Pelvic inflammatory disease in the United States: incidence and trends in private practice. Sexually Transmitted Diseases 8: 56–61

St John R K, Jones O G, Blount J H, Zaidi A A 1981b Pelvic inflammatory disease in the United States: epidemiology and trends among hospitalized women. Sexually Transmitted Diseases 8: 62–66

Senanayake P, Kramer D G 1980 Contraception and the etiology of pelvic inflammatory disease. American Journal of Obstetrics and Gynecology 138: 852–860

Siegler A M 1979 Evaluation of tubal factors in infertility and management of tubal obstruction. Clinics in Obstetrics and Gynaecology 22: 81–91

Studdiford W E, Casper W A, Scandron E N 1938 The persistence of gonococcal infections in the adnexa. Surgery in Gynecology and Obstetrics 67: 176–186

Sundén B 1959 The results of conservative treatment of salpingitis diagnosed at laparotomy and laparoscopy. Acta Obstetrica et Gynecologica Scandinavica 38: 286–296

Svensson L 1983 Chlamydial salpingitis. Thesis: Institute of Obstetrics and Gynecology, University of Lund, Sweden

Svensson L, Mårdh P-A, Weström L 1983 Infertility after acute salpingitis with special reference to Chlamydia trachomatis. Fertility and Sterility 40: 322–329

Svensson L, Weström L, Mårdh P-A 1984 Contraceptives and acute salpingitis. Journal of the American Medical Association 251: 2553–2555

Sweet R L, Gibbs R S 1985a Pelvic abscess. In: Infectious diseases of the female genital tract. Williams & Wilkins,

Baltimore, pp 161–180

Sweet R L, Gibbs R S 1985b Sexually transmitted diseases. in: Infectious diseases of the female genital tract. Williams & Wilkins, Baltimore, pp 17–52

Sweet R L, Draper D, Hadley W K 1981 Etiology of acute salpingitis: influence of episode number and duration of symptoms. Obstetrics and Gynecology 58: 62–68

Sweet R L, Schachter J, Robbie M O 1983 Failure of β-lactam antibiotics to Chlamydia trachomatis in the endometrium despite apparent clinical cure of acute salpingitis. Journal of the American Medical Association 250: 2641–2645

Teisala K, Heinonen P K, Aine R, Punnonen R, Paavonen J 1987 Second-look laparoscopy after treatment of acute pelvic inflammatory disease. Obstetrics and Gynaecology 69: 343–346

Thomas H H 1962 Tests for tubal patency. Clinics in Obstetrics and Gynecology 5: 791–798

Urquhart J 1979 Effect of the venereal disease epidemic on the incidence of ectopic pregnancy—implications for the evaluation of contraceptives. Contraception 19: 455–480

Urquhart J 1984 Epidemiology of ectopic pregnancy—1984 update. Personal communication presented at International Congress on Ectopic Pregnancy, Kiawah Island, South Carolina, September

Vasquez G, Winston R M L, Boeckx W, Gordts S, Brosens I A 1983 The epithelium of human hydro salpinges: light optical and scanning electron microscopic study. British Journal of Obstetrics and Gynaecology 90: 764–770

Viberg L 1964 Acute inflammatory conditions of the uterine adnexa. Acta Obstetrica et Gynecologica Scandinavica 43 (suppl 4)

Weström L 1975 Effect of acute pelvic inflammatory disease on fertility. American Journal of Obstetrics and Gynecology 121: 707–713

Weström L 1976 Diagnosis, aetiology, and prognosis of acute salpingitis. Thesis, Studentlitteratur, Lund, Sweden

Weström L 1980a Reproductive events after acute salpingitis. Sexually transmitted diseases, status report, NIAID STD study group, NIH Publications No 81-2213, pp 43–54

Weström L 1980b Incidence, prevalence and trends of acute pelvic inflammatory disease and its consequences in industrialized countries. American Journal of Obstetrics and Gynecology 138: 880–892

Weström L 1985a Epidemiology of PID. Abstract presented at Xth World Congress of Gynecology and Obstetrics, West Berlin 15–20 September

Weström L 1985b Influence of sexually transmitted diseases on sterility and ectopic pregnancy. Acta Europaea Fertilitates 16: 21–24

Weström L, Mårdh P-A 1983a Chlamydial salpingitis. British Medical Bulletin 39: 145–150

Weström L, Mårdh P-A 1983b Pelvic inflammatory disease: epidemiology, diagnosis, clinical manifestations, and sequelae. In: Holmes K K, Mårdh P-A (eds) International perspectives on neglected sexually transmitted diseases. Western Hemisphere Publishing, Washington DC, pp 235–249

Weström L, Mårdh P-A 1984a Salpingitis. In: Holmes K K, Mårdh P-A, Sparling PF, Wiesner P J (eds) Sexually transmitted diseases. Mc Graw Hill Book Company, New York, pp 615–632

Weström L, Mårdh P-A 1984b Current views on the concept of pelvic inflammatory disease. Australian and New Zealand Journal of Obstetrics and Gynaecology 24: 98–105

Weström L, Bengtsson L Ph, Mårdh P-A 1976 The risk of pelvic inflammatory disease in women using intra-uterine contraceptive devices as compared to non-users. Lancet ii: 221–224

Weström L, Iosif S, Svensson L, Mårdh P-A 1979 Infertility after acute salpingitis: results of treatment with different antibiotics. Current Theory and Research 26: 752–759

Weström L, Bengtsson L Ph, Mårdh P-A 1981 Incidence, trends and risks of ectopic pregnancy in a population of women British Medical Journal 282: 15–18

Weström L, Svensson L, Wölner-Hanssen P, Mårdh P-A 1982 Chlamydial and gonococcal infections in a defined population of women. Scandinavian Journal of Infectious Diseases 32: 157–162S

WHO 1975 The epidemiology of infertility. Report of a WHO scientific group. WHO Technical Report, Series 582

WHO 1981 Non-gonococcal urethritis and other sexually transmitted diseases of public health importance. WHO Technical Report, Series 660: 98–100

Wölner-Hanssen P, Mårdh P-A 1985 Chlamydial periappendicitis. Surgery in Gynecology and Obstetrics 106: 304–306

Wölner-Hanssen P, Weström L 1983 Second-look laparoscopy after acute salpingitis. Obstetrics and Gynecology 61: 702–704

Wölner-Hanssen P, Weström L, Mårdh P-A 1980 Perihepatitis and chlamydial salpingitis. Lancet i: 901–904

Wölner-Hanssen P, Svensson L, Mårdh P-A, Weström L 1985 Laparoscopic findings and contraceptive use in women with signs and symptoms suggestive of acute salpingitis. Obstetrics and Gynecology 66: 1–6

Wright N, Laemmle P 1968 Acute pelvic inflammatory disease in an indigent population. American Journal of Obstetrics and Gynecology 101: 779–790

Appendix

Human immunosuppressive and hepatitis viruses
M J Hare

INFECTIONS FOR WHICH THE GENITAL TRACT IS A PORTAL OF ENTRANCE OR EXIT: THE HEPATITIS AND AIDS VIRUSES

There are certain viruses which may enter or leave the body through the genital tract, and, whilst causing severe and sometimes fatal systemic disease, have never been linked with lower genital tract upset. It is possible that cytomegalovirus infection is in this category, but this infection has been covered in the chapter on herpesvirus. This appendix will be concerned with the viruses causing Hepatitis and the Acquired Immune Deficiency Syndrome (Aids). Strictly there is no need to include them as they do not cause localised disease; however the anxiety over them that is universal at present justifies this short account. This will be confined solely to the question of infectiousness; clinical manifestations will not be discussed.

Hepatitis A

The virus of Hepatitis A is an enterovirus, and is spread by the oral route under normal circumstances. Although sexual spread amongst homosexuals has been demonstrated, probably as a consequence of oro-anal sex (Corey & Holmes 1980), heterosexual controls followed in the same study did not acquire this disease. Urine is also infected, and Bannister (1982) described probable passage of infection between male homosexuals in the practice of mutual urination or 'golden rain'. Obviously female urine may just as well be infected as male urine, and sexual practices involving contamination with urine or faeces are potential methods of virus transfer, but the lower genital tract seems not to be infectious or at risk from infection.

Hepatitis B

Hepatitis B virus is a hepatotrophic DNA virus. It is spread by blood contamination, and hence is commonly passed between drug addicts by the sharing of needles and syringes, and between male homosexuals. However the virus is also found in seminal fluid (Heathcote et al 1974) and there is some evidence that transmission by heterosexual intercourse can occur. Thus Bradley (1946) reported jaundice developing in the wives of two men who had had hepatitis two to three months previously and Hersh et al (1971) described six cases of heterosexual transmission from males to their female sexual partners. Pattison et al (1973) found evidence of Hepatitis B infection in the wives of haemodialysis patients more frequently than in other family members, and Heathcote and Sherlock (1973) thought that about a quarter of Hepatitis B patients might have acquired the disease by heterosexual coitus.

The viral antigen has been demonstrated in menstrual blood (Mazzur 1973) and vaginal secretions (Darani and Gerher 1974) and so female to male transmission by sexual intercourse is theoretically possible. Inaba et al (1979) described eight couples where the infection appeared to have been sexually transmitted from wife to husband; they considered that the risk of infection was greatest if intercourse took place just after the menstrual period.

No experiments have been reported showing the experimental transfer of Hepatitis B by deposition of infected semen in the vagina of female animal models, nor by the contamination of male genitalia by infected blood or vaginal secretions, and as Zuckerman (1977) pointed out, those who share a bed share many other things intimately. Nevertheless, the possibility of the genital tract as a source of infection remains, and patients and clinicians must be aware of it.

Aids

The primary cause of the acquired immune deficiency syndrome (Aids) is a human retrovirus, and has been known during its short period of recognition variously as human immunosuppressive virus (HIV), human T-lymphotrophic virus type III (HTLV-III), lymphadenopathy associated virus (LAV) and Aids related virus (ARV). The nature of the virus and the natural history of the infection have been well described by Melbye (1986). It must be remembered that the full blown Aids is the end result of infection, and this may not occur until many years after acquisition of the virus, if it occurs at all. In this appendix what is discussed is the acquisition of infection as demonstrated by sero-conversion, not the development of the clinical syndrome.

At the time of writing (March 1987) and in the United Kingdom heterosexual intercourse appears to be the method of acquisition of HIV for only a small minority of cases. Thus of 4471 cases of antibody positive persons known in England, Wales and Northern Ireland to the end of March 1987, 4227 were males, 214 females and in 30 cases the sex had not been reported (CDSC 1987). Most positive males were homosexual or bisexual (2377) or haemophiliacs (950) and about half of the women were intravenous drug abusers (95). Seventy men and 80 women were thought to have acquired the infection by heterosexual intercourse, and these include women who were the consorts of males in the high risk groups and men and women who had recently returned from high risk areas such as parts of Africa where heterosexual transmission appears to be important. Thus in these parts of the United Kingdom only 3.8% of cases to date appear to have been acquired by this means.

There seems little room for doubt, however, that the female genital tract can receive and pass on this infection. Artificial insemination with semen from HIV positive donors provoked antibody development in half the women exposed (Stewart et al 1985) and the virus has been identified in semen. Francis (reported by Melbye 1986) reported that atraumatic intravaginal innoculation experiments performed on chimpanzees have demonstrated HIV sero-conversion. Men with Aids or the Aids related complex infect their female sexual partners (Reedfield et al 1985), and HIV positive haemophiliacs pass on the infection in similar fashion. Of 36 female sexual partners of men with haemophilia A tested by Jones et al (1985), 3 were HIV positive, although one of these had recently had a blood transfusion. Although Melbye et al (1985) suggest that anal rather than vaginal intercourse was the true mode of infection in such cases, other authors have not confirmed this theory.

The female can also be the source of infection through vaginal intercourse. Vogt et al (1986) reported that 4 of 14 women with serological evidence of HIV infection had the virus identified in cervical secretion. Wofsy et al (1986) showed the virus to be present in endocervical cells and cell free vaginal secretions in 4 of 8 HIV positive women, although in every case the titre of virus was reported to be very low. Higher titres were observed in the increased vaginal secretions of one woman who masturbated to orgasm. The potential for female-male heterosexual transmission therefore exists, and although in the Western world this does not seems to be of maximum importance, elsewhere patterns of spread may be different. Piot et al (1984) reported an almost equal male to female ratio in Aids cases in Zaire, and stated that homosexuality, drug abuse and blood transfusions were not risk factors in these groups. Clumeck et al (1985) found a strong link between Aids and heterosexual promiscuity; 10 of 42 African women suffering from Aids or the Aids related complex were prostitutes and the group of 58 men with the same conditions had a far higher number of female sexual partners than a group of matched controls, and were much more likely to regularly have intercourse with prostitutes. Similar findings have been reported from Haiti.

The knowledge concerning Aids is increasing by the month, and until all the basic facts are known there will be widespread worry and alarm amongst patients and those who care for them. At present it seems that the genital tract in women can be the portal of entry for HIV, and, when the woman is infected, she can release infectious HIV particles in her cervical and vaginal secretions. These would seem to be at a relatively low level of infectiousness, but regular partners especially are at risk. From the point of view of health care workers the avoidance of needle-stick injuries would seem the most important consideration. As always gloves should be worn when examining moist genital surfaces, and gowns and eye protection are probably wise for more complex procedures such as suturing after delivery.

REFERENCES

Bannister B 1982 Hepatitis in homosexual men: possibility of urinary transmission. British Medical Journal 285: 223–224

Bradley W H 1946 Homologous serum jaundice. Proceedings of the Royal Society of Medicine 39: 649–654

CDSC (Communicable Disease Surveillance Centre) Reports 1987. Public Health Laboratory Service, London

Clumeck N, Van de Perre P, Carael M, Rouvroy D, Nzaromba D 1985 Heterosexual promiscuity amongst African patients with AIDS. New England Journal of Medicine 313: 182–183

Corey L, Homes K K 1980 Sexual Transmission of Hepatitis A in homosexual men. New England Journal of Medicine 302: 435–438

Darani M, Gerker M 1974 Hepatitis B antigen in vaginal secretions. Lancet ii: 1008

Heathcote J, Sherlock S 1973 Spread of acute Hepatitis B in London. Lancet i: 1468–1470

Heathcote J, Cameron C H, Dare D S 1974 Hepatitis B antigen in saliva and serum. Lancet i: 71–73

Hersh T, Melnick J L, Goyal R K, Hollinger F B 1971 Non-parenteral transmission of viral hepatitis type B. New England Journal of Medicine 285: 1363–1364

Inaba N, Ohkawa R, Matsuvra A, Kudoh J, Takamizawa H 1979 Sexual transmission of hepatitis B surface antigen. British Journal of Venereal Diseases 55: 366–368

Jones P, Hamilton P J, Bird G et al 1985 AIDS and haemophilia: morbidity and mortality in a well defined population. British Medical Journal 291: 695–699

Mazzur S 1973 Menstrual blood as a vehicle of Australian antigen transmission. Lancet i: 749

Melbye M 1986 The natural history of human T lymphotropic virus III infection, the cause of AIDS. British Medical Journal 292: 5–12

Melbye M, Ingerssley J, Biggar R J et al 1985 Anal intercourse as a possible factor in heterosexual transmission of HTLV-III to spouses of haemophiliacs. New England Journal of Medical 313: 857

Pattison C P, Berqvist K R, Maynard J E and Webster H M 1973 Serological and epidemiological studies of hepatitis B in haemodialysis units. Lancet ii: 172–174

Piot P, Taelman H, Minlangu K B et al 1984 AIDS in a heterosexual population in Zaire. Lancet ii: 65–69

Reedfield R R, Markham P D, Salahuddu S Z et al 1985 Frequent transmission of HTLV III among spouses of patients with AIDS related complex and AIDS. Journal of the American Medical Association 253: 1571–1573

Stewart G H, Tyler J P P, Cunningham A L 1985 Transmission of human T. cell lymphotropic virus type III by artificial insemination by donor. Lancet ii: 581–584

Vogt M W, Witt D J, Craven D E et al 1986 Isolation of HTLV-III/LAV from cervical secretions of women at risk for AIDS. Lancet i: 525–527

Wofsy C B, Cohen J B, Hauer L B 1986 Isolation of AIDS assoicated retrovirus from genital secretions of women with antibodies to the virus. Lancet i: 527–529

Zuckerman A J 1977 Sexual transmission of hepatitis B. Nature 266: 14–15

Index